Colour Atlas on
Colposcopy and
Cytology

Colour Atlas on
Colposcopy and
Cytology

Priya Ganesh Kumar

MBBS DGO MD

Senior Gynaecologist and Colposcopist
WHO/IARC Trainer for Colposcopy in India
FOGSI Colposocpy Course Convenor
Master Trainer for State Govt of Madhya Pradesh,
GOI for Colposcopy and cervical cancer prevention
PhD guide at University of Bhartiya Vidhyapeeth, Pune

Venkateswaran K Iyer

MD

Professor, Department of Pathology
AIIMS, New Delhi

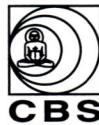

CBS

CBS Publishers & Distributors Pvt Ltd

New Delhi • Bengaluru • Chennai • Kochi • Kolkata • Mumbai

Bhopal • Bhubaneswar • Hyderabad • Jharkhand • Nagpur • Patna
• Pune • Uttarakhand • Dhaka (Bangladesh) • Kathmandu (Nepal)

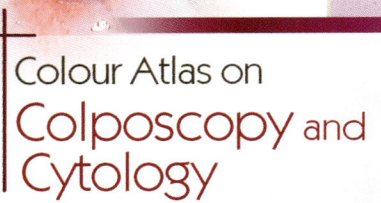

Colour Atlas on
Colposcopy and
Cytology

ISBN: 978-93-89688-60-3

Published by Satish Kumar Jain and produced by Varun Jain for

CBS Publishers & Distributors Pvt Ltd
4819/XI Prahlad Street, 24 Ansari Road, Daryaganj, New Delhi 110 002
Ph: 011-23289259, 23266861, 23266867   Fax: 011-23243014   Website: www.cbspd.com
e-mail: delhi@cbspd.com; cbspubs@airtelmail.in

Corporate Office: 204 FIE, Industrial Area, Patparganj, Delhi 110 092
Ph: 011-4934 4934   Fax: 011-4934 4935   e-mail: publishing@cbspd.com; publicity@cbspd.com

Branches

- **Bengaluru:** Seema House 2975, 17th Cross, KR Road, Banasankari 2nd Stage, Bengaluru 560 070, Karnataka
  Ph: +91-80-26771678/79   Fax: +91-80-26771680   e-mail: bangalore@cbspd.com
- **Chennai:** 7, Subbaraya Street, Shenoy Nagar, Chennai 600 030, Tamil Nadu
  Ph: +91-44-26260666, 26208620   Fax: +91-44-42032115   e-mail: chennai@cbspd.com
- **Kochi:** 42/1325, 1326, Power House Road, Opp KSEB Power House, Eranakulam 682 018, Kochi, Kerala
  Ph: +91-484-4059061-65   Fax: +91-484-4059065   e-mail: kochi@cbspd.com
- **Kolkata:** No. 6/B, Ground Floor, Rameswar Shaw Road, Kolkata-700014 (West Bengal), India
  Ph: +91-33-2289-1126, 2289-1127, 2289-1128   e-mail: kolkata@cbspd.com
- **Mumbai:** 83-C, Dr E Moses Road, Worli, Mumbai-400018, Maharashtra
  Ph: +91-22-24902340/41   Fax: +91-22-24902342   e-mail: mumbai@cbspd.com

Representatives

• **Bhopal**	0-8319310552	• **Bhubaneswar**	0-9911037372	• **Hyderabad**	0-9885175004
• **Jharkhand**	0-9811541605	• **Nagpur**	0-9421945513	• **Patna**	0-9334159340
• **Pune**	0-9623451994	• **Uttarakhand**	0-9716462459	• **Dhaka (Bangladesh)**	01912-003485
• **Kathmandu (Nepal)**	977-9818742655				

Printed at: Nutech Print Services, Faridabad, Haryana, India

to

All those cervical cancer patients who could have been saved from this deadly disease, had they been detected at the earliest precancerous stage where their treatment could have been very effective and simple, thus avoiding mortality and morbidity due to cervical cancer

and

womanhood

Foreword

The recent decision by the Indian Government to develop a cervical screening programme represents a great advance.

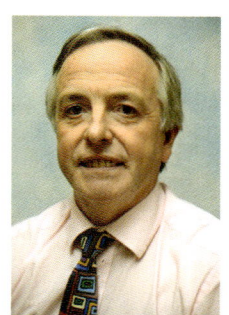

I encourage you to read this new 'Colour Atlas on Colposcopy and Cytology' by Dr Priya Ganesh Kumar and prof Iyer. The book is well written with many high quality images both from colposcopy, cytology and histopathology. The images are annotated to describe the features present and help the colposcopist and pathologist to obtain greater insight into the various clinical and pathological issues relating to the detection of cervical neoplasia. There are helpful chapters on the role of VIA and VILI along with a selection of formative images. A unique section in this atlas is the chapter on nomenclature and scoring systems with helpful illustrations on the practical use of the Swede score. Further chapters include the various techniques that can be used to treat CIN. Finally there is a useful chapter on congental variation of the cervix. The section on cytology has important chapters illustrating the clinical criteria used to assessing cervical cytology samples and making a diagnosis on histologic samples.

Cervical cancer remains a great health burden in the world with many women presenting with advanced cervical cancer and in many countries having poor access to healthcare and treatment.

This book is a practical manual and will of value to not only to a busy gynaecologist running a colposcopic clinic but any doctor training in colposcopy and cervical pathology.

John Tidy
MD FRCOG
Past President, British Society of Colposcopy and Cervical Pathology
Honorary Professor and Consultant Gynaecological Oncologist
Sheffield Teaching Hospital NHS Foundation Trust, UK

Foreword

It is with great pleasure that I write this foreword for an important publication that promises to make a difference to the practice of gynecology.

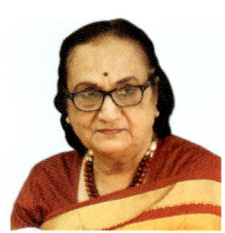

Cervical cancer continues to be the commonest cancer in women in most parts of the developing world. It was in 1967 that WHO announced and classified it as a preventable disease and suggested strategies to be implemented the world over. We have come a long way since those days. It gave rise to a new field of 'preventive oncology' and it applied to many cancers include Breast + Endometrium which affect women.

We have also learned some lessons; we talked and worked on 'cure of cancer'. Finally, we realized that it is not within our reach. Then we came down to a practical approach 'control of cancer'. We accepted it as a chronic disease where mortality and morbidity can be reduced. From that, in 2018, WHO made a big step in announcing that all nations must work towards 'Elimination of Cervical Cancer by 2030'. This is now possible because of the introduction of cervical cancer vaccine.

Pap smear, colposcopy and histopathology have been standard diagnostic tools. They have stood the 'test of time'. In the developed world, incidence of mortality has been drastically reduced due to the liberal use of the above tests. Coupled with available HPV diagnostic tests and vaccinations, the road is now clear for elimination.

This new book will certainly contribute to that goal.

First 8 chapters written by Dr Priya, a senior colposcopist which cover several issues. The importance of correct reporting, understanding the patients need and to help plan the correct line of treatment based on all the evidence gathered through investigations.

I quote,   *"As in our Pathology, So in our Practice"*
                                                                        —Sir William Osler (1849-1919)

In keeping with this, there are chapters from Dr Iyer, an eminent pathologist, which make all readers familiar with cytology and histopathology of pre and early cancers.

This book will give confidence to all those working in the field. Also more doctors will get inducted into mass screening and treatment of pre-cancerous lesions.

If the knowledge gained from this book translates into good clinical practice and prevents some invasive cancers, the authors will feel that they have not toiled in vain.

We live in interesting times. The future holds many opportunities to strengthen health systems for women and children. New partnerships will develop between gynecologists, pediatricians and pathologists, public health and research workers. Global players will come in with financing and administrative strategies. In a sense, the world will come together!

Congratulations and best wishes to the authors, publishers and all those who have contributed to this effort.

Finally, cervical cancers may actually get eliminated. We may say 'Good Bye' to it as we have said to smallpox and polio.

Happy reading and best wishes!

Usha B Saraiya
Past President, Indian Academy of Cytologists MOGS FOGSI AMWI
Medical Women's International Association
Vice President Central Asia 2013-2016
Conferred honorary membership in 2019
Colposcopy Recognition Award by American Society of Colposcopy and Cervical Pathology
Executive Member of IFCPC 1993-1996
Hon. Member of Polish Society of Colposcopy and Cervical Pathology
Conferred Hon. Fellowship by RCOG in 2012
Award for 'Outstanding Woman Obstetrician and Gynaecologist' at FIGO 2003
Lifetime Achievement Award by AOGIN India in September 2017
Zur Hausen Oration delivered at Cuttack in March 2018

Preface

India tops the globe in cervical cancers.

Ironically, it is the most preventable cancer in woman. Colposcopy and guided biopsy is the gold standard for the diagnosis of cervical precancerous lesions, as per the statement released by Singer and Monaghan 2000.

Colposcopy is the science of understanding the morphology of cervix and its precancerous lesions. The knowledge of performing colposcopy, its interpretations, undertaking a good cervical biopsy along with efficient therapeutic procedure is very essential for a colposcopist, also understanding of the cytopathology of the specimen provided, gives the ultimate clarity of subject of precancerous lesions.

This atlas gives a bird's-eye view of the cervical precancerous lesions from the perspective of colposcopy and histopathology.

Section I covers the subject of colposcopy with all its nuances, do's and don'ts to achieve at a diagnosis, which will help the readers to upgrade the skills of colposcopy, with various images, case discussions to arrive at right scoring system, case dilemmas sorted out by thorough understanding of the subject along with tissue knowledge.

The 8 chapters in this section have been very thoughtfully scripted to elucidate the subject in an illustrative manner with plenty of images from authors' encyclopaedia collection of original work of around 50,000 colposcopy cases.

Happy Reading!

Priya Ganesh Kumar

Preface

Knowledge of cervical pathology and cytology is essential for a colposcopist. This atlas is being written in a simple and systematic fashion to explain details of pathology to a colposcopist who would have done pathology at an undergraduate level but not much since then.

Tissue sections from excision specimens and biopsies are used for illustration of histopathology. They are photomicrographs of hematoxylin and eosin stained slides, where the hematoxylin stains the nucleus and eosin stains the cytoplasm.

Cytology smears are made by scraping the superficial surface of the stratified squamous epithelium. They are stained using the Papanicolaou or Pap stain. The Pap stain also stains the nucleus using hematoxylin. However, it is a special hematoxylin which accentuates the nuclear details, making screening easier. Pap stain also has eosin as a cytoplasmic stain but in addition has two other stains—Light Green which stains intermediate cell cytoplasm and Orange G which stains the keratin in cytoplasm, if present.

The Pap stain helps in staining different types of cells in different colours, helping in screening of cervical smears. Superficial cells are pink with eosin, intermediate cells are green due to Light Green and keratinized cells are orange with Orange G.

The atlas is arranged systematically. Initially the normal cervical histology is explained in text and illustrations. Photographs of the histology are described using labels and arrows. Then the atlas follows with more photographs having labels. Text is reduced. After histology, the corresponding cytology follows. Each abnormal histopathology is similarly dealt with in the form of a written description having a representative photograph, followed by the atlas. After each histopathologic abnormality, corresponding cytology follows in a similar fashion.

Some of these pictures would have been used in the colposcopy section. These same pictures as well as further photographs of the same lesion and with different labelling are used in this section for more detailed explanation.

Venkateswaran K Iyer

Acknowledgements

We are privileged and honored to get this atlas reviewed by Dr Partha Basu, Head, Screening (SCR) Group, Early Detection and Prevention Section (EDP), International Agency for Research on Cancer, World Health Organization (WHO), France. We thank and acknowledge Dr Partha for sparing his valuable time to review all the chapters and to suggest a few alterations and corrections. Those suggestions have been incorporated at suitable places.

Our sincere thanks to Prof John Tidy, Past President, British Society of Colposcopy and Cervical Pathology, eminent gynaecological oncologist, Sheffield Teaching Hospital NHS Foundation Trust, UK for the precious Foreword for the Atlas. This has truly boosted our confidence in presenting "State of Art" literature to the scientific community.

A very thoughtful foreword from Dr Usha B Saraiya, stalwart and pioneer in the field of colposcopy and preventive oncology, has been received as blessings for the Atlas. We are truly indebted to her.

Dedicated team of CBS Publishers and Distributors has worked relentlessly to get this atlas in the most appealing flawless format. We would like to thank Mr YN Arjuna, Ms Ritu Chawla, Mr Ramesh Krishnamachari Iyengar, Mr Sanju, Ms Jyoti and all others from the CBS for their contribution in bringing this atlas in appropriate time.

The success of any book lies with the acceptance by the scientific world and its end users.

We sincerely acknowledge and admire our readers who have been our constant inspiration to churn out the best from us. Suggestions from our worthy readers are most welcome and you can mail us on drpriyagk@gamil.com.

Writing a book consumes a lot of time and sacrifices of family members and near and dear ones.

We sincerely and wholeheartedly acknowledge our respective family who allowed us to squeeze time from family hours to pursue and complete our atlas work.

Nothing is possible in this world without the blessings of Almighty.

Gurur Brahma Guru Vishnu Gurur Devo Maheshwara
Gurur Sakshat Parabrahma Tasmaye Shree Guruvey Namaha.

We humbly bow to Guru and Almighty, who is the power, essence and ink of the pen who wrote the book.

Last but not the least we thank our patients, staff members and each and everyone who have been with us in this journey of creating this atlas.

Priya Ganesh Kumar
Venkateswaran K Iyer

Contents

Section II: Cytology

Section I

Colposcopy

CHAPTER

1

Introduction

Colposcopy (ancient Greek word, *Kolpos*—'sheath, vagina' and *skopein*—'to look at') is a diagnostic procedure to have a magnified view of cervix and vagina. Many precancerous and cancerous lesions of the cervix have discernible characteristics which can be easily detected by using colposcopy.

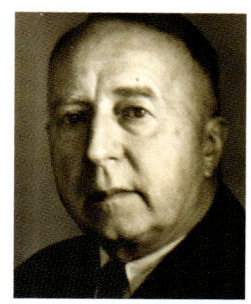

HISTORY OF INVENTION OF COLPOSCOPE

Father of colposcopy is Hans Hinselmann. He was born on 6th August 1884 at Neumunster, Germany. In the year 1908, he qualified for practicing colposcopy and he developed interest in gynecology. He later became an Associate Professor in 1921 at University of Hamburg. Here he started a very thorough research in order to examine the portio and vulva better firstly with von Eicken's frontal lens with magnification of 1, 2 and then with the help of Leitz's technique. He improved the instrument now called *colposcope*. Initially, it was difficult to perform colposcopy due to the distance from focus was not more than 80 mm; he tried to pull out the uterine cervix for examination, which was clumsy. This made Hinselmann to create a colposcope with focal distance of 150 mm (Leitz) and then of 190 mm (Zeiss). Those days, the concept of precancerous lesions was not very clear. A size of pigeon's egg was considered an early cervical cancer. By means of his instrument, Hinselmann was able to dedicate himself to detect cervical cancer in the form of a point. In 1928, Walter Schiller, histologist, found that dysplasia and carcinomatous structures do not contain glycogen and this led to the method of detecting an early carcinoma by smearing the portio with Lugol iodium iodurate solution (Auguste Lugol 1788–1851). This solution is till date used as Lugol's solution. Hinselmann incorporated this in his colposcopy procedure.

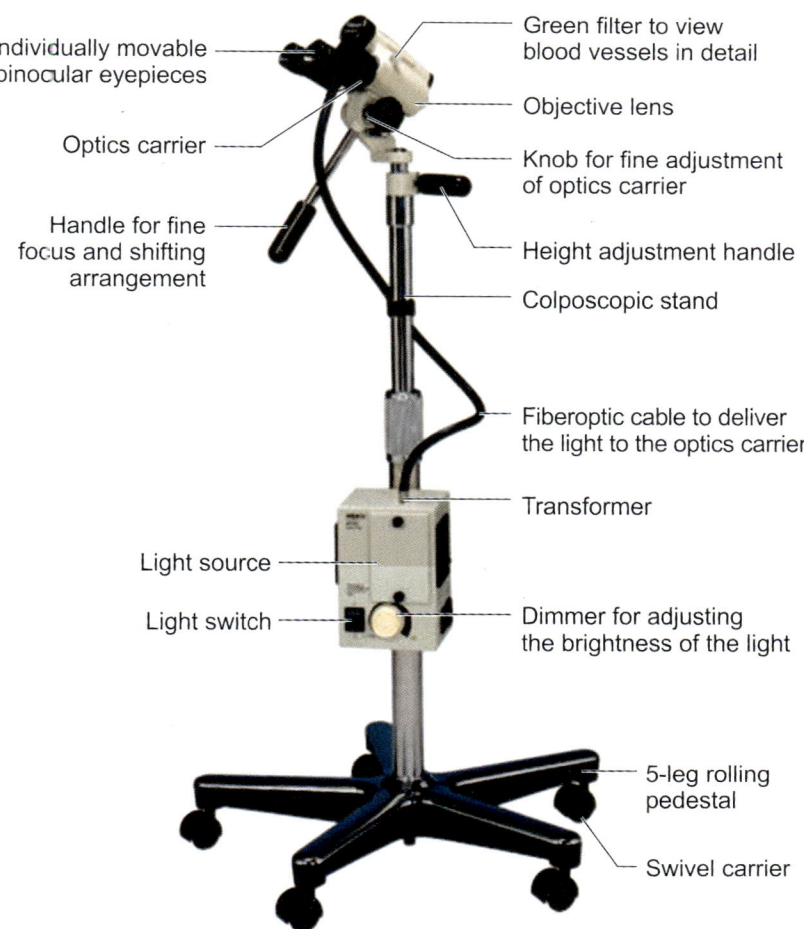

Individually movable binocular eyepieces

Optics carrier

Handle for fine focus and shifting arrangement

Green filter to view blood vessels in detail

Objective lens

Knob for fine adjustment of optics carrier

Height adjustment handle

Colposcopic stand

Fiberoptic cable to deliver the light to the optics carrier

Transformer

Light source

Light switch

Dimmer for adjusting the brightness of the light

5-leg rolling pedestal

Swivel carrier

Fig. 1.1: Binocular colposcope

COLPOSCOPE (Fig. 1.1)

A colposcope is a low power, stereoscopic binocular field microscope with a powerful variable intensity light source that illuminates the area being examined. The colposcope first discovered had binocular lens, a light source, green or blue filter, and objective lens.

The filter is used to remove red light so as to facilitate the visualization of blood vessels by making them appear dark.

DIGITAL VIDEO COLPOSCOPE (Fig. 1.2)

Nowadays we are using a video colposcope which is useful for real-time teaching and documentation.

With a modern CCD camera attached to a digitalizing port, it is possible to create high resolution digital images of the colposcopy findings. Magnification used is up to 40×, lower magnification yields a wider view and greater depth of field for examination of cervix. With higher magnification, the field of view becomes smaller, but reveals finer features such as abnormal blood vessels. A focal distance of 250 to 300 mm is adequate.

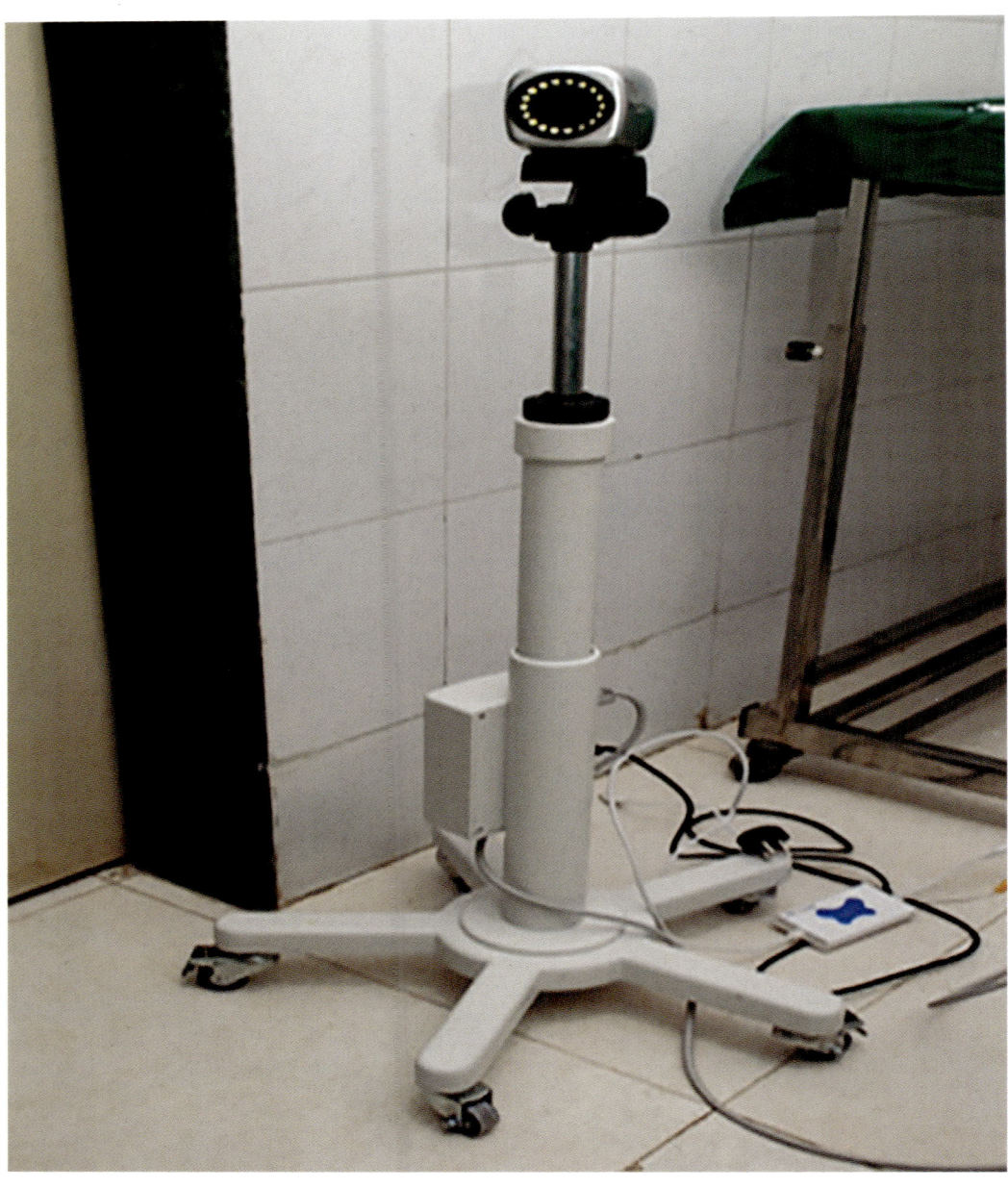

Fig. 1.2: Digital video colposcope

Indications for Colposcopy

1. Suspicious looking cervix
2. LSIL or HSIL on cytology
3. Persistent low-grade abnormality on cytology
4. Persistent unsatisfactory report on cytology
5. Infection with oncogenic HPV
6. VIA (visual inspection on acetic acid) positives
7. VILI (visual inspection on Lugol's iodine) positives
8. Hyperkeratosis on cervix (thick white patch)
9. Condyloma

Patient Selection

Inclusion criteria:
- Incurable leucorrhoea
- Postmenopausal bleeding
- Intermenstrual spotting
- Postcoital bleeding
- Early sexual exposure
- Immunocompromised status
- Abnormal cytology
- High-risk HPV infection

Exclusion criteria: Menstruation.

Patient Evaluation

A detailed history of the patient is mandatory which includes:
- Age of marriage
- Age of first sexual intercourse
- Number of pregnancies including abortions, live births, fetal demises, etc.
- Last menstrual period
- Menstrual history
- Any previous cytology/HPV report
- Allergies
- Any significant medical history
- Type of discharge whether foul smelling, itching
- Any history of dyspaneuria
- History of burning micturition
- History of vaginal douching
- Other medications
- Prior cervical procedure
- History of smoking

Instruments and Procedures

INSTRUMENT TROLLEY (Fig. 2.1)

- Cusco's self-retaining vaginal speculum of different sizes
- Endocervical speculum
- Sponge holder
- Normal saline
- 5% acetic acid
- Lugol's iodine
- Cervical punch biopsy forceps
- ECC (endocervical curettage)
- Container with formalin for the biopsy specimen
- Gloves
- Cotton balls
- Monsel's paste (to stop bleeding).

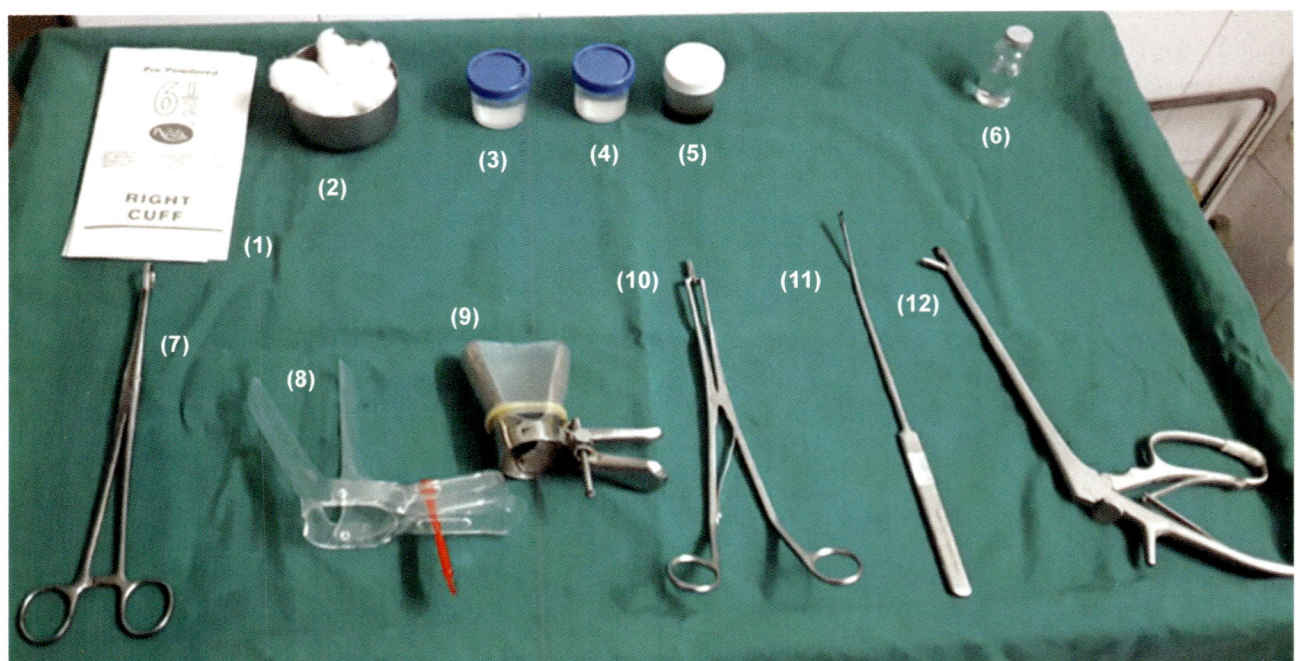

Fig. 2.1: Instruments used for colposcopy: (1) Gloves, (2) cotton ball, (3) normal saline, (4) 5% acetic acid, (5) Lugol's iodine, (6) specimen collection bottle, (7) sponge holder, (8) disposable speculum used in camps, (9) Cusco's speculum with condom for lax vagina, (10) cervical speculum, (11) endocervical curettage (ECC), and (12) Tischler's punch biopsy forceps

PROCEDURE

The following steps are followed:

1. Position of the Patient

Patient is given dorsal lithotomy position. Legs are in stirrups and the buttocks are to the lower edge of table.

2. Insertion of Vaginal Self-retaining Cusco's Speculum

Bivalve self-retaining Cusco's speculum is inserted in the vagina and fixed in such a manner that the cervix is localized in the center.

Tips to be followed:

a. Many a times, it has been observed that in multiparous women with lax vagina, the visualization of cervix is not easy due to the laxity of the vaginal mucosa. This can be corrected by using a Cusco's speculum (Fig. 2.2) with a cover of latex condom whose tip is cut, which serves to keep the vaginal mucosa away from the point of visualization.

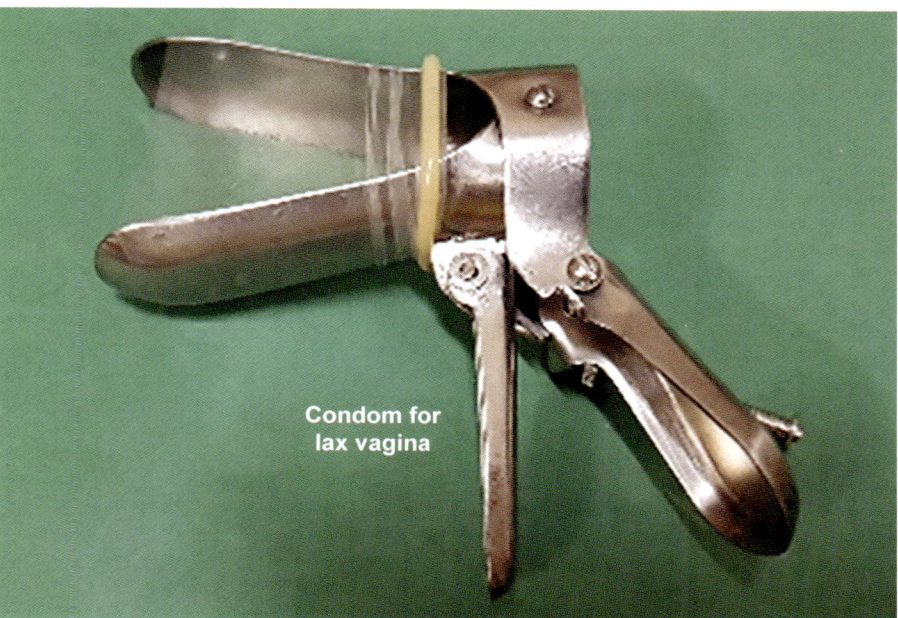

Fig. 2.2: Cusco's speculum

b. Due to the varied positions of uterus, the localization and fixing of the cervix is many a times difficult, especially so in multiparous woman, anxious woman keeping her vagina tight, nulliparous woman with tight vagina muscles, pervious surgeries leading to adhesions, and pulling up of the uterus. In such cases, it is advisable to use different sizes of speculum (Fig. 2.3).

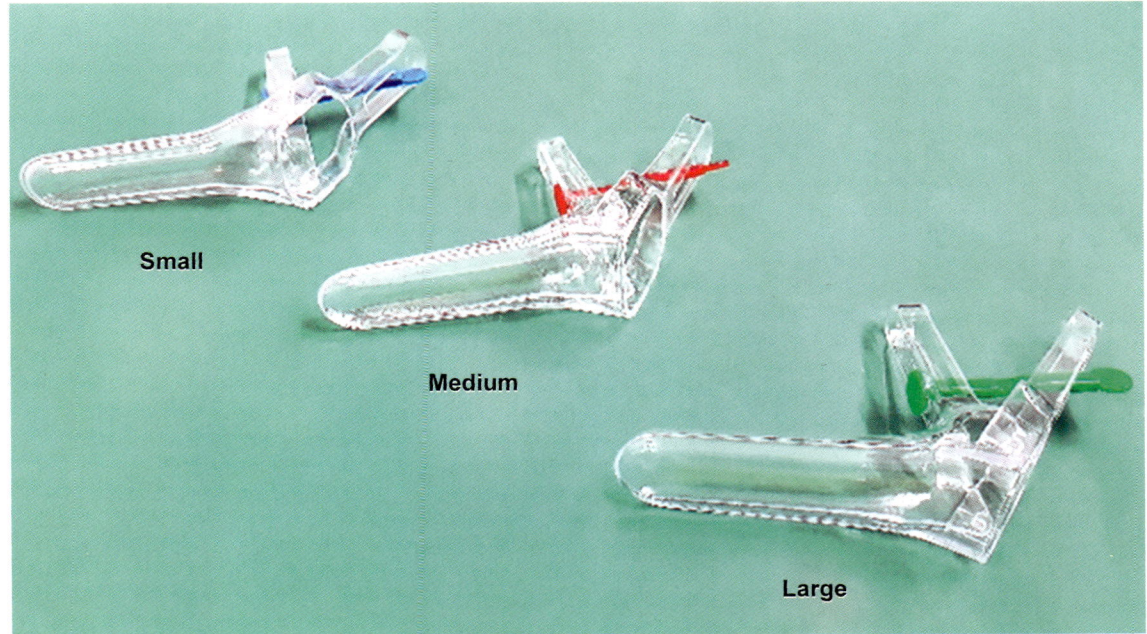

Fig. 2.3: Different sizes of speculum

c. Maneuvering and pushing the vaginal fornix to the side where you want to localize the cervix with blunt instrument say tip of sponge holder (Fig. 2.4), further helps in getting the desirable view of the cervix. Never maneuver by gripping the cervix, as there is a possibility of disturbing the epithelial cells of the cervix. For proper central fixation, give a gentle push on the contralateral fornix without touching the cervix thereby causing minimum damage to the cervical cells.

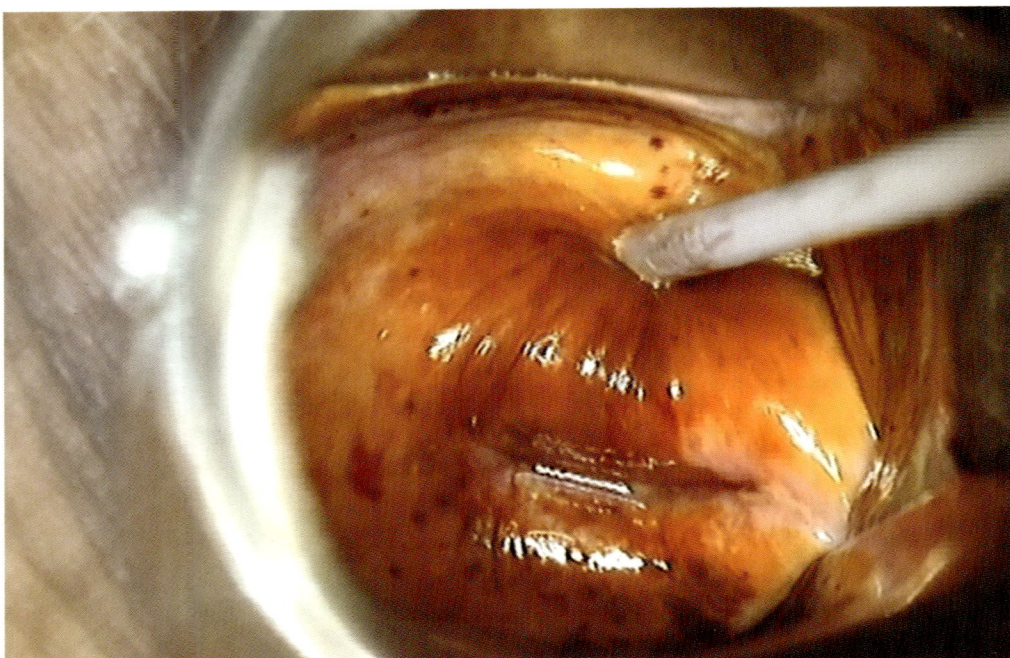

Fig. 2.4: Maneuvering the vaginal fornix

d. Be very gentle in opening the blades of the Cusco's speculum. Many a times, iatrogenic trauma (Fig. 2.5) and bleeding of the cervix have been encountered, especially in case of grade 1 prolapse of the uterus, supravaginal elongation of cervix.

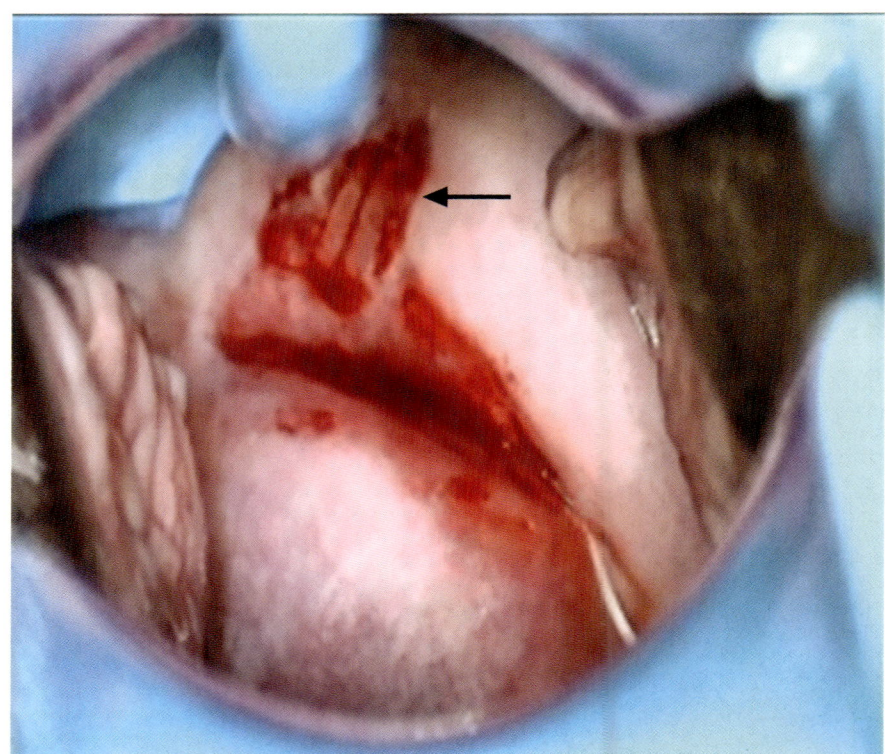

Fig. 2.5: Iatrogenic trauma while inserting Cusco's speculum

Do not start the procedure, if the entire cervix is not visualized properly, or else we can miss out many important findings (Fig. 2.6). Proper fixation is very important for correct visualization of cervix and central fixation.

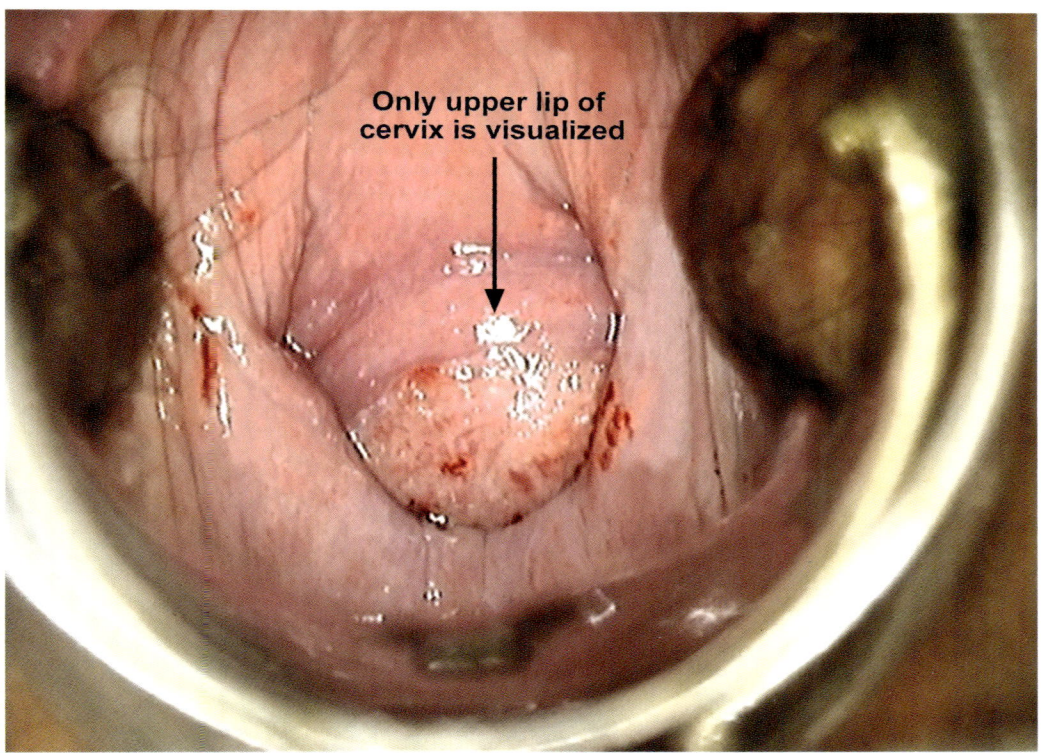

Fig. 2.6: Visualization of incomplete cervix

e. Correct magnification is necessary (Fig. 2.7).

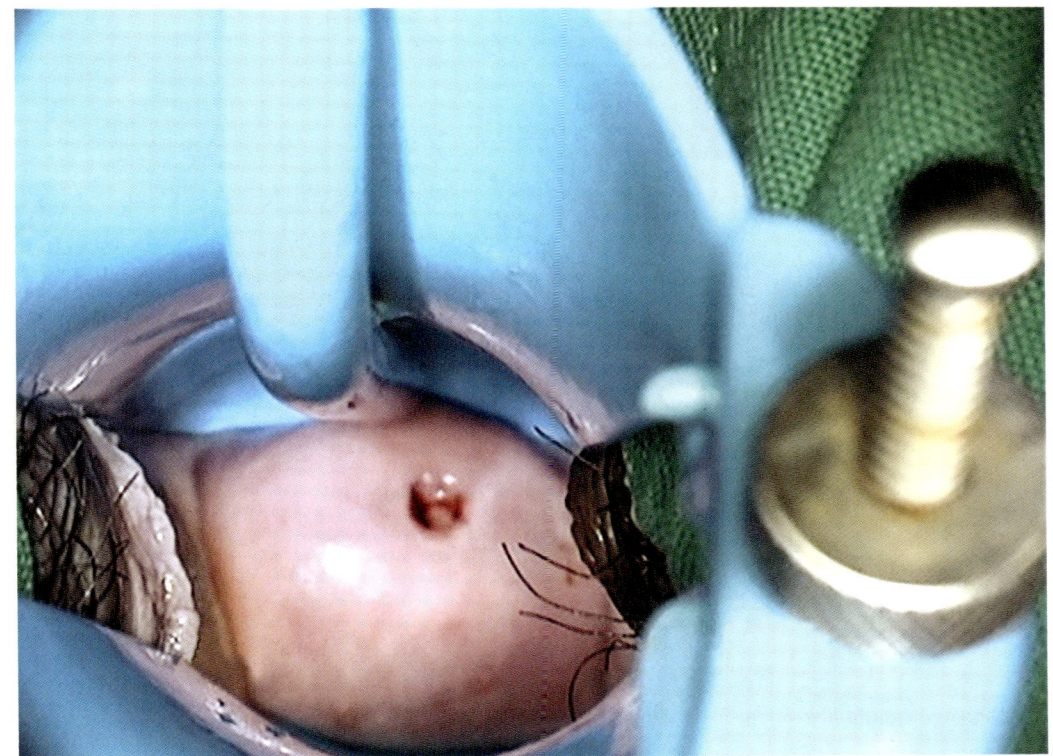

Fig. 2.7: Correct zoom in of the picture with right magnification for good quality study. Always the rim of the speculum should be minimally visualized in video colposcopy

f. Central fixation of cervix is very important before starting the procedure. The common images found during the fixing of the cervix are shown in Figs 2.8a to c.

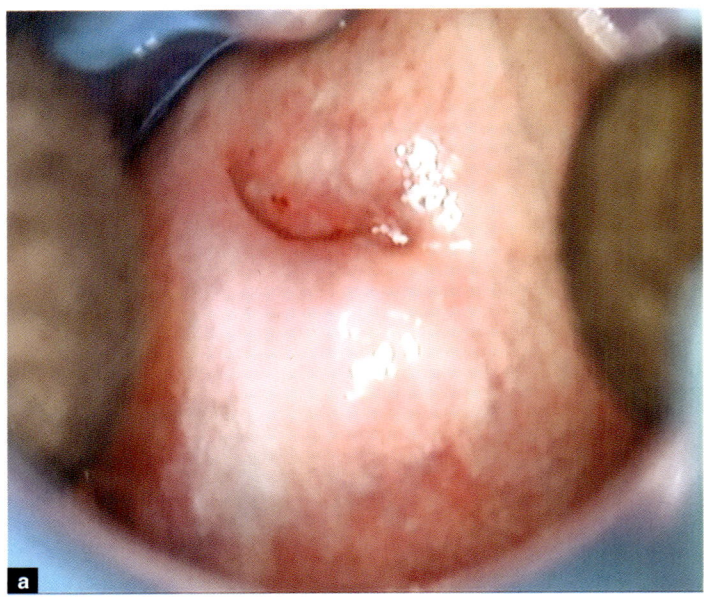

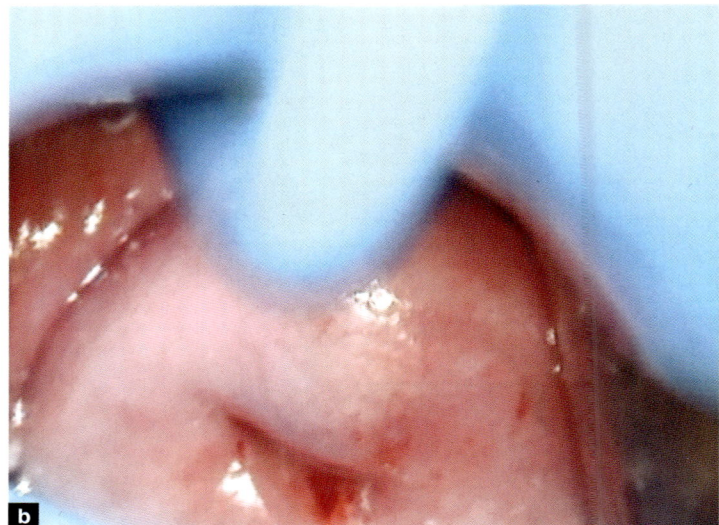

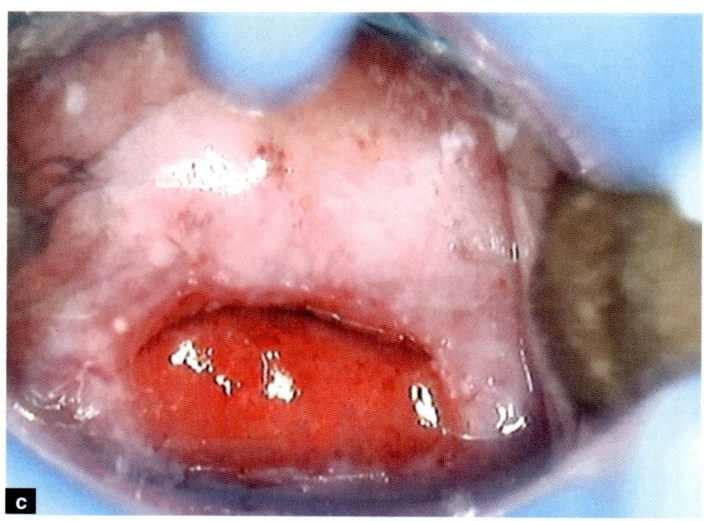

Figs 2.8a to c: (a) Central fixation of cervix with both lips of cervix well visualized; (b) Improper fixation of cervix, lower lip not seen; (c) Lower lip is not seen

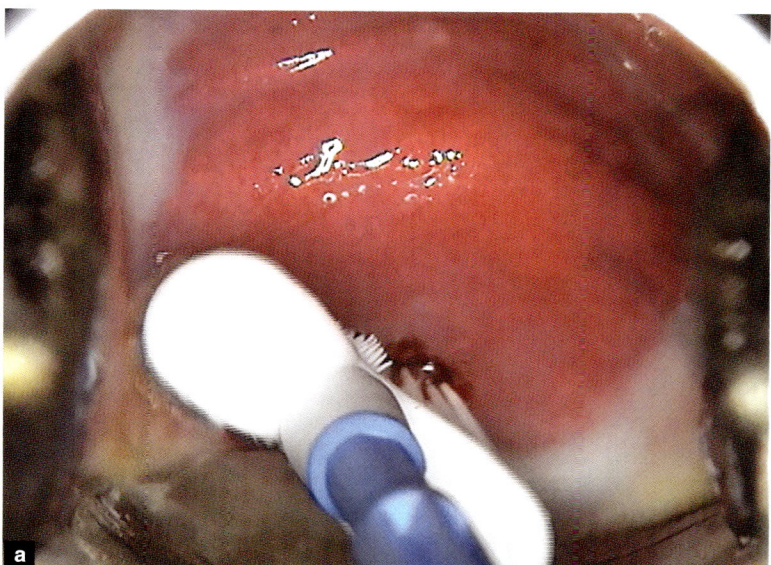

g. Cervical scrape can be taken before doing colposcopy for HPV, cytology (Figs 2.9a to c).

Tips: Usually slight-to-moderate bleeding is observed after cervical scraping, hence it is advisable to gently scrape the cervical epithelium with the cervical cell sampler brush.

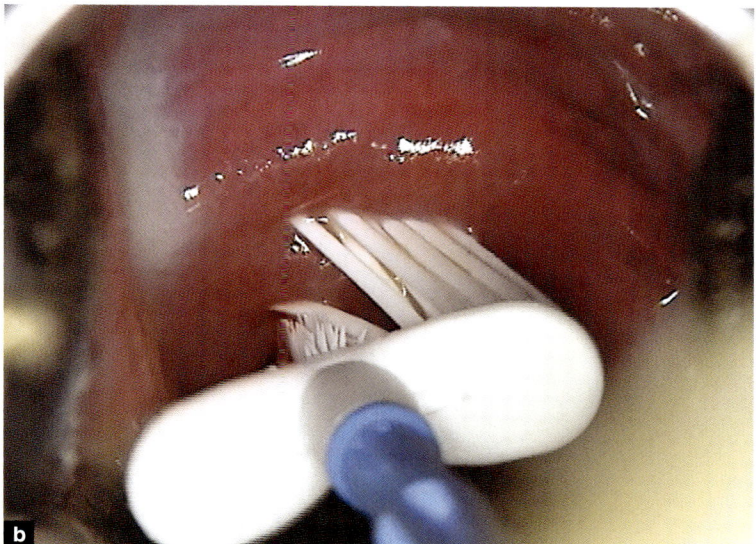

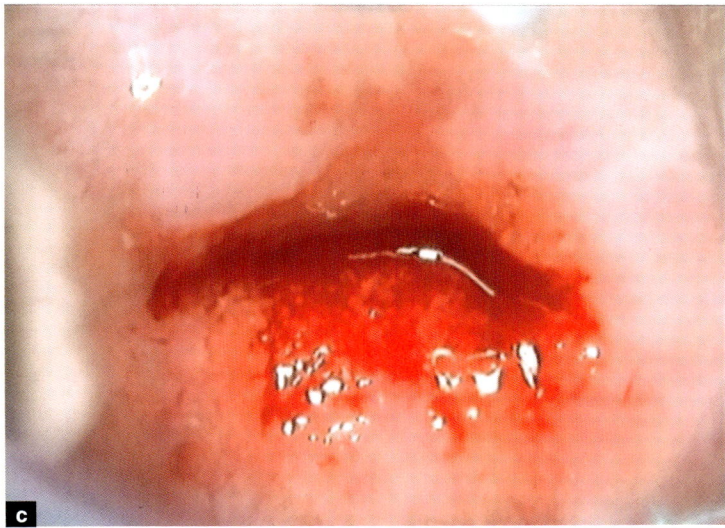

Figs 2.9a to c: Cervical scrape

h. Cleaning the cervix gently with normal saline to remove the cervical discharge. The extra fluid that is accumulated has to be removed (Figs 2.10a and b).

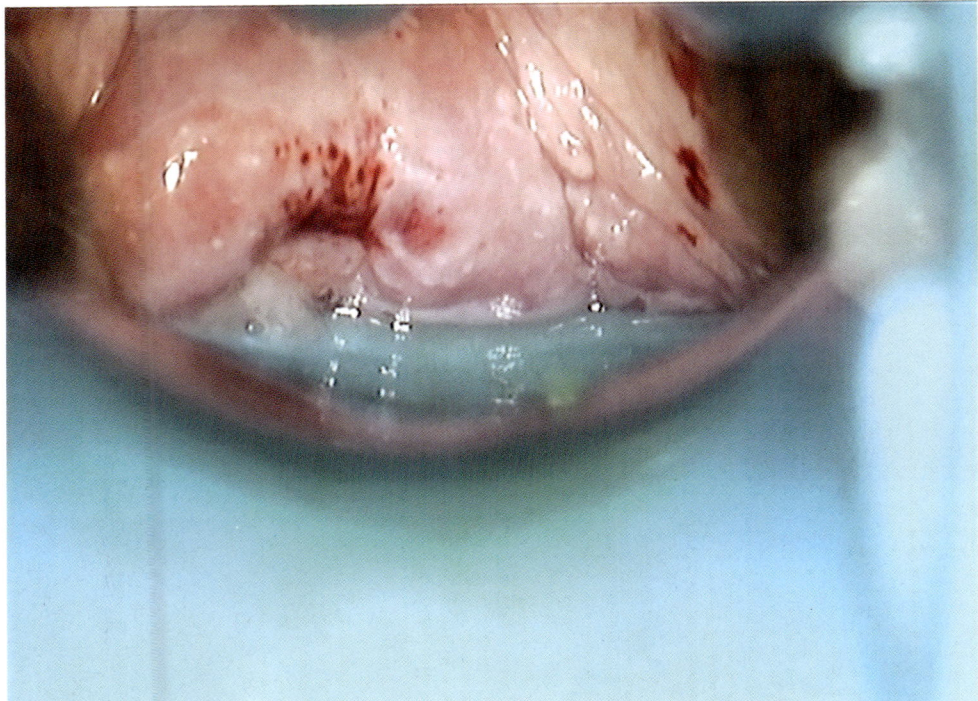

Fig. 2.10a: Improper fixation. Cervix has to be fixed in the centre and the extra fluid should be removed

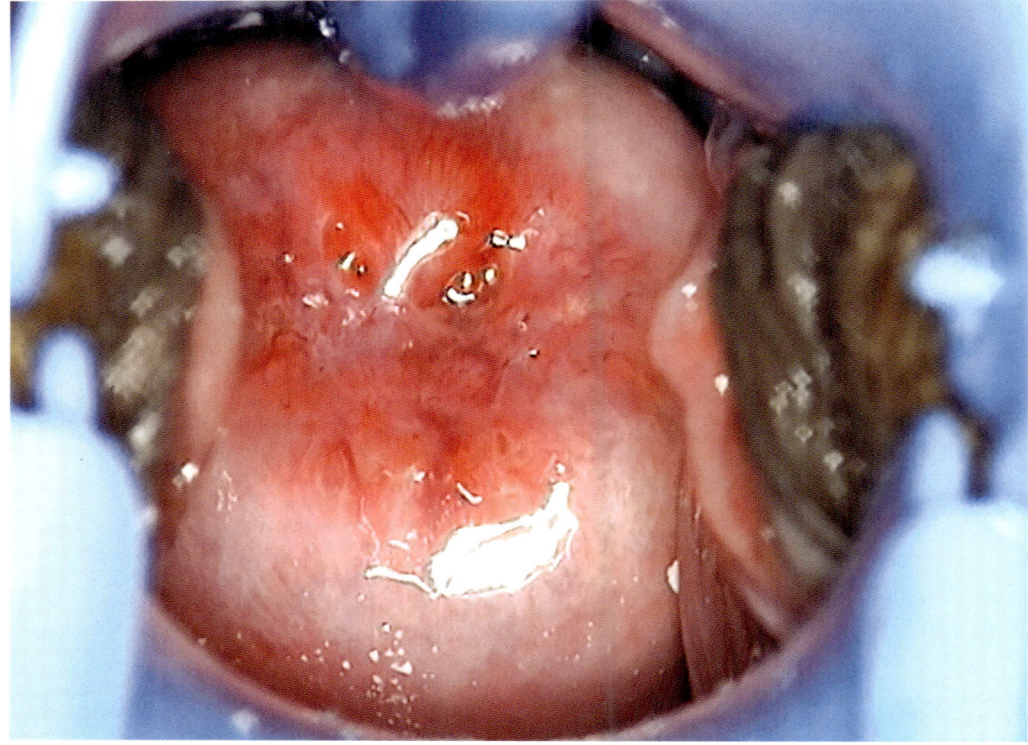

Fig. 2.10b: Central fixation of cervix

3. On Cleaning with Normal Saline

Following features are seen (Fig. 2.11):

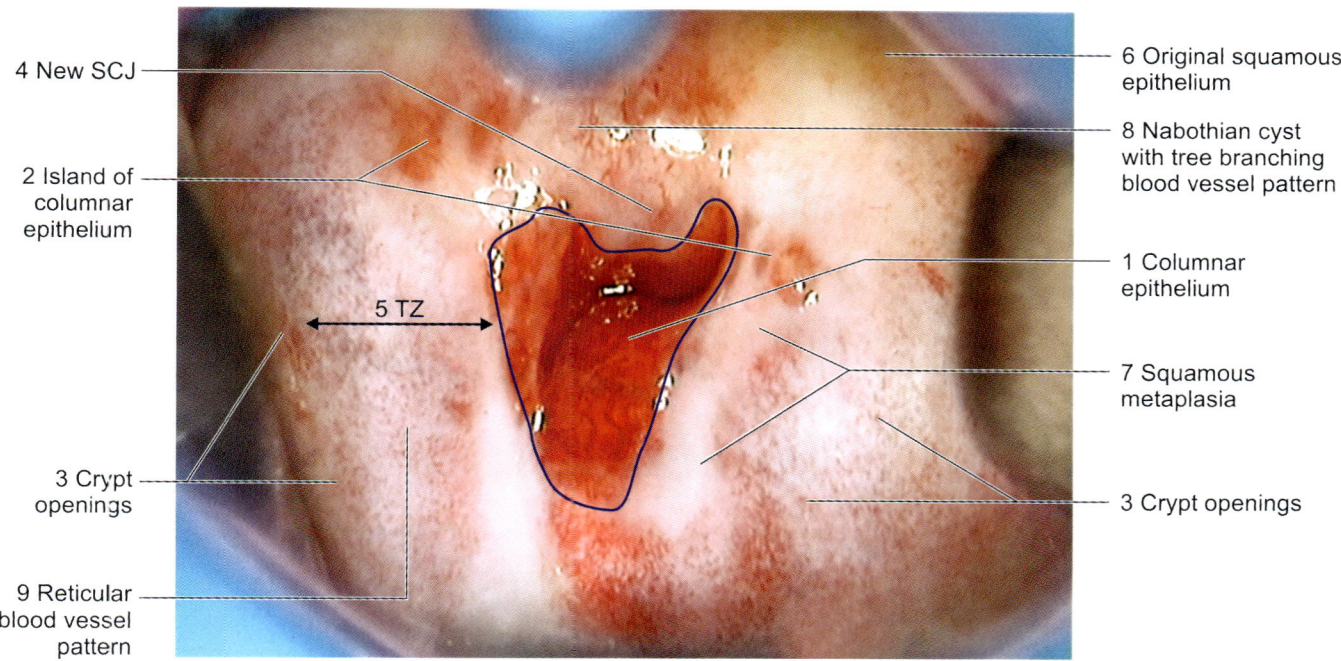

Fig. 2.11: Procedure with normal saline

1. *Columnar epithelium:* This appears as grape-like reddish epithelium. Since columnar epithelia are single-layered, the underlying stromal blood vessels are clearly visible as reddish colour.
2. *Islands of columnar epithelium* are sometimes visible as small patch of columnar epithelium, identified by its colour and grape like texture.
3. *Crypt opening:* To identify the original SCJ, we have to look out for distal crypt opening which appears as depression. Arbitrarily joining the distal crypts gives us an idea of old/original SCJ prior to occurrence of metaplasia.
4. *New SCJ:* Appears as sharp demarcation boundary between the columnar and squamous epithelia. The new SCJ is more highlighted as white line on application of acetic acid (Fig. 2.12).
5. *Transformation zone (TZ):* Between the original arbitrary SCJ and new SCJ. This signifies the metaplastic epithelium. More will be dealt in the terminology chapter (Chapter 3).
6. *Original squamous epithelium:* Squamous epithelium being multilayered appears pinkish red. The original squamous epithelium is usually located distal to the distal crypt openings.
7. *Squamous metaplasia:* Appears thin translucent whitish highlighted more on application of 5% acetic acid.
8. *Nabothian cyst:* Several retention cysts are seen on the cervix at the area of metaplastic epithelium, called nabothian cysts. These retention cysts develop as a result of the occlusion of the endocervical crypt openings by the overlying metaplastic squamous epithelium. The buried columnar cells in the endocervical crypts continue to secrete mucus, which later develops into retention cysts called nabothian cysts (Figs 2.13a and b). They appear as whitish swellings on the ectocervix.
9. *Reticular blood vessel pattern:* The stromal blood vessels appear as reticular mesh pattern seen usually on the squamous epithelium, near SCJ.

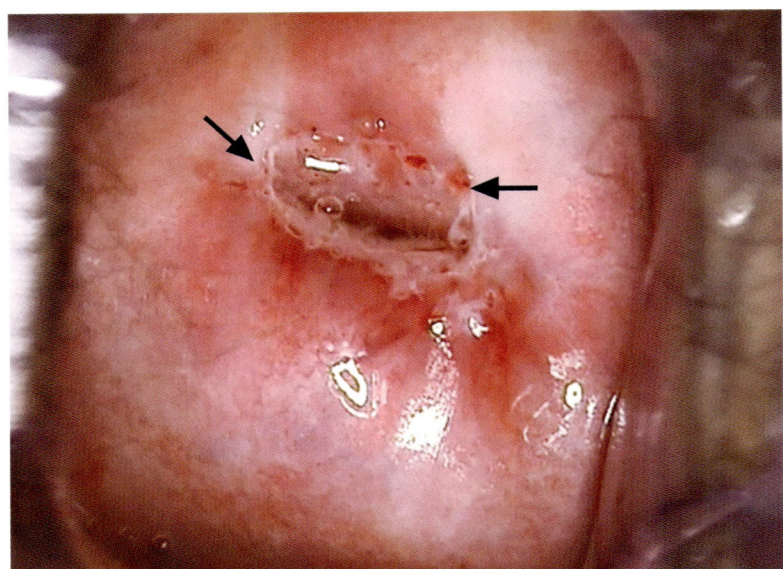

Fig. 2.12: Squamocolumnar junction (SCJ) (on acetic acid application) seen as whitish line around the external os

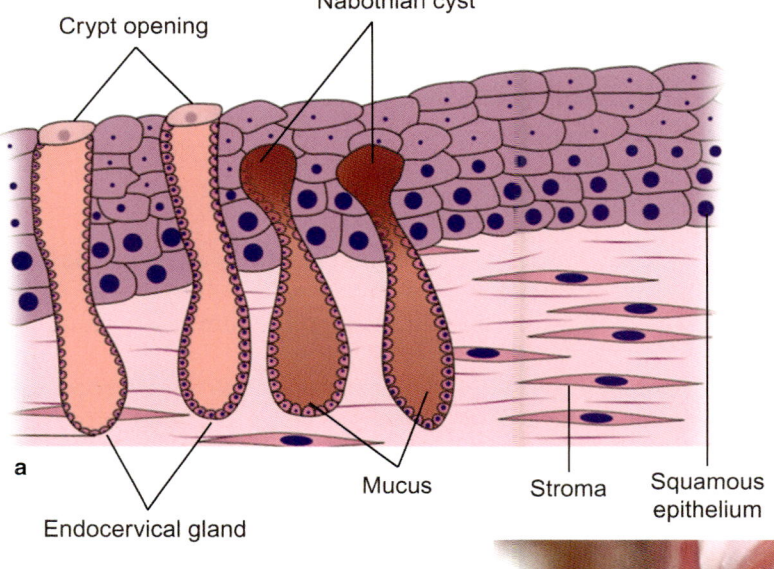

Crypt opening

Nabothian cyst

Endocervical gland

Mucus   Stroma   Squamous epithelium

a

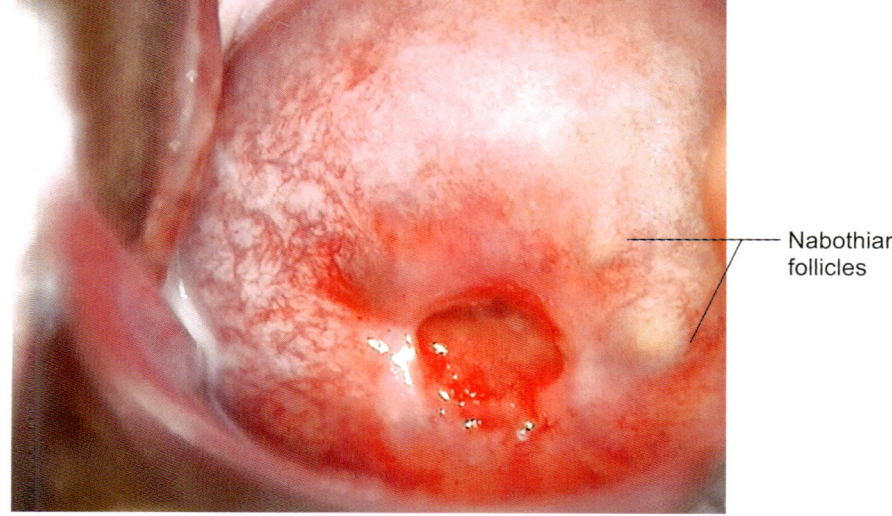

Nabothian follicles

b

Figs 2.13a and b: Nabothian cyst

4. Blue-Green Filter

The blood vessel pattern gets perfectly highlighted with blue-green filter (Fig. 2.14). Usually, a typical blood vessel pattern is noted on the cervix, the knowledge of which is important to identify the abnormal vascular

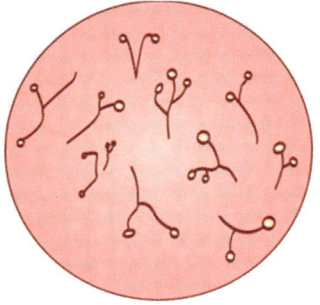

Staghorn-like capillaries—
trichomoniasis infection

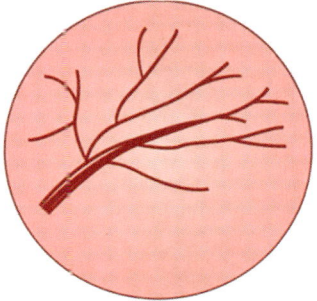

Regular branching patteren with
gradual decrease in caliber—
near immature metaplasia

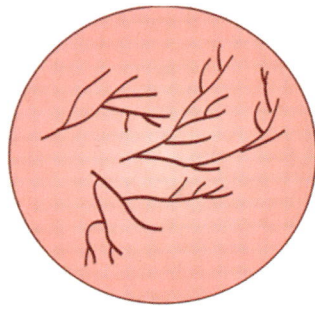

Tree branching patteren
over the nabothian follicle

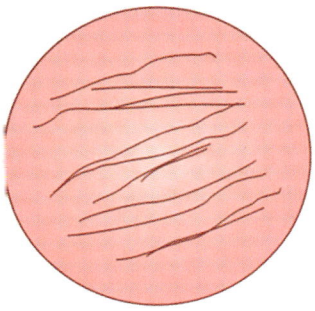

Healing CIN

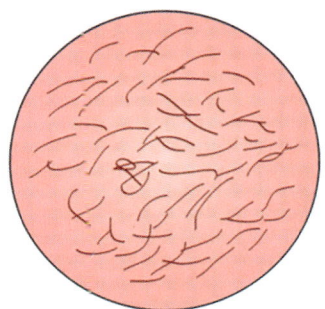

Reticular network capillaries near
original SCJ—mature metaplasia

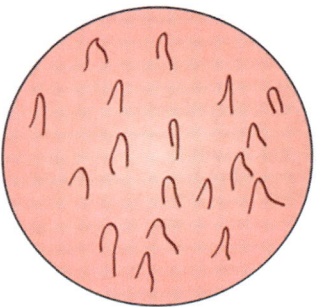

Hairpin capillaries
near original SCJ

Fig. 2.14: Vascular patterns

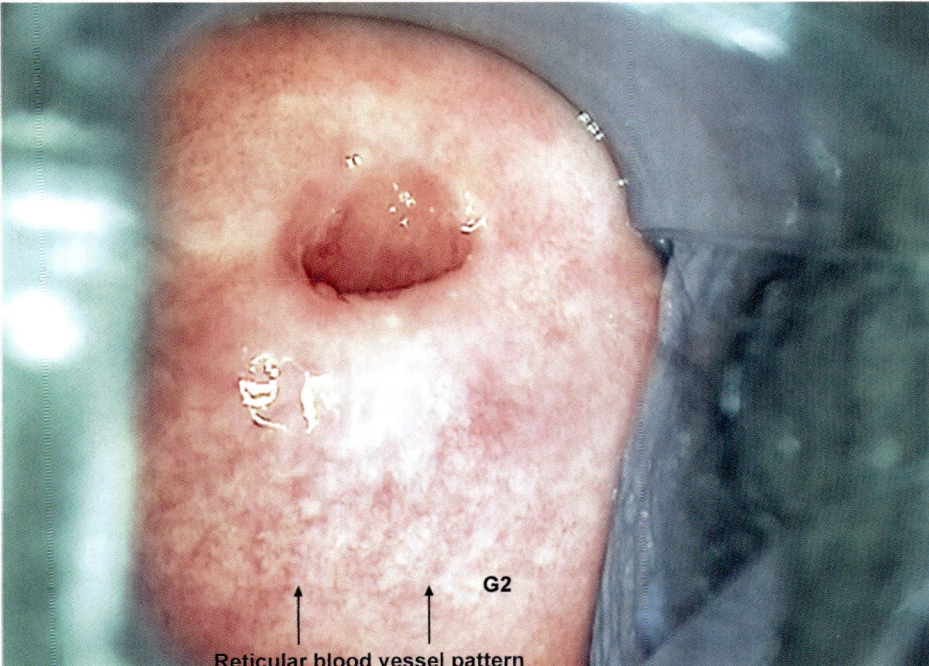

G2

Reticular blood vessel pattern

Fig. 2.15: Reticular blood vessel pattern

pattern. These are the stromal blood vessels forming a pattern. They are highlighted in blue-green filter. The two common types of vascular patterns noted are reticular (Fig. 2.15) and hairpin-shaped patterns (Fig. 2.16). Regular tree branching pattern (Figs 2.17 and 2.18) is seen on the nabothian follicles. Parallel vascular pattern (Figs 2.19a and b) is seen on the healing tissues. In infection with trichomoniasis (Fig. 2.20), the hairpin shape vessels assumes staghorn-like shapes.

Irregular blood vessels on blue-green filter: Mosaics and punctations are to be appreciated and noted. The explanation with images are shown in separate chapter.

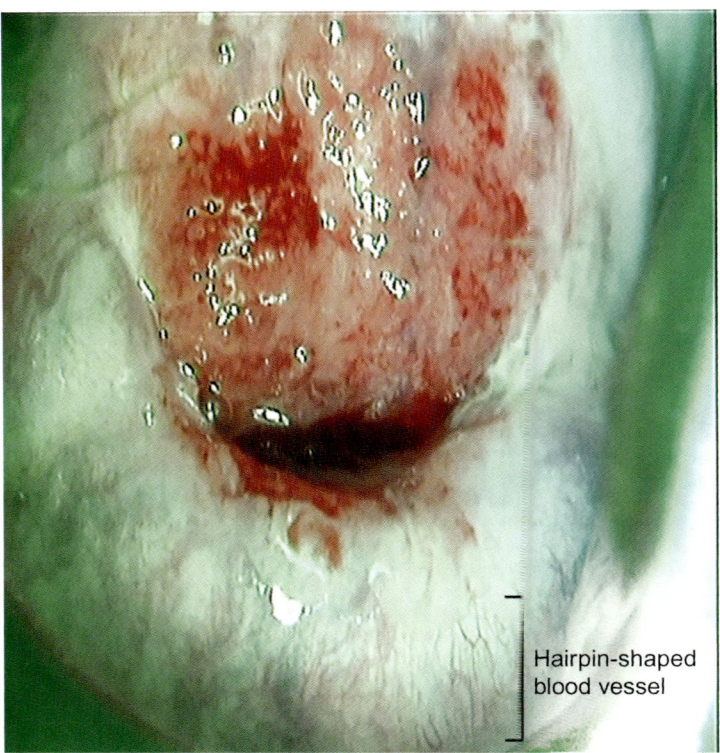

Hairpin-shaped
blood vessel

Fig. 2.16: Hairpin blood vessel pattern

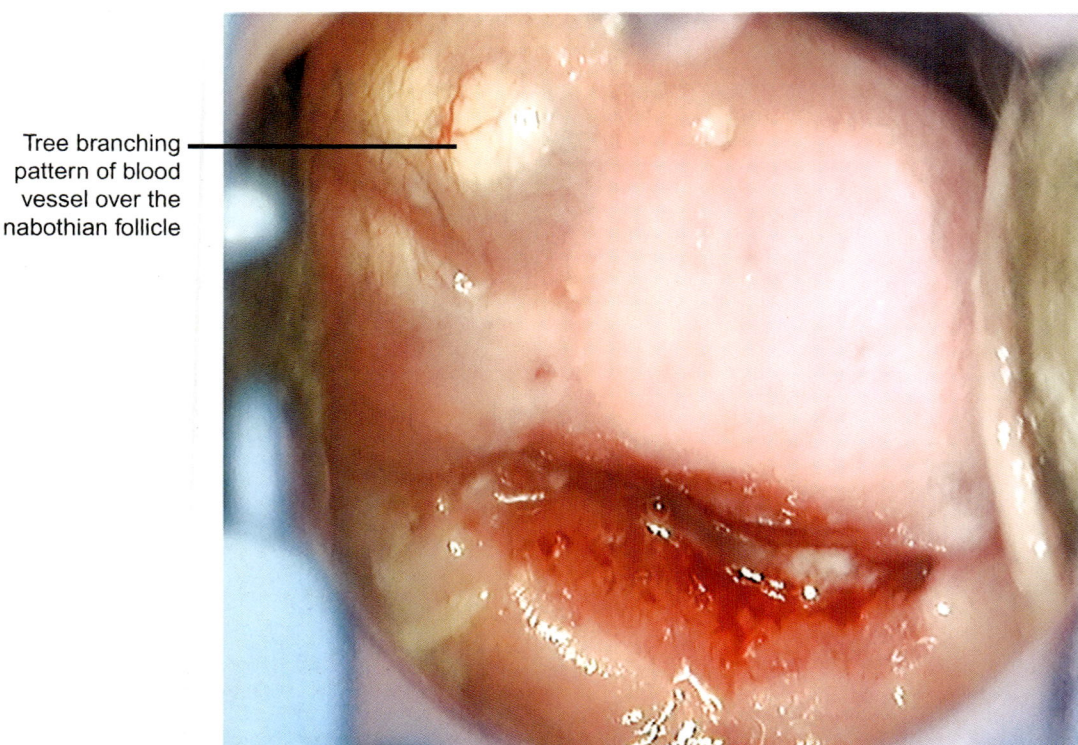

Tree branching
pattern of blood
vessel over the
nabothian follicle

Fig. 2.17: Tree branching pattern

Elicited more clearly
on blue-green filter

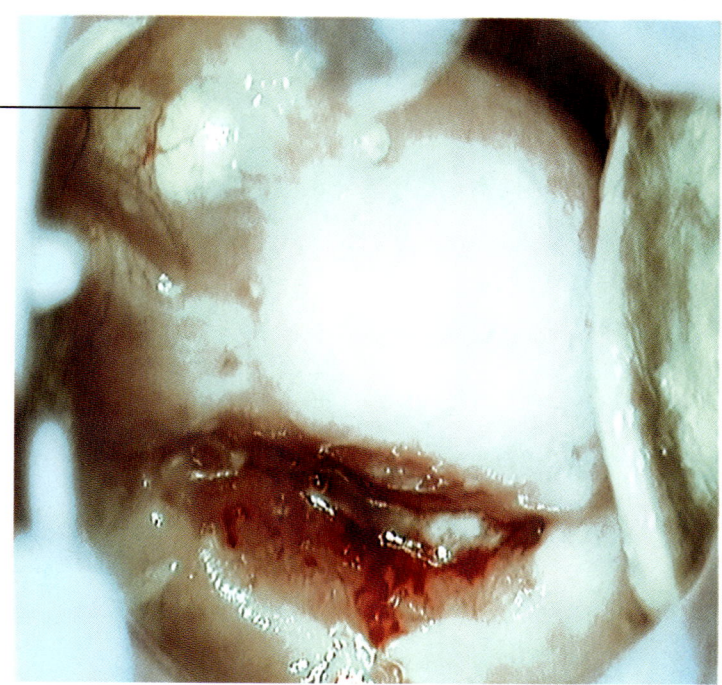

Fig. 2.18: Tree branching pattern

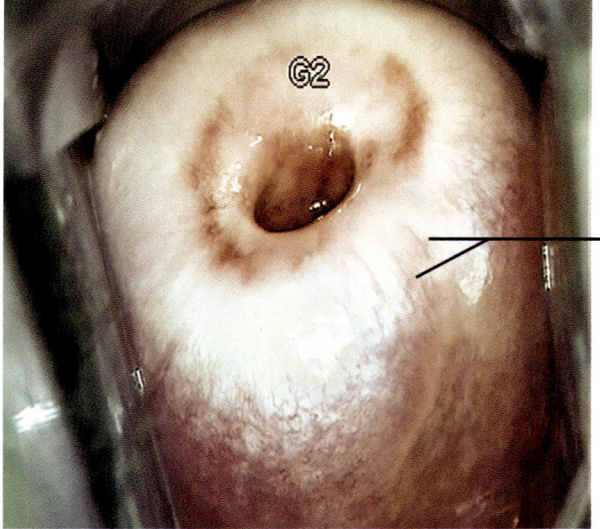

Fig. 2.19a: Parallel vascular pattern

Healing parallel
blood vessel pattern
seen usually in the
healing tissue.
This is a case of post-
cryotherapy follow-up

Healing
parallel blood
vessel
pattern—post-
LEEP treatment

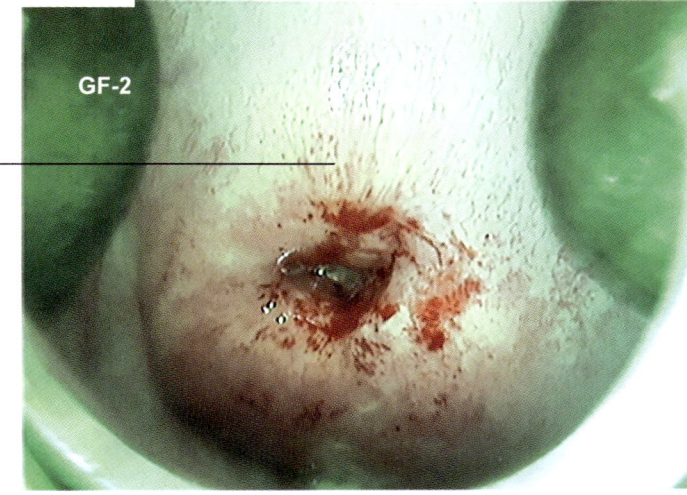

Fig. 2.19b: Healing blood vessels in blue-green filter

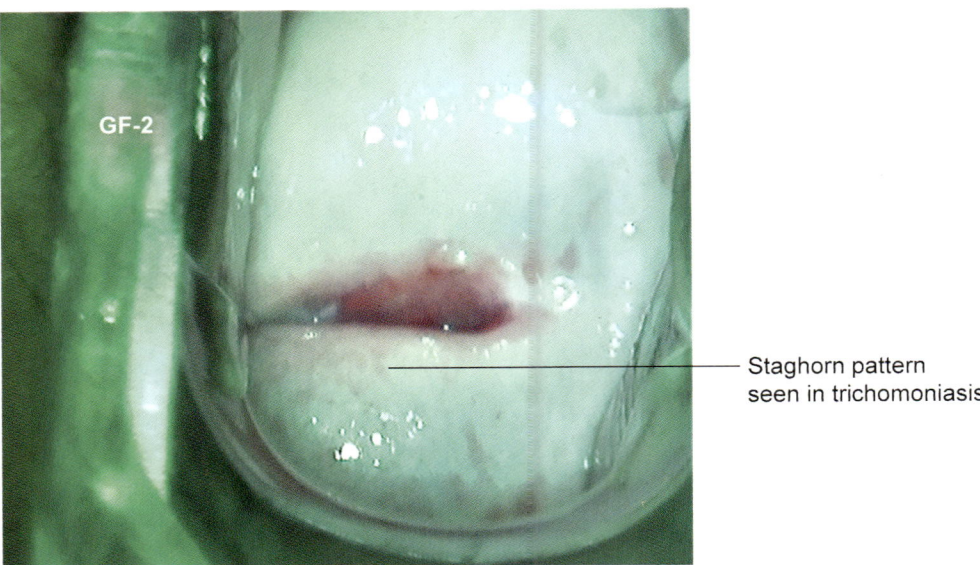

Staghorn pattern
seen in trichomoniasis

Fig. 2.20: Trichomoniasis infection

Abnormal Blood Vessel Patterns

On HSIL and microinvasive lesion, we often see abnormal vessel pattern (Fig. 2.21a).

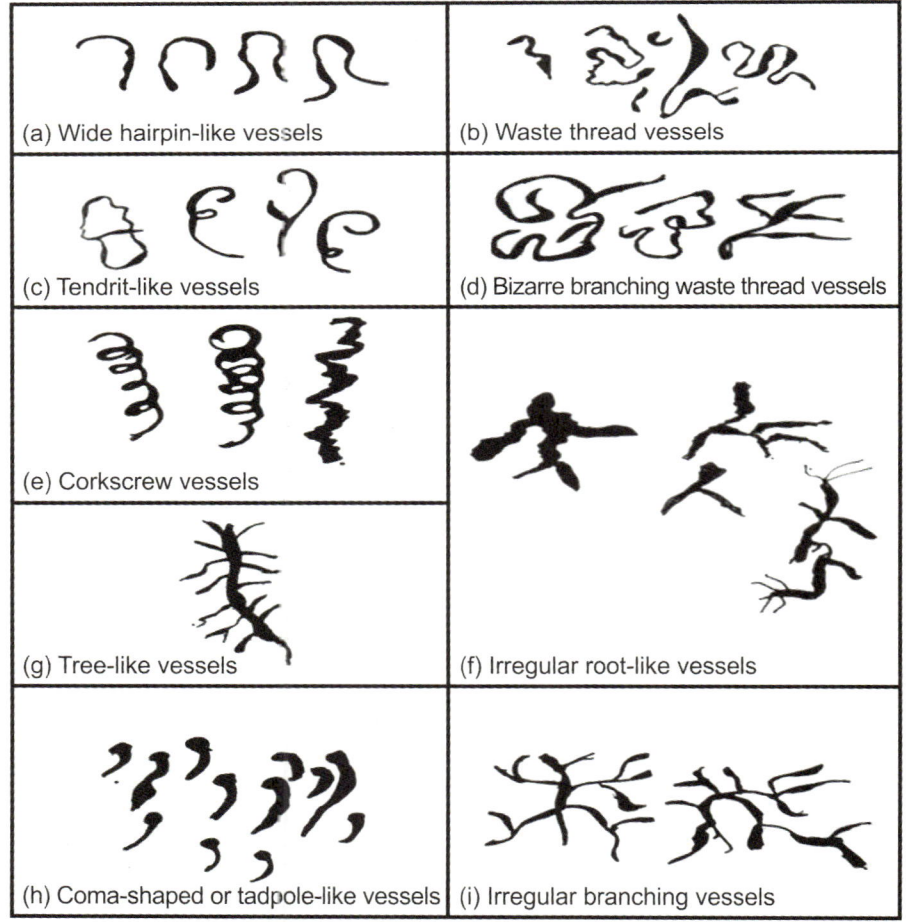

(a) Wide hairpin-like vessels	(b) Waste thread vessels
(c) Tendrit-like vessels	(d) Bizarre branching waste thread vessels
(e) Corkscrew vessels	(f) Irregular root-like vessels
(g) Tree-like vessels	
(h) Coma-shaped or tadpole-like vessels	(i) Irregular branching vessels

Fig. 2.21a: Abnormal blood vessel patterns

Different types of abnormal blood vessel patterns (Figs 2.21b to f)

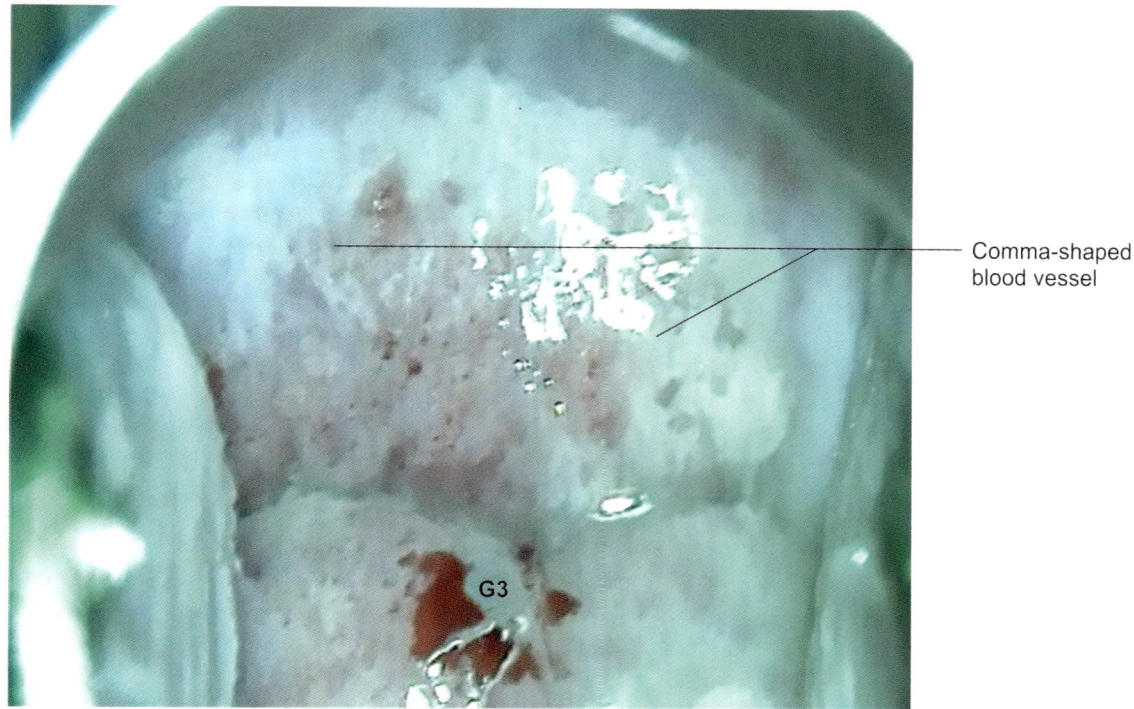

Comma-shaped
blood vessel

G3

Fig. 2.21b: Coma-shaped abnormal vessel

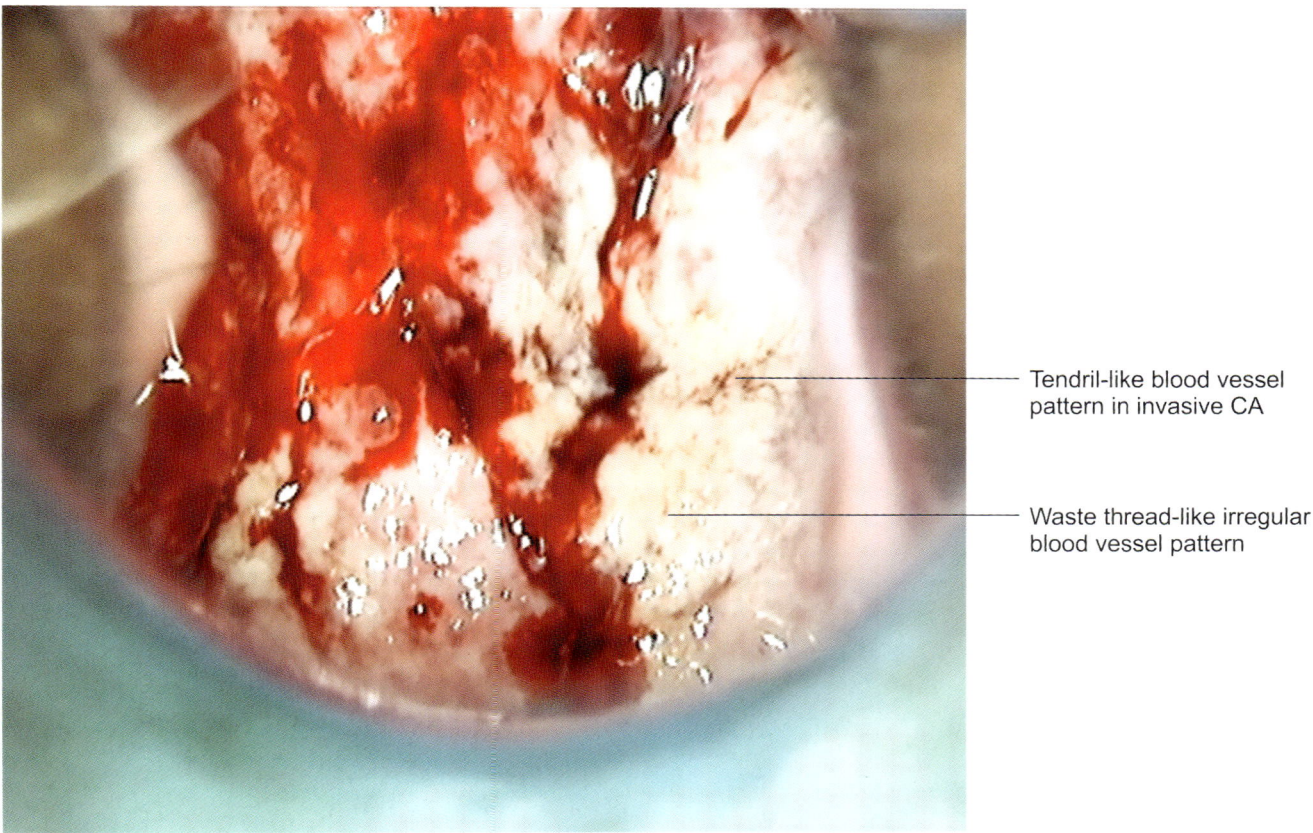

Tendril-like blood vessel
pattern in invasive CA

Waste thread-like irregular
blood vessel pattern

Fig. 2.21c: Tendril-like vessel

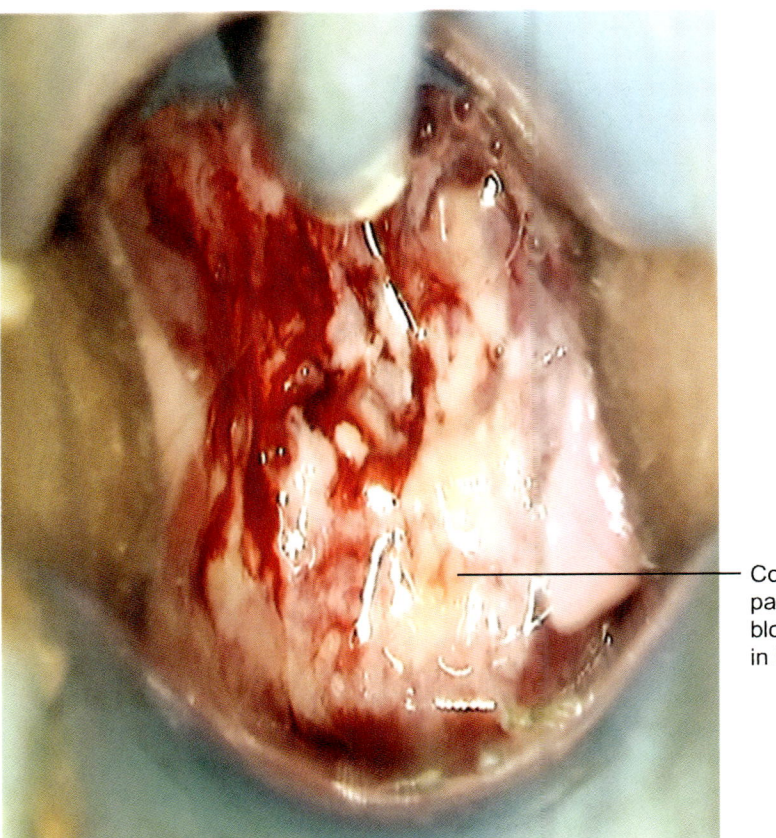

Corkscrew
pattern of
blood vessel
in invasive CA

Fig. 2.21d: Corkscrew blood vessel

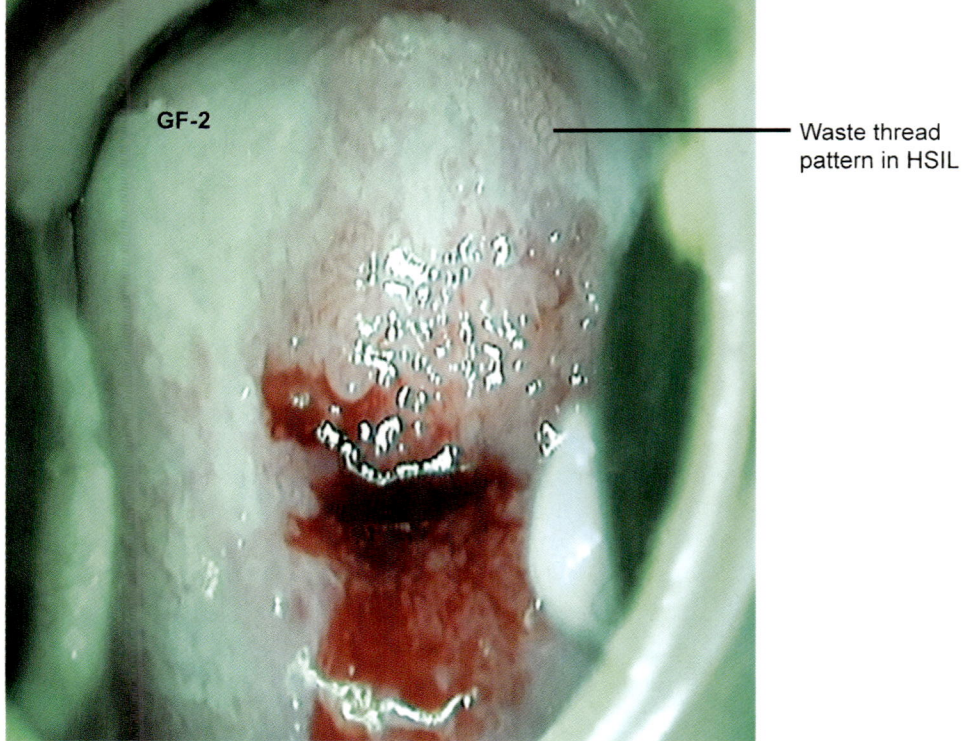

GF-2

Waste thread
pattern in HSIL

Fig. 2.21e: Waste thread blood vessel

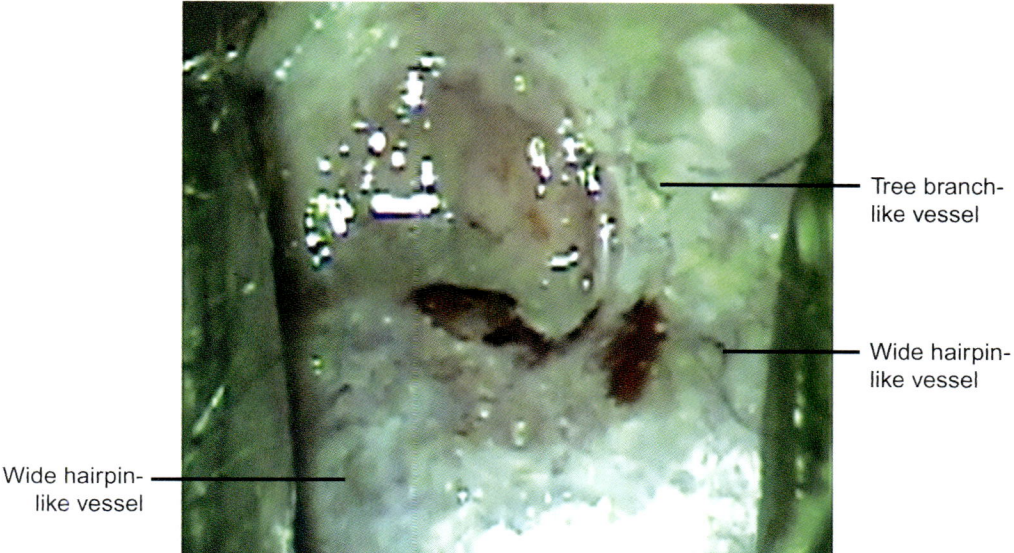

Wide hairpin-like vessel

Tree branch-like vessel

Wide hairpin-like vessel

Fig. 2.21f: Tree branch and hairpin blood vessel

5. 5% Acetic Acid Application

Acetic Acid Test

3–5% acetic acid is gently applied on the cervix. There should be a generous and liberal application of acetic acid all around the cervix for about one complete minute. The cervix should be literally bathed in the pool of acetic acid using cotton balls soaked with acetic acid and held with a sponge holder (Fig. 2.22). Observation should be for next one minute, so total of 2 minutes—1 min for application and 1 min for observation.

Preparation of 5% acetic acid—1 ml glacial acetic acid with 19 ml distilled water for routine OPD purpose. For camp setting—5 ml glacial acetic acid with 95 ml distilled water. It should be a fresh preparation and has to be discarded after 24 hrs

Points to Observe

- New SCJ, which is very nicely noticed as a sharp line or margin
- Distal crypt openings to mark the limit of original SCJ
- Metaplastic epithelium
- Transformation zone

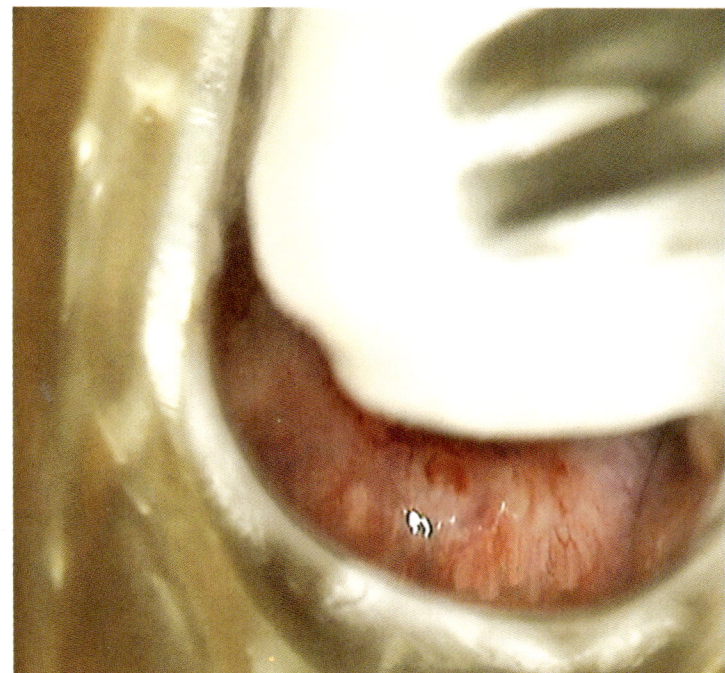

Fig. 2.22: Application of 5% acetic acid

- Abnormal acetowhite lesions (if any): Its margins, its position with respect to new SCJ and TZ, its surface contour, texture, its luster, how soon has it become acetowhite and how long does it retains its acetowhiteness, intensity of acetowhiteness whether pale white, oyster egg white, or chalk white, density of the lesion, whether any lesions within the lesions or umbilication noted, any cuffed crypt noted.
- Columnar epithelium

Tips

a. After application of acetic acid, patients experience a slight burning sensation. Patients have to be adequately counselled prior to the application of acetic acid to avoid discomfort.
b. Some colposcopists have adopted the practice of spraying the cervix with acetic acid using a syringe fitted with wide bore long needle. It is very useful in camps to avoid autoclaving of the instruments used.

c. In postmenopausal woman, due to the thin atrophic epithelium, the cervix appears pale white. The reporting can be misleading due to tiny petechial hemorrhage developed after application of acetic acid. One should have an adequate experience in performing colposcopy in postmenopausal women before reporting the case to avoid over or under reporting.

Principle

Acetic acid coagulates the intracellular proteins thus obscuring the passage of light, thus turning acetowhite.

Columnar epithelium, mature squamous metaplasia and original squamous epithelium do not turn acetowhite since there are very less intracellular proteins.

In case of immature squamous metaplasia, the cells are dividing cells with high nucleocytoplasmic ratio. On application of 5% acetic acid, immature metaplastic tissue turns acetowhite, which is thin, transparent, shiny, without any geographical pattern with finger-like or feathery margins. They can arise focally anywhere on the columnar epithelium. The acetowhiteness disappears very quickly.

In case of CIN lesions, the acetowhite lesions have set geographical pattern arising from SCJ within the transformation zone distributed centrifugally. Low grade lesions have feathery but distinct margins. They are milky white. High grade lesions have distinct margins, sometimes elevated rolled out margins, with distinct oyster egg white or chalky white. Low grade lesions appear late and disappears fast, whereas the high grade lesions appear instantly and disappear late.

Sometimes the columnar epithelium appears white due to the metaplastic changes occurring on them. SCJ appears as a distinct thin acetowhite line.

Physiological VIA positive conditions (Figs 2.23a to g):

1. NEW SCJ
2. Metaplastic epithelium
3. Columnar epithelium covered with squamous metaplasia.
4. Satellite lesions, which is acetowhite within or outside the TZ zone.
5. Congenital TZ
6. Hyperkeratotic patches.

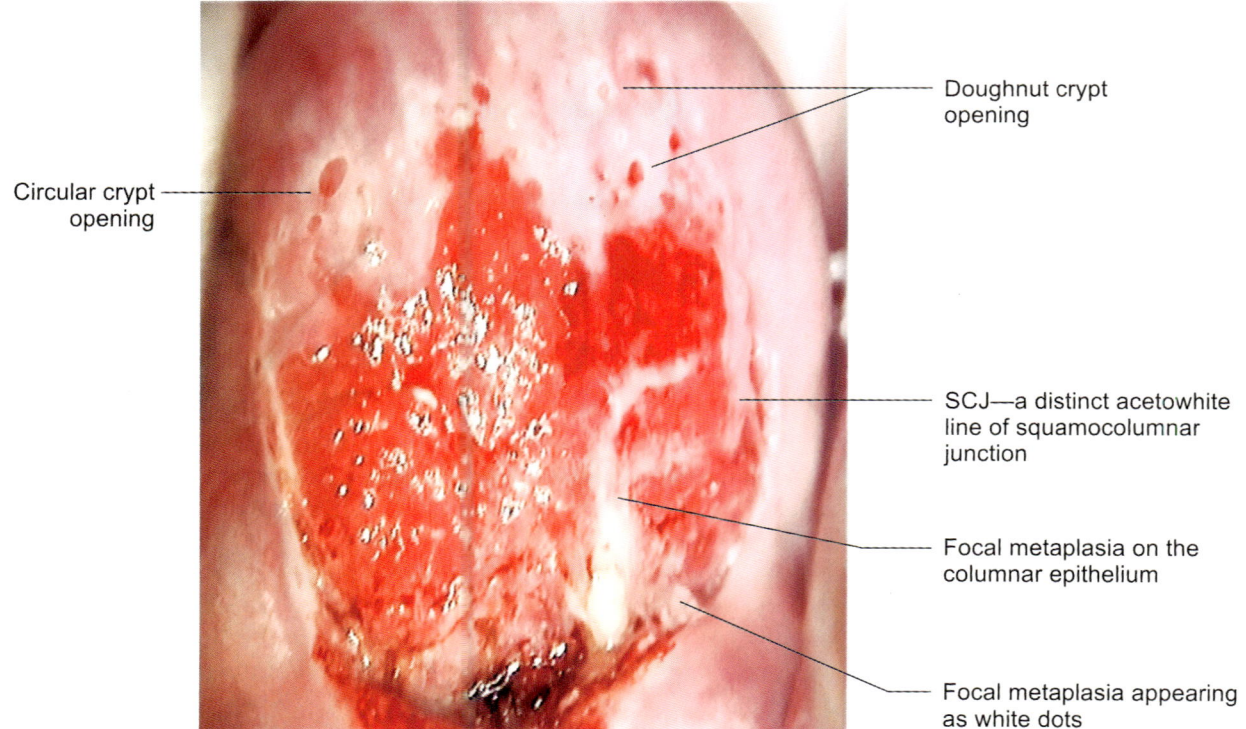

Circular crypt opening — Doughnut crypt opening — SCJ—a distinct acetowhite line of squamocolumnar junction — Focal metaplasia on the columnar epithelium — Focal metaplasia appearing as white dots

Fig. 2.23a

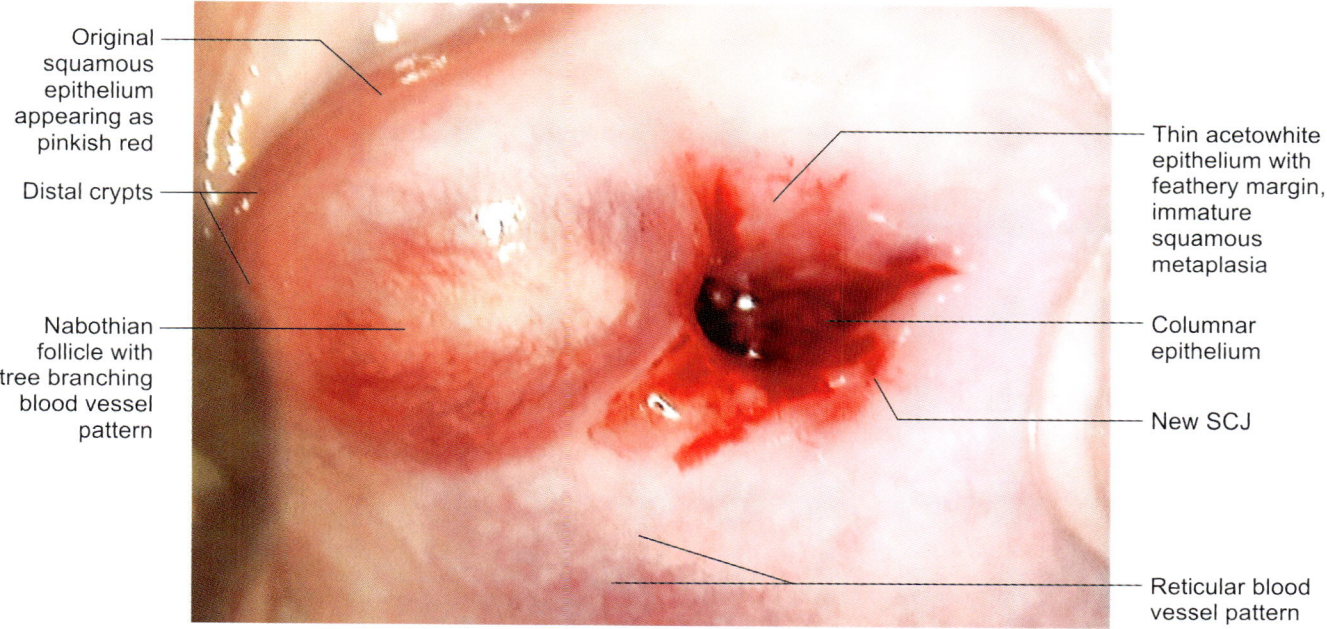

Original squamous epithelium appearing as pinkish red

Distal crypts

Nabothian follicle with tree branching blood vessel pattern

Thin acetowhite epithelium with feathery margin, immature squamous metaplasia

Columnar epithelium

New SCJ

Reticular blood vessel pattern

Fig. 2.23b

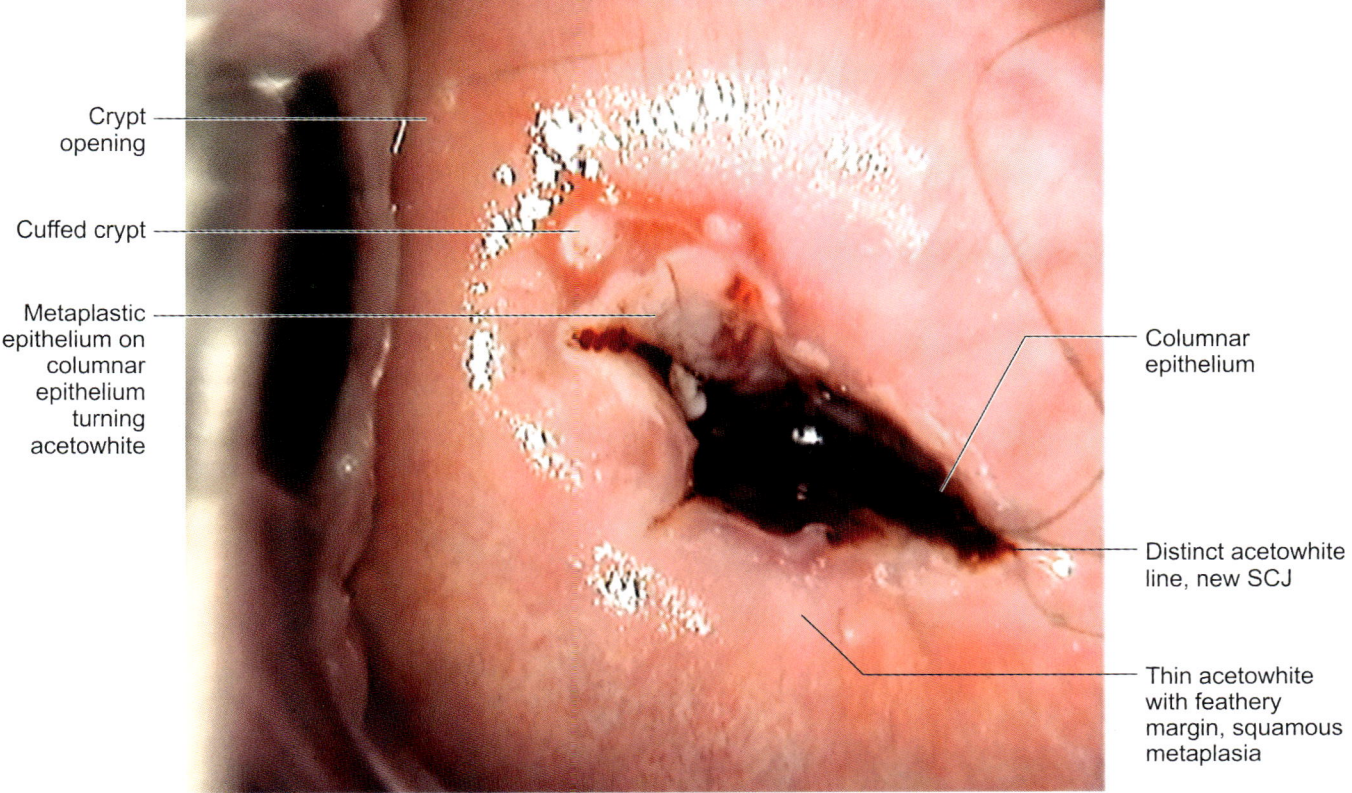

Crypt opening

Cuffed crypt

Metaplastic epithelium on columnar epithelium turning acetowhite

Columnar epithelium

Distinct acetowhite line, new SCJ

Thin acetowhite with feathery margin, squamous metaplasia

Fig. 2.23c: Cuffed crypts may be a pathagnomonic features of HSIL, hence better to take biopsy to r/o lesions

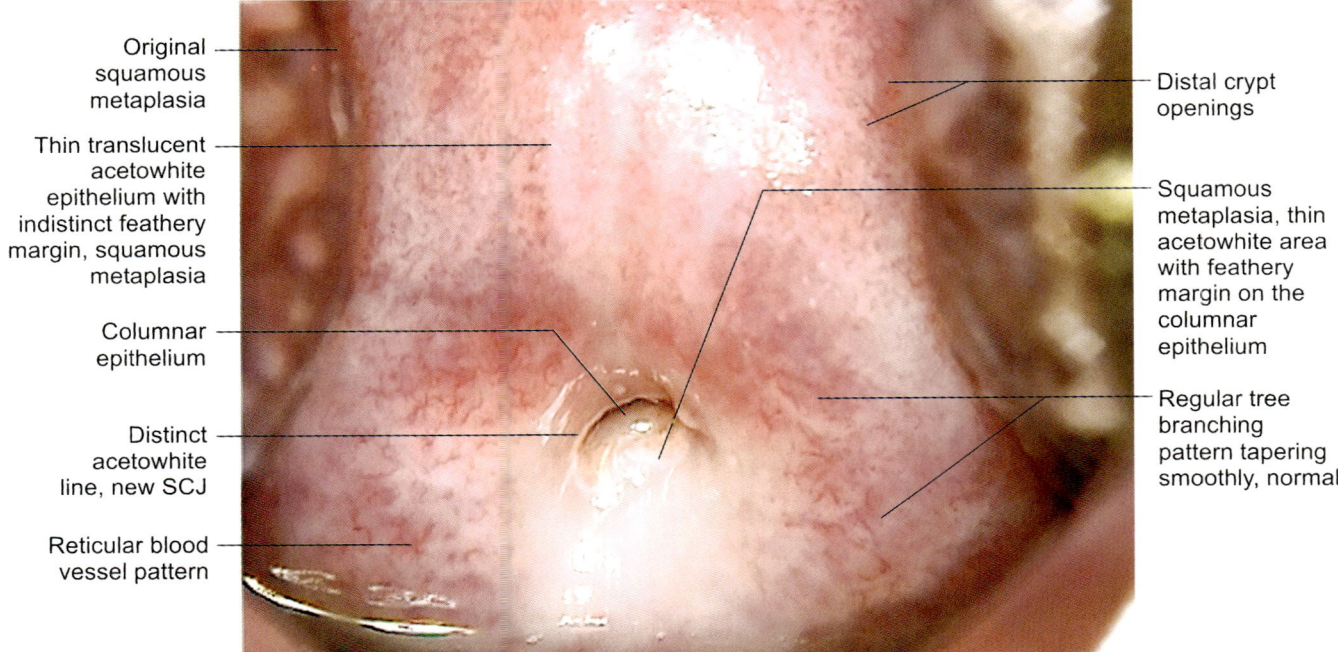

Original squamous metaplasia

Thin translucent acetowhite epithelium with indistinct feathery margin, squamous metaplasia

Columnar epithelium

Distinct acetowhite line, new SCJ

Reticular blood vessel pattern

Distal crypt openings

Squamous metaplasia, thin acetowhite area with feathery margin on the columnar epithelium

Regular tree branching pattern tapering smoothly, normal

Fig. 2.23d

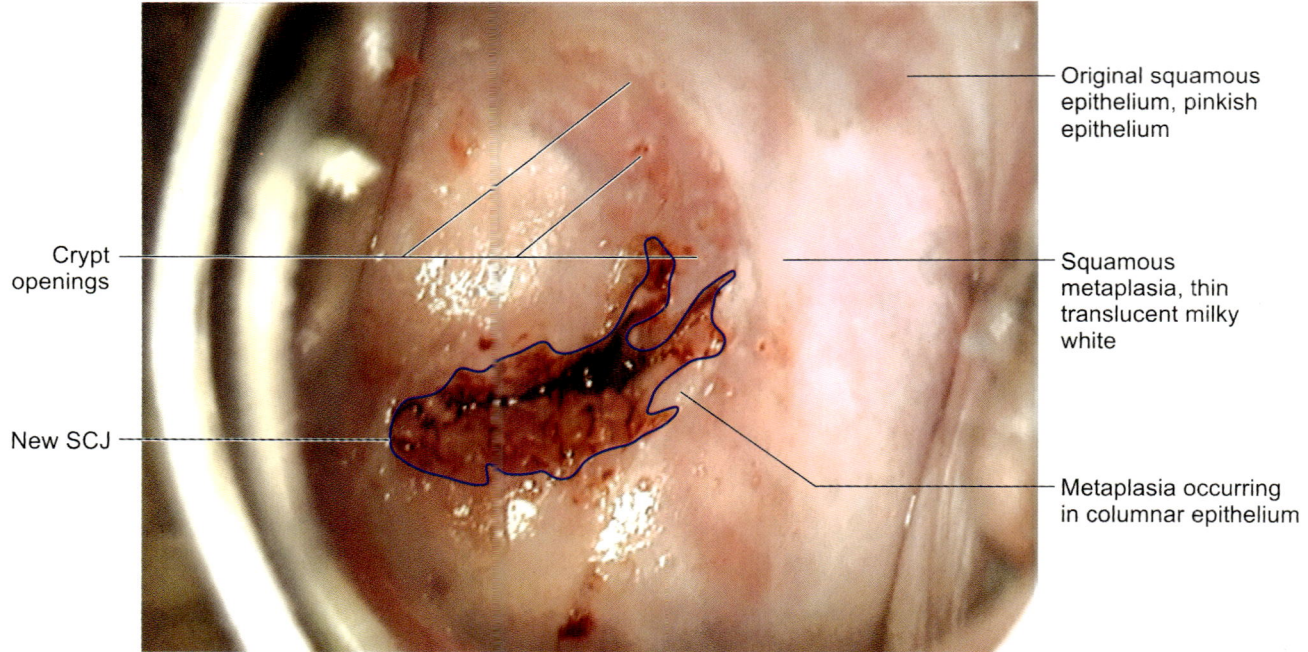

Crypt openings

New SCJ

Original squamous epithelium, pinkish epithelium

Squamous metaplasia, thin translucent milky white

Metaplasia occurring in columnar epithelium

Fig. 2.23e

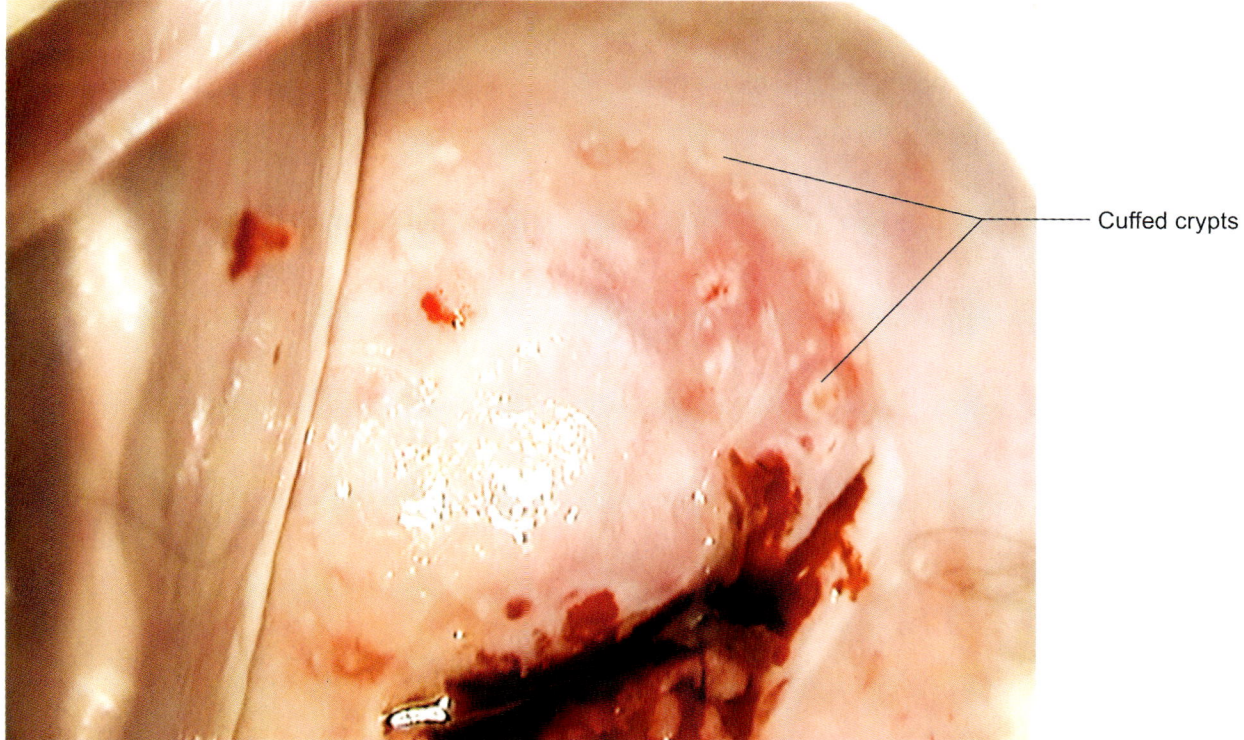

Cuffed crypts

Fig. 2.23f

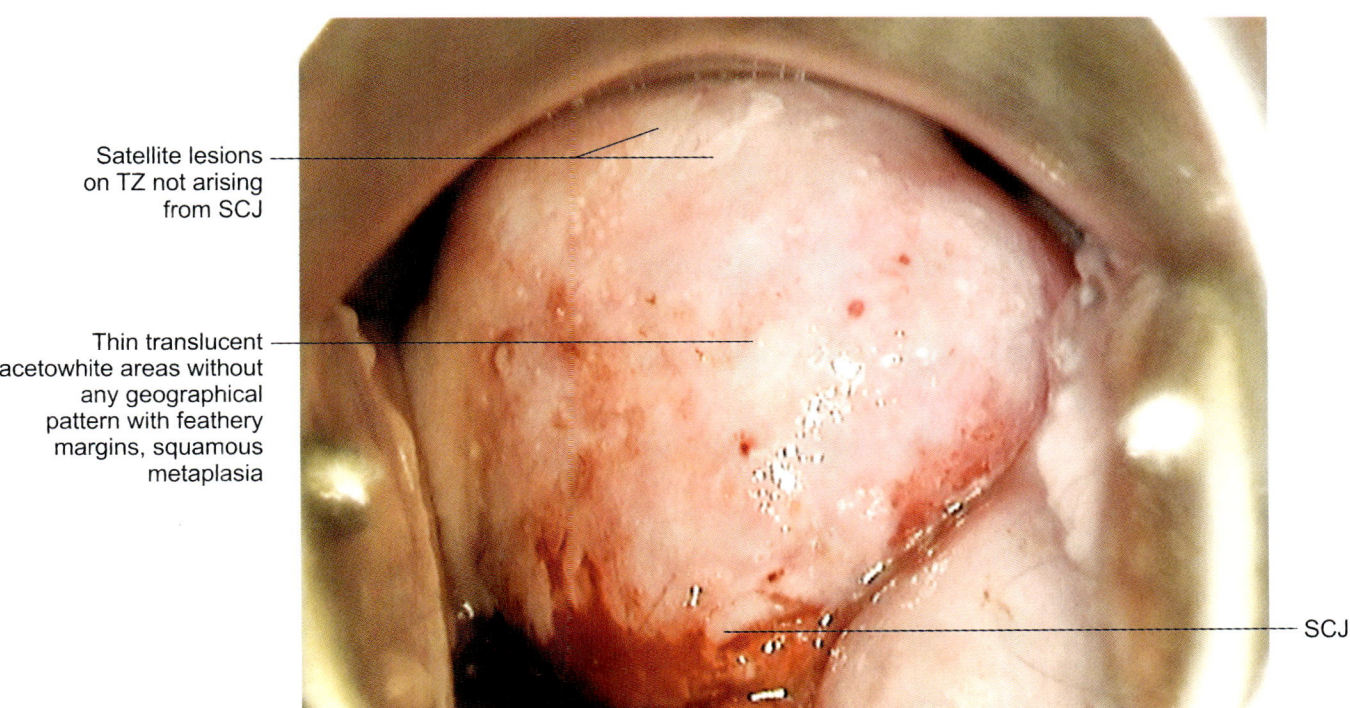

Satellite lesions on TZ not arising from SCJ

Thin translucent acetowhite areas without any geographical pattern with feathery margins, squamous metaplasia

SCJ

Fig. 2.23g

Pathological VIA positive conditions (Figs 2.24a to f):

1. LSIL   3. Invasive CA
2. HSIL   4. Microcondylomatous lesion

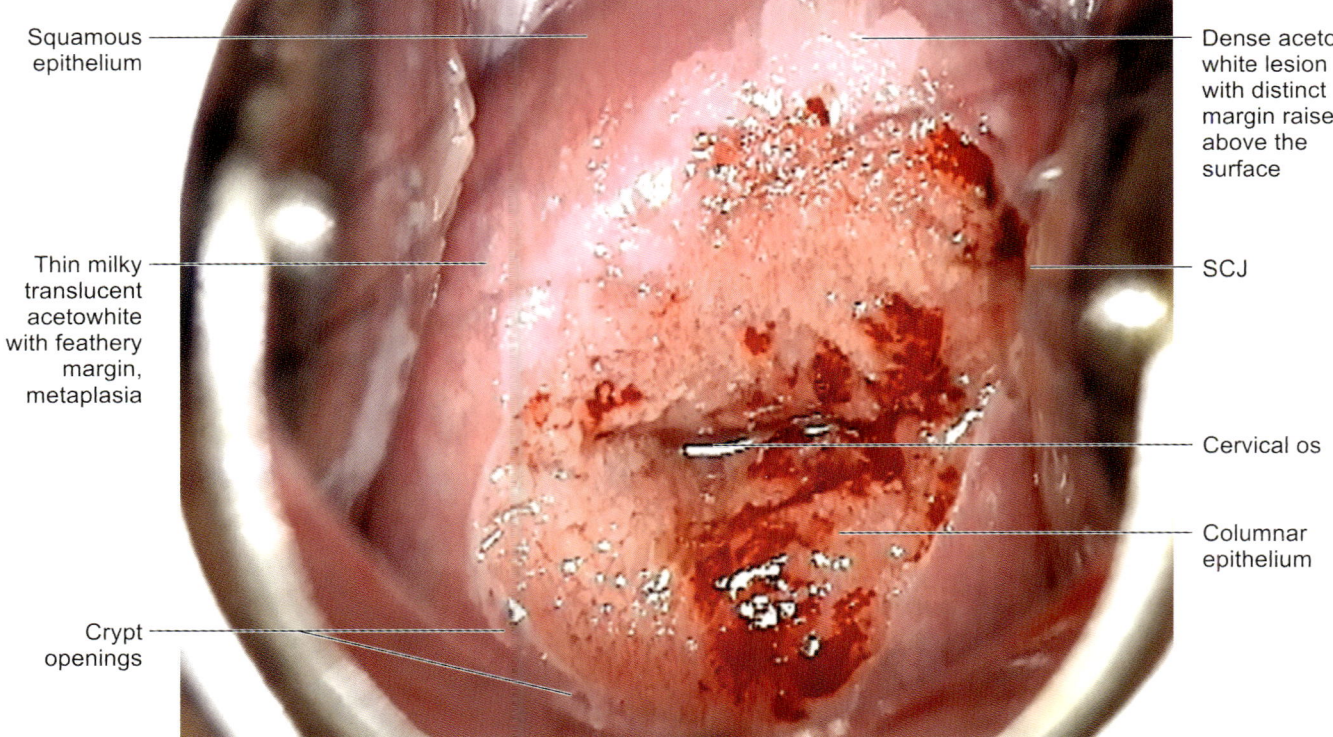

Squamous epithelium

Dense aceto-white lesion with distinct margin raised above the surface

Thin milky translucent acetowhite with feathery margin, metaplasia

SCJ

Cervical os

Columnar epithelium

Crypt openings

Fig. 2.24a: Lesion at 1 O'clock position

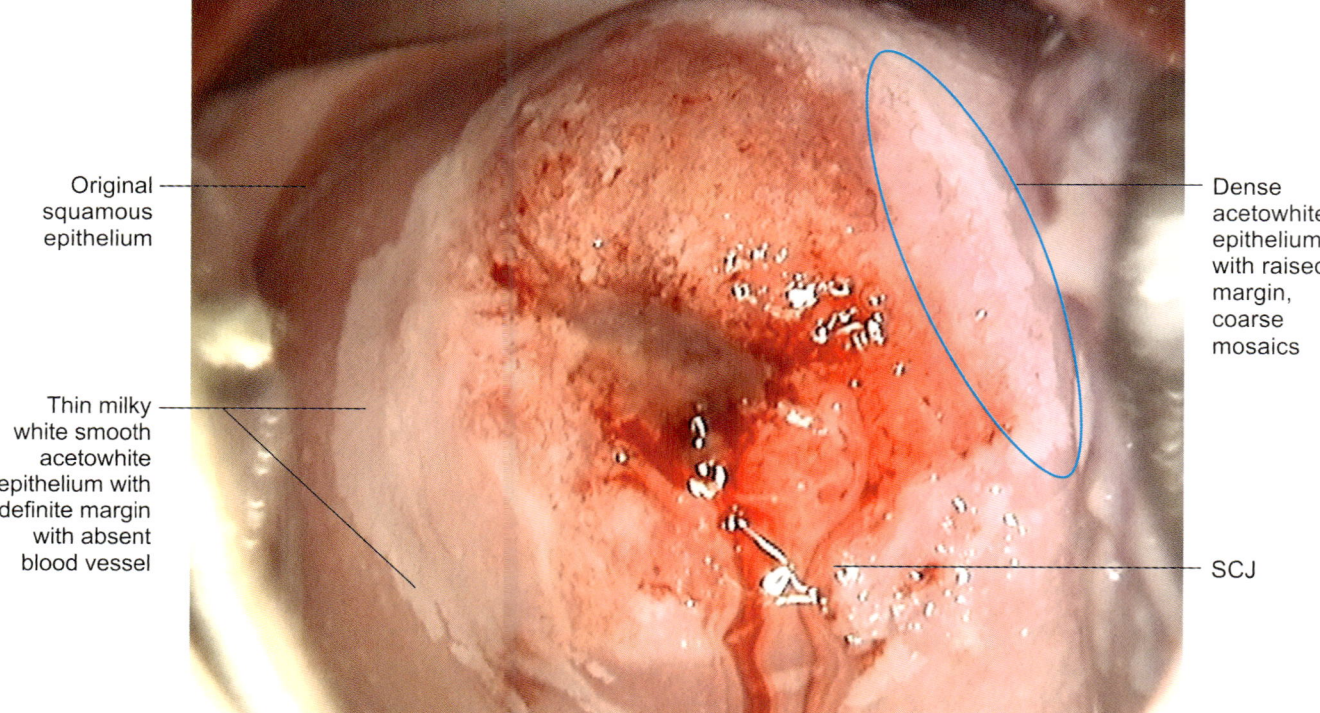

Original squamous epithelium

Dense acetowhite epithelium with raised margin, coarse mosaics

Thin milky white smooth acetowhite epithelium with definite margin with absent blood vessel

SCJ

Fig. 2.24b: Circumferential lesions

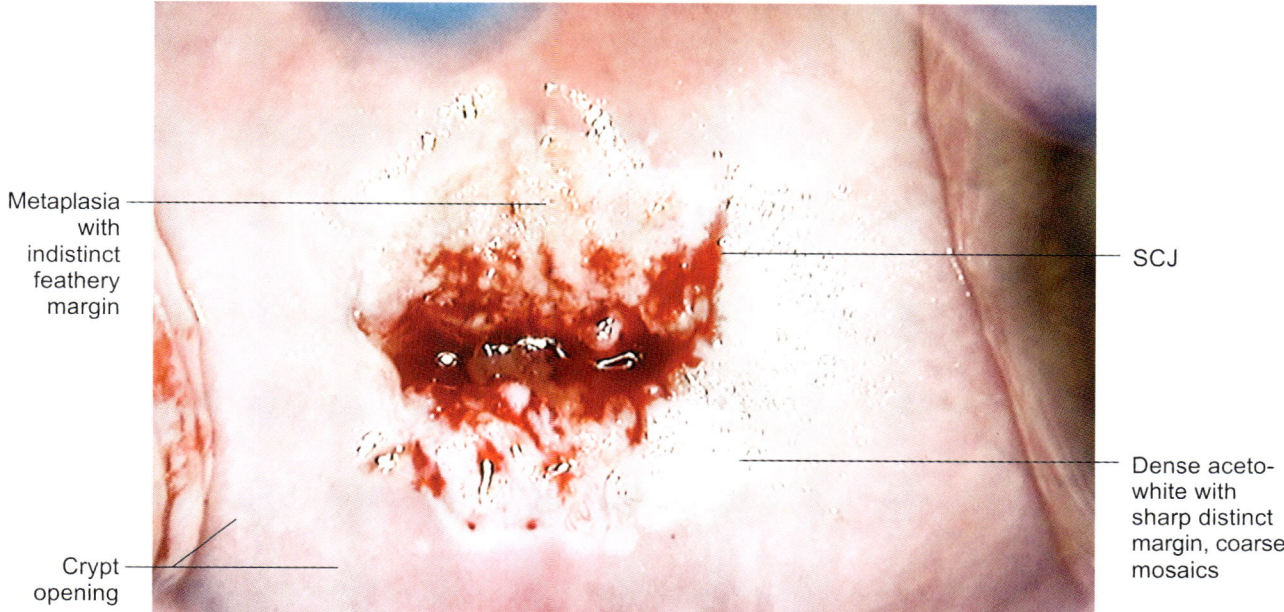

Metaplasia with indistinct feathery margin

SCJ

Crypt opening

Dense aceto-white with sharp distinct margin, coarse mosaics

Fig. 2.24c: Lesion at 5 O'clock position

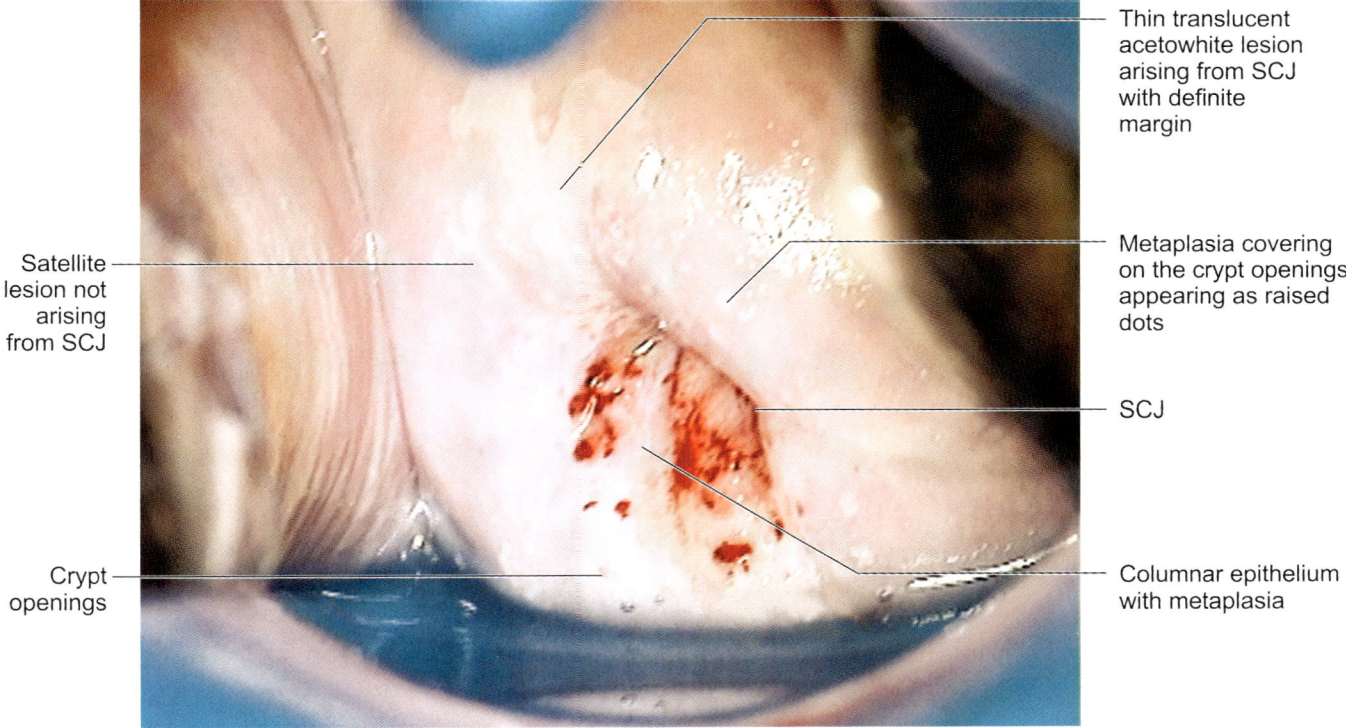

Satellite lesion not arising from SCJ

Crypt openings

Thin translucent acetowhite lesion arising from SCJ with definite margin

Metaplasia covering on the crypt openings appearing as raised dots

SCJ

Columnar epithelium with metaplasia

Fig. 2.24d: Lesion at 12 O' clock position and satellite lesion

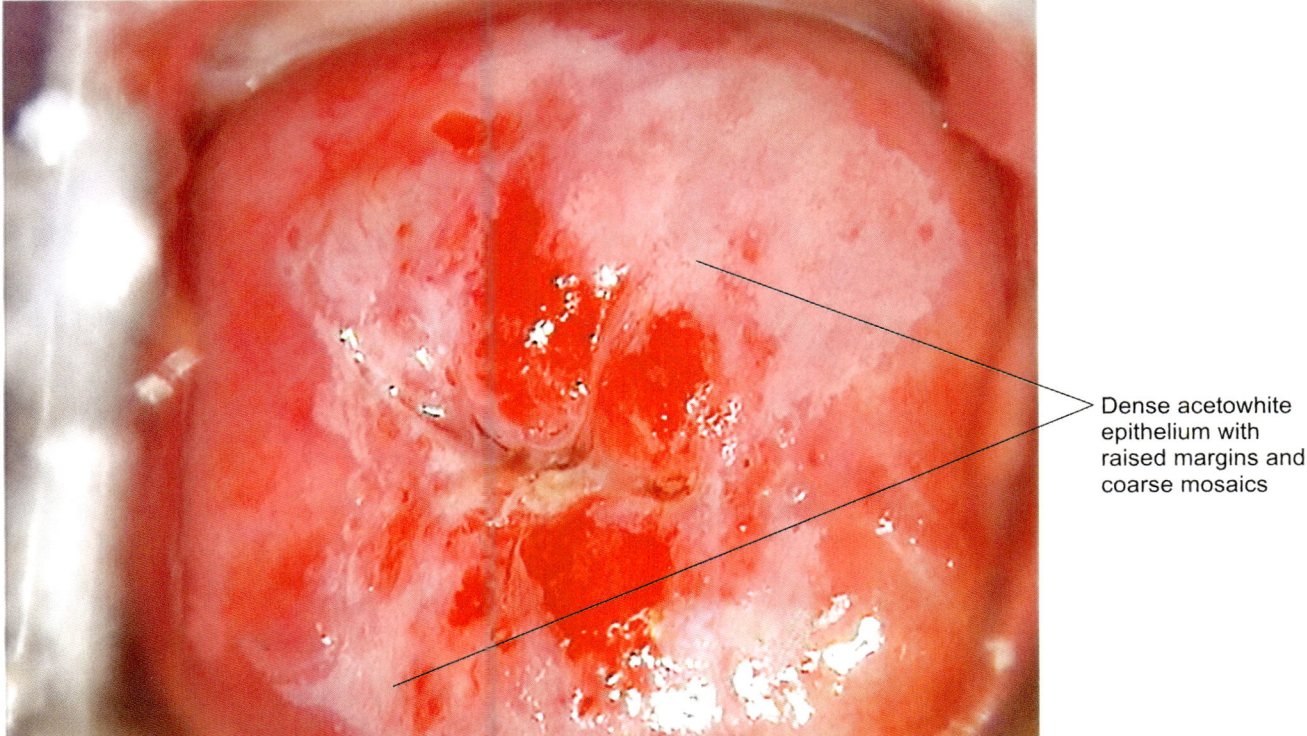

Dense acetowhite epithelium with raised margins and coarse mosaics

Fig. 2.24e: HSIL lesion

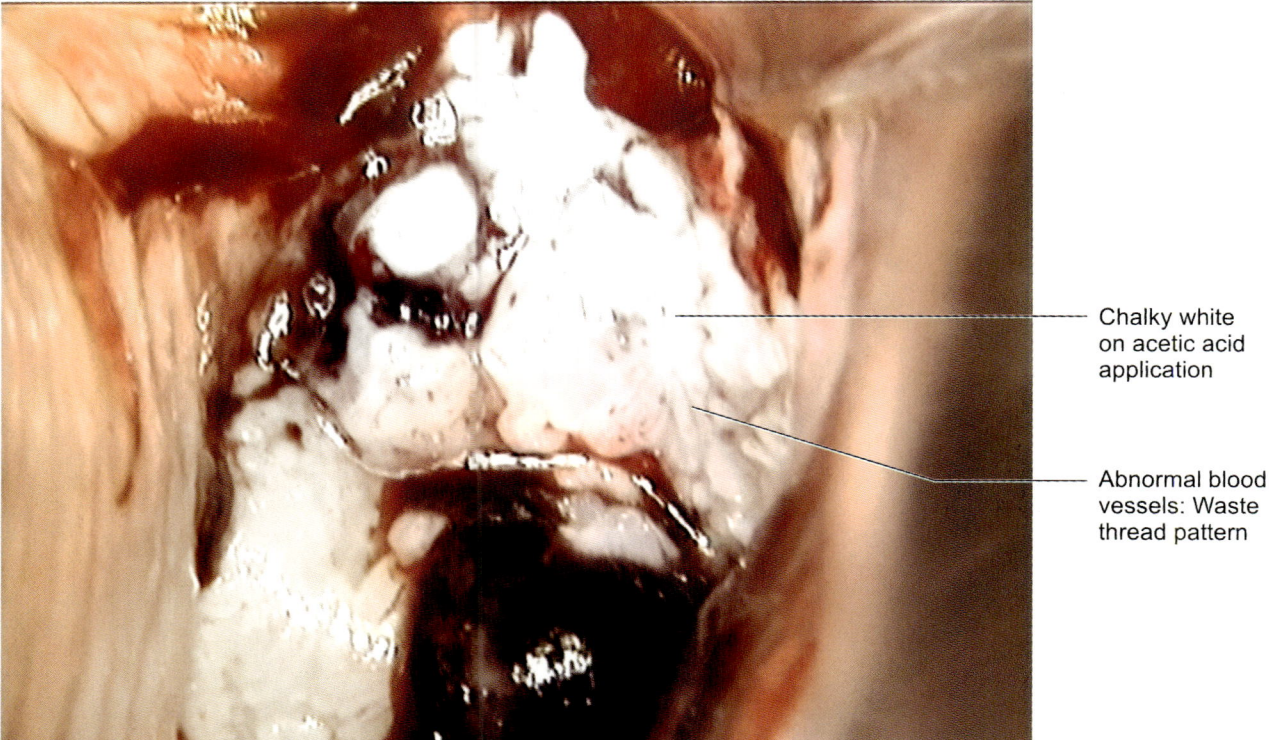

Chalky white on acetic acid application

Abnormal blood vessels: Waste thread pattern

Fig. 2.24f: Rags sign seen in invasive SCC

6. Lugol's Iodine Application

Principle

Stratified squamous epithelia have glycogen in their superficial cells. On application of Lugol's iodine, these cells take up iodine and turn mahogany brown or dark brown. The cells which do not contain glycogen do not turn brown, they remain unstained or variegated patchy appearance.

Physiological conditions where Lugol's iodine is taken up and turns mahogany brown—original squamous epithelium, mature squamous metaplasia.

Physiological conditions where Lugol's iodine is not taken up—columnar epithelium, immature squamous epithelium, nabothian follice, menopausal epithelium (Figs 2.25a to f).

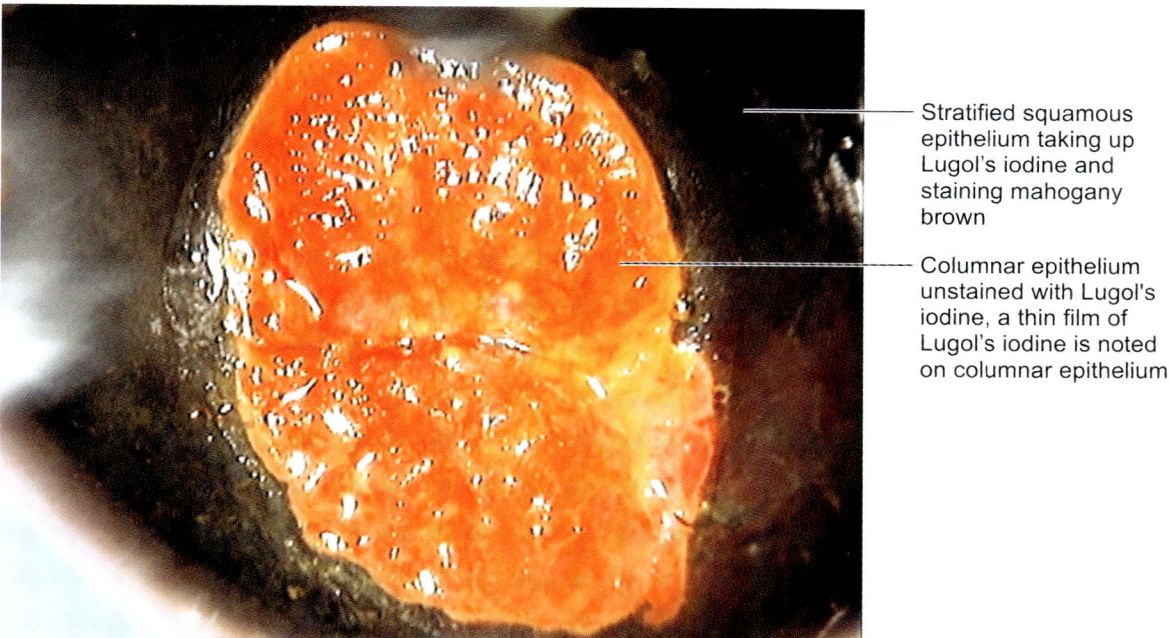

Stratified squamous epithelium taking up Lugol's iodine and staining mahogany brown

Columnar epithelium unstained with Lugol's iodine, a thin film of Lugol's iodine is noted on columnar epithelium

Fig. 2.25a: VILI negetive

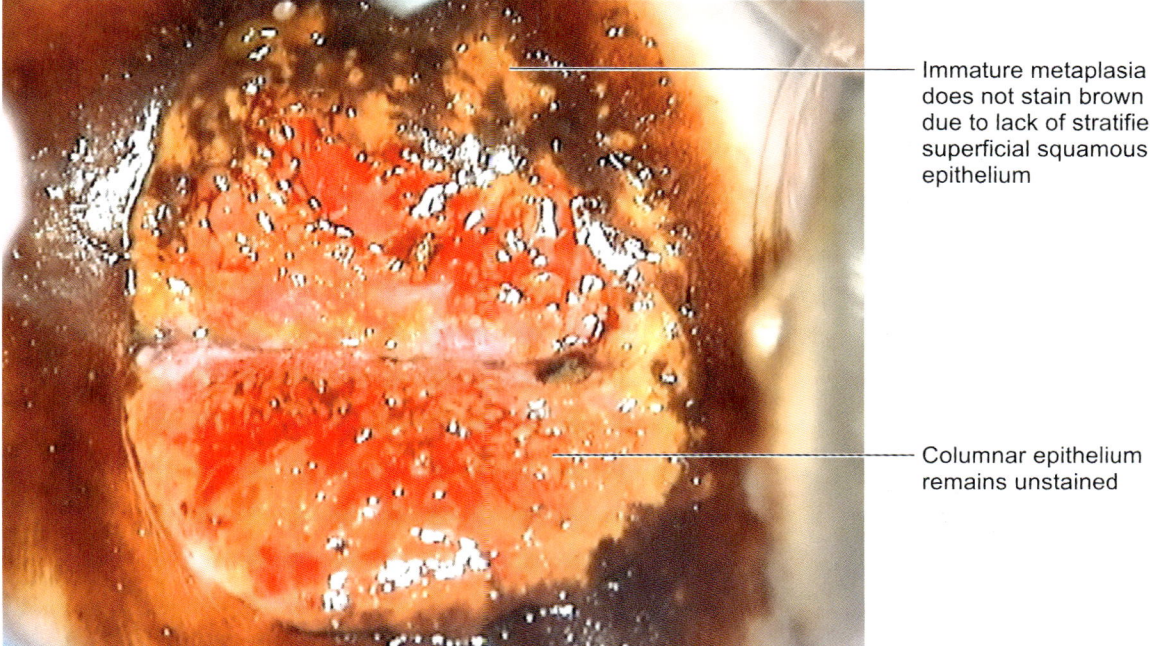

Immature metaplasia does not stain brown due to lack of stratified superficial squamous epithelium

Columnar epithelium remains unstained

Fig. 2.25b: Physiological VILI positive due to immature squamous metaplasia

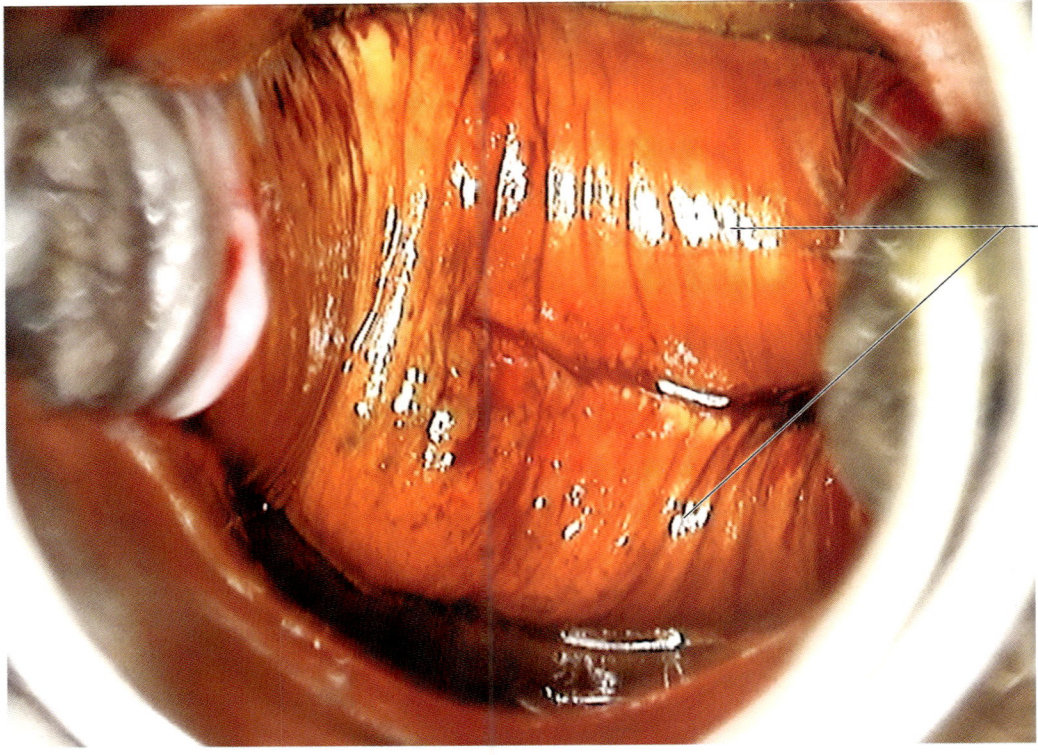

Unstained with Lugol's iodine due to lack of stratified superficial layer in the squamous epithelium in case of menopause

Fig. 2.25c: Physiological VILI positive in menopausal age group

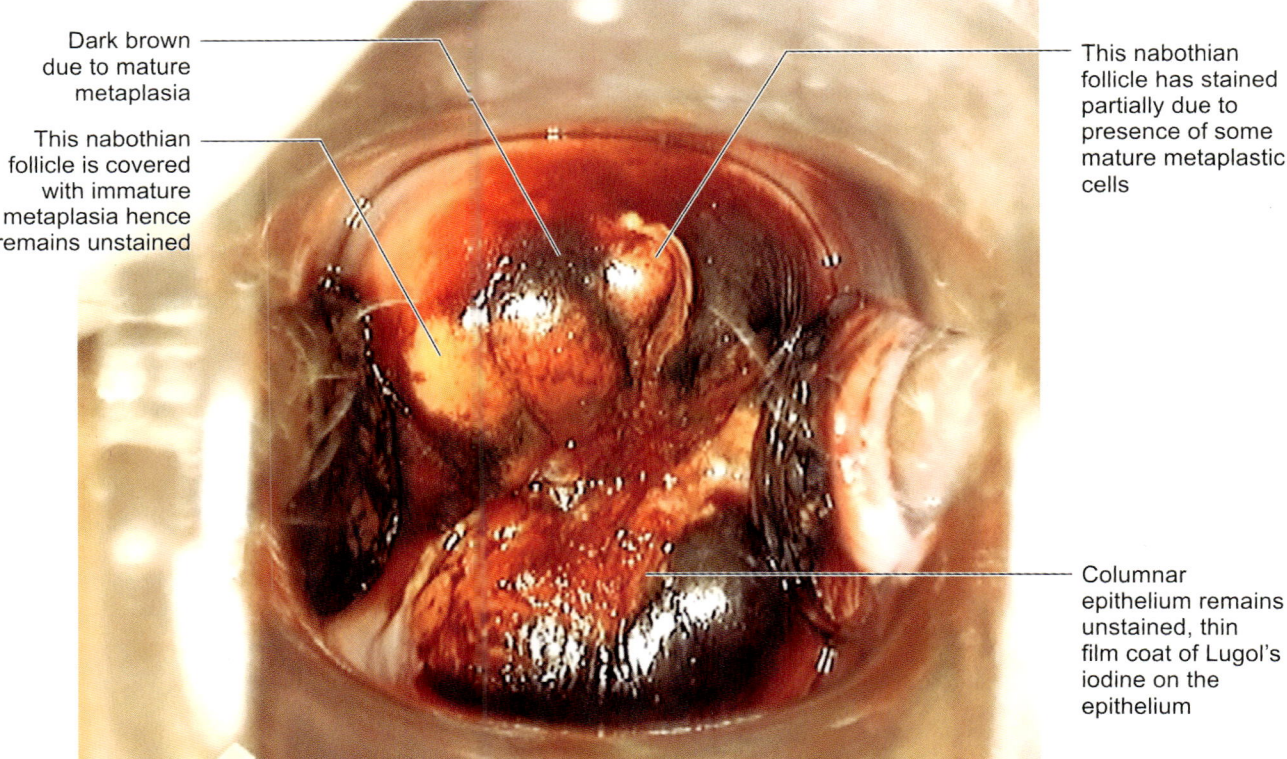

Dark brown due to mature metaplasia

This nabothian follicle is covered with immature metaplasia hence remains unstained

This nabothian follicle has stained partially due to presence of some mature metaplastic cells

Columnar epithelium remains unstained, thin film coat of Lugol's iodine on the epithelium

Fig. 2.25d: Nabothian follicles

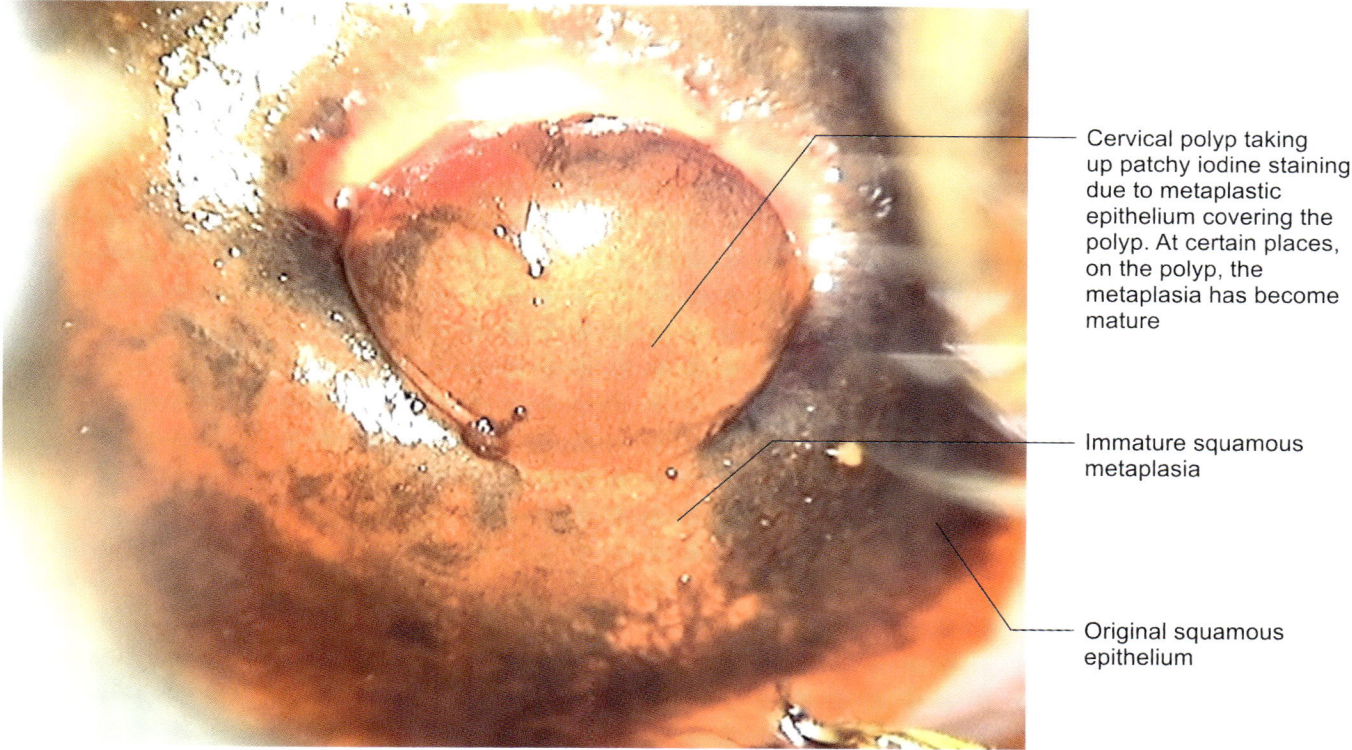

Cervical polyp taking up patchy iodine staining due to metaplastic epithelium covering the polyp. At certain places, on the polyp, the metaplasia has become mature

Immature squamous metaplasia

Original squamous epithelium

Fig. 2.25e: Cervical polyp

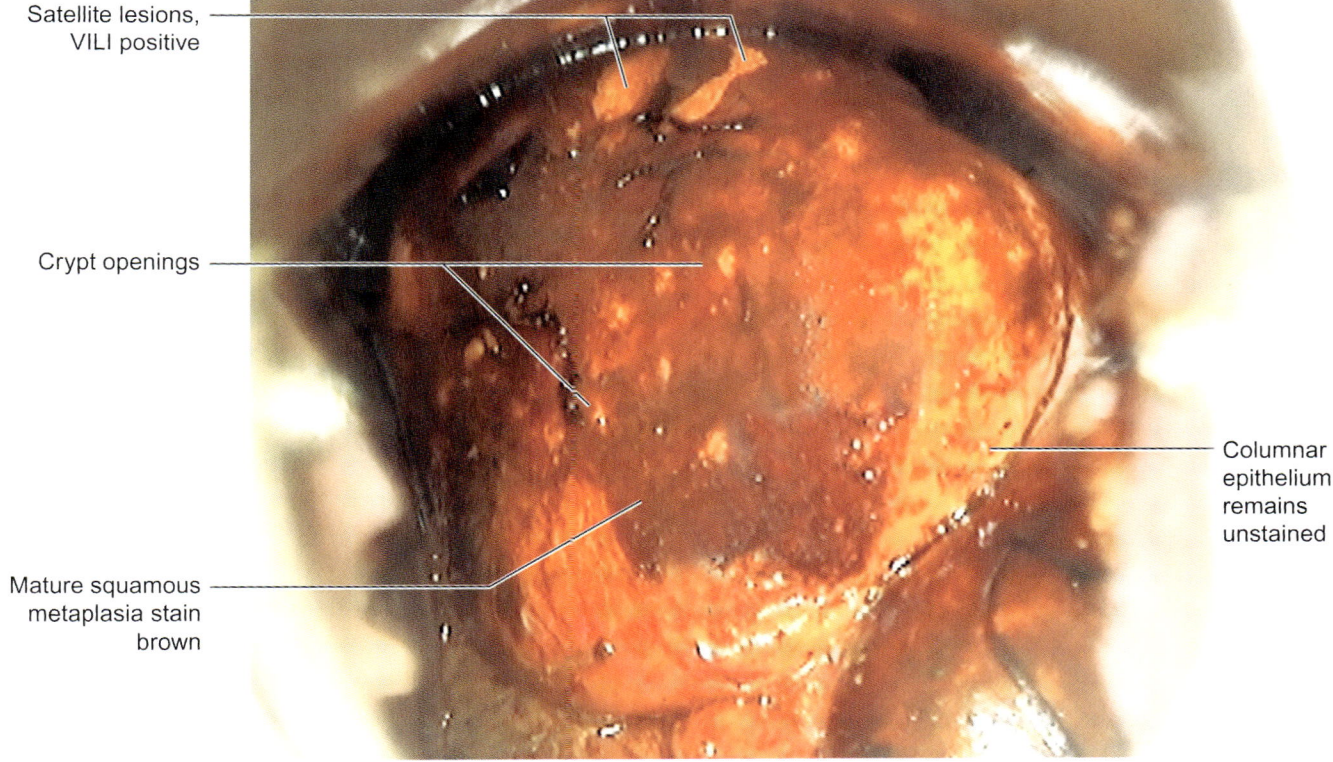

Satellite lesions, VILI positive

Crypt openings

Mature squamous metaplasia stain brown

Columnar epithelium remains unstained

Fig. 2.25f: Satellite lesions not taking up Lugol's iodine

Pathological conditions not taking up Lugol's iodine (VILI positive): CIN lesions—due to the lack of superficial stratified cells in the dividing cells of CIN lesions which are usually basal, parabasal or intermediate cells, these lesions do not stain brown. Depending on the severity of the CIN lesions, they either remain unstained or take up partial variegated Lugol's stains, higher grade lesions, such as microinvasive CA, stain as mustard yellow.

Trichomonial infections cause denudation of the superficial cells which do not get stained giving rise to leopard skin pattern.

Satellite lesions, not arising from SCJ within or away from TZ, do not stain with Lugol's iodine and are VILI positive (Figs 2.26a to i).

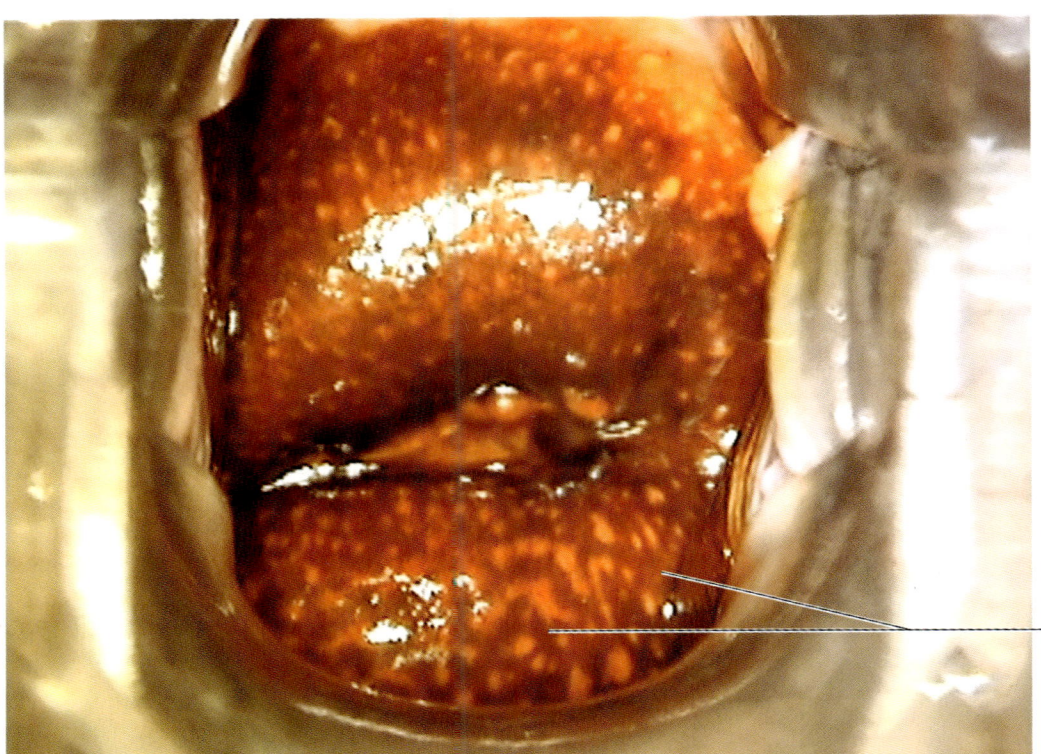

Trichomonial infection, leopard skin pattern

Fig. 2.26a: Leopard skin patches

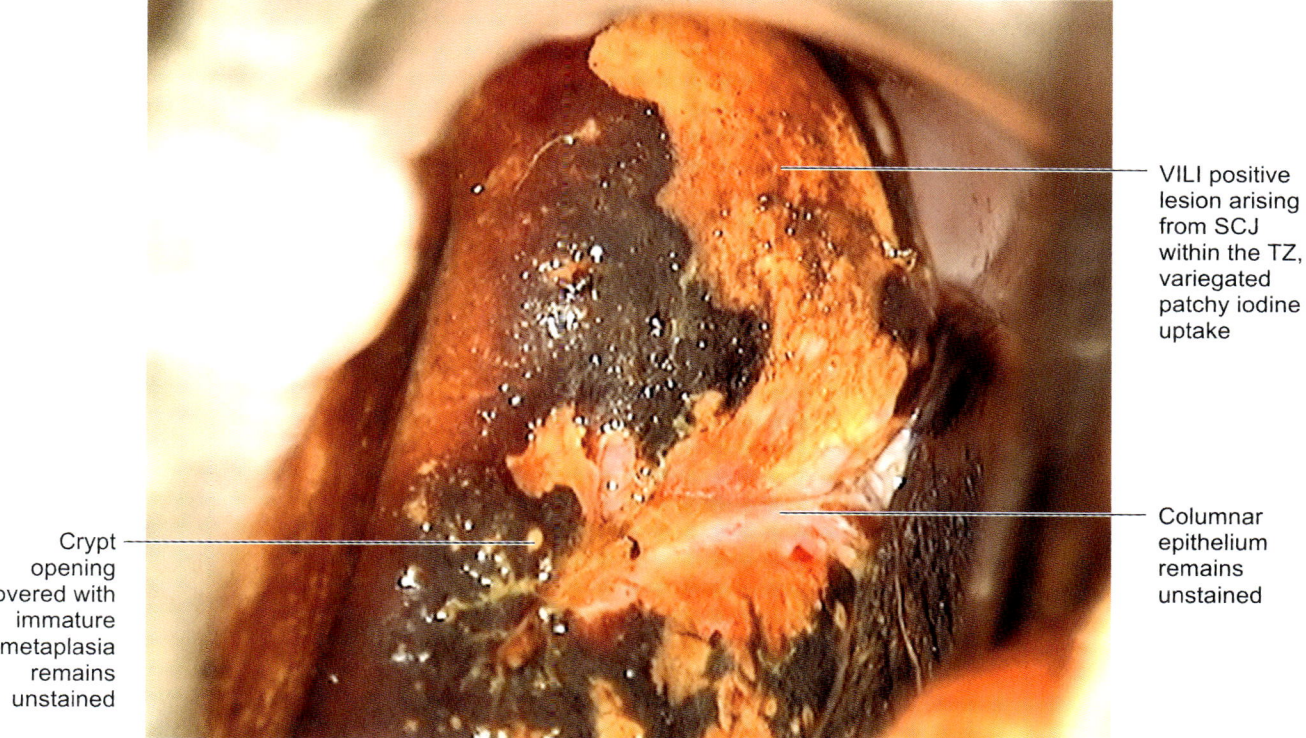

VILI positive lesion arising from SCJ within the TZ, variegated patchy iodine uptake

Columnar epithelium remains unstained

Crypt opening covered with immature metaplasia remains unstained

Fig. 2.26b: VILI positive

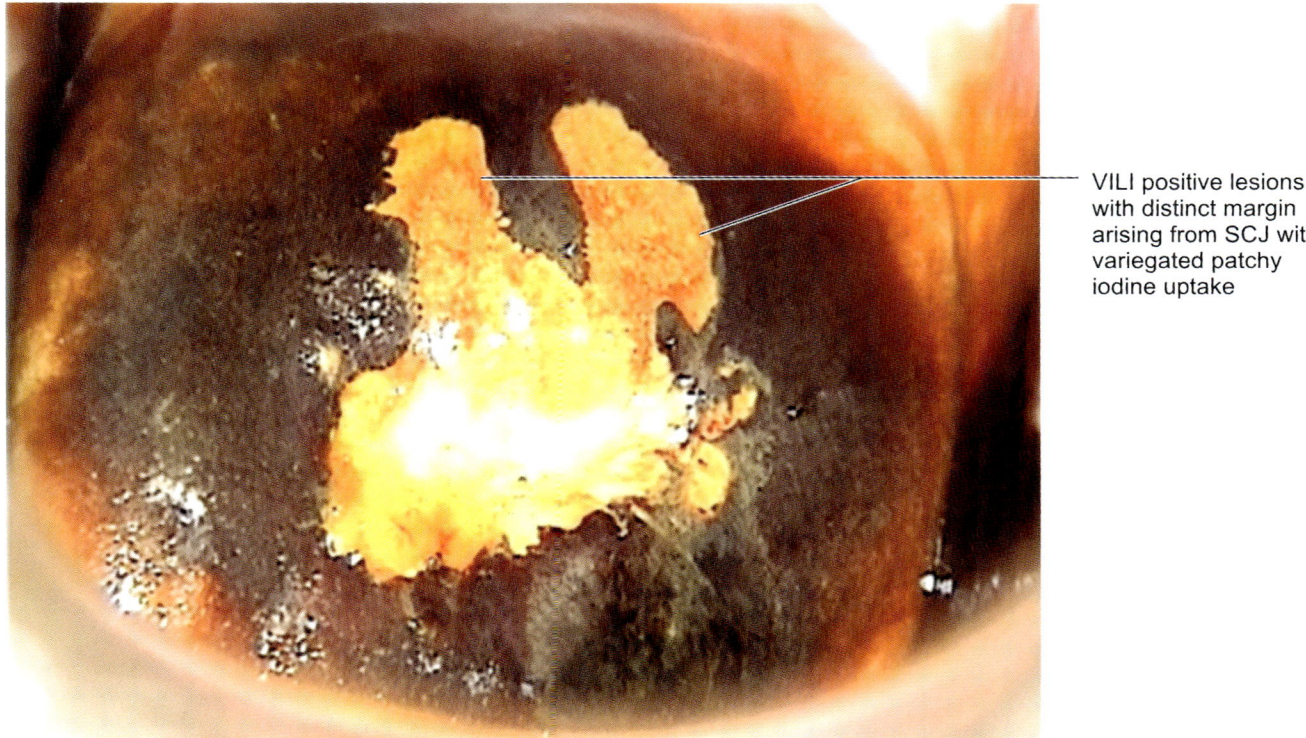

VILI positive lesions with distinct margin arising from SCJ with variegated patchy iodine uptake

Fig. 2.26c: VILI positive

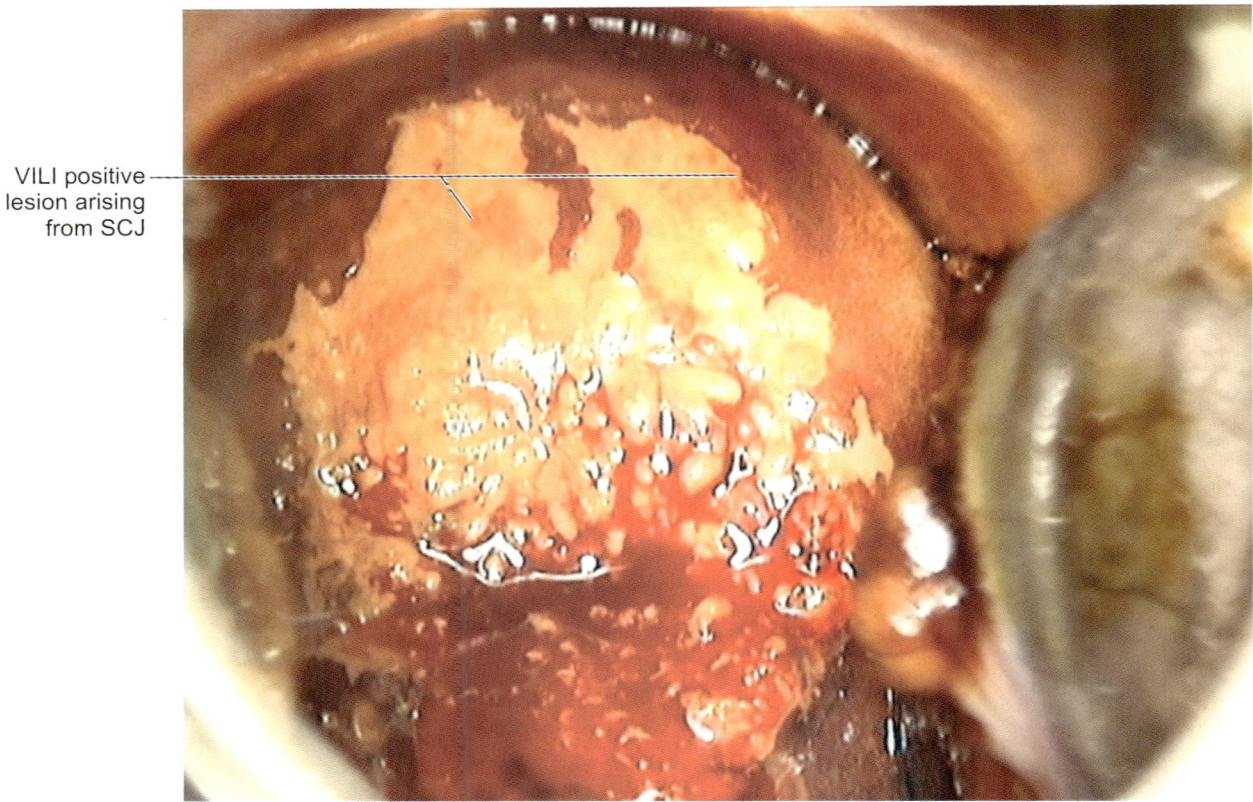

VILI positive
lesion arising
from SCJ

Fig. 2.26d: VILI positive

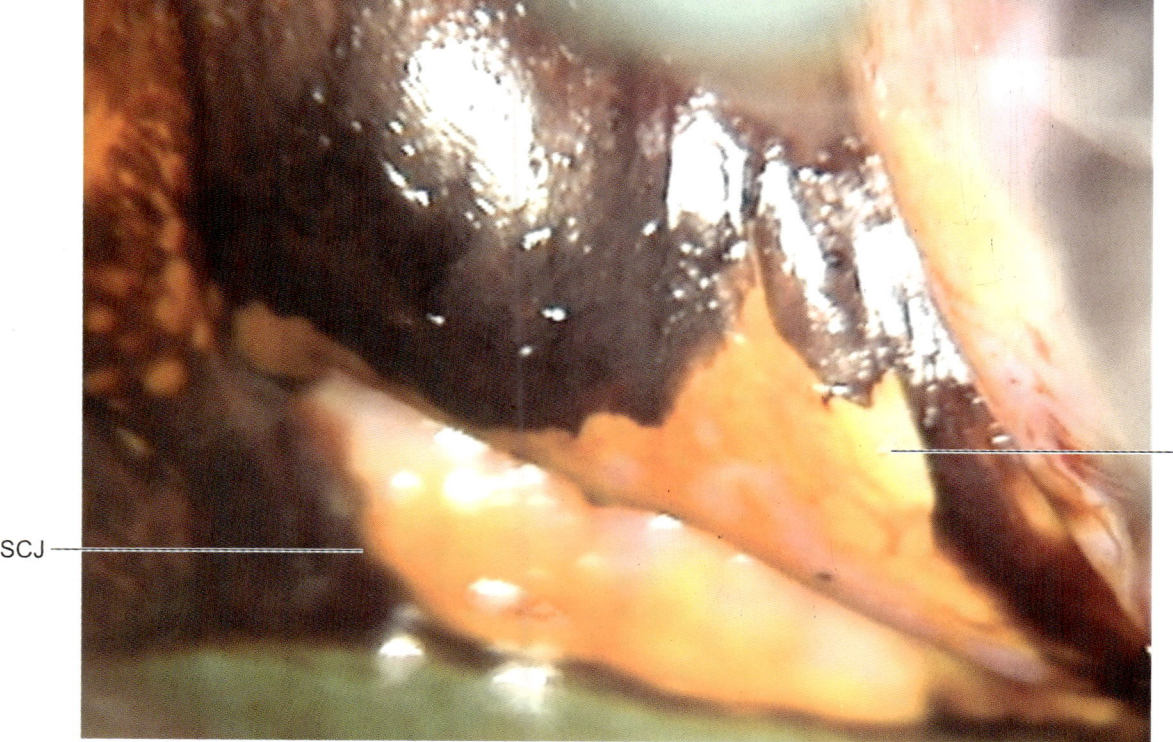

SCJ

VILI positive
lesion from
SCJ with
distinct margin
and absent
iodine uptake

Fig. 2.26e: VILI positive

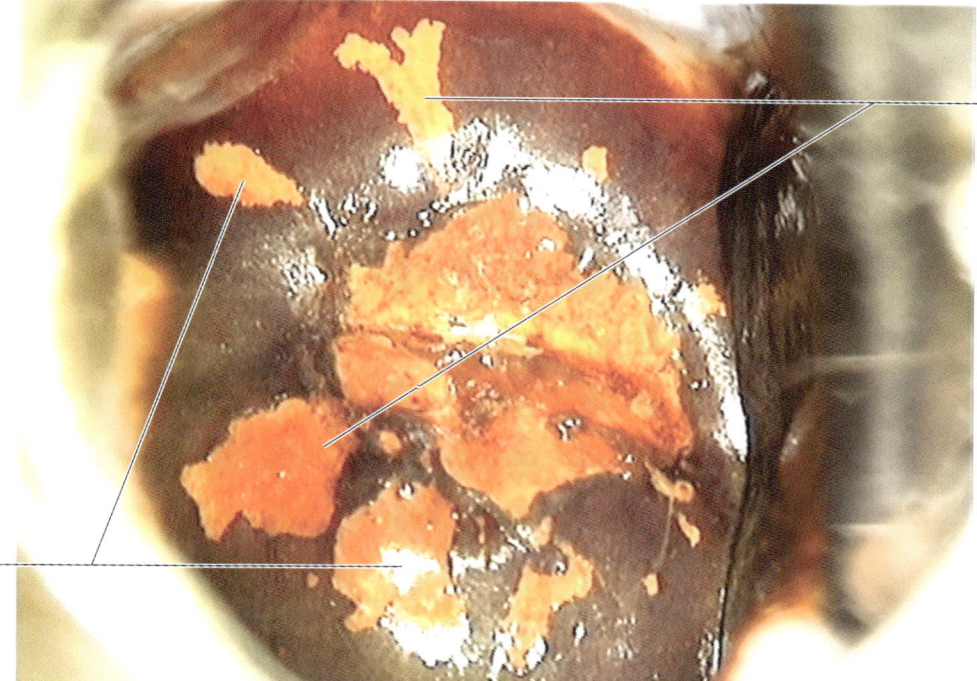

VILI positive lesions arising from SCJ in TZ with distinct margin and Variegated patchy iodine uptake

VILI positive satellite lesions not arising from SCJ within TZ

Fig. 2.26f: VILI positive

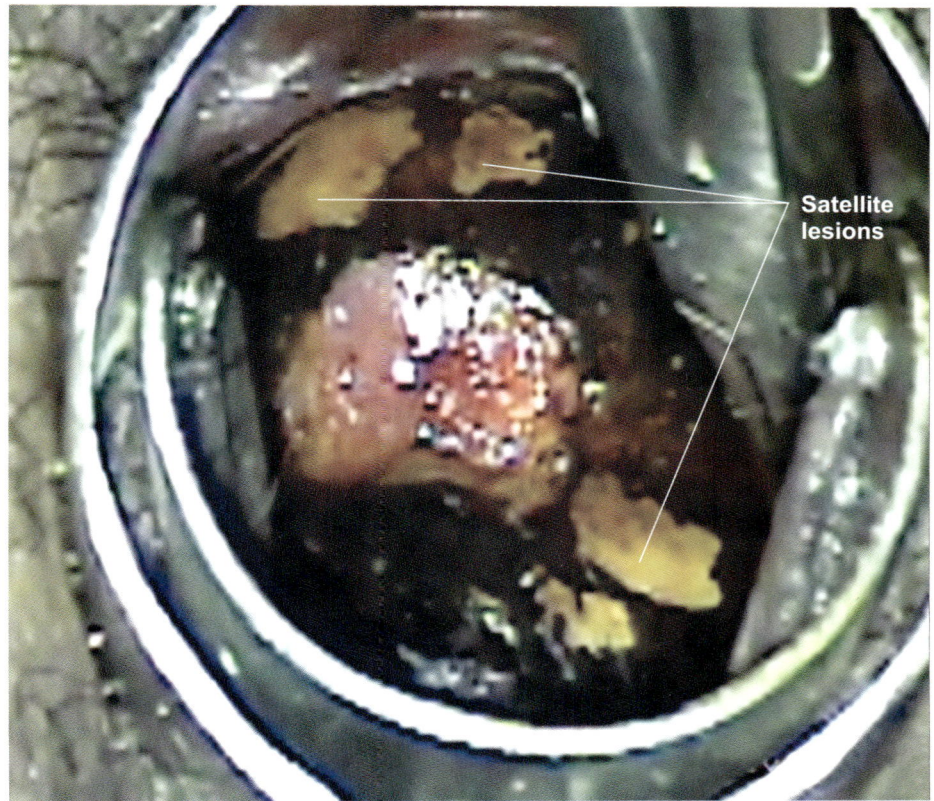

Satellite lesions

Fig. 2.26g: Satellite lesions

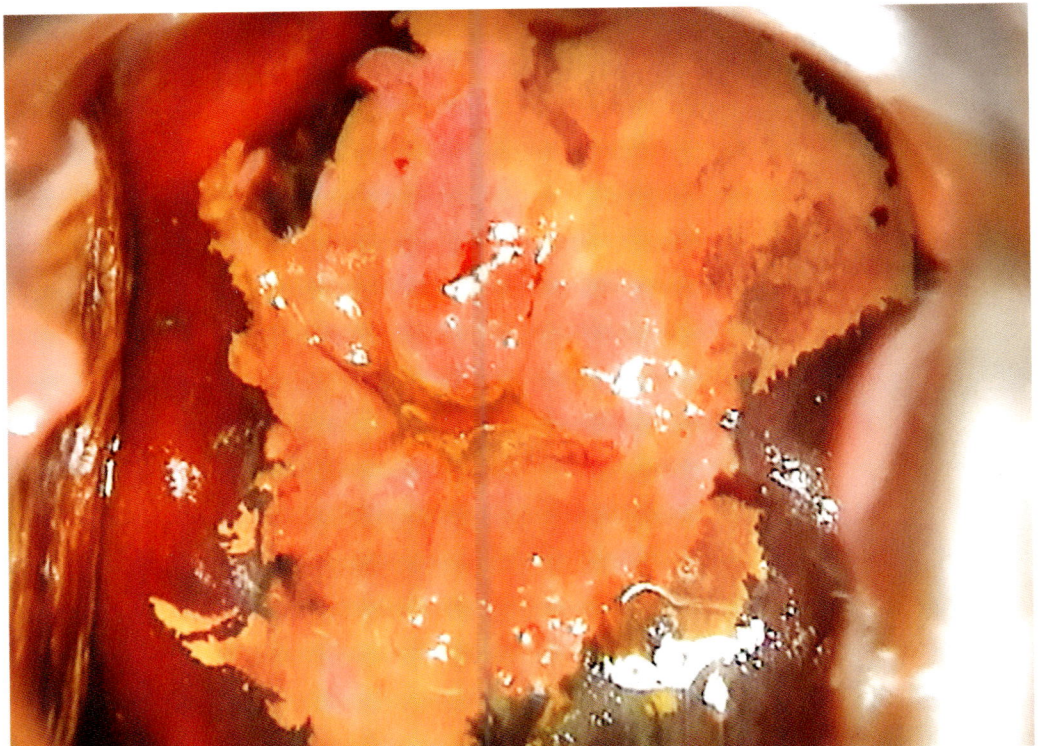

Fig. 2.26h: Mustard staining in invasive cancer

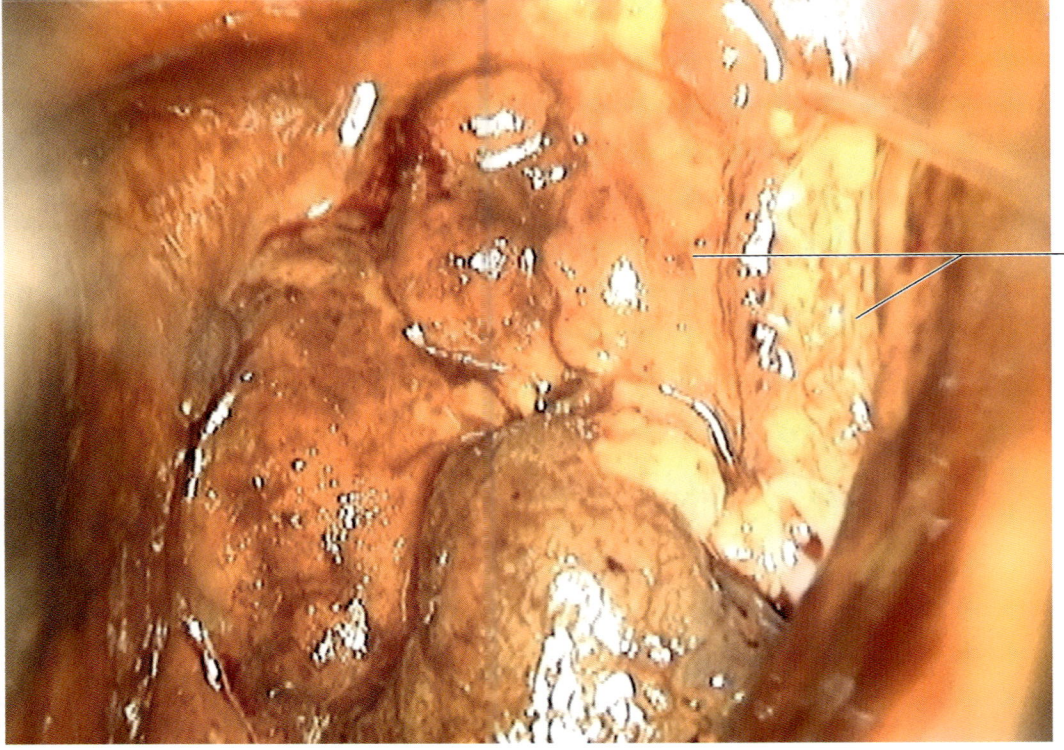

Invasive CA with mustard yellow staining with Lugol's iodine

Fig. 2.26i: Mustard staining in invasive cancer

Thus to sum up the terminology:
- *VILI negative:* Uptake of Lugol's iodine to turn into mahogany brown colour.
- *VILI positive:* There is no Lugol's iodine uptake hence they remain unstained or turn yellow, seen in physiological or pathological conditions.

3

Explanations of Different Terminologies

1. SQUAMOUS EPITHELIUM

A mature stratified squamous epithelium is composed of four layers (Figs 3.1a and b): (1) Basal layer; (2) parabasal layers; (3) intermediate layer; and (4) superficial layer.

Basal and parabasal cells are round cells with large nucleus in comparison to cytoplasm, intermediate cells are polygonal in shape with abundant cytoplasm and small round nuclei forming basket weave pattern, superficial cells are flattened with pyknotic nuclei and transparent cytoplasm.

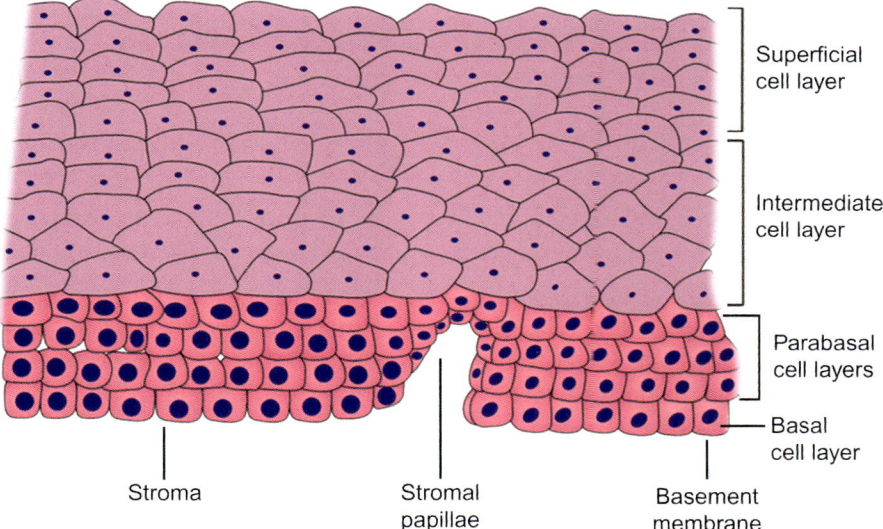

Superficial cell layer

Intermediate cell layer

Parabasal cell layers

Basal cell layer

Stroma

Stromal papillae

Basement membrane

Fig. 3.1a: Stratified squamous epithelium

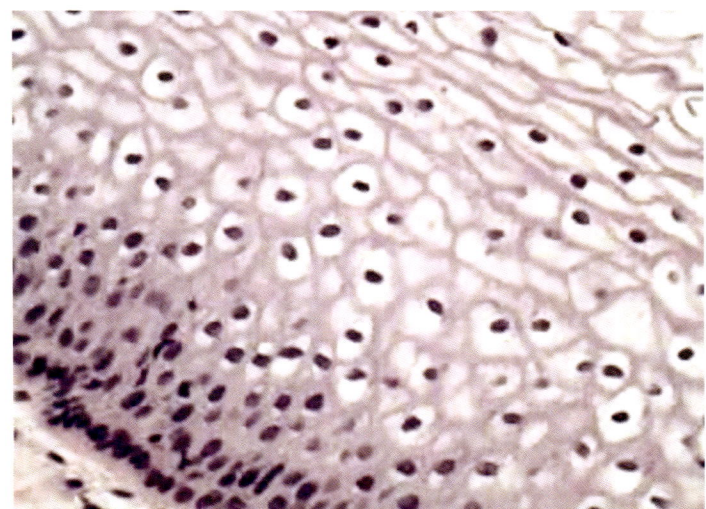

Fig. 3.1b: Histology of squamous epithelium

Basal layer: It is a single layer of round basal cells with a large dark staining nuclei and a little cytoplasm. It rests on the basement membrane, which separates epithelial layer from stroma containing connective tissue and blood vessels. Usually, the basement membrane is straight, but sometimes it has short projections called stromal papillae into the epithelial cells. These stromal papillae carry along with them branches of blood vessels. The stromal papillae (Figs 3.1a and b) are found at regular intervals.

The part of epithelium between the two papillae is called the rete pegs (Fig. 3.2). Rete pegs carries importance and significance in the pathology of CIN in identifying the mosaic pattern.

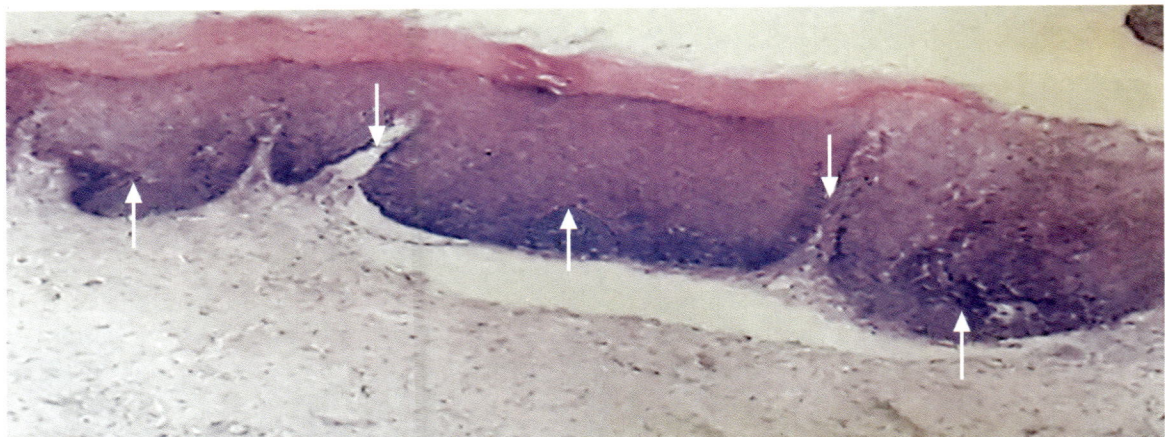

Fig. 3.2: Rete pegs (arrows upward) and stromal papillae (arrows downward)

Parabasal layers: These are two to three layers situated above the basal layer. They are relatively rounded and have dark staining nuclei with basophilic cytoplasm.

Intermediate layer: The parabasal layer further differentiates into intermediate layer of polygonal cells with abundant cytoplasm and small round nuclei. They form a basketweave pattern. They contain glycogen in their cytoplasm.

Superficial layer: The cells of the intermediate layer matures to form large markedly flattened cells with dense pyknotic nuclei and transparent cytoplasm. There is increase in size of the cells with reduction of nuclear size. The superficial cell layer has abundant glycogen in the cytoplasm, responsible for staining as dark mahogany brown on application of Lugol's iodine and magenta with periodic acid-Schiff stain in histological sections.

Stratification of the intermediate and superficial cell layers occurs with inclusion of glycogen in the cellular cytoplasm, this is sign of maturation. Hence, mature squamous epithelium is called stratified squamous epithelium. It is estrogen dependent. Usually, the cytoplasm of the epithelial cells does not have keratin, so-called stratified nonkeratinized squamous epithelium. Many a times, we find keratin inclusion bodies in the cytoplasm of the superficial cells; this is called stratified keratinized squamous epithelium. Sometimes due to irritation to some objects or chemicals, we find hyperkeratotic thick white patch on the cervix which can be covering the high grade lesion beneath it. Hence, every white patch has to be thoroughly scrutinized.

Usually, ectocervix appears pink, shiny, and smooth. Due to multilayered cellular structure, the underlying stroma is very less visible giving it a pink colour. Since maturation of the superficial layer is estrogen dependent; the cervix during early reproductive age group will show all the features of stratified squamous epithelium.

The epithelium of premenopausal and menopausal women will appear dull, opaque and less shiny, lusterless as the epithelium lack superficial and intermediate cell layers with only basal and parabasal cell layers. Due to lack of estrogen, they are fragile and atrophic; more prone to trauma and giving rise to tiny petechial hemorrhage while taking smear or doing colposcopy examination.

2. COLUMNAR EPITHELIUM

Usually, the endocervix is lined by columnar epithelium. It is made up of single layer of tall cells with dark staining nuclei close to the basement membrane. This layer is thrown into multiple folds within the lumen of the cervical canal giving rise to papillary projections. The invagination of the columnar epithelium gives rise to crypts. The mouth of crypts is called crypt opening. These crypts are, many a times, referred to as endocervical glands which secretes mucus.

The cervical mucus secretion is secreted by the cells and is released into the endocervical canal from the crypt opening. Since the columnar epithelium is single layered, the stroma along with its blood vessels underneath the cells is clearly visible in red color. Also the layer is thrown into manifold giving it a grape-like appearance. The cell cytoplasms do not have glycogen, so they remain unstained on Lugol's iodine test (Figs 3.3a and b).

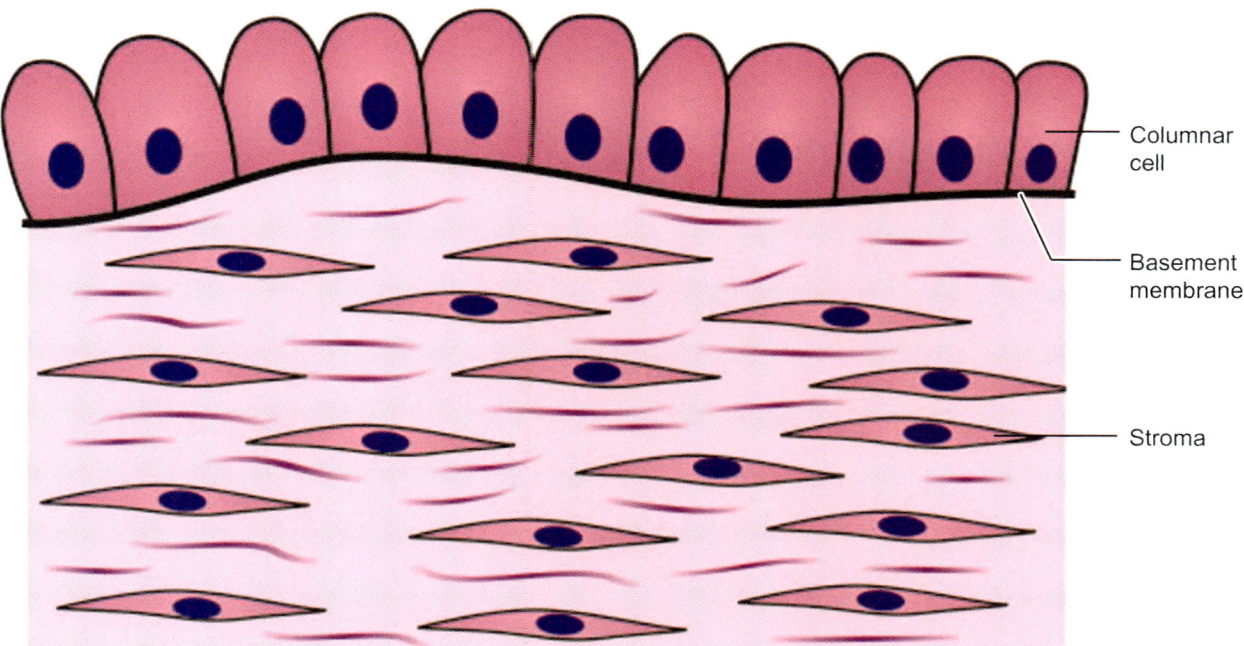

Fig. 3.3a: Columnar epithelium

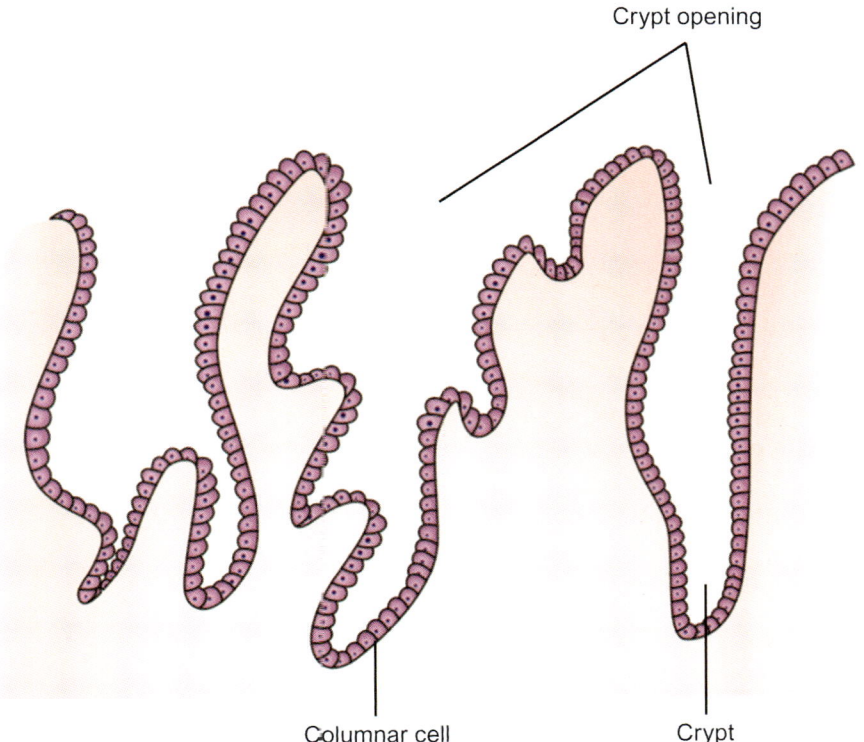

Fig. 3.3b: Columnar epithelium thrown into folds to form crypts

3. SQUAMOCOLUMNAR JUNCTION (SCJ) (Fig. 3.4)

This is the junction of squamous epithelium and columnar epithelium.

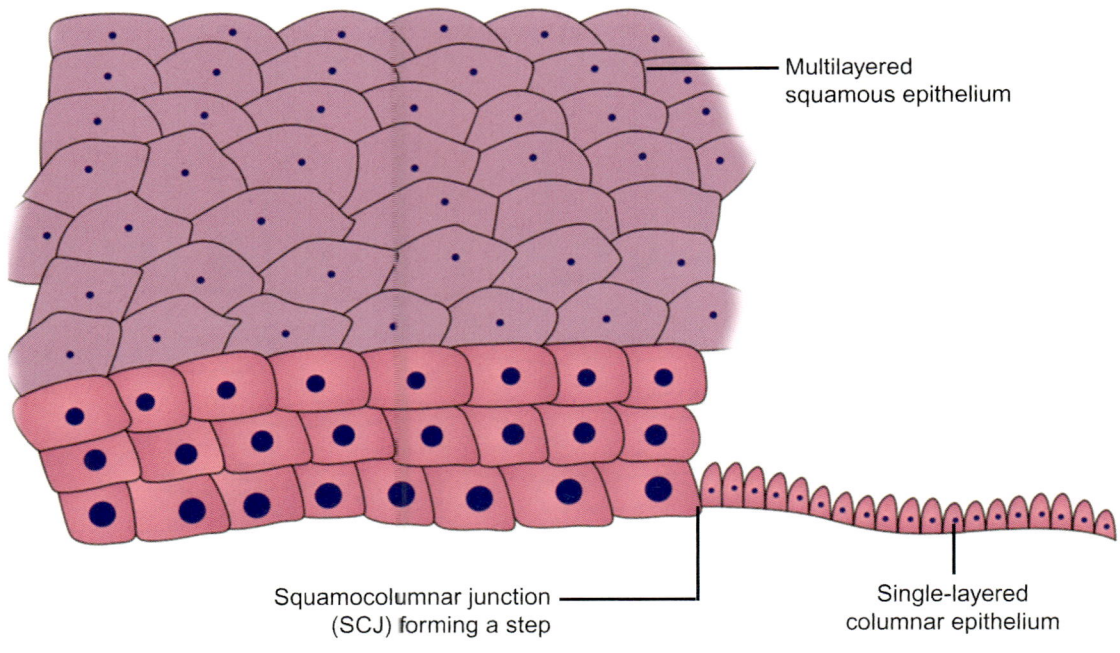

Fig. 3.4: Squamocolumnar junction (SCJ)

Prepubertal

Usually, the original SCJ is located within the cervical canal during the prepubertal period (Figs 3.5a and b).

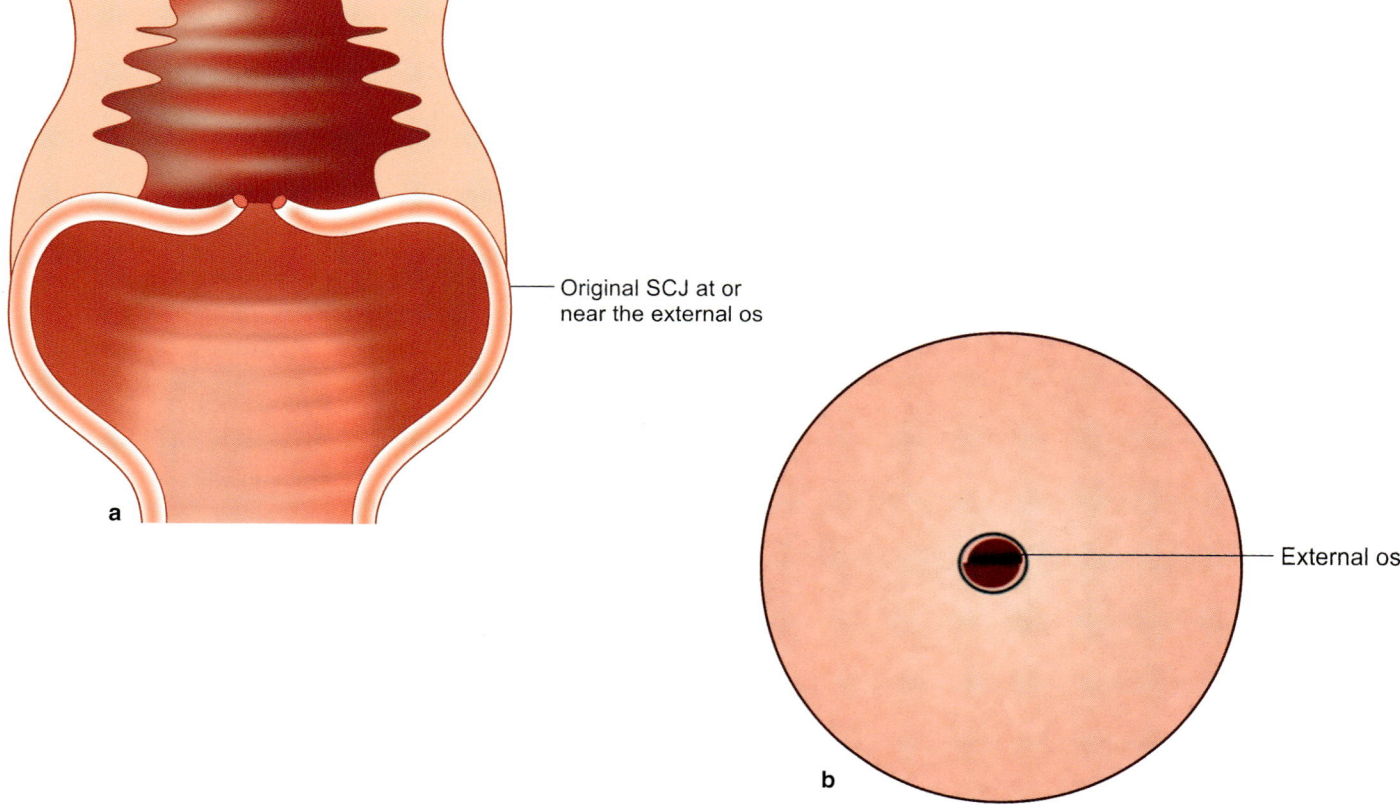

Figs 3.5a and b: Prepubertal SCJ

Pubertal

During menarche, due to influence of estrogen hormones, there is growth of endocervical columnar epithelium. This overgrowth of columnar epithelium leads to eversion of the columnar cells on the ectocervix. The SCJ shifts to periphery (Figs 3.6a to c).

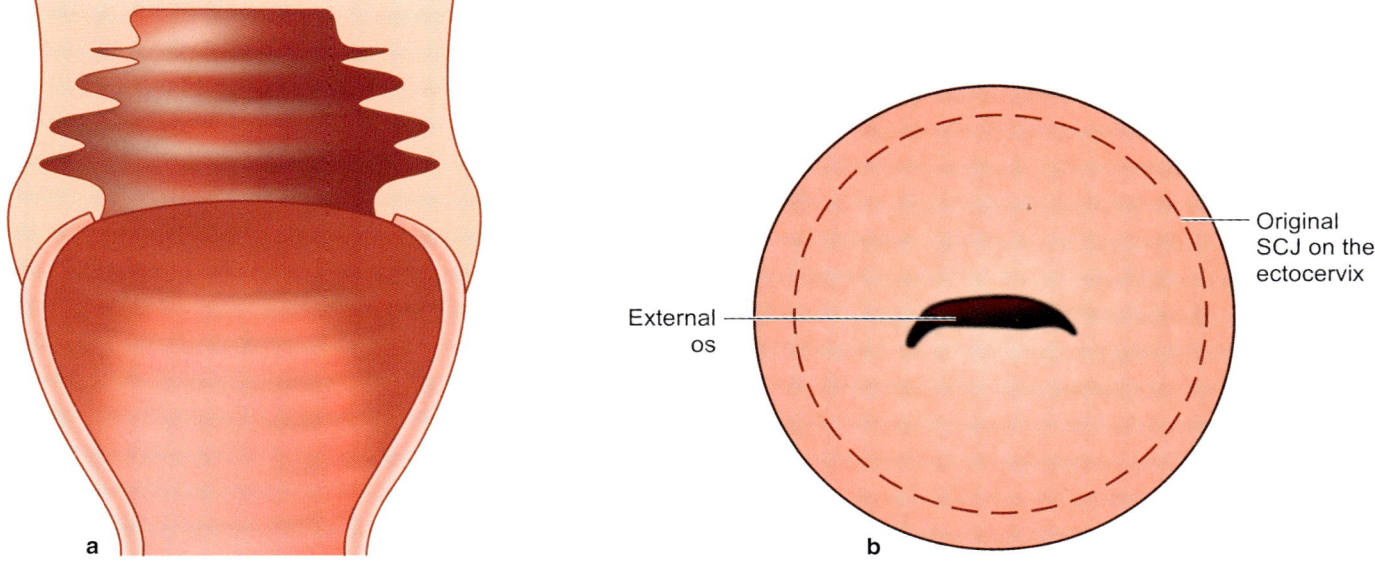

a

b

External os

Original SCJ on the ectocervix

Figs 3.6a and b: Pubertal SCJ

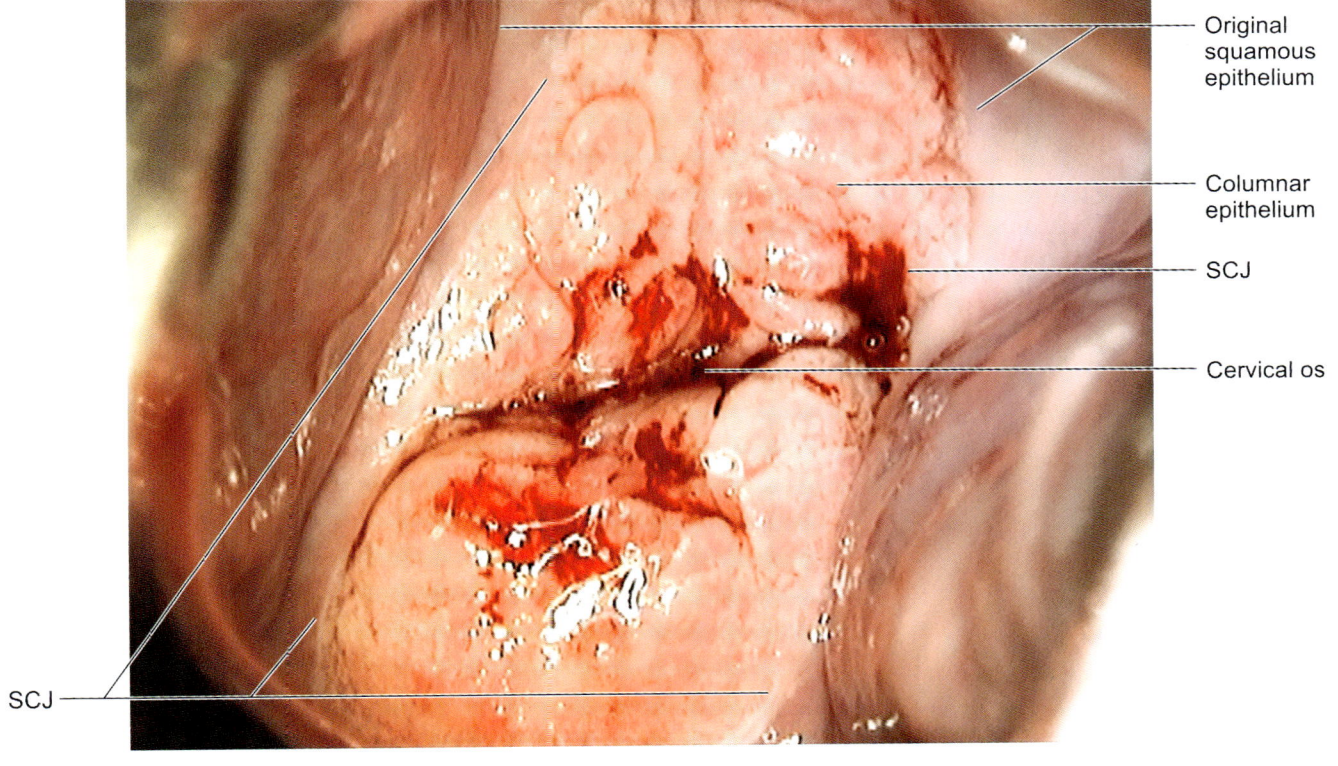

Original squamous epithelium

Columnar epithelium

SCJ

Cervical os

SCJ

Fig. 3.6c: Ectopy cervix

Reproductive Age Group (Figs 3.7a to c)

Columnar epithelium, being single layered, cannot withstand the brunt of acidic pH. The reserve cells, which are pluripotent cells located beneath the columnar epithelium, become active and start multiplying to create multilayered squamous epithelium, thus the single-layered columnar epithelium is transformed to multilayered squamous epithelium. This phenomenon is called metaplasia.

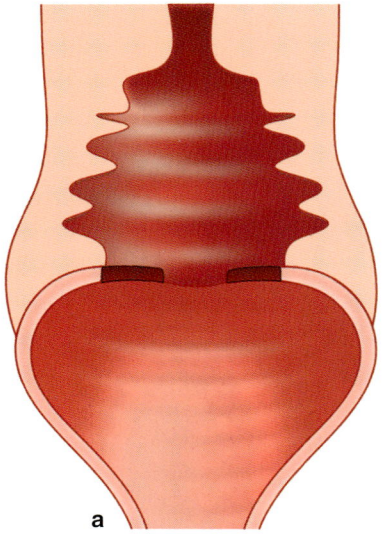

a

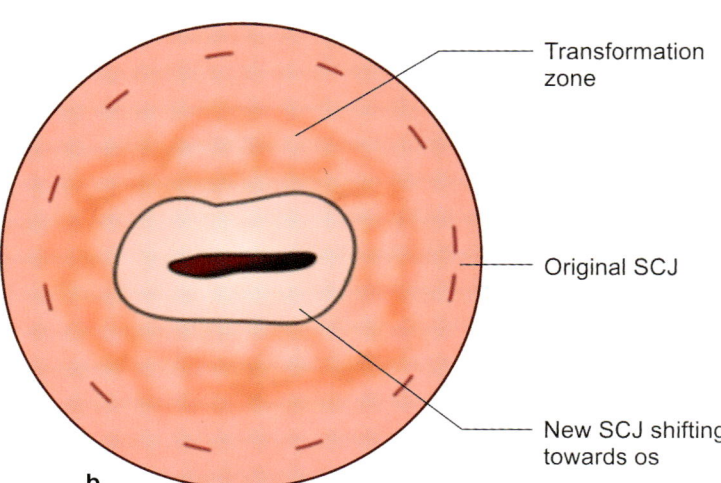

Transformation zone

Original SCJ

New SCJ shifting towards os

b

Figs 3.7a and b: Reproductive age SCJ

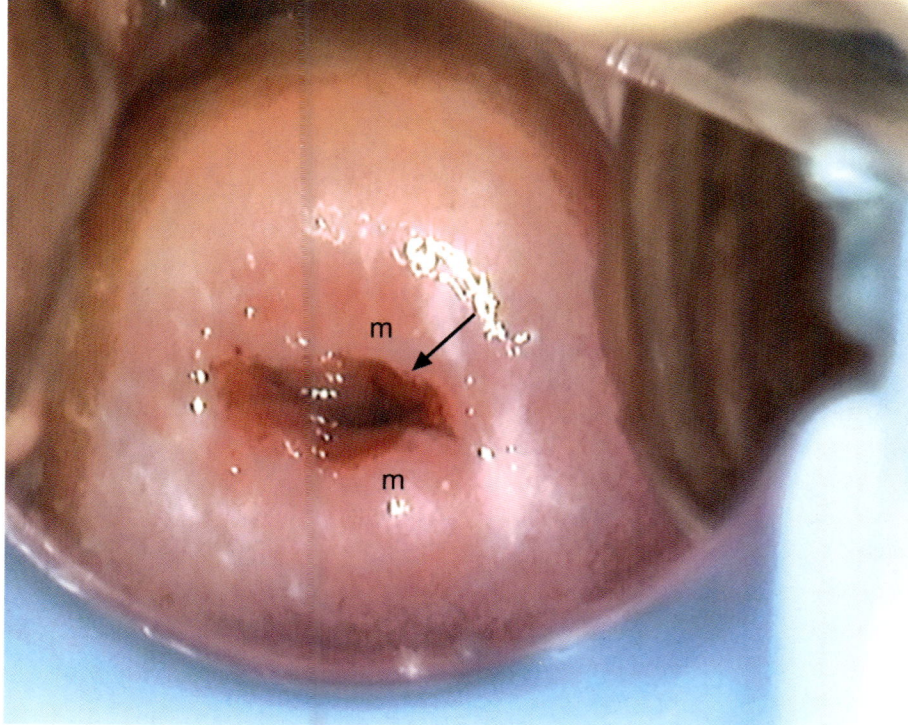

Fig. 3.7c: Reproductive age: SCJ (→) can be seen nearing the os, with columnar epithelium appearing reddish, metaplasia (m) as thin translucent finger-like projections pointing centripetally.

Perimenopausal (Figs 3.8a to c)

The new SCJ is at the external os.

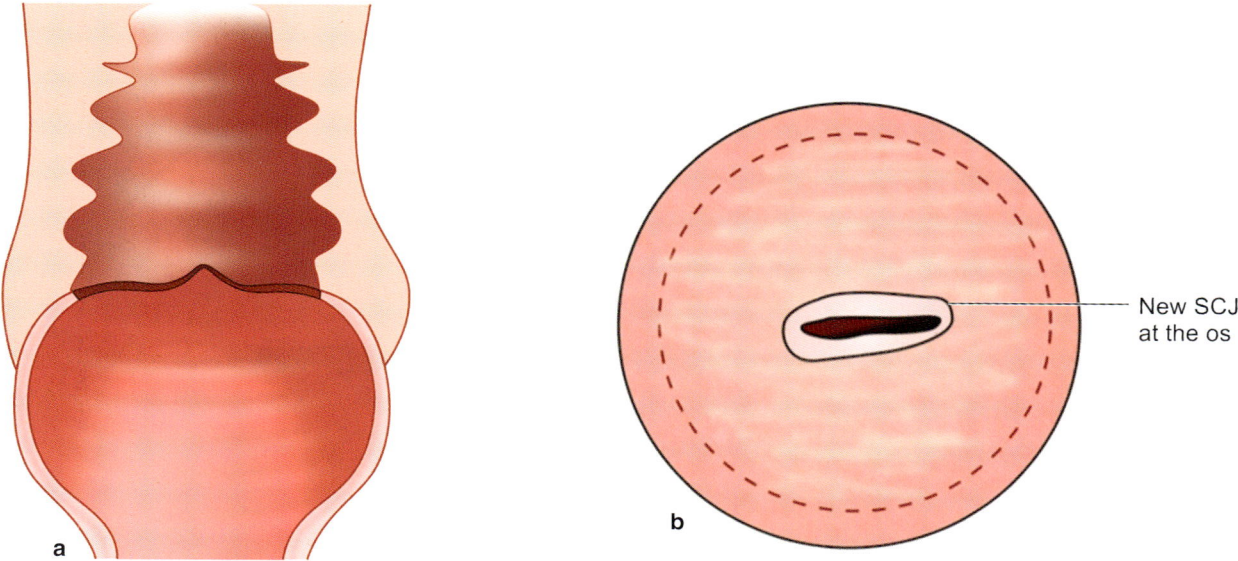

Figs 3.8a and b: Perimenopausal SCJ

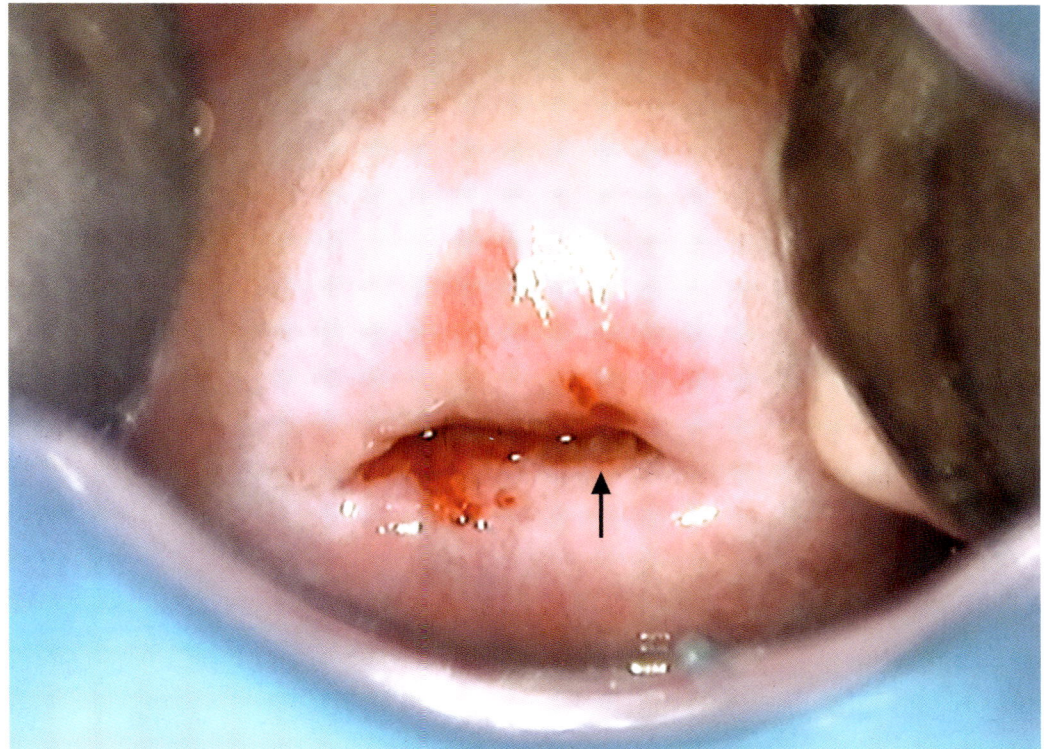

Fig. 3.8c: Perimenopausal age SCJ (→) seen completely at the os

Menopausal Age (Figs 3.9a to d)

The new SCJ is receded into the endocervical canal and is not visible. Sometimes we have to use an endocervical speculum to locate and trace it. Usually, at this age, the ectocervix is covered by mature metaplastic squamous epithelium.

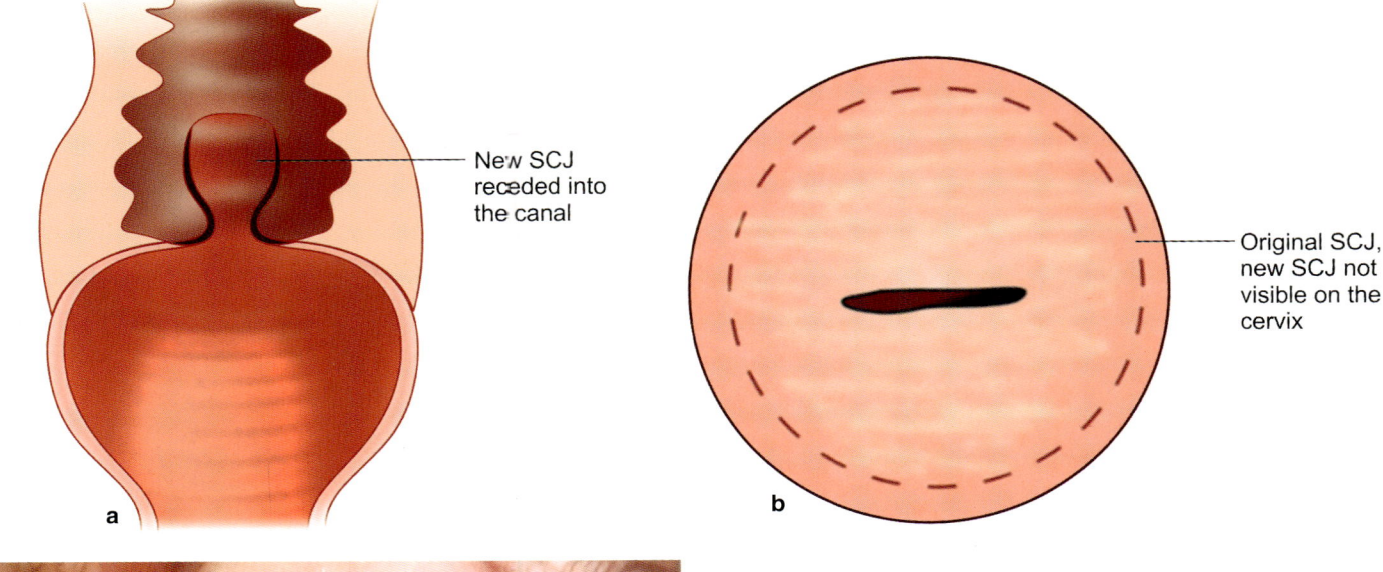

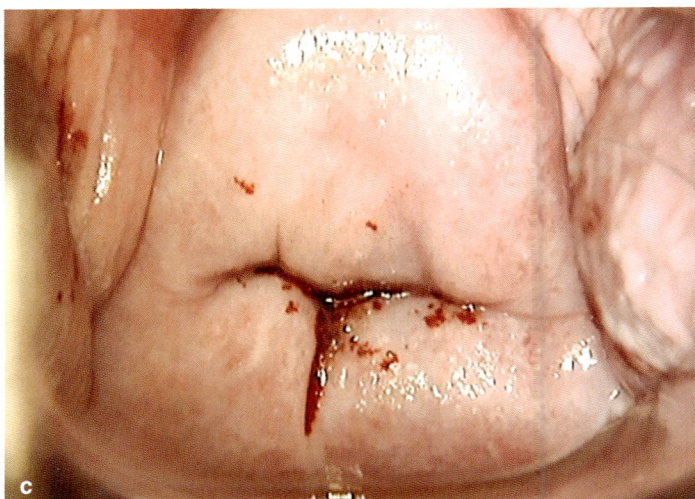

Figs 3.9a to c: Menopausal age SCJ

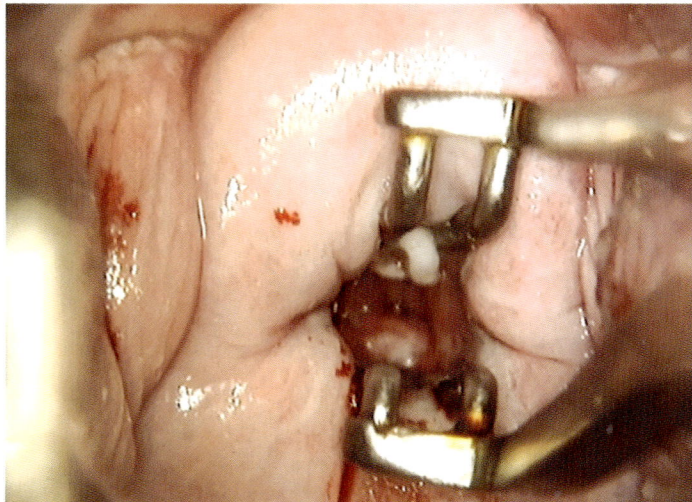

Fig. 3.9d: TZ 3, SCJ visualized on endocervical speculum examination in menopausal age

4. ORIGINAL SCJ/OLD SCJ

Original SCJ/old SCJ is the junction of squamous and metaplastic epithelium. It can be delineated by identifying the distal crypt opening on the ectocervix and tracing them.

5. NEW SCJ

New SCJ is the junction of squamous metaplastic epithelium and columnar epithelium. It is always seen shifting towards the external os.

6. TRANSFORMATION ZONE (TZ)

It is the area between the original/old SCJ and the new SCJ.

Different Types of TZ

TZ type 1: When the new SCJ is completely visible on the ectocervix.

TZ type 2: When the new SCJ is visible on or near the cervical os and is partially visible. Slight maneuvering is required for complete visibility of SCJ.

TZ type 3: When the new SCJ has regressed into the endocervix and is usually not visible even on endocervical speculum examination.

Transformation Zone Type 1 (Figs 3.10a to g)

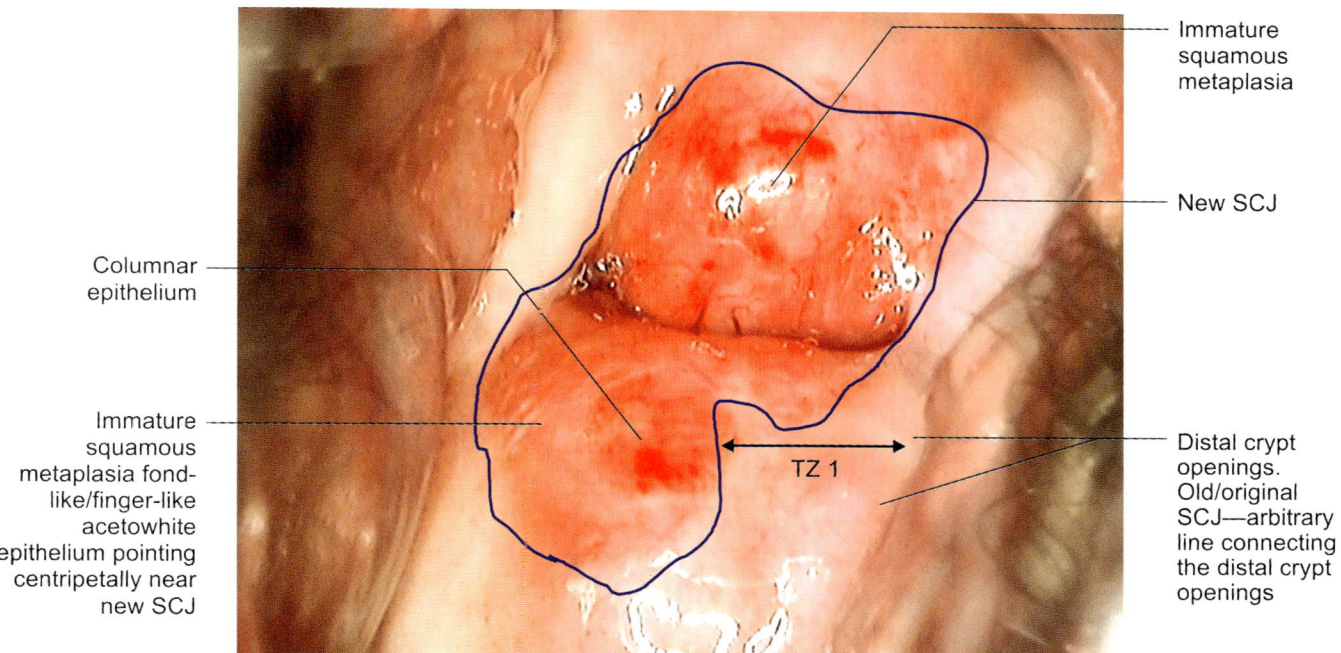

Fig. 3.10a

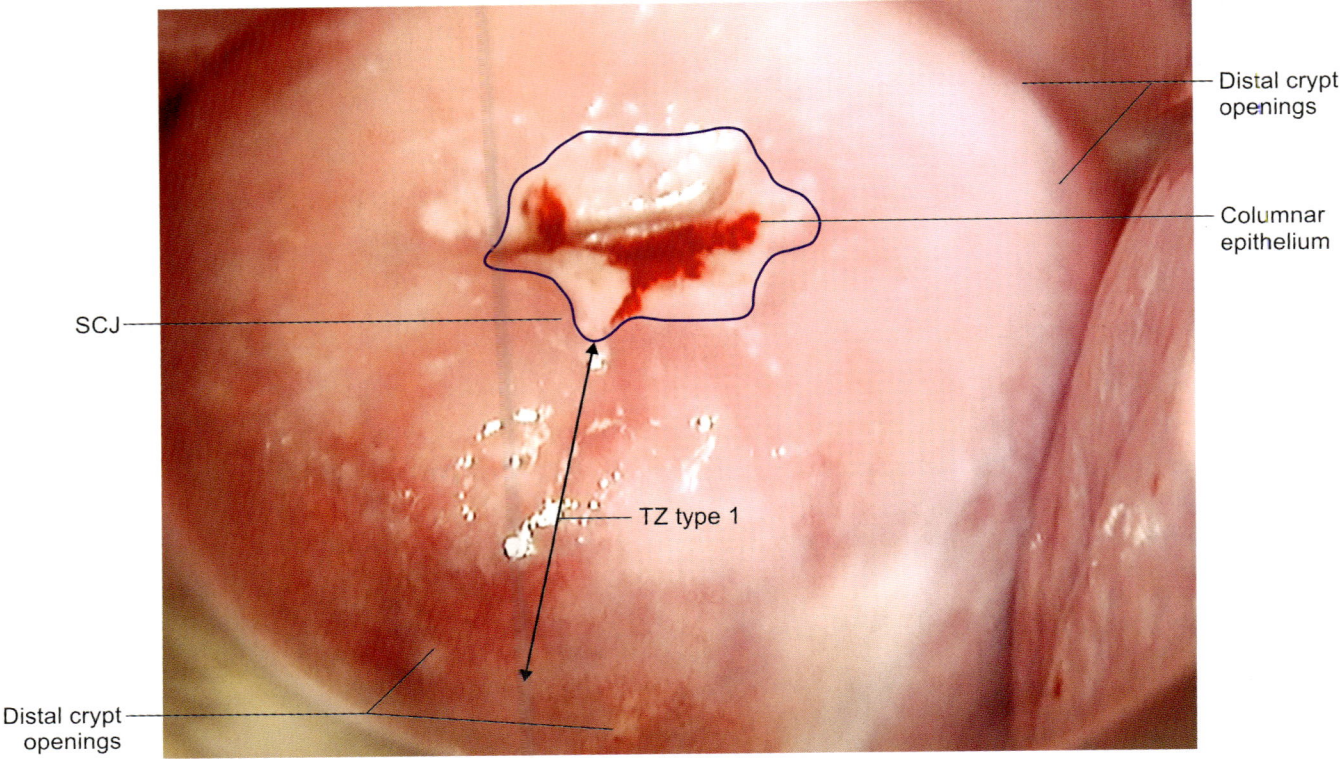

SCJ

Distal crypt openings

Distal crypt openings

Columnar epithelium

TZ type 1

Fig. 3.10b

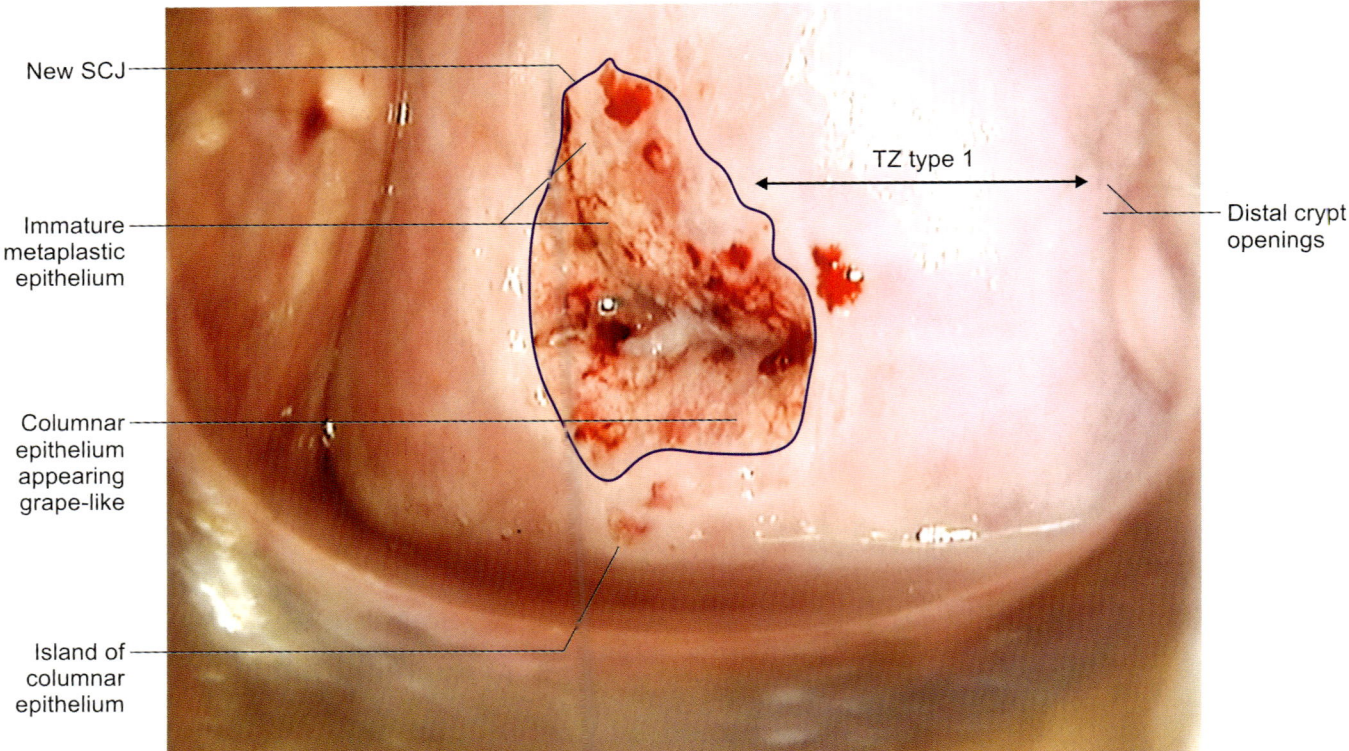

New SCJ

Immature metaplastic epithelium

Columnar epithelium appearing grape-like

Island of columnar epithelium

TZ type 1

Distal crypt openings

Fig. 3.10c

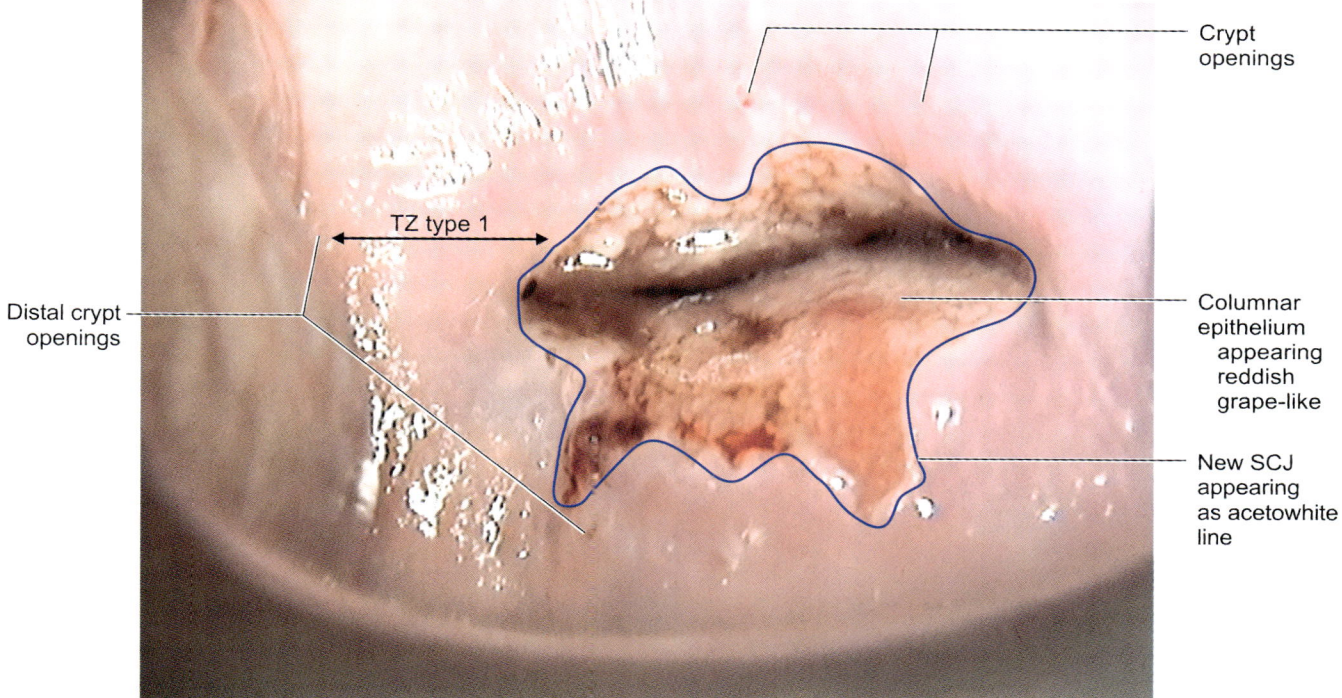

Crypt openings

Columnar epithelium appearing reddish grape-like

New SCJ appearing as acetowhite line

TZ type 1

Distal crypt openings

Fig. 3.10d

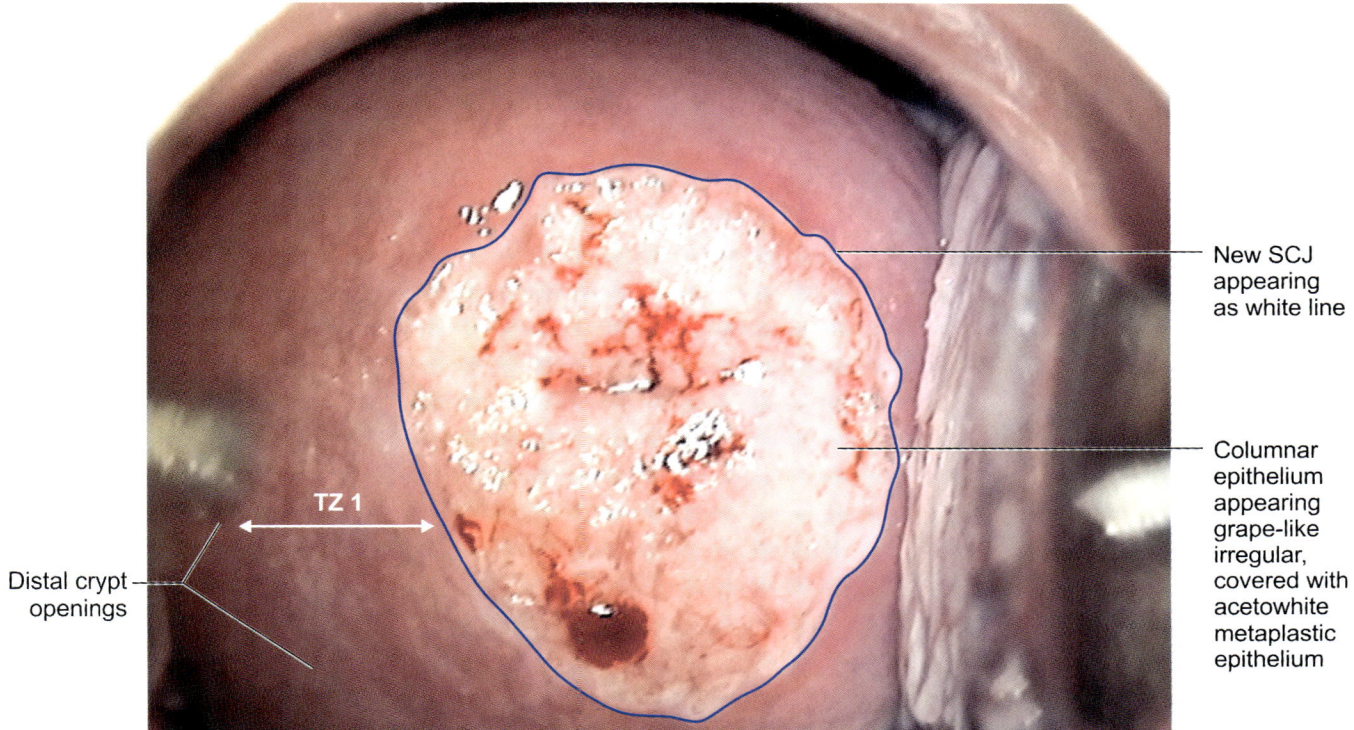

New SCJ appearing as white line

Columnar epithelium appearing grape-like irregular, covered with acetowhite metaplastic epithelium

TZ 1

Distal crypt openings

Fig. 3.10e

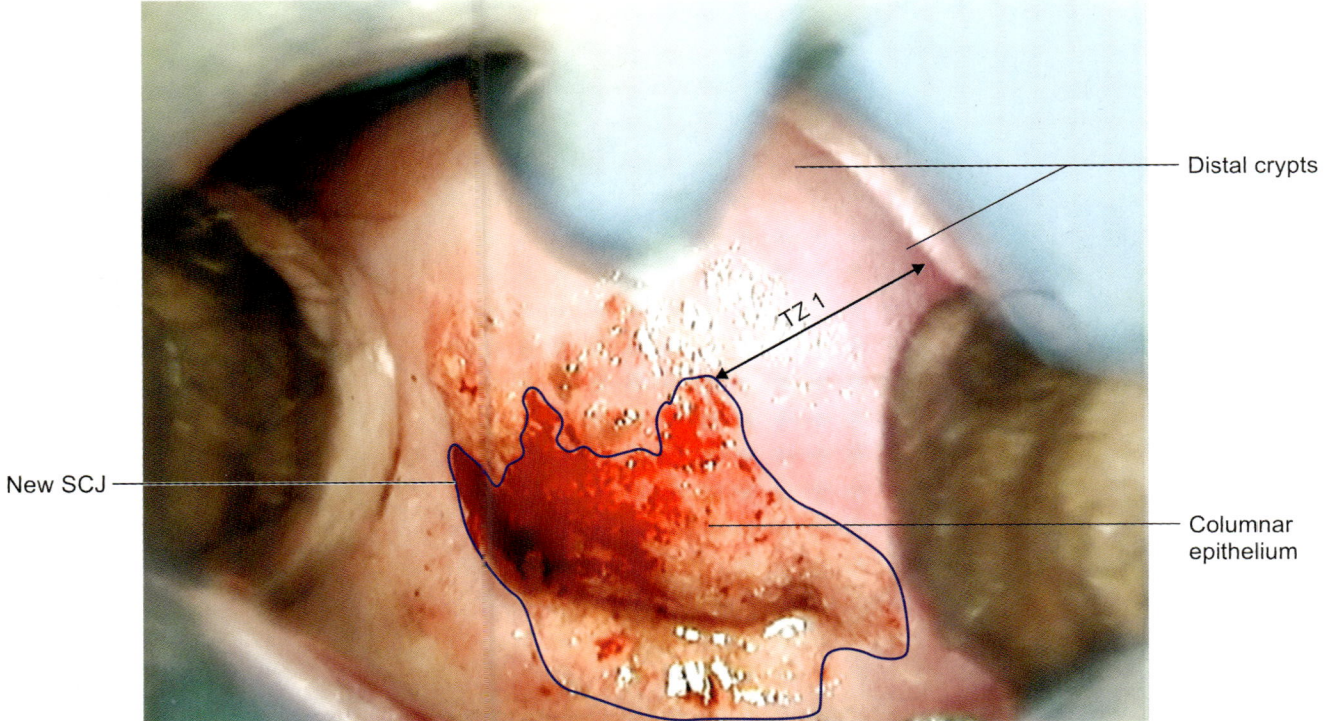

Distal crypts

New SCJ

TZ 1

Columnar epithelium

Fig. 3.10f

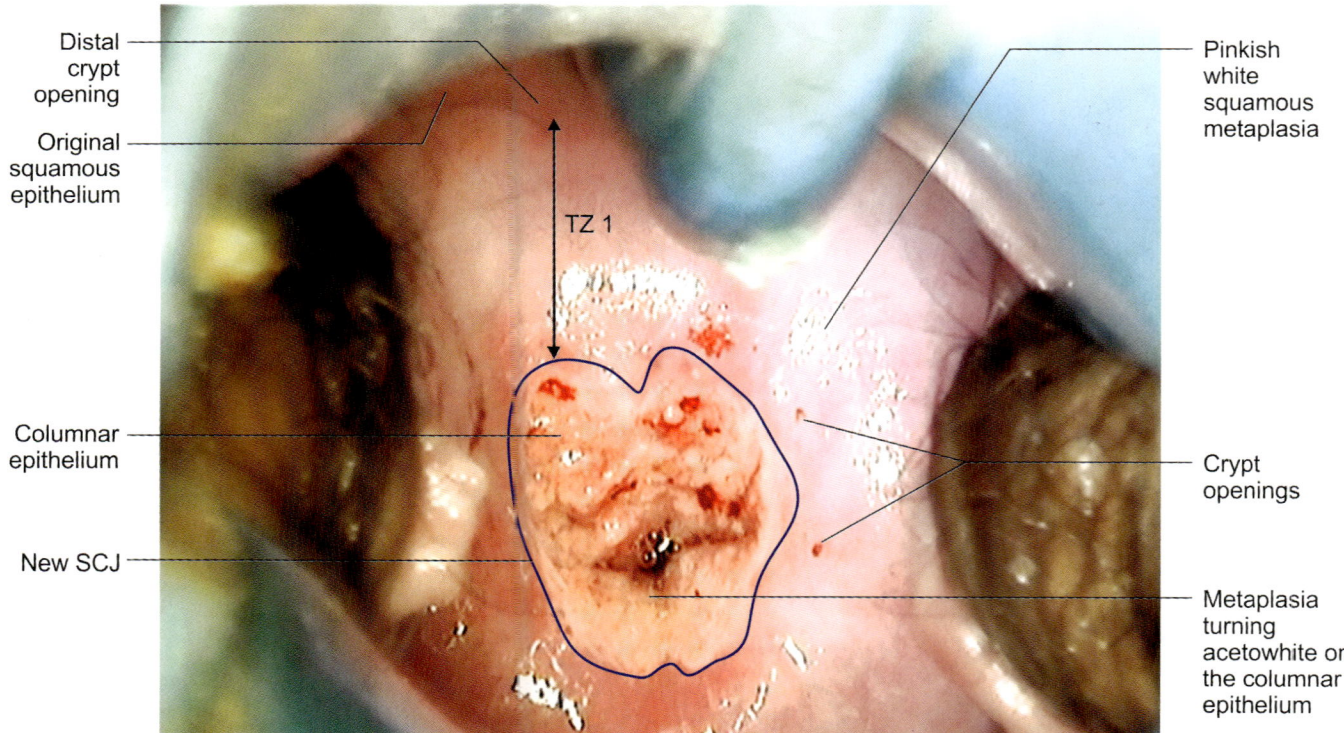

Distal crypt opening

Original squamous epithelium

Pinkish white squamous metaplasia

TZ 1

Columnar epithelium

New SCJ

Crypt openings

Metaplasia turning acetowhite on the columnar epithelium

Fig. 3.10g

Transformation Zone Type 2 (Figs 3.11a to h)

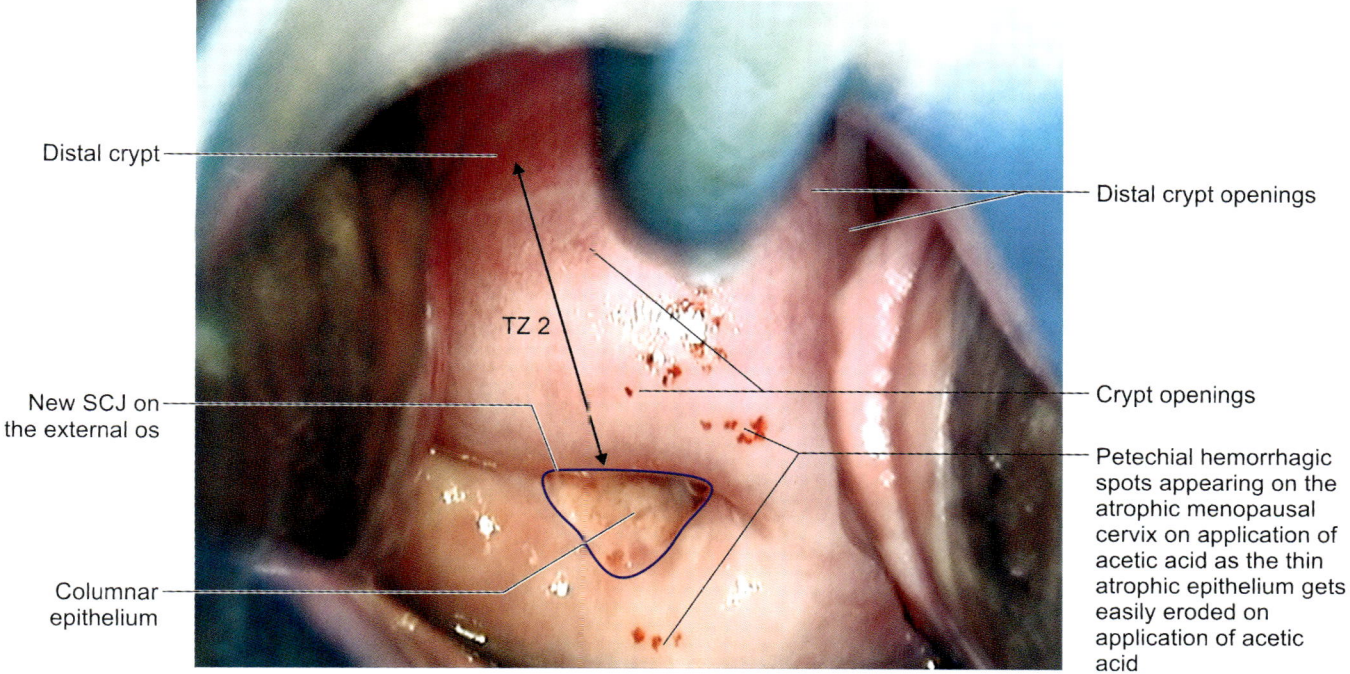

Distal crypt

Distal crypt openings

TZ 2

New SCJ on the external os

Crypt openings

Petechial hemorrhagic spots appearing on the atrophic menopausal cervix on application of acetic acid as the thin atrophic epithelium gets easily eroded on application of acetic acid

Columnar epithelium

Fig. 3.11a

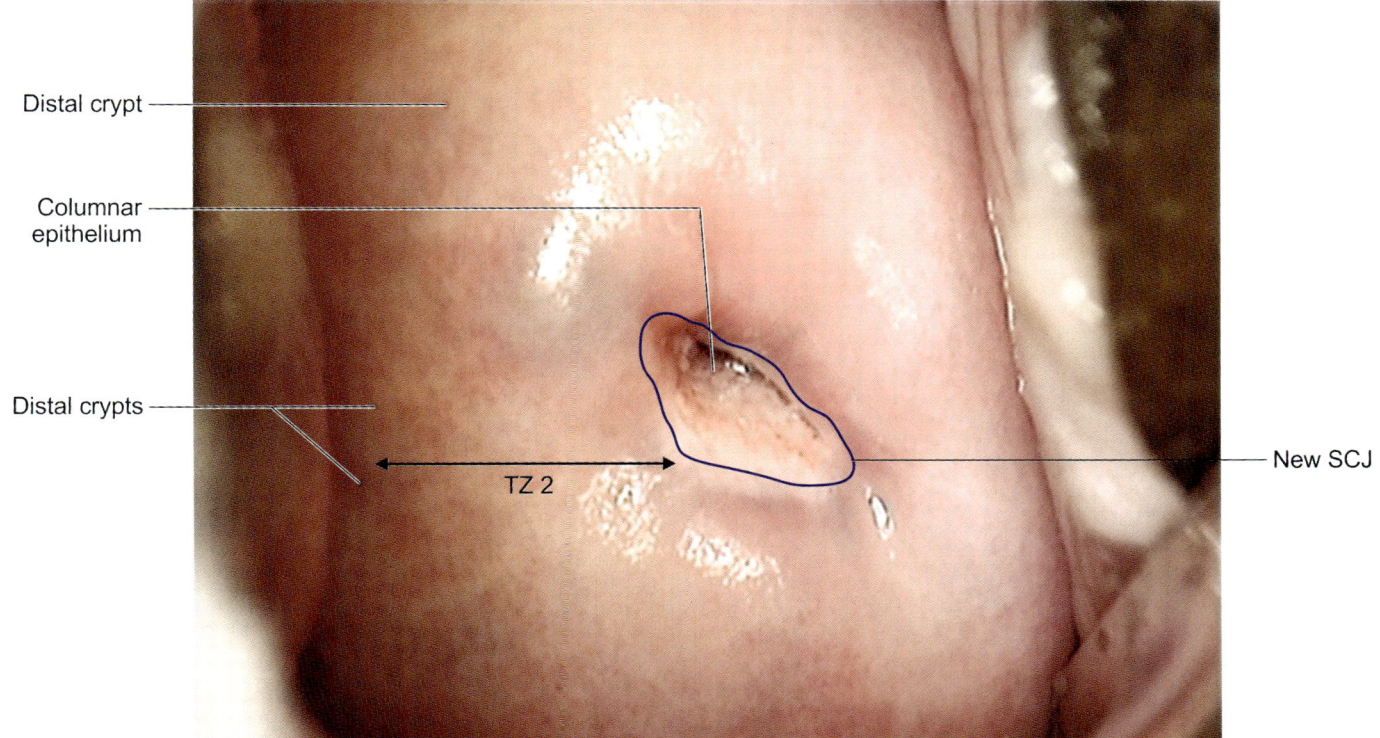

Distal crypt

Columnar epithelium

Distal crypts

TZ 2

New SCJ

Fig. 3.11b

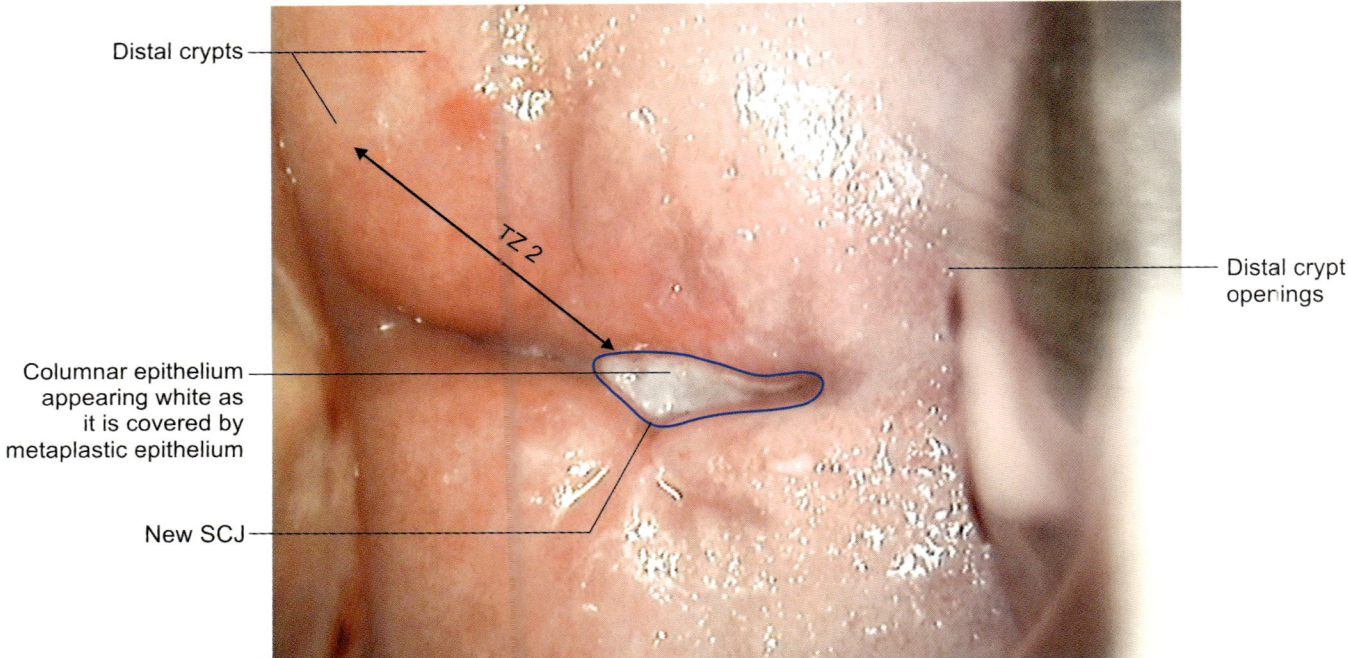

Distal crypts

Distal crypt openings

TZ 2

Columnar epithelium appearing white as it is covered by metaplastic epithelium

New SCJ

Fig. 3.11c

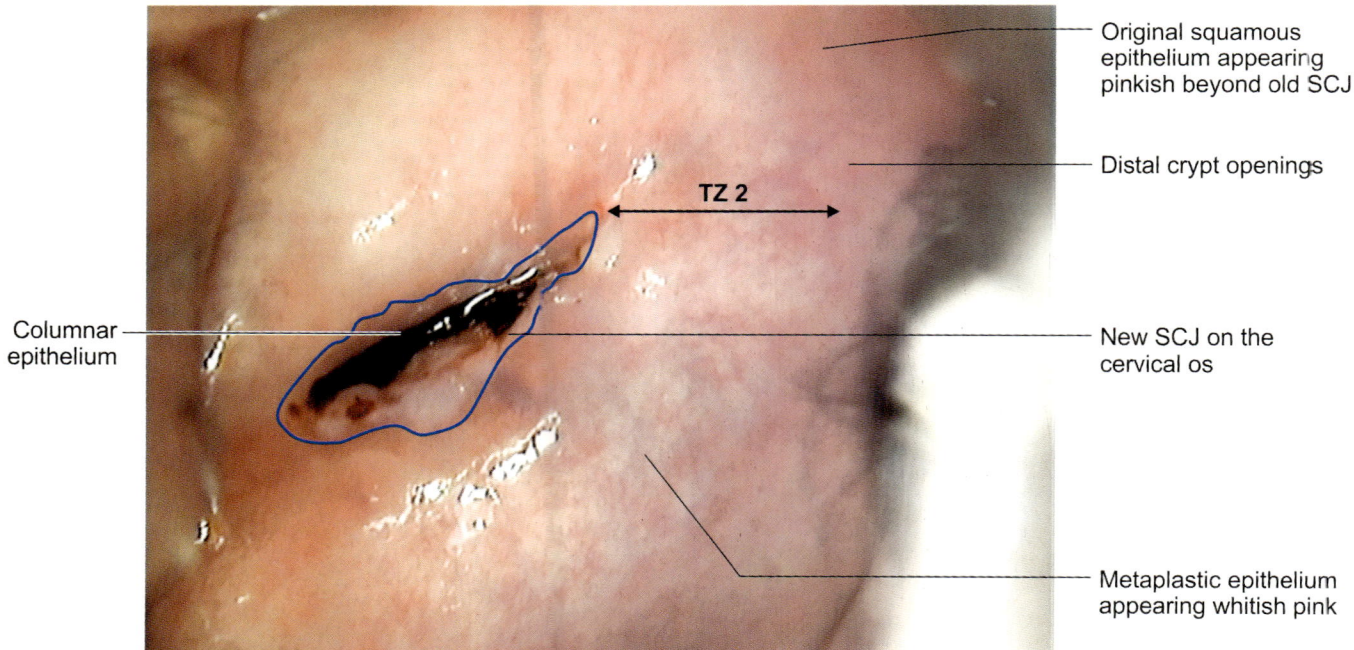

Original squamous epithelium appearing pinkish beyond old SCJ

Distal crypt openings

TZ 2

Columnar epithelium

New SCJ on the cervical os

Metaplastic epithelium appearing whitish pink

Fig. 3.11d

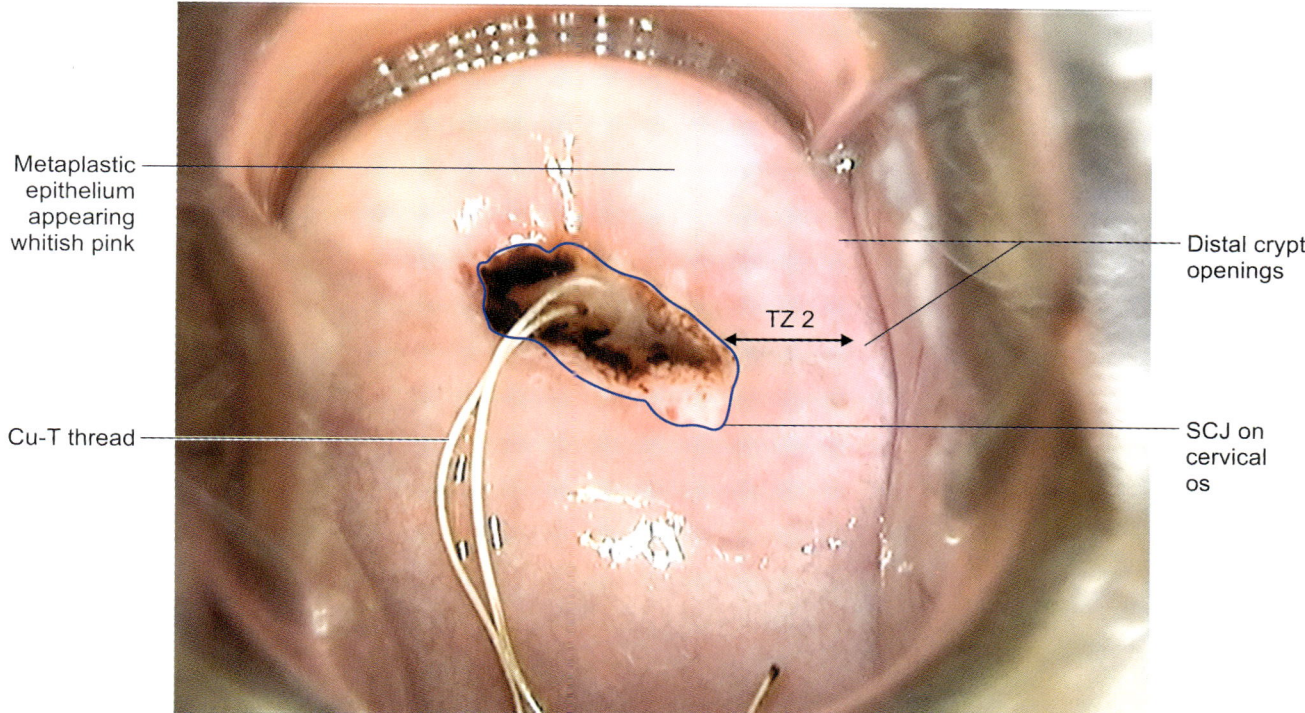

Metaplastic epithelium appearing whitish pink

Distal crypt openings

TZ 2

Cu-T thread

SCJ on cervical os

Fig. 3.11e

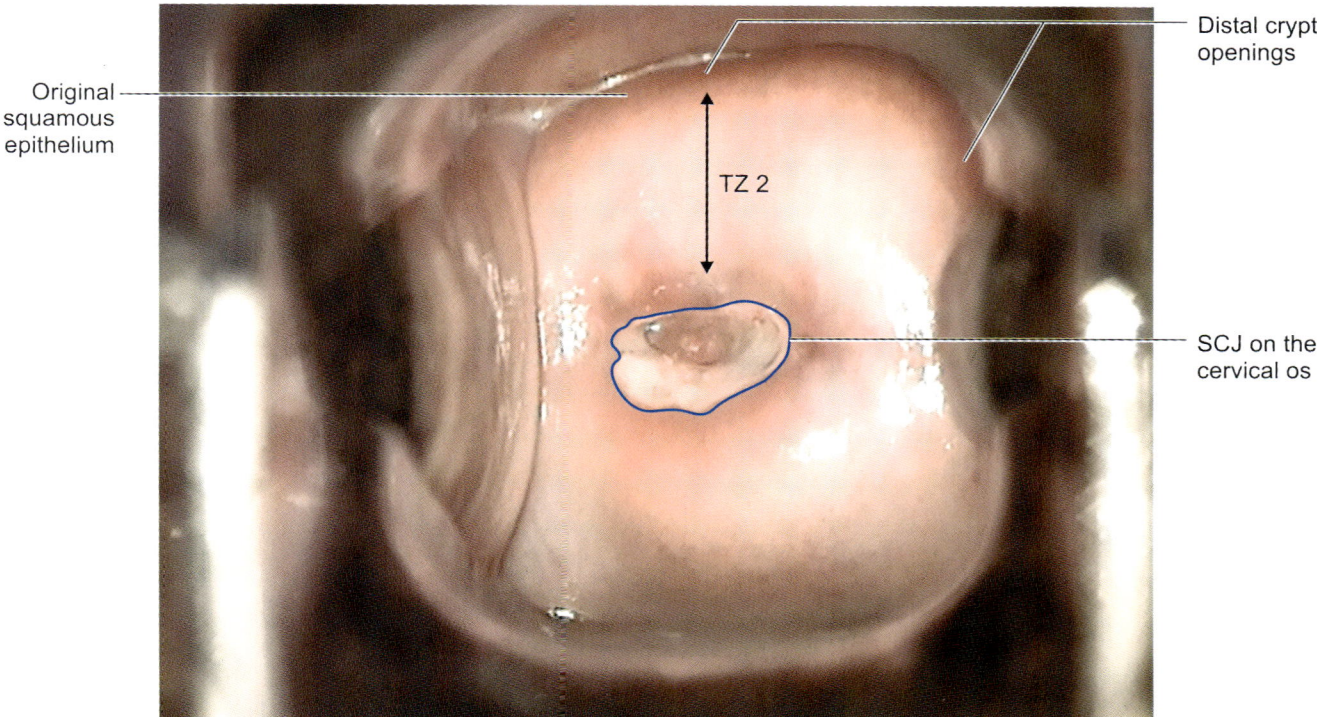

Distal crypt openings

Original squamous epithelium

TZ 2

SCJ on the cervical os

Fig. 3.11f

Original
squamous
epithelium
appearing
pinkish red

Distal crypt
openings

TZ 2

SCJ on the
cervical os

Columnar
epithelium

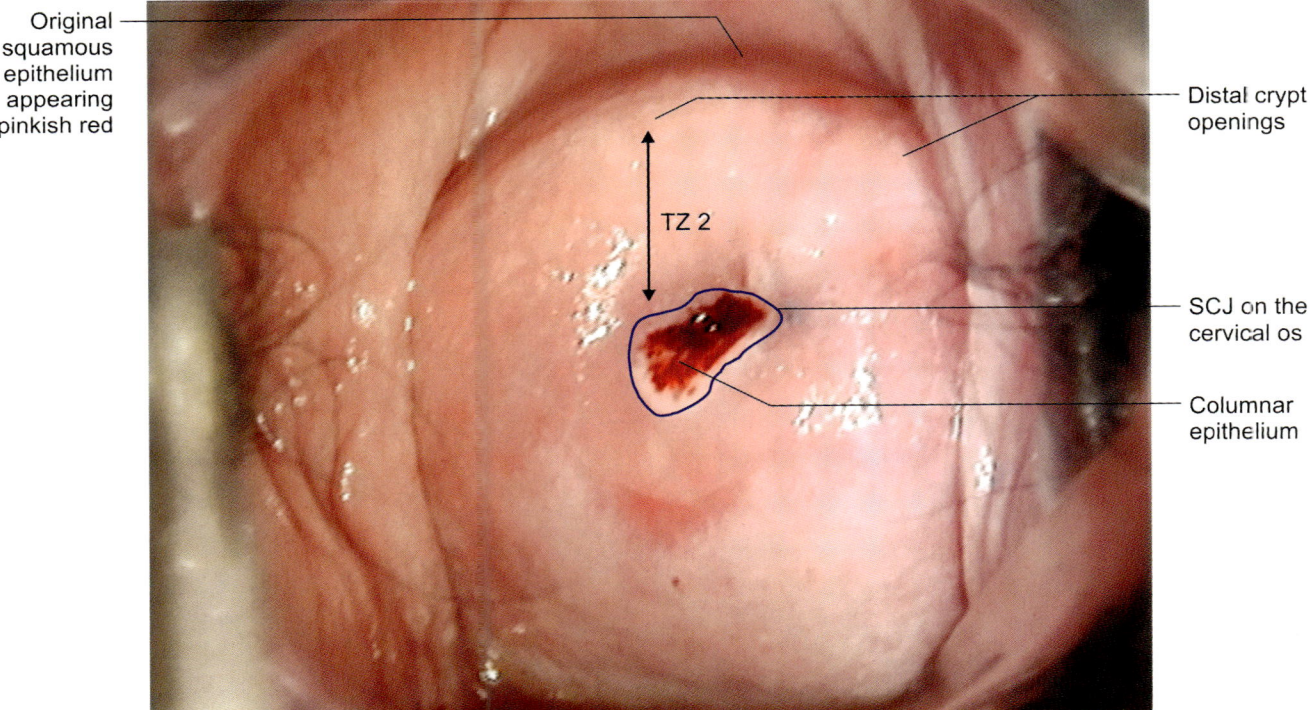

Fig. 3.11g

Original
squamous
epithelium

TZ 2

Distal crypt
openings

Columnar
epithelium

SCJ as thin
white line
on the os

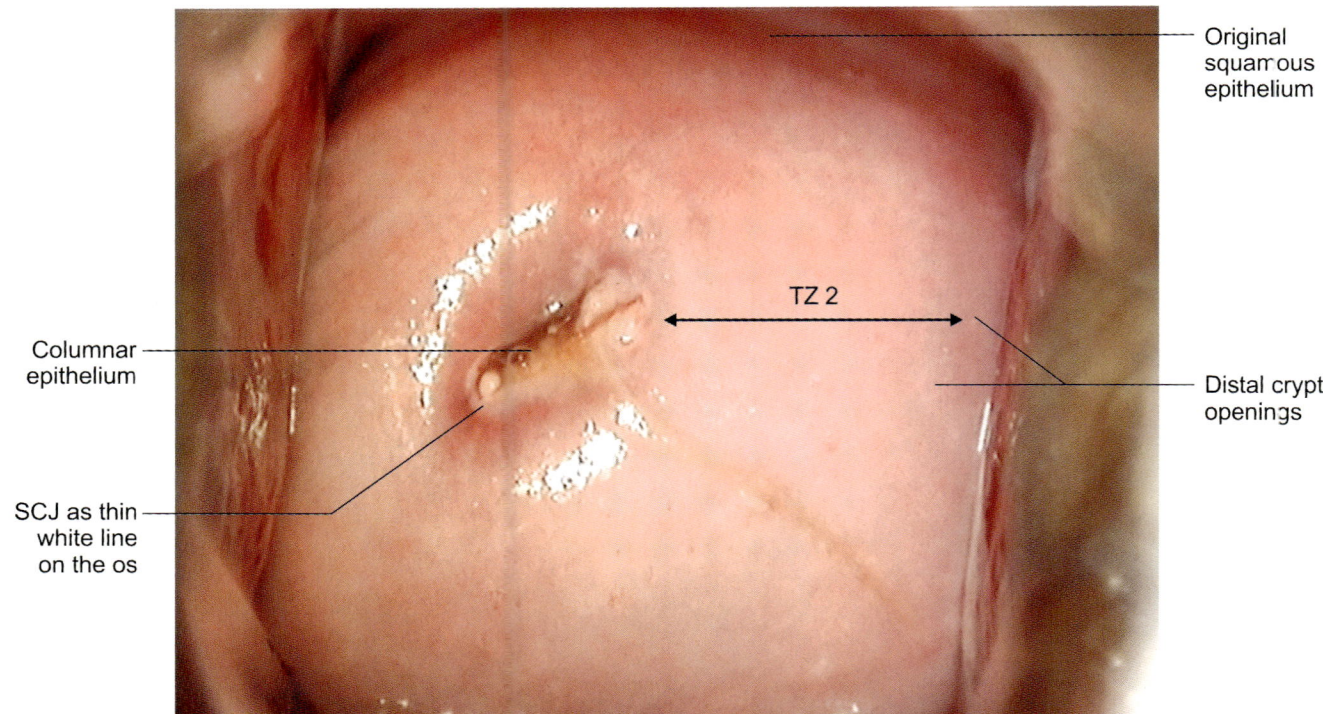

Fig. 3.11h

Transformation Zone Type 3 (Figs 3.12a to h)

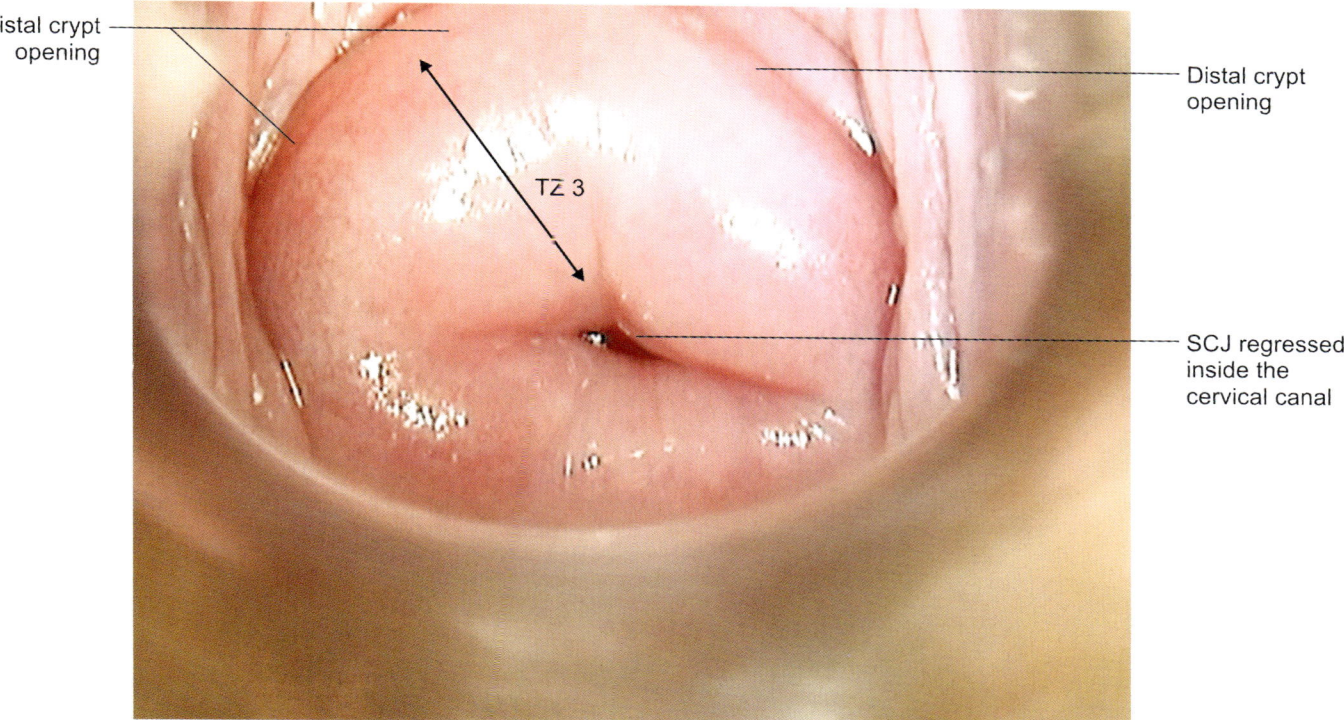

Distal crypt opening

Distal crypt opening

TZ 3

SCJ regressed inside the cervical canal

Fig. 3.12a

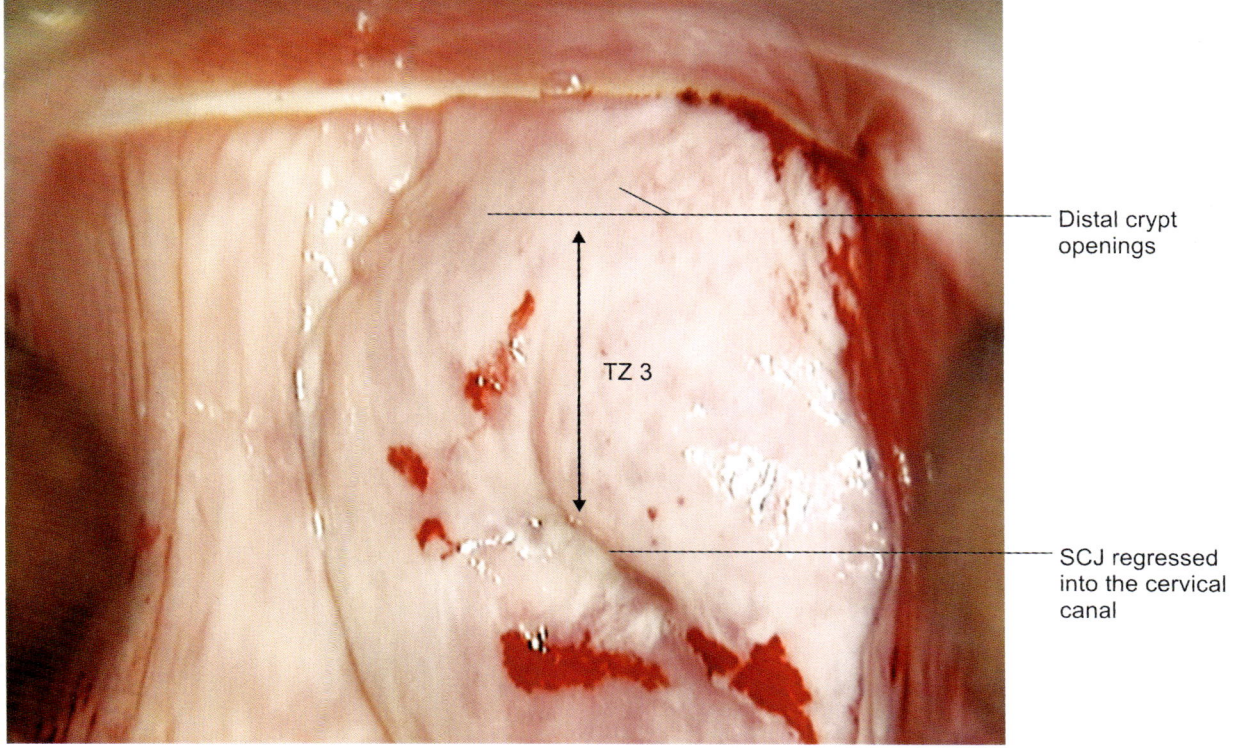

Distal crypt openings

TZ 3

SCJ regressed into the cervical canal

Fig. 3.12b

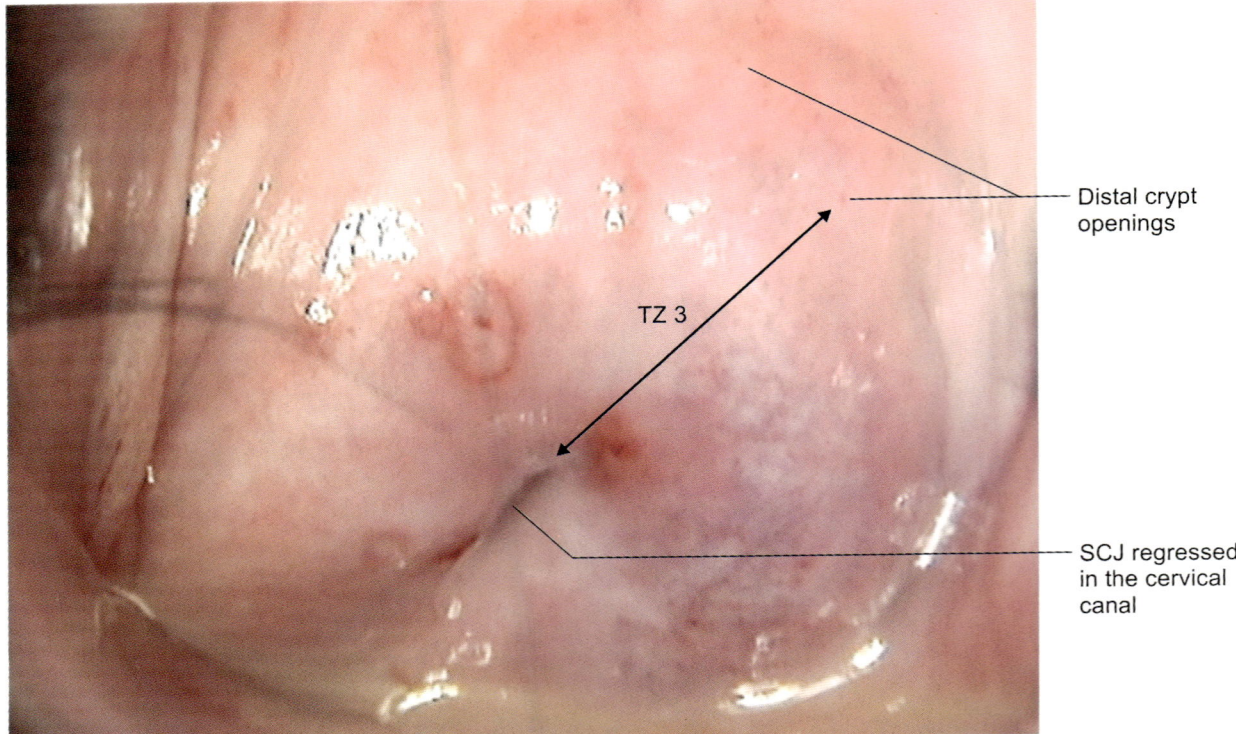

Distal crypt openings

TZ 3

SCJ regressed in the cervical canal

Fig. 3.12c

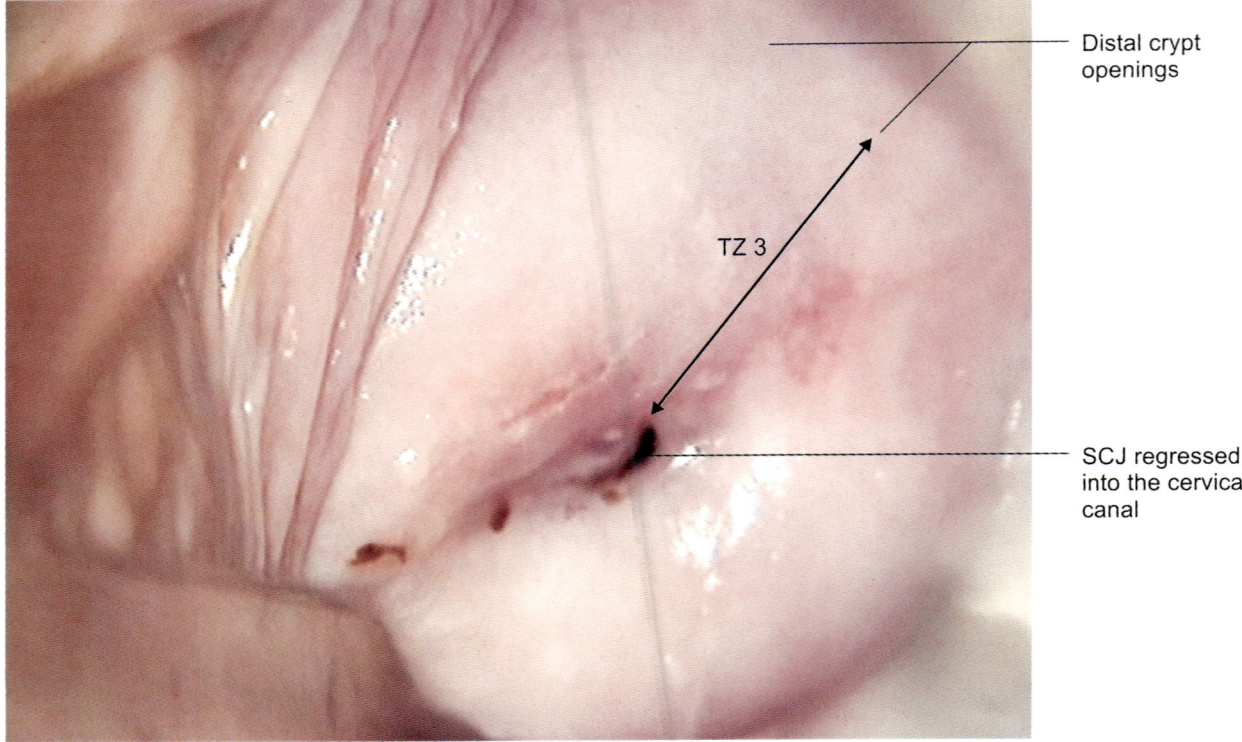

Distal crypt openings

TZ 3

SCJ regressed into the cervical canal

Fig. 3.12d

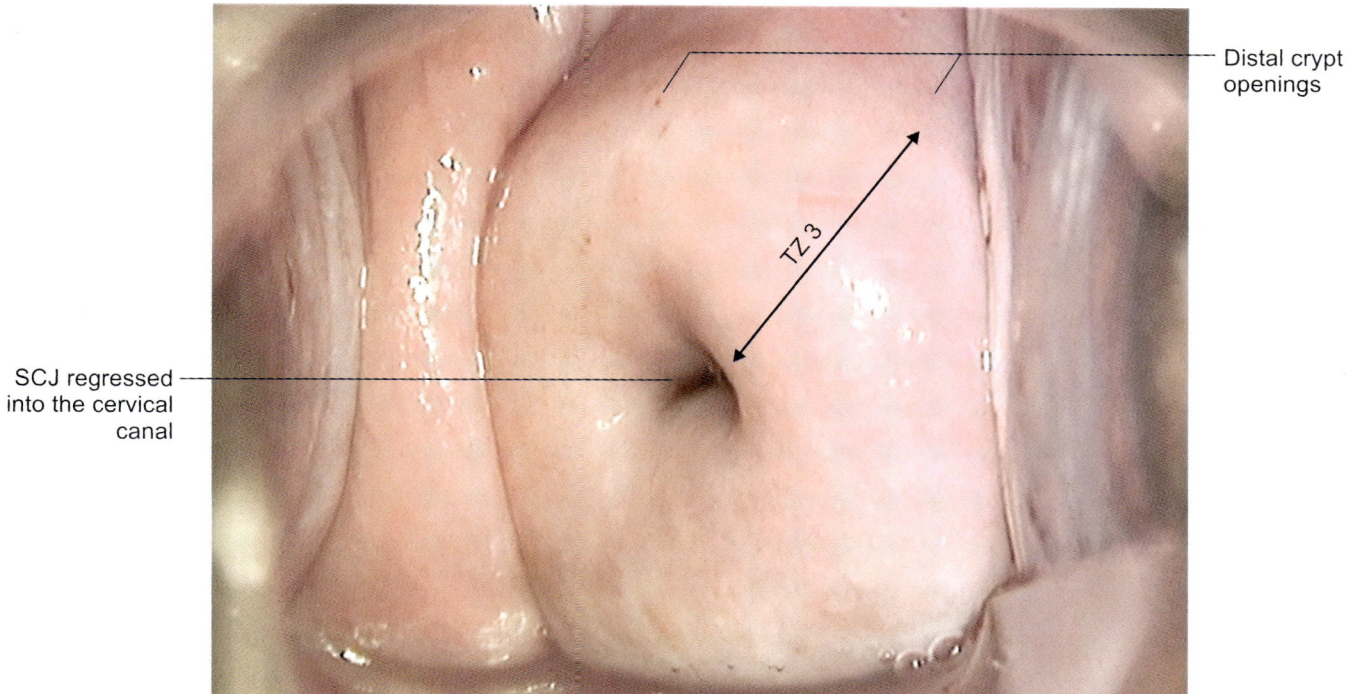

Distal crypt openings

TZ 3

SCJ regressed into the cervical canal

Fig. 3.12e

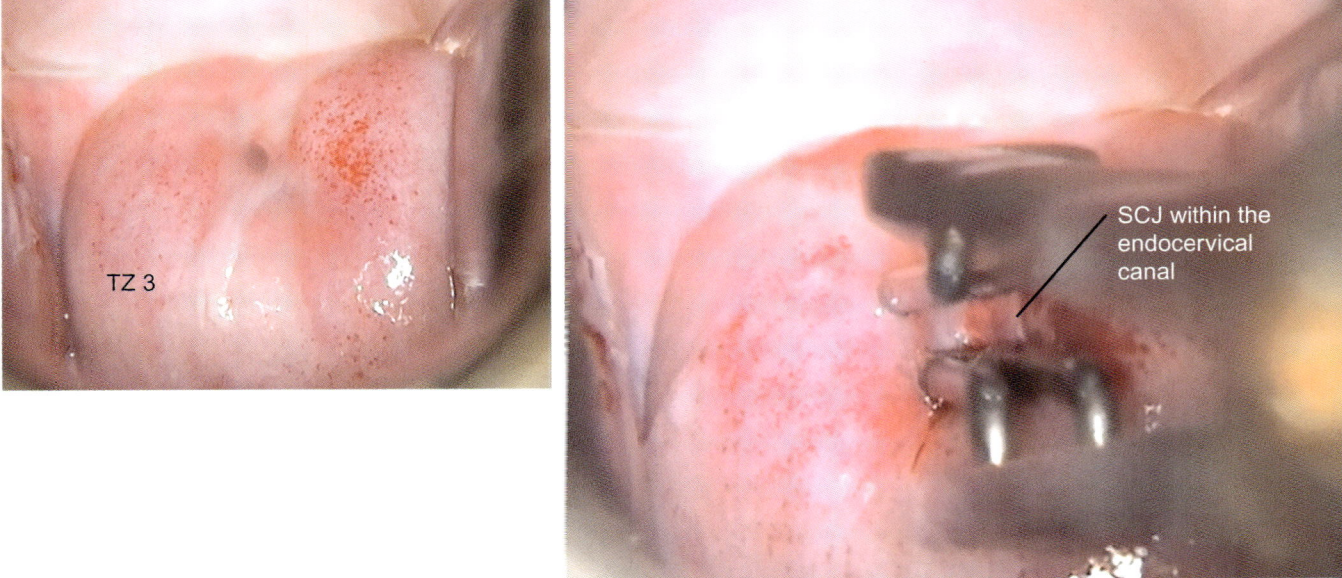

TZ 3

SCJ within the endocervical canal

Fig. 3.12f: TZ 3 endocervical speculum examination

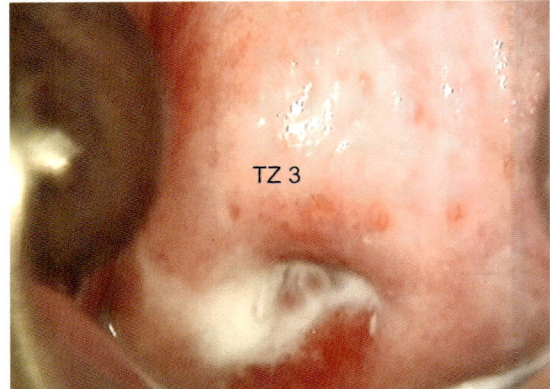

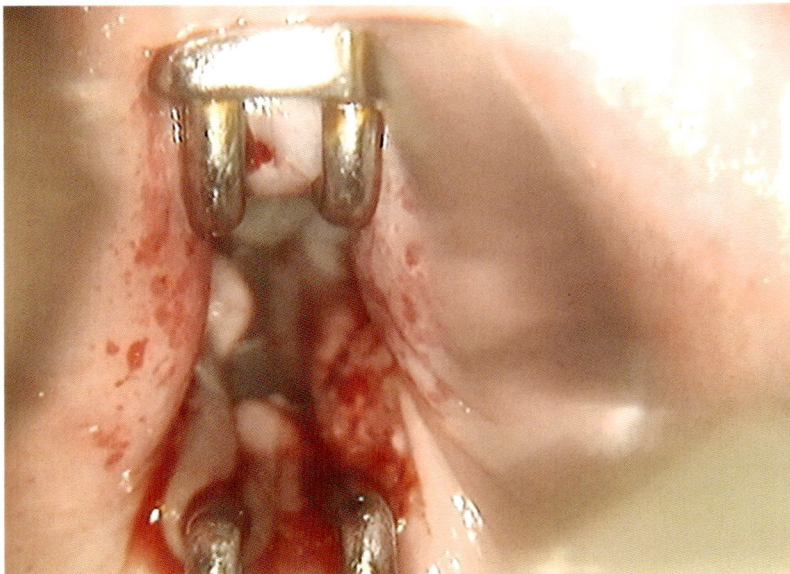

Fig. 3.12g

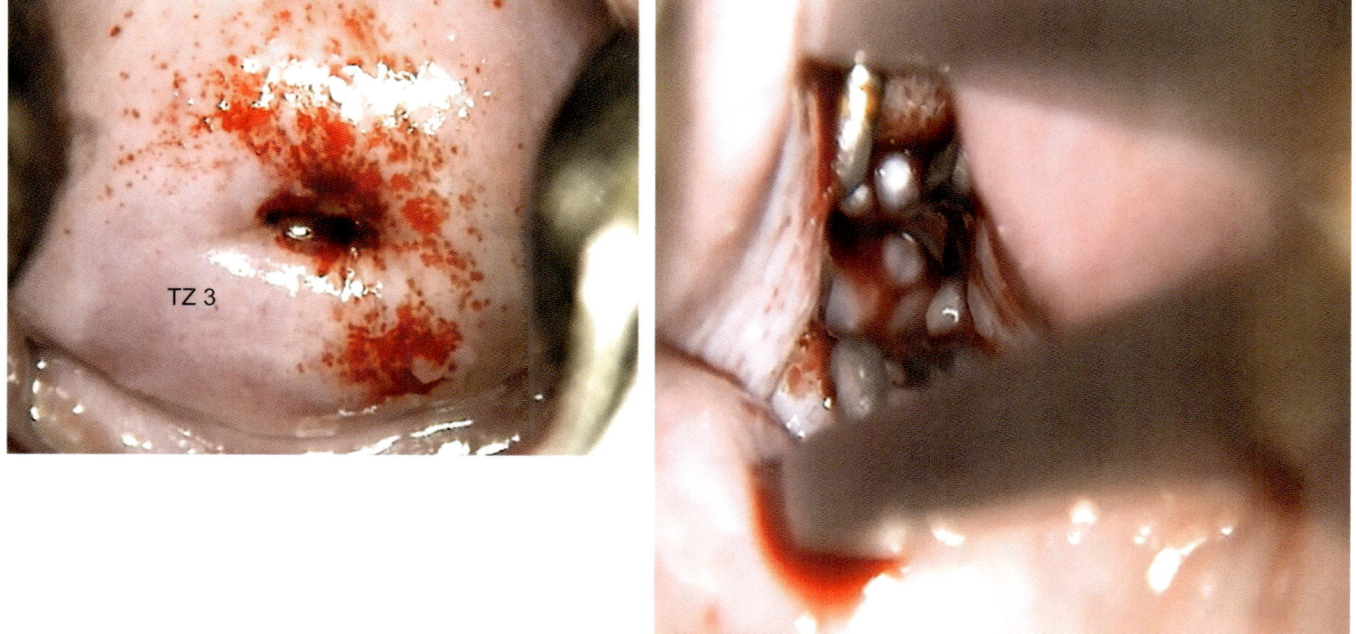

Fig. 3.12h: TZ 3 endocervical speculum examination

7. ECTOPY (Figs 3.13a to f)

In the early reproductive age group, due to influence of estrogen hormones, the columnar epithelium is everted on the squamous epithelium. Due to the influence of acidic vaginal pH, the reserve cells get activated and metaplasia, i.e. transformation of columnar epithelium to squamous epithelium, takes place.

Sometimes this process of metaplasia is not initiated and hence the cervix appears reddish due to columnar epithelium. This is, many a times, termed as ulcer or erosions by many.

When the columnar epithelium covers more than two-thirds of the cervix, it is termed as ectopy.

Usually, the ectopy causes excessive repeated white discharge. This can be treated with electrocauterization, cryo or thermal ablation also.

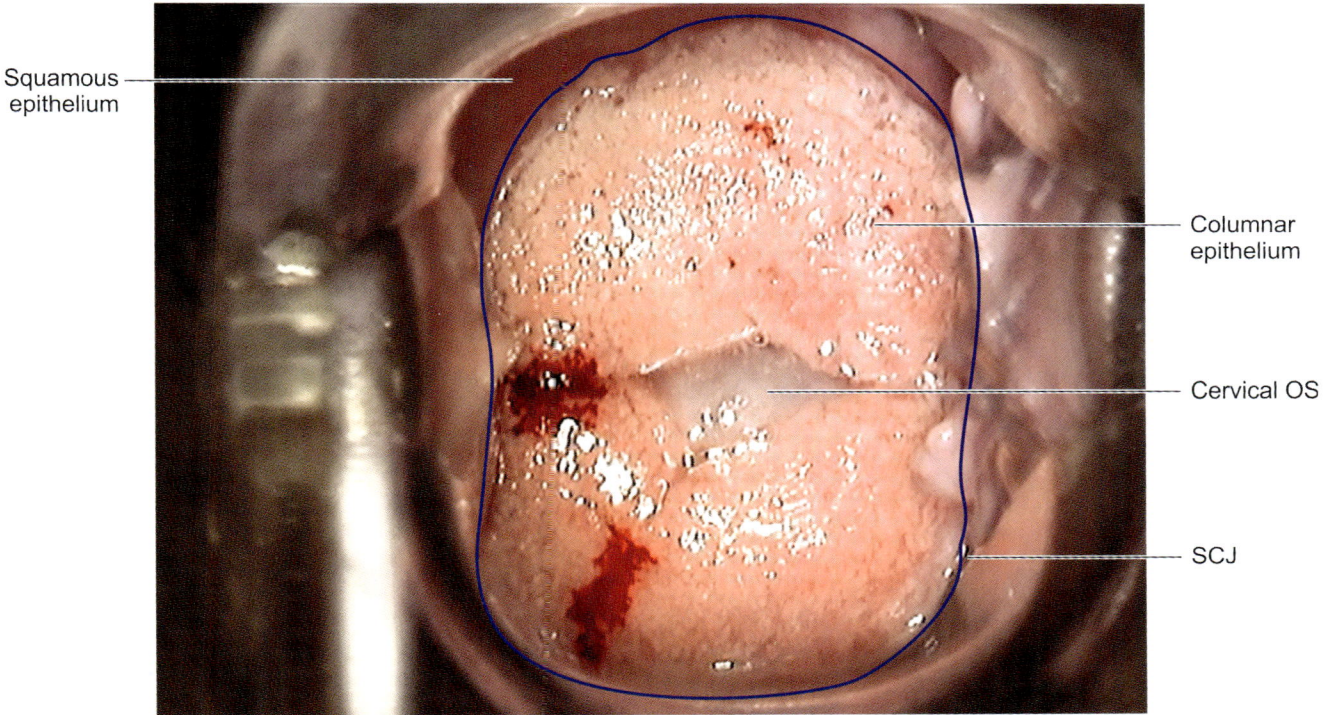

Fig. 3.13a

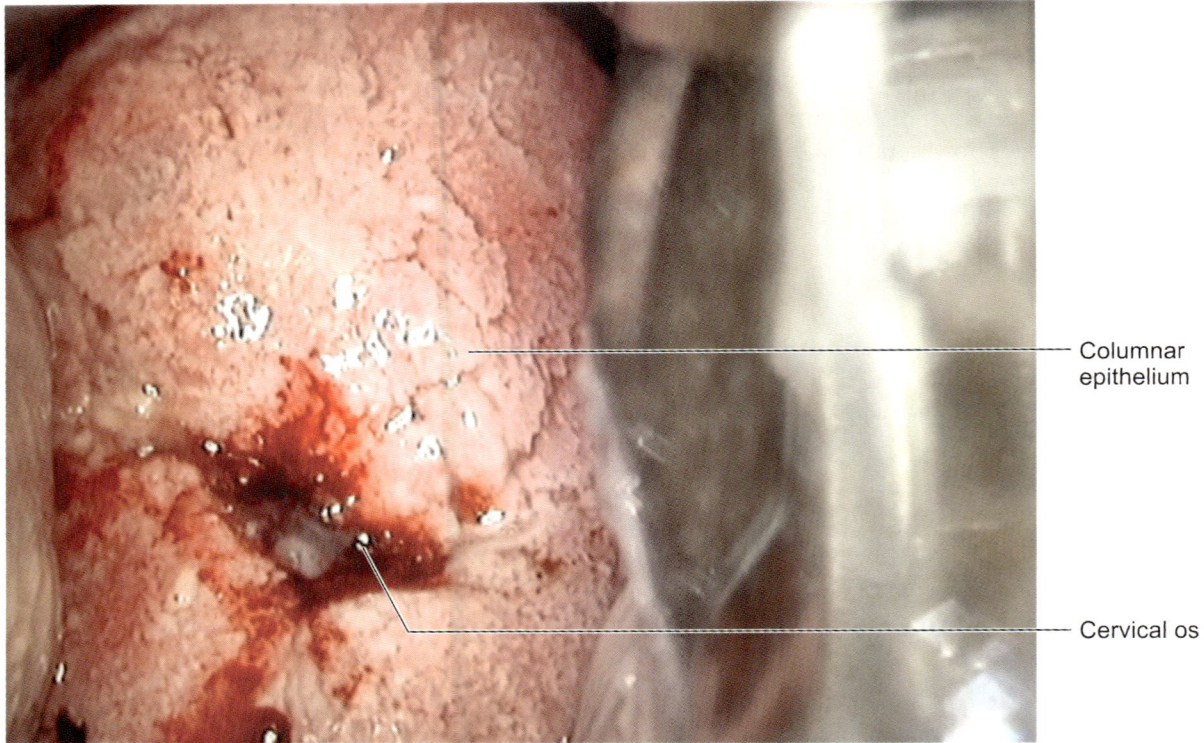

Columnar epithelium

Cervical os

Fig. 3.13b

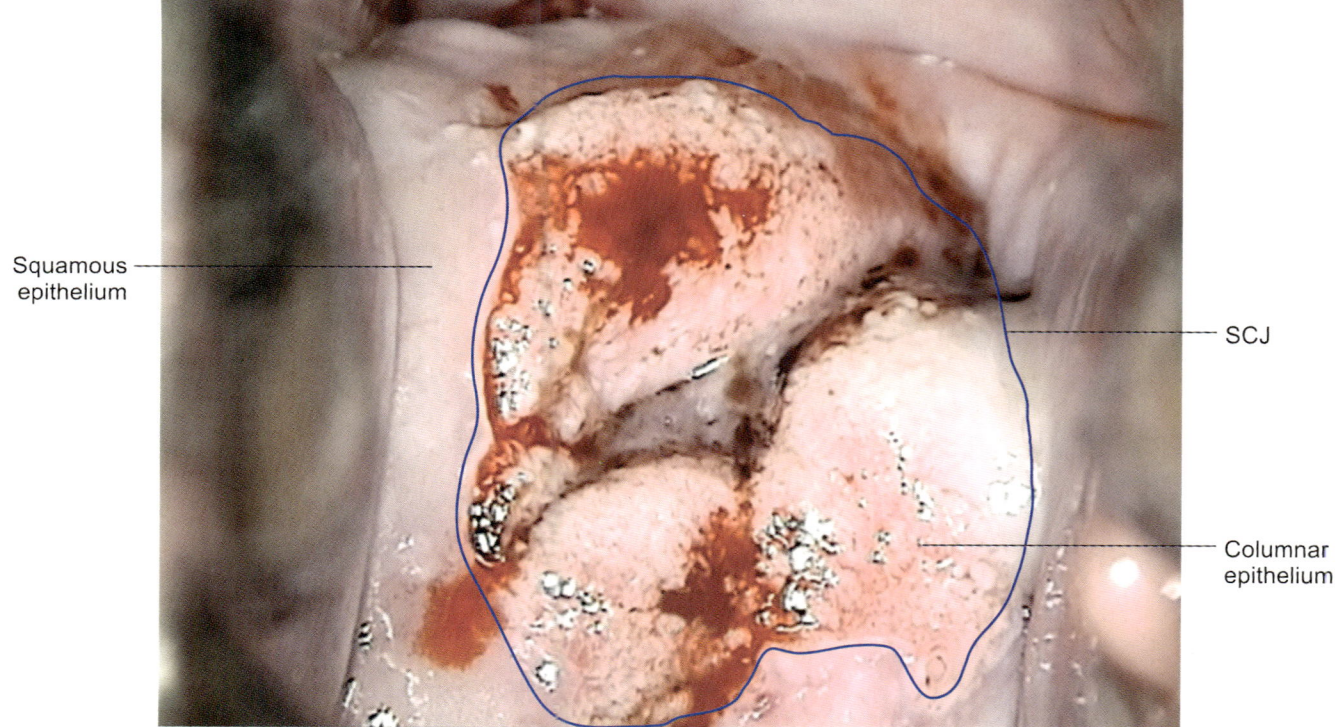

Squamous epithelium

SCJ

Columnar epithelium

Fig. 3.13c

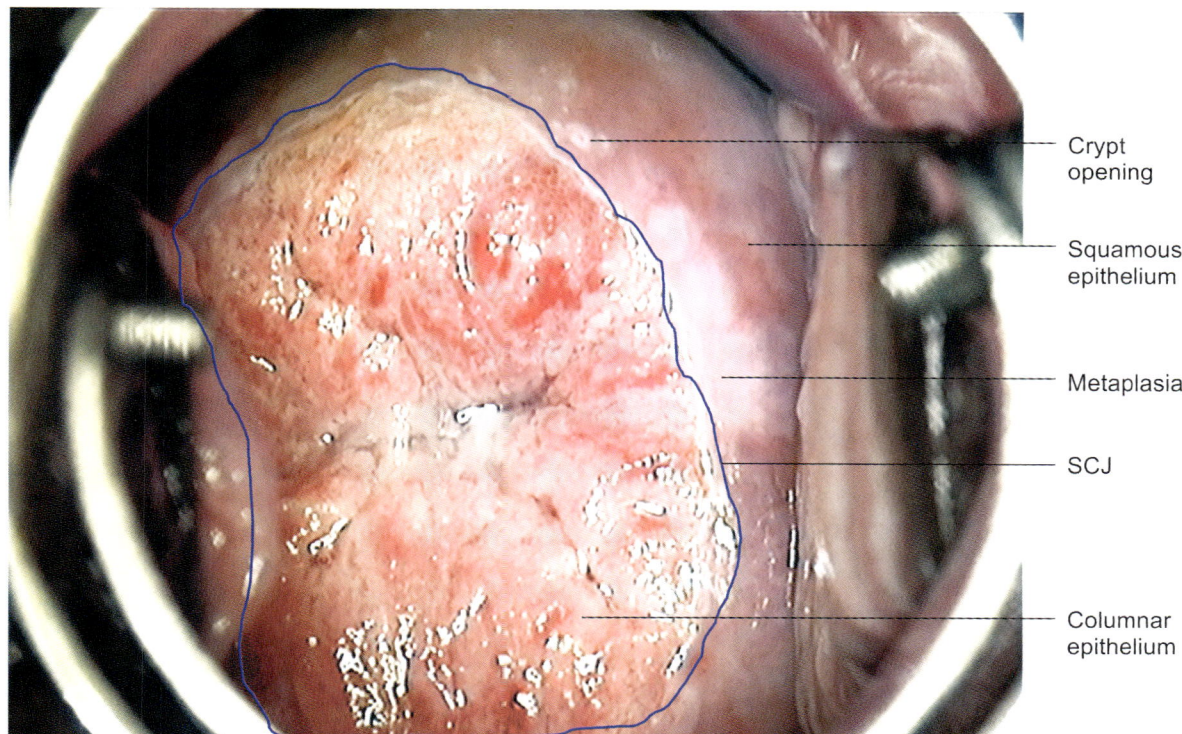

Crypt opening

Squamous epithelium

Metaplasia

SCJ

Columnar epithelium

Fig. 3.13d

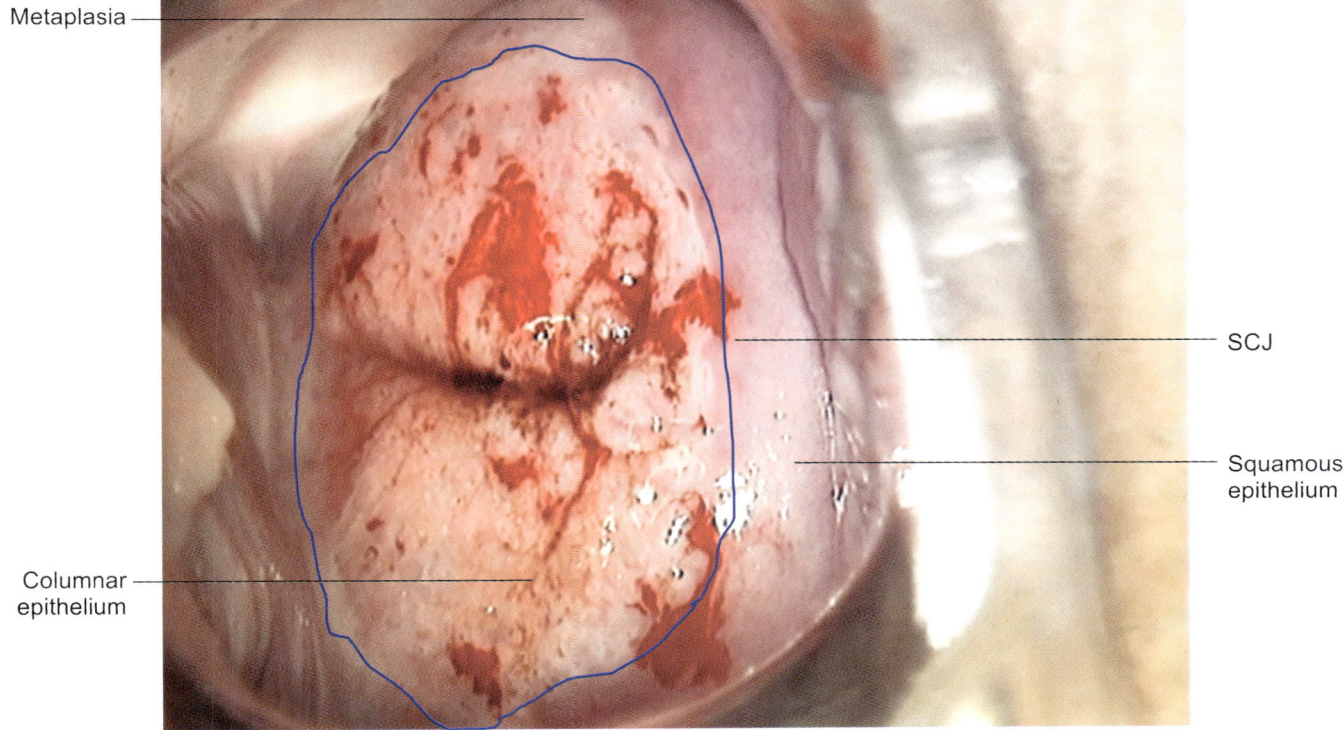

Metaplasia

SCJ

Columnar epithelium

Squamous epithelium

Fig. 3.13e

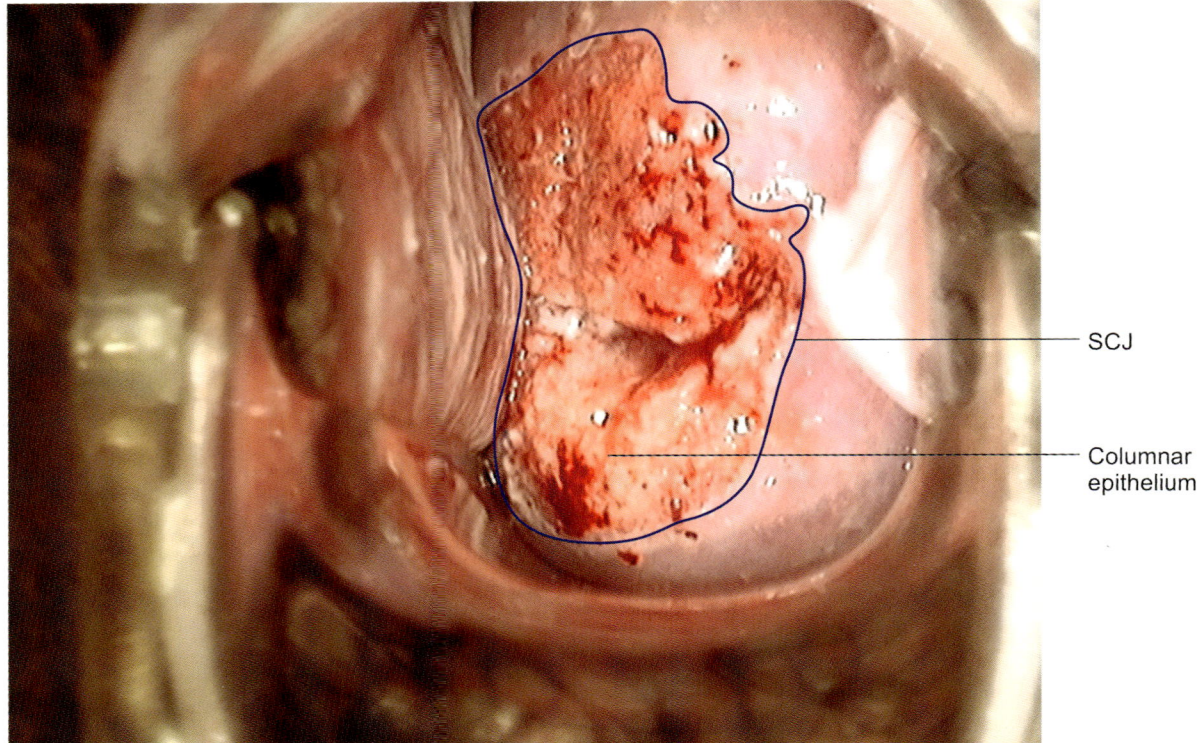

SCJ

Columnar
epithelium

Fig. 3.13f

Ectopy can be corrected by electrocauterization with ball cautery (Figs 3.14a and b).

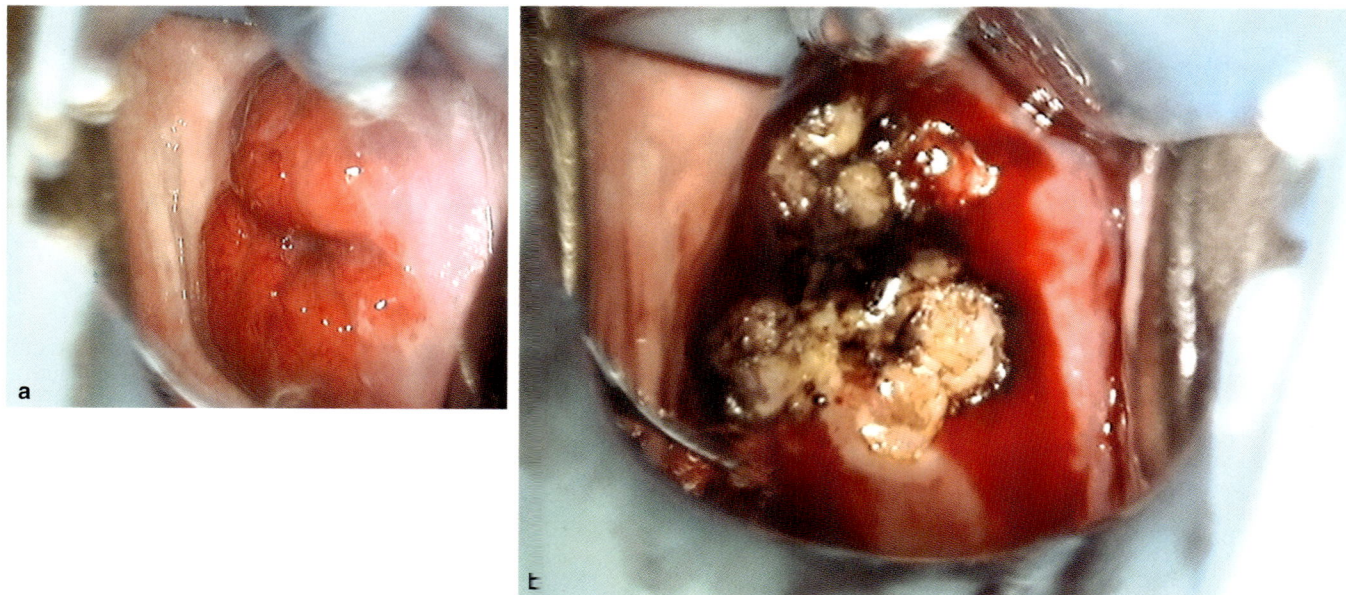

Figs 3.14a and b: Electrocauterization with ball cautery

8. CONGENITAL TZ (Figs 3.15a and b)

During embryonic life, the cuboidal epithelium of vaginal tube is replaced by the squamous epithelium, which begins at the caudal end of the dorsal urogenital sinus. This process is completed well before birth. So during birth, the vaginal epithelium and the ectocervix is covered by squamous epithelium. With this normal epithelialization, the original SCJ is located at the external os at the time of birth. If for some reason, this process is arrested, the original SCJ will be located distal to the external os or may be rarely found on vaginal wall and the cuboidal epithelium persists all throughout the lifetime giving rise to congenital transformation zone (TZ).

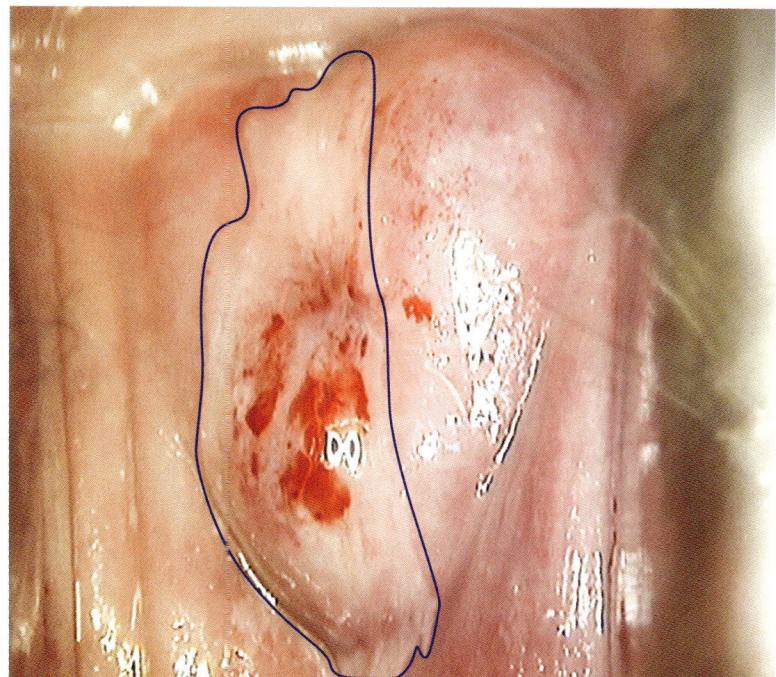

Fig. 3.15a: Acetowhite area covering the entire ectocervix more on the anterior and posterior regions extending till the vagina

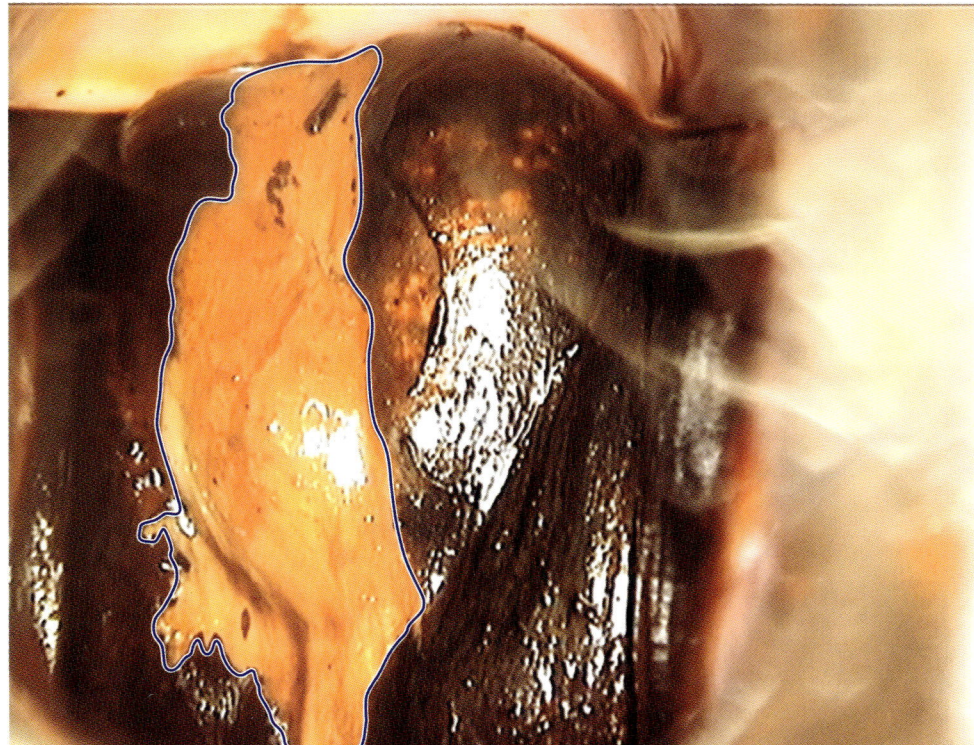

Fig. 3.15b: The entire area not taken up iodine, Lugol's negative, extending till the vagina

9. METAPLASIA (Figs 3.16a and b)

As discussed, metaplasia is transformation of one type of epithelium to another.
  Squamous metaplasia is conversion of columnar epithelium to squamous epithelium.

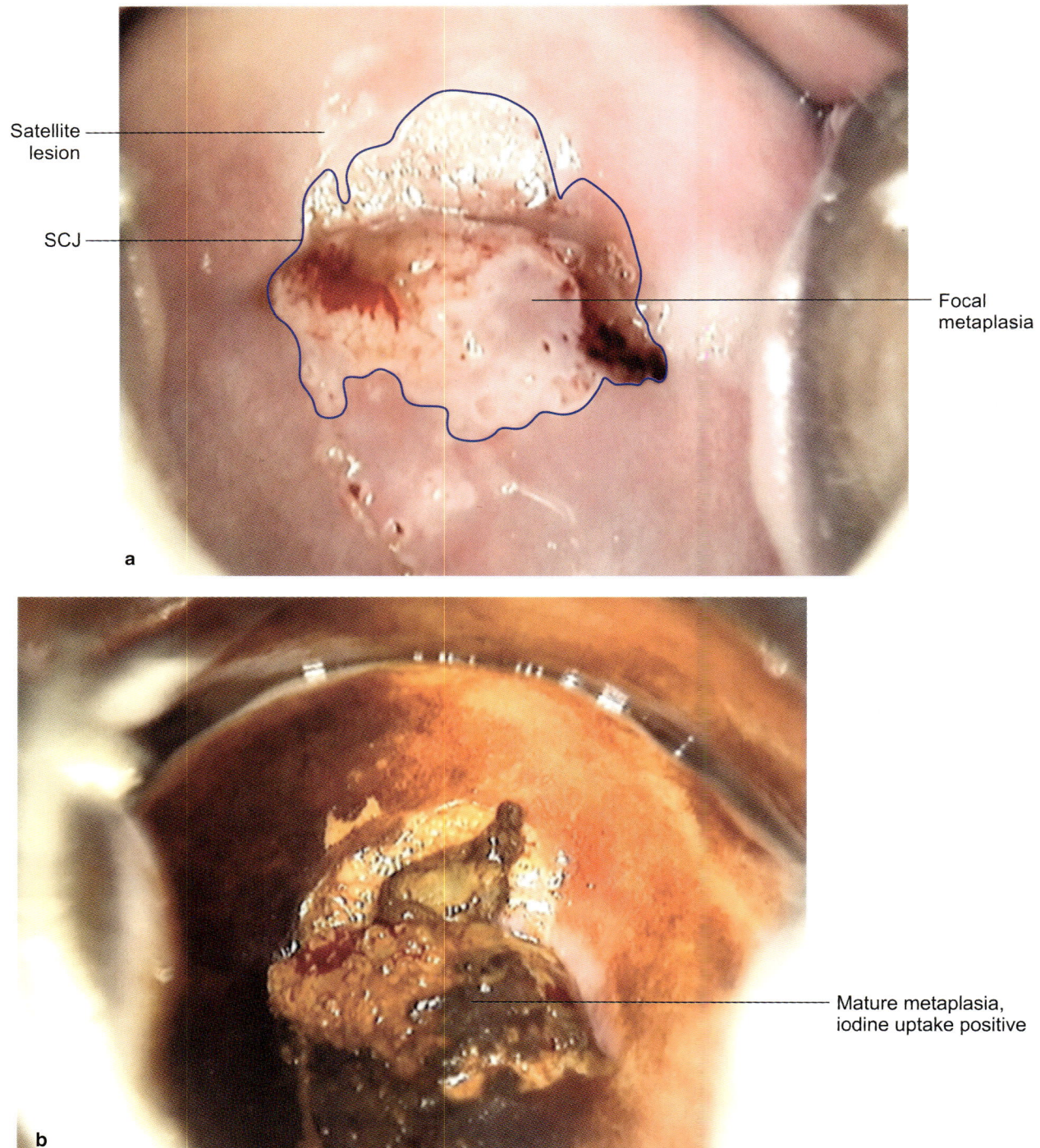

Satellite lesion

SCJ

Focal metaplasia

a

Mature metaplasia, iodine uptake positive

b

Figs 3.16a and b: Squamous metaplasia can begin focally from any area on the columnar epithelium. They appear as thin translucent acetowhite area without any geographical margin, initially immature slowly turning to mature metaplasia. Iodine uptake is negative during immature metaplasia and takes mahogany brown after mature metaplasia

Immature squamous metaplasia (Fig. 13.17). This term is used when the upper layer of superficial squamous metaplastic epithelium has yet not stratified, i.e. does not have intracellular glycogen. This stains acetowhite on 5% acetic acid application as thin translucent shiny acetowhite with feathery margins. On Lugol's iodine application, the immature metaplasia does not stain brown.

Mature squamous metaplasia: The immature metaplastic epithelium eventually matures, i.e. the upper superficial layers stratify, i.e. there is intracellular accumulation of glycogen. This epithelium appears pinkish white as compared to the original squamous epithelium which appears more pinkish. Mature metaplasia turns mahogany brown on application of Lugol's iodine.

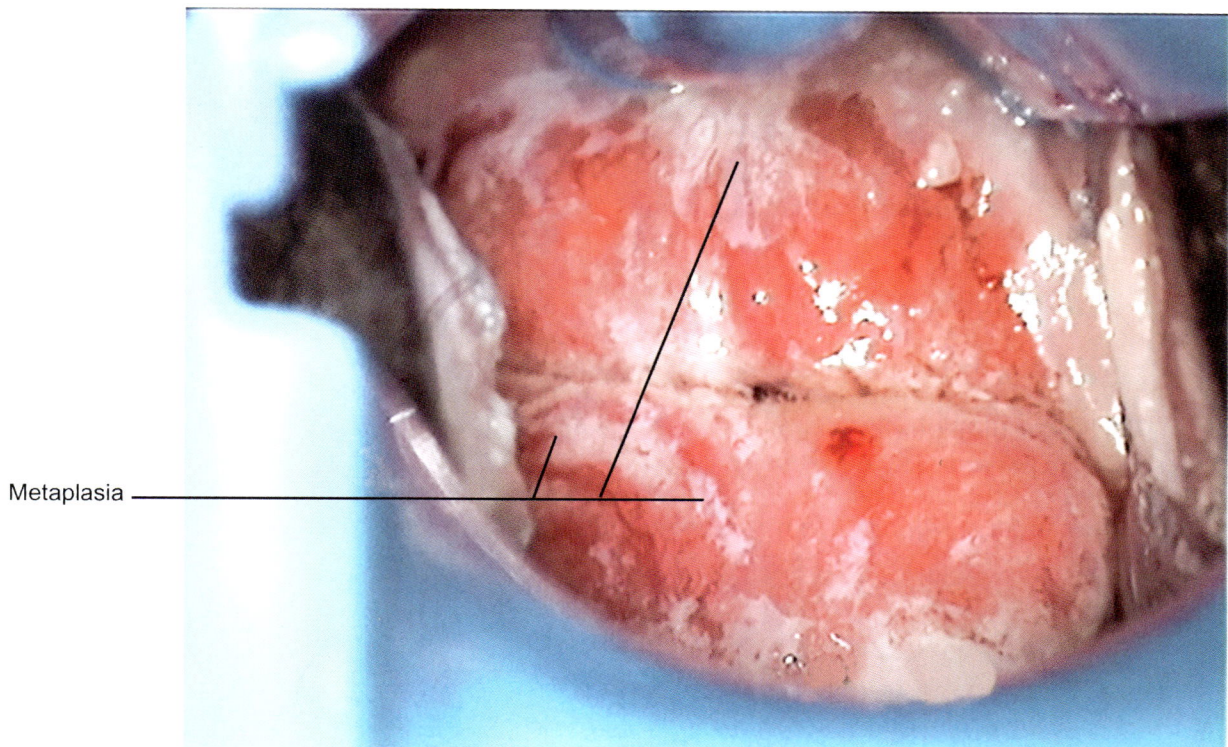

Metaplasia

Fig. 3.17: Thin transparent acetowhite with finger-like/fond-like projection pointing centripetally on the columnar epithelium

10. DYSPLASIA

Dysplasia is the pathological deviation from the normal course of metaplasia, where the columnar cells while getting converted to squamous cells become abnormal, irregular in size and shape with disproportion in the nuclear cytoplasmic ratio due to infection of the cells.

11. MOSAICS AND PUNCTATIONS

This terminology is very important in describing the lesions.

The basement membrane of the squamous epithelium is not straight but thrown into folds called stromal papillae. The stroma along with the blood vessels is invaginated within the stromal papillae. These blood vessels supply nutrition to the dividing cells. The areas between two stromal papillae are called rete pegs (Fig. 3.18). The blood vessels appear as punctations on the cross-sectional head on view. In case of normal epithelium, the blood vessels are of normal caliber which appear as small dots or fine punctations. They can be easily located.

In case of pathological dividing cells as in case of CIN lesions, the stromal blood vessels develop into high caliber blood vessels to feed the rapidly dividing cells (Fig. 3.19). In case of higher lesions as in c/o CIN 2/3, the dividing cells with bizarre nucleocytoplasmic ratio, occupy many layers, thus the stromal papillae along with the stromal blood vessels are invaginated and stretched further towards the surface, which are easily visible as larger dots, i.e. coarse punctations on head on view of cervix.

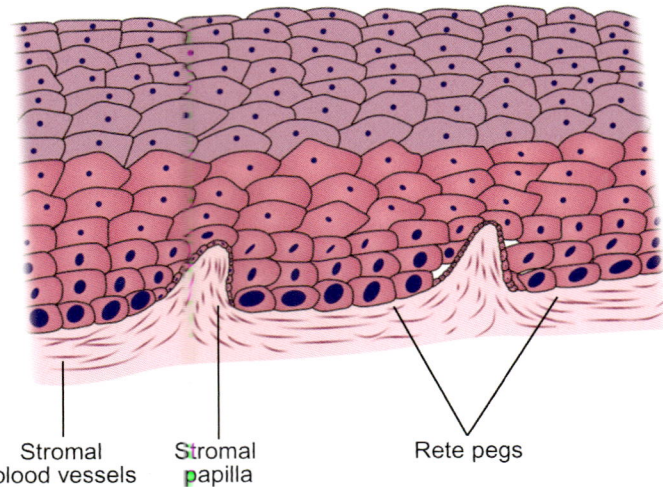

Stromal   Stromal   Rete pegs
blood vessels   papilla

Fig. 3.18: Rete pegs

The dividing cells occupy the rete pegs. On head-on view, the interconnecting stromal vessels supplying these cells form a mosaic tile pattern, polygonal in shape. Usually these mosaic patterns are fine mosaics. In case of lesions, the rete pegs get widened due to accumulation of the dividing cells within the rete pegs. Hence, the mosaic pattern now appears as large tiled mosaic pattern. Thus, we see large mosaics (Fig. 3.20) within the lesions detected on colposcopy.

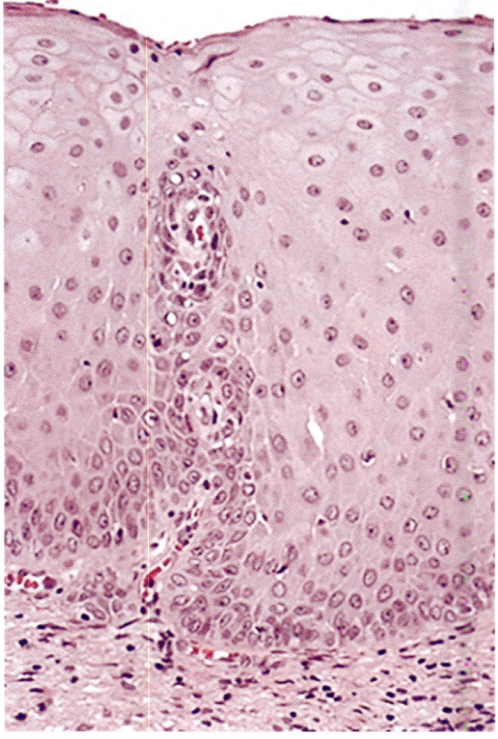

Fig. 3.19: Stretched vessels in stromal papilla

Punctation   Mosaic   Punctation

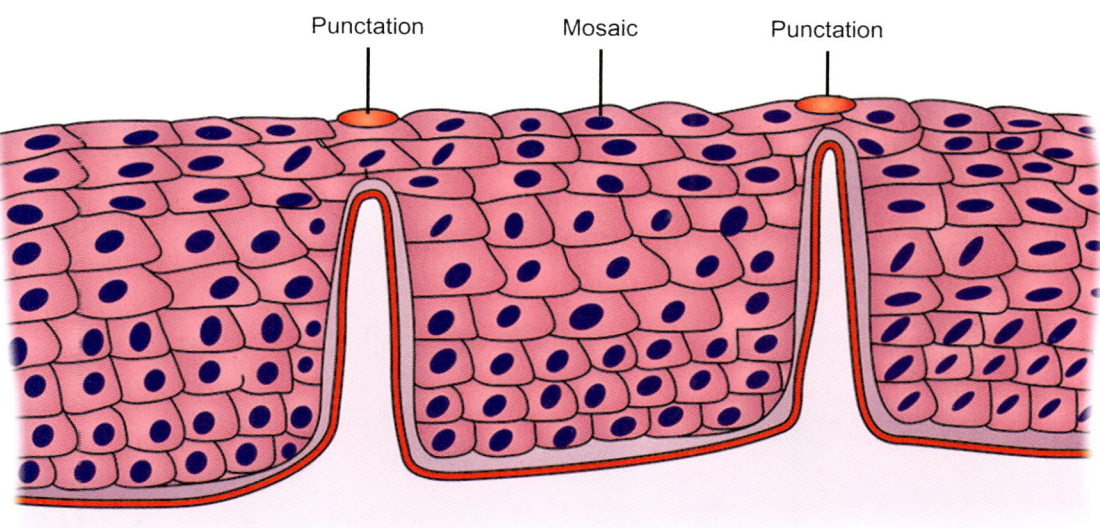

Fig. 3.20: Stretched blood vessels in the stromal papillae in CIN lesion giving rise to punctation and mosaic on colposcopic examination

Fine Mosaics and Punctations (Figs 3.21a to g)

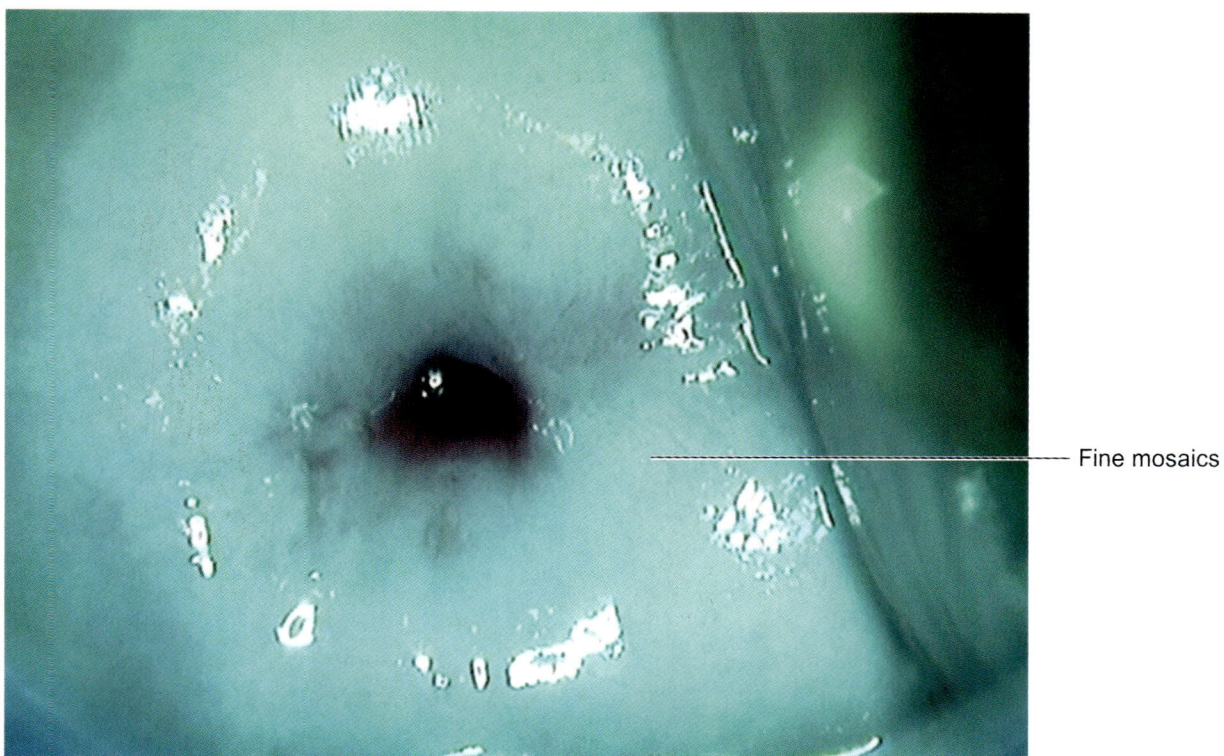

Fine mosaics

Fig. 3.21a

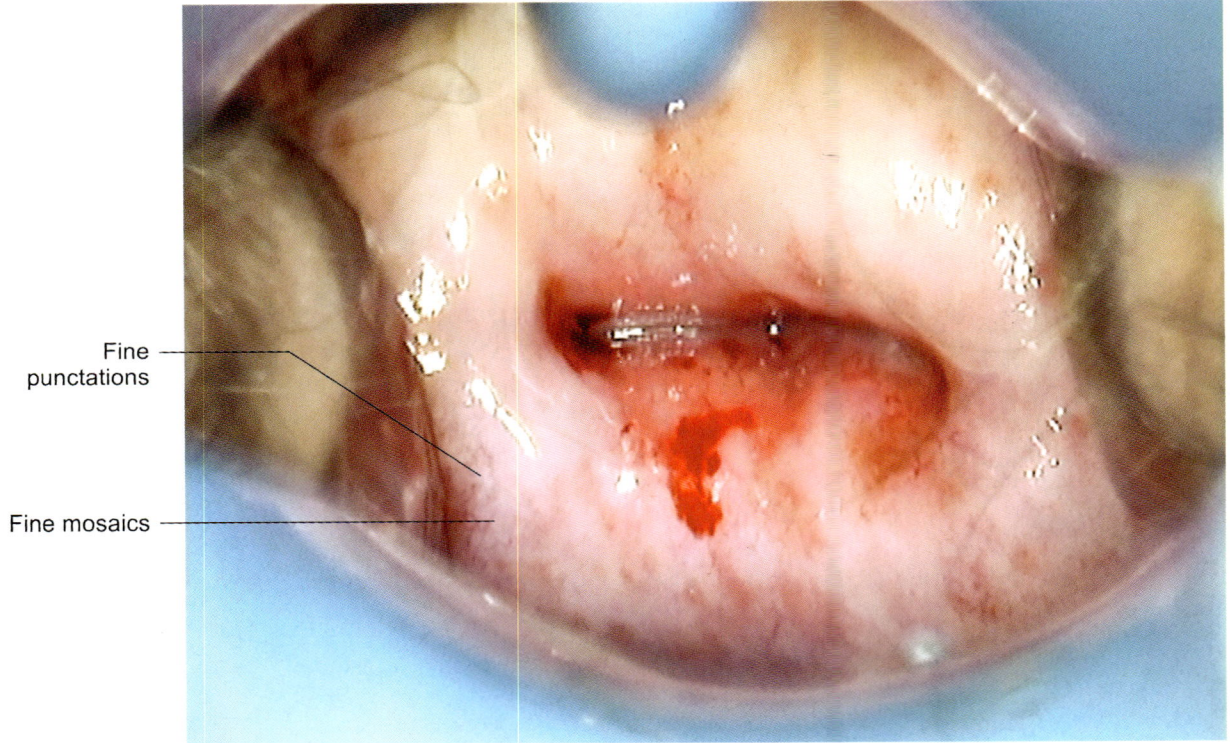

Fine punctations

Fine mosaics

Fig. 3.21b

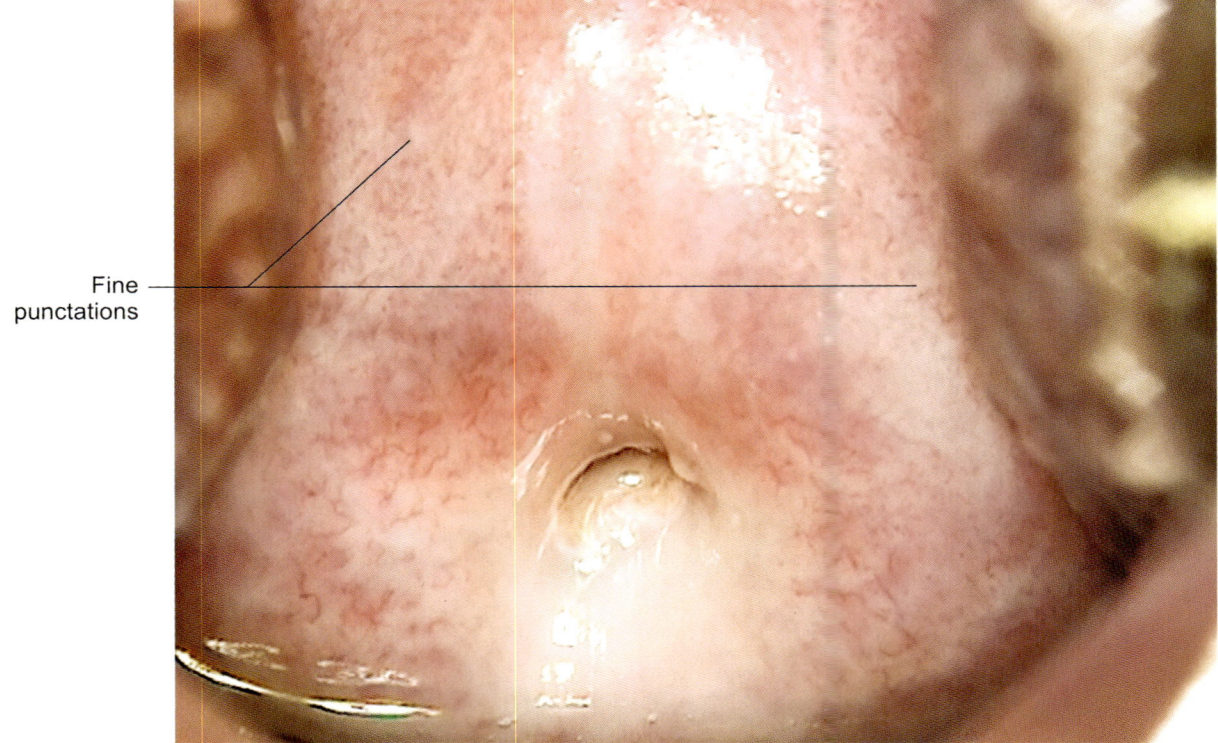

Fine punctations

Fig. 3.21c

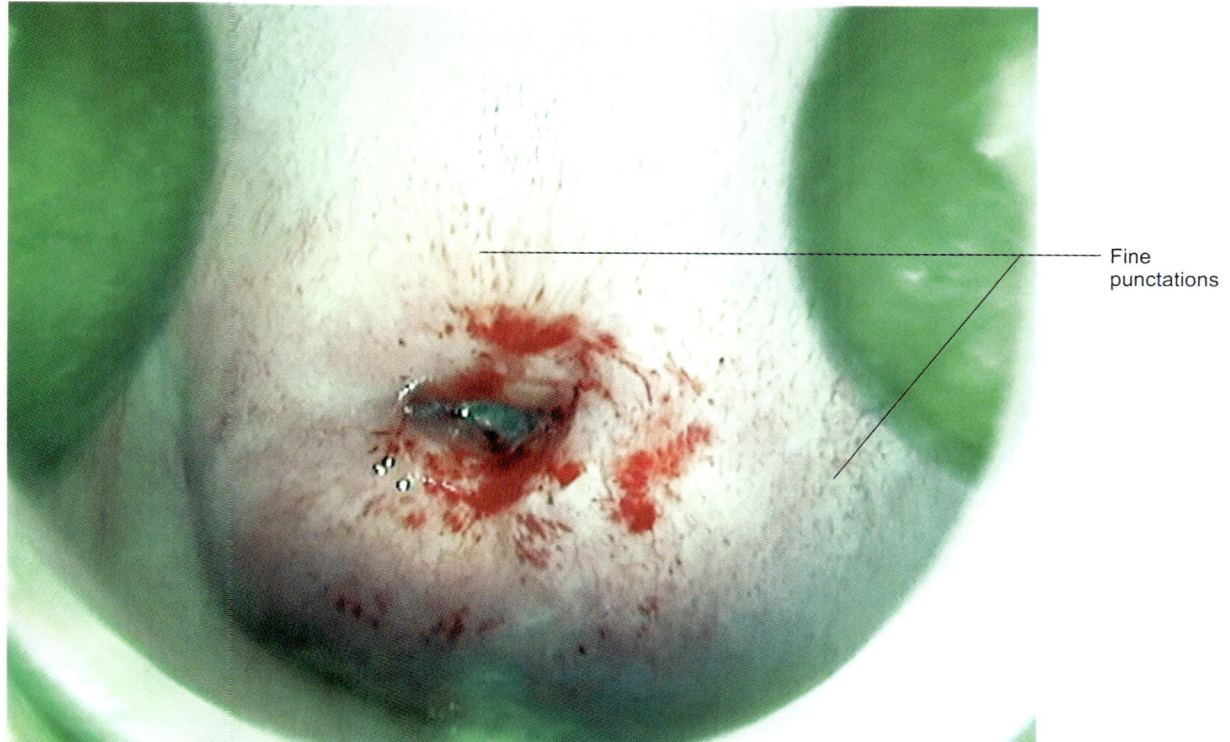

Fine
punctations

Fig. 3.21d

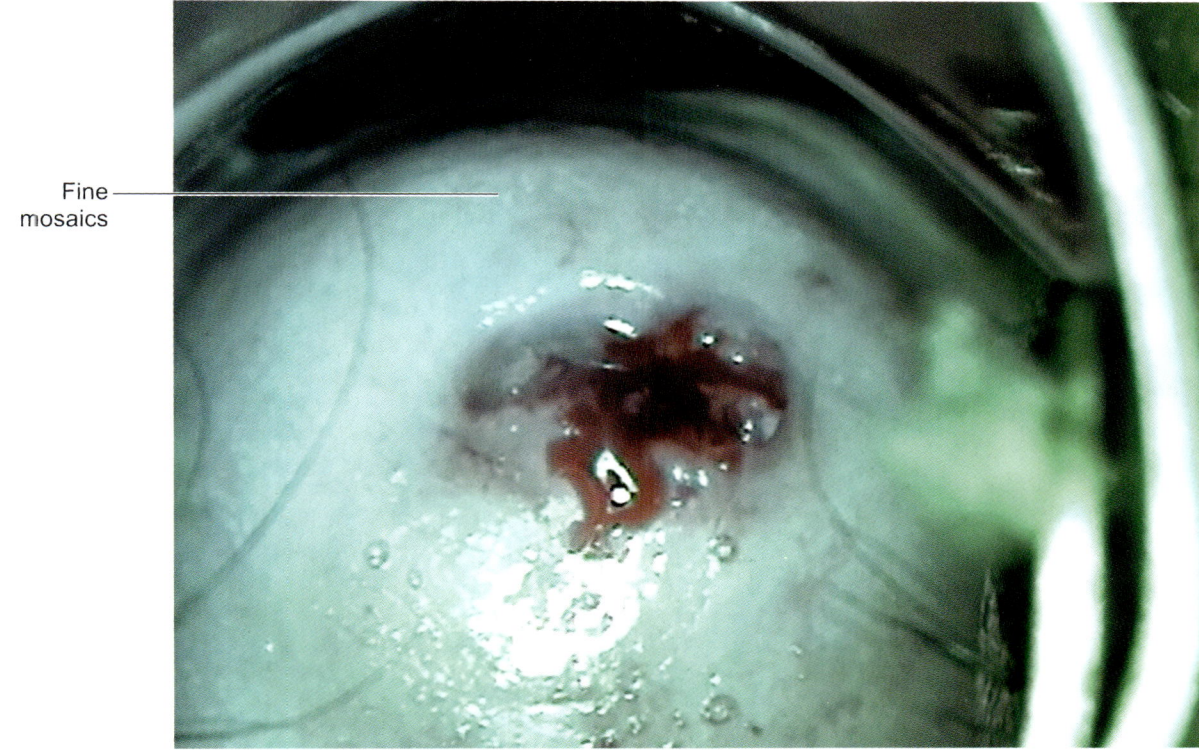

Fine
mosaics

Fig. 3.21e

Fine mosaics

Fine punctations

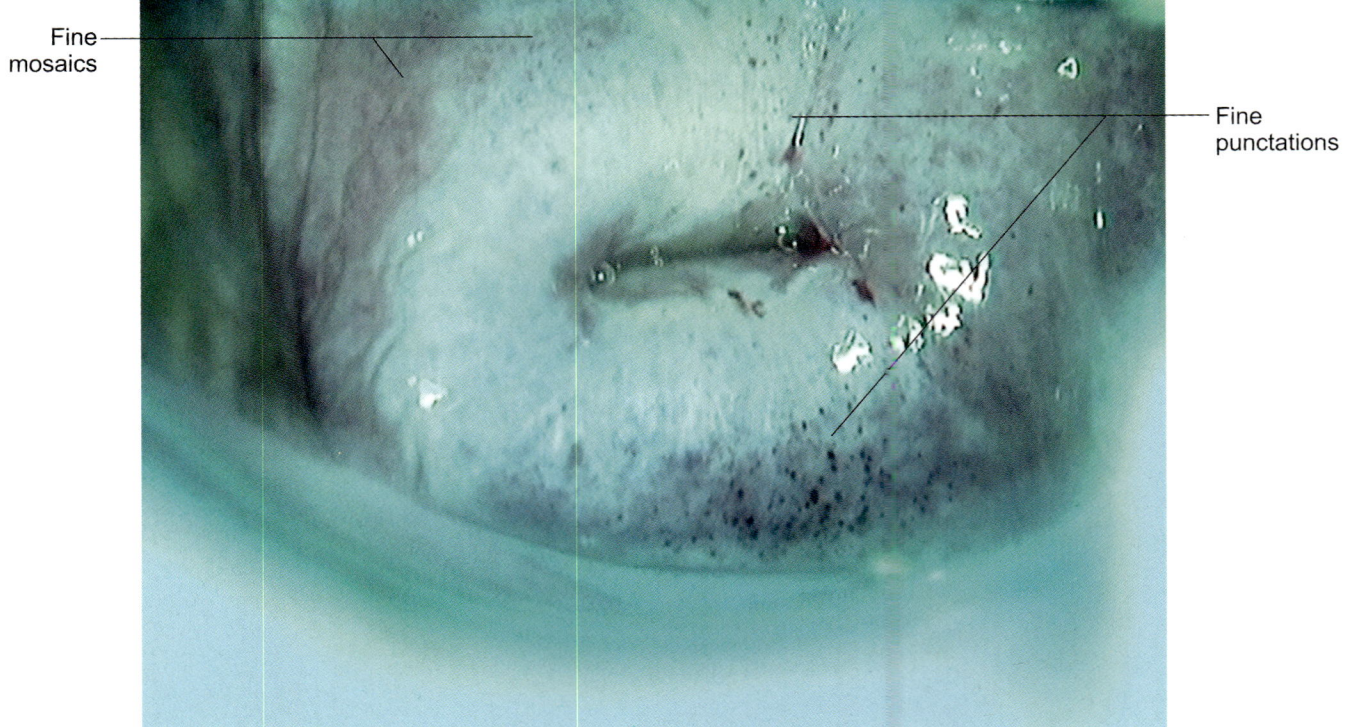

Fig. 3.21f

Fine mosaics

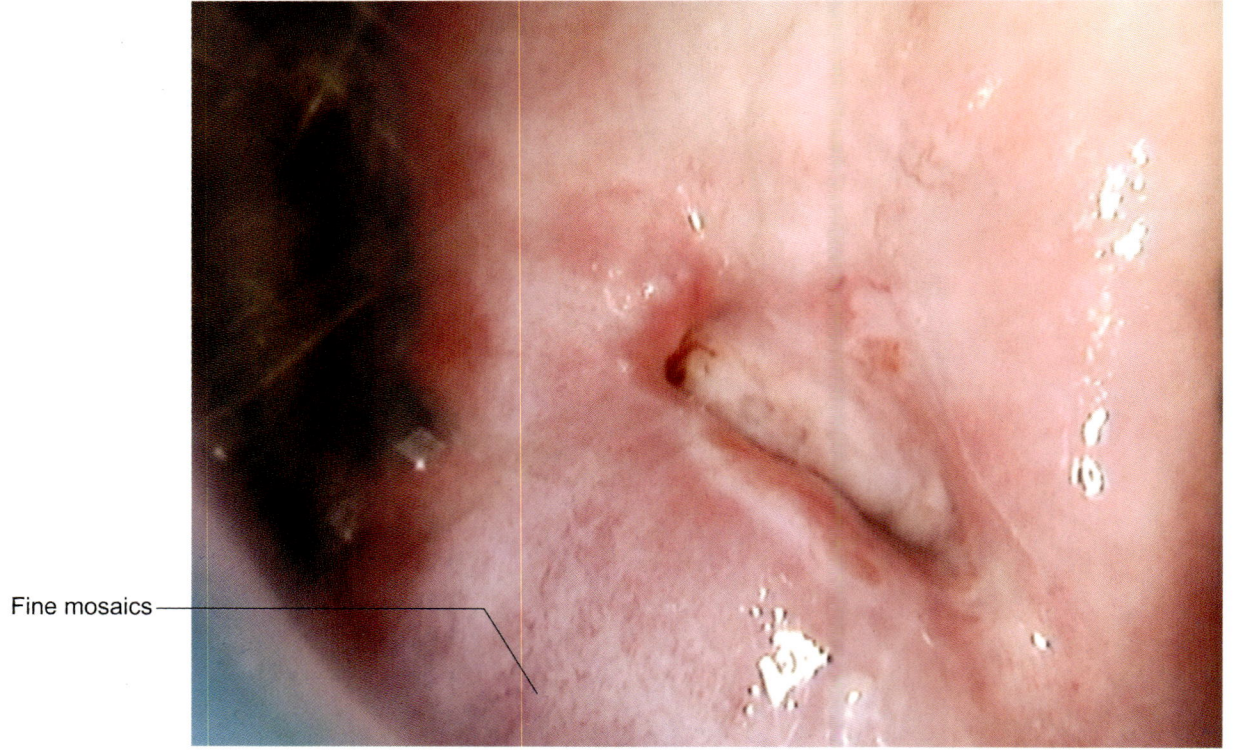

Fig. 3.21g

Coarse Mosaics and Punctations (Figs 3.22a to g)

Coarse punctations are seen on cross-sectional head-on view as large dots. They are observed due to high caliber blood vessels and neovascularization supplying the rapidly dividing neoplastic cells.

Coarse mosaics are noticed as large tiled pattern. They are due to stretching of rete pegs with the dividing cells surrounded by stromal papillae.

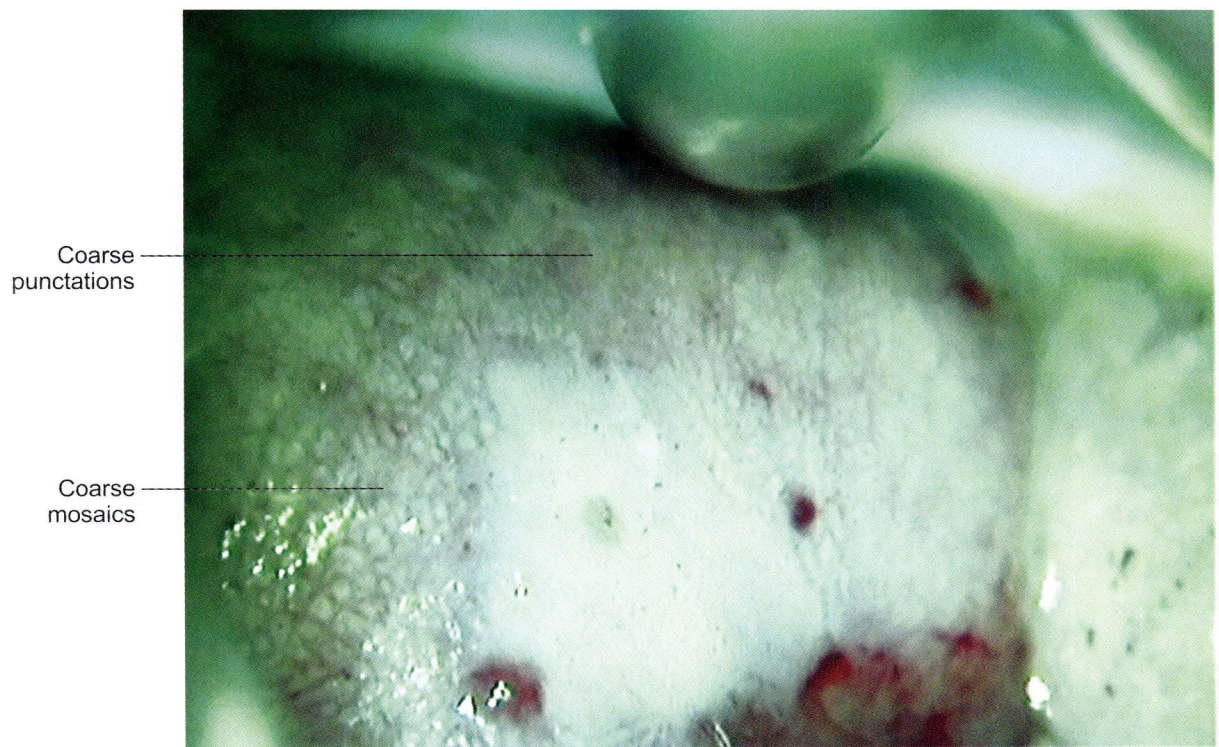

Coarse punctations

Coarse mosaics

Fig. 3.22a

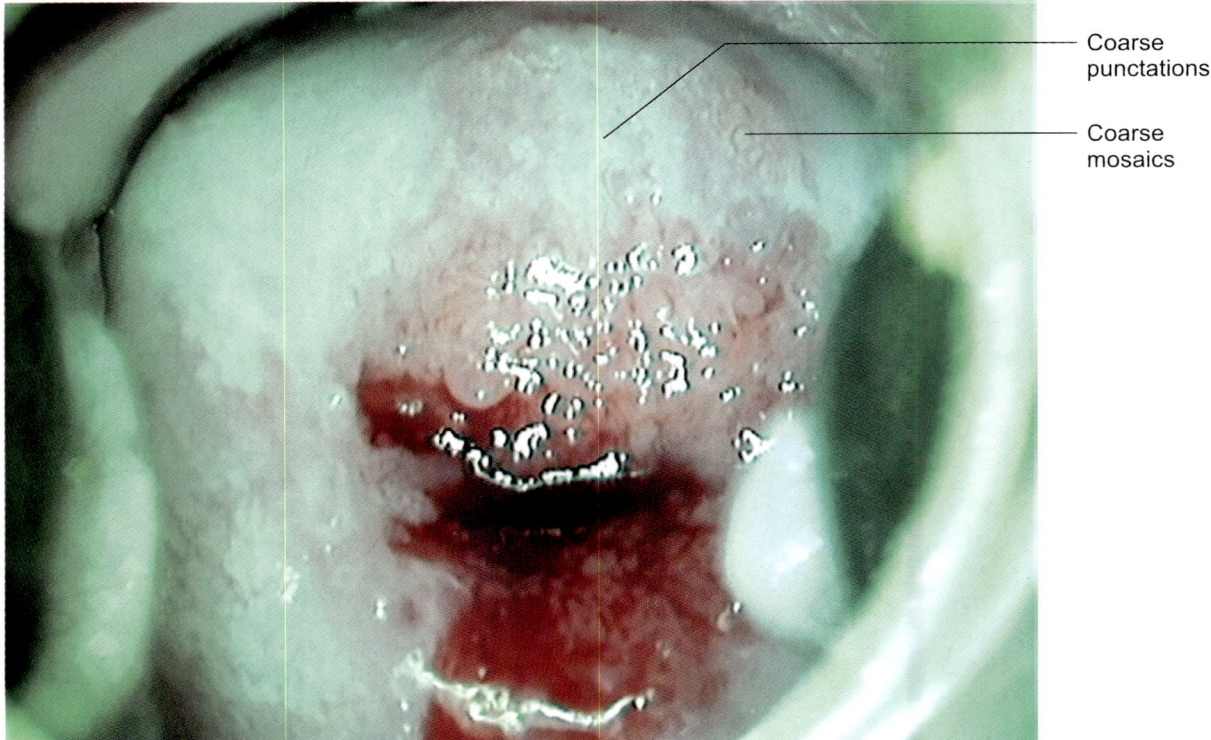

Coarse punctations

Coarse mosaics

Fig. 3.22b

Coarse mosaic

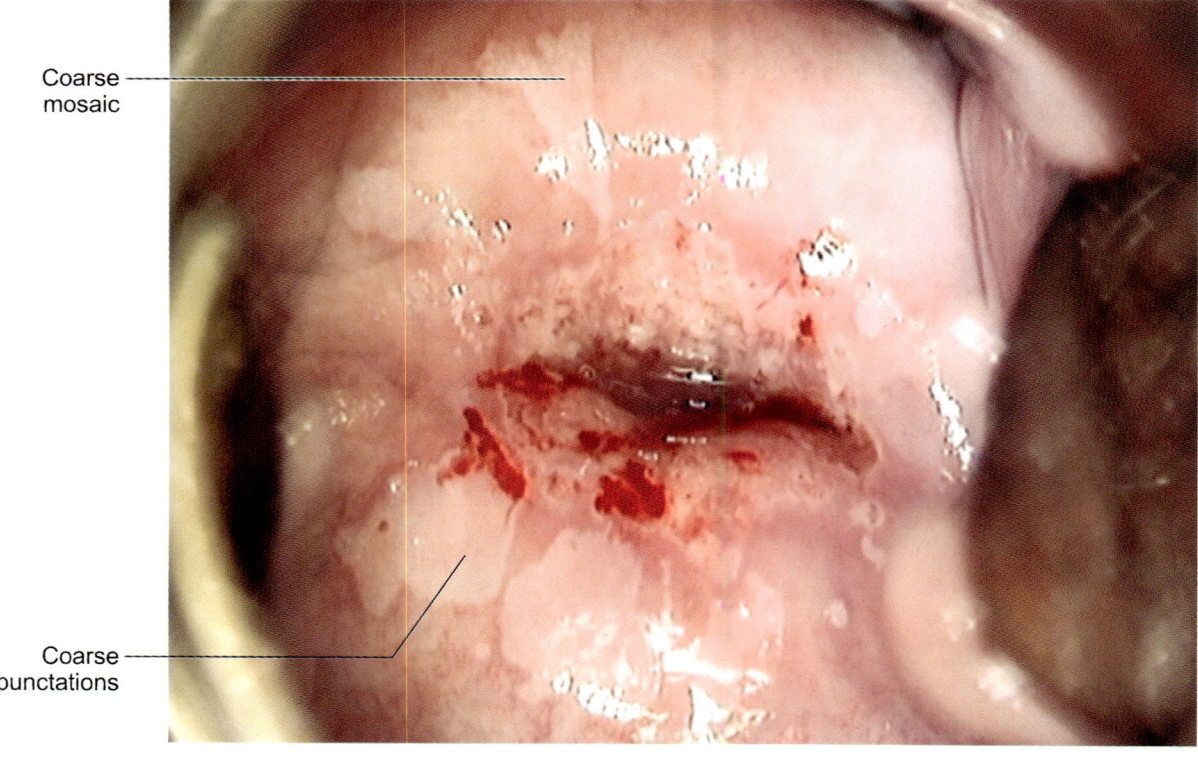

Coarse punctations

Fig. 3.22c

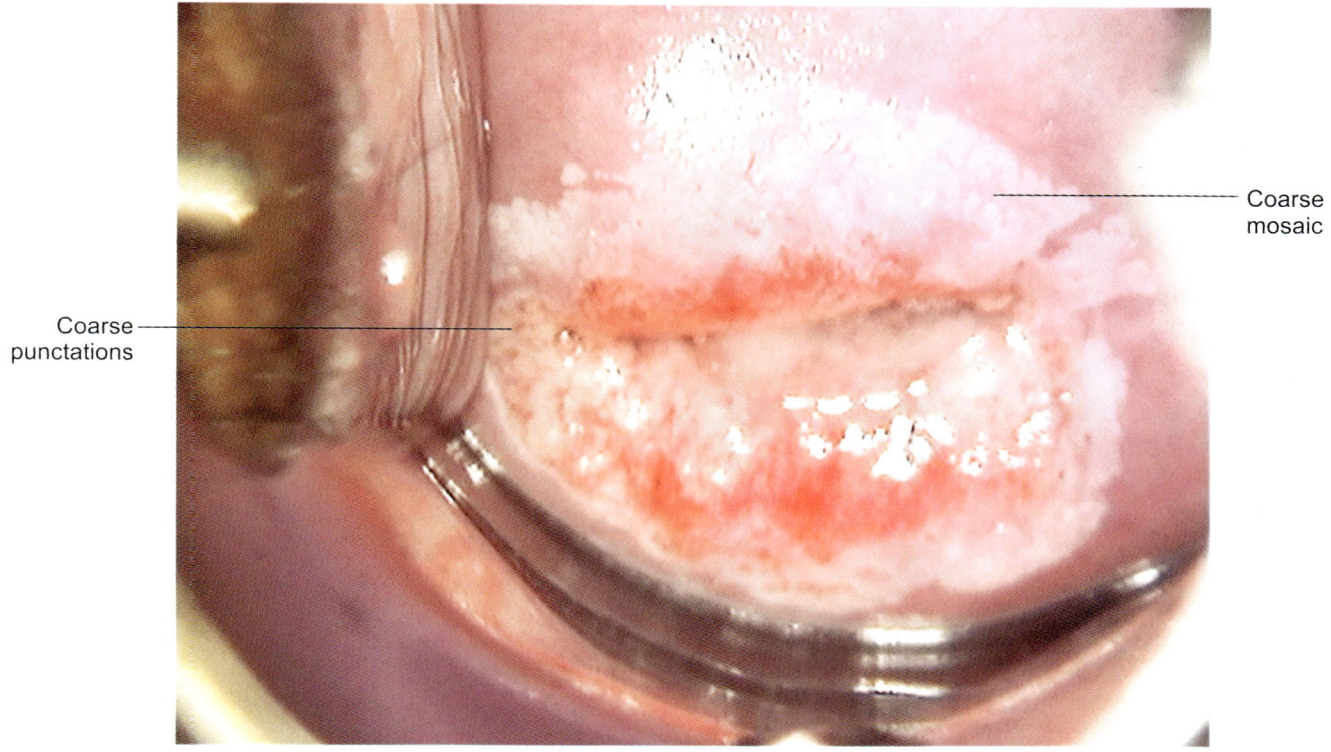

Coarse mosaic

Coarse punctations

Fig. 3.22d

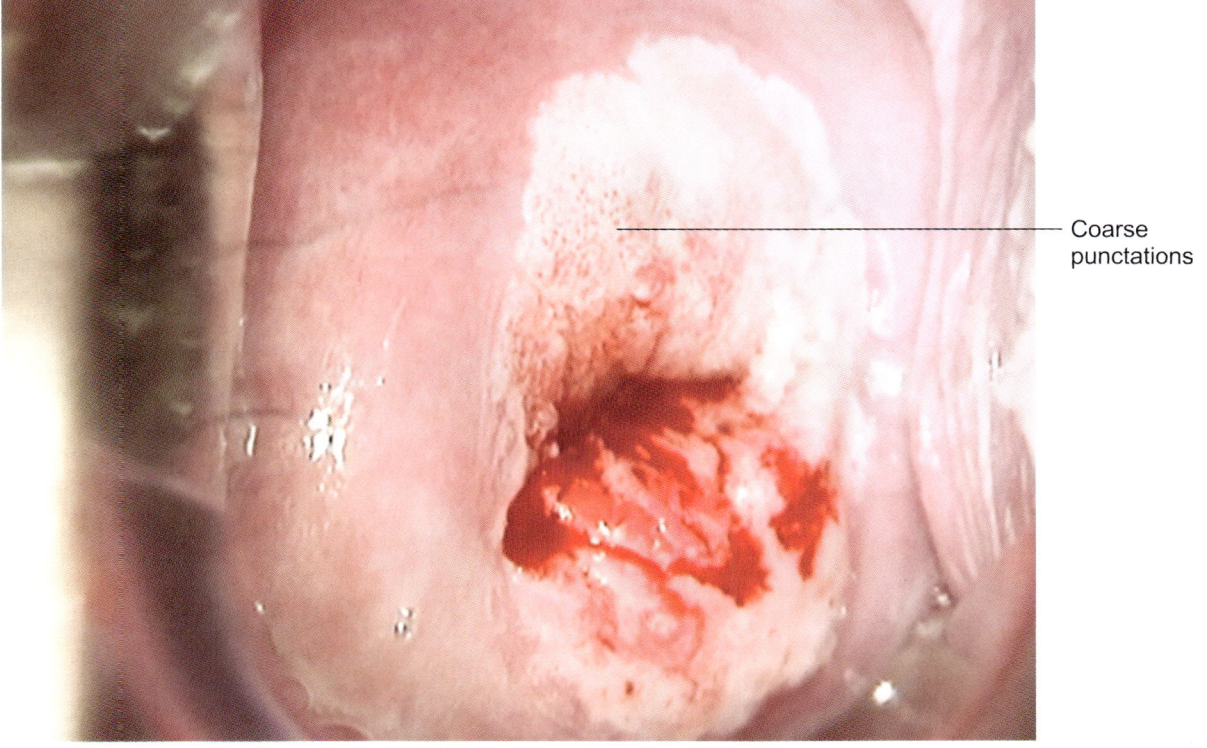

Coarse punctations

Fig. 3.22e

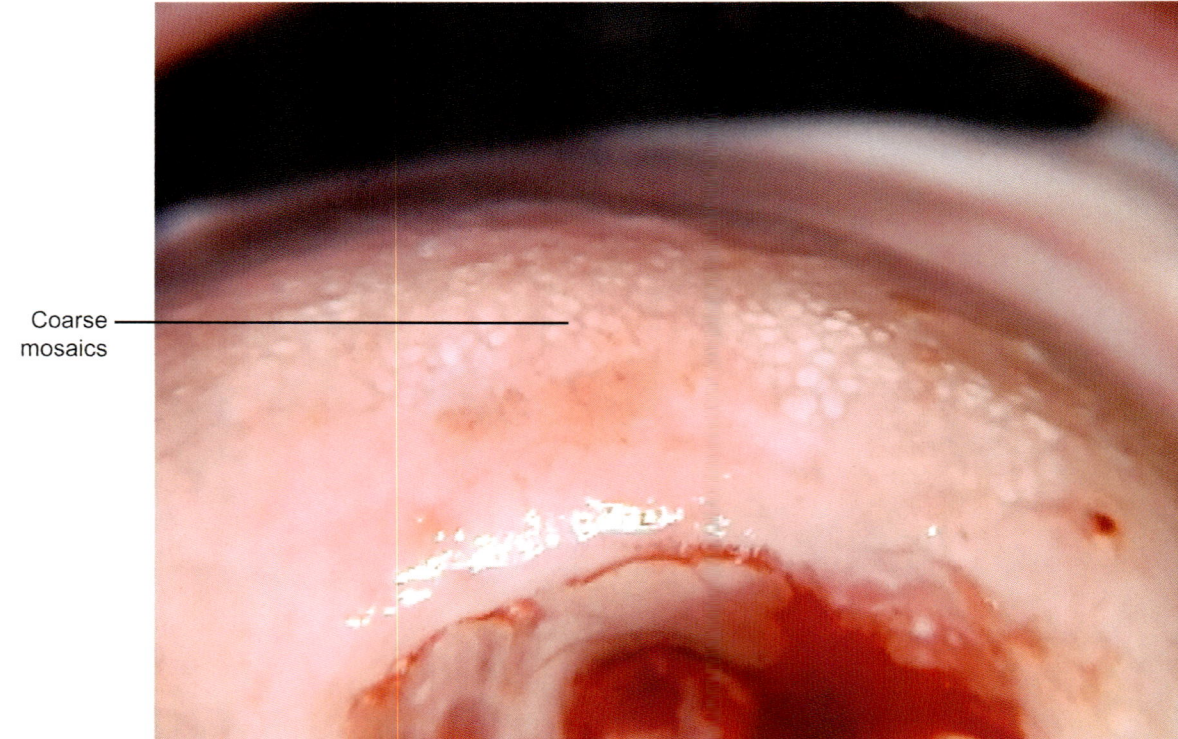

Fig. 3.22f

Fig. 3.22g

4

Cervical Intraepithelial Neoplasia (CIN)

Invasive cervical cancers are usually preceded by a long phase of clinically identifiable precancerous phase called cervical intraepithelial neoplasia (CIN) phase. CIN, as the name suggests, is a neoplasia (neo—new; plasia—cellular division) within the epithelial cells of the cervix. This precancerous phase is characterized microscopically as a spectrum of cellular abnormalities progressing from cellular atypia to CIN further progressing to cervical cancer.

Depending on the concept, that there is a continuous spectrum of disease process, whereby the normal epithelium turns into precancerous lesions and then into invasive cancerous lesions, Richart, et al in 1968 coined the term cervical intraepithelial neoplasia (CIN), to describe the progressive staging of cellular atypia confined to the epithelium.

CIN is further graded as CIN 1, 2, 3. In 1980, condylomatous atypical koilocytic changes due to HPV infection were recognized and described. Thus a newer grading system was evolved as per modified Richart classification in 1980, i.e. low grade CIN comprising of abnormalities consistent with koilocytic changes and CIN 1; and high grade CIN comprising of CIN 2, and CIN 3. In 1989, the US National Cancer Institute (NCI) workshop's report on newer methodology for pathological reporting was published. The recommendations from this workshop and the subsequently one held in 1991 gave rise to The Bethesda System (TBS). This simplified the reporting system even further by creating a two-tier classification system, viz. squamous intraepithelial lesions (SIL) of low grade (LSIL) and high grade (HSIL). LSIL included condylomatous changes and CIN 1. HSIL included CIN 2 and CIN 3.

LOW GRADE LESIONS (LSIL)

Low grade lesions appear as thin opaque acetowhite areas with clear cut geographical pattern arising from SCJ, directing centrifugally within the transformation zone. The lesions appear as thin milky white neither transparent nor opaque with feathery finger-like projections arising from SCJ within the TZ . They appear late and fades away fast within minutes. They show fine punctations and fine mosaic. On application of Lugol's iodine, low grade lesions do not take up iodine or partially take up iodine giving it a variegated appearance.

Condylomas: Condylomas are due to low grade HPV infections. Flat condylomas (Fig. 4.1) arise anywhere within or outside transformation zone away from SCJ. They appear as satellite lesions.

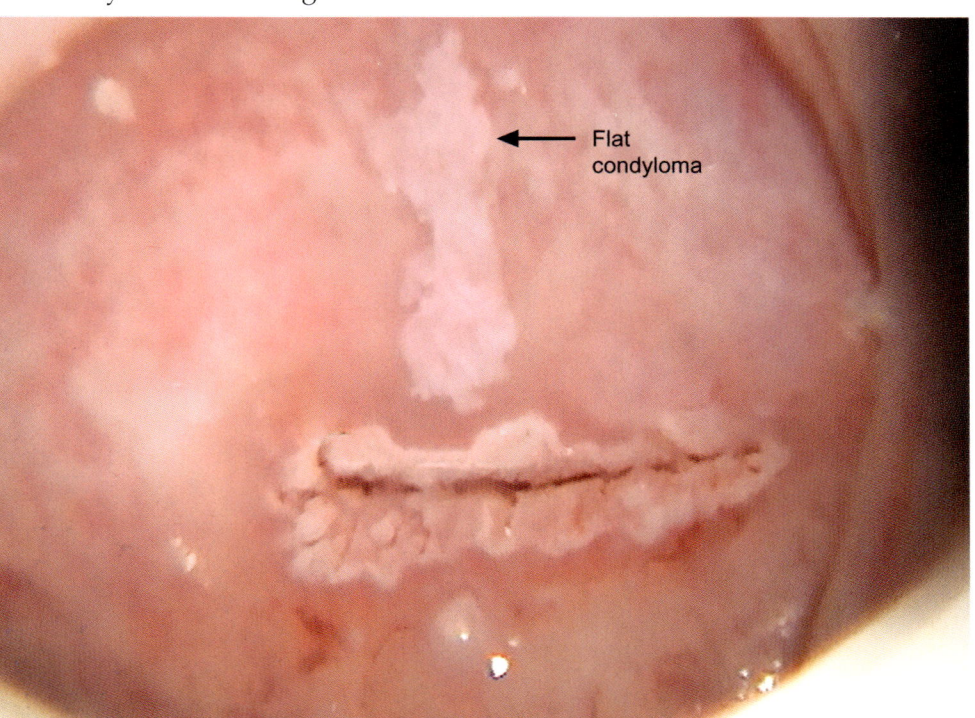

Flat condyloma

Fig. 4.1: Flat condyloma

Condylomatous condylomas or exophytic condylomata accuminata turn acetowhite immediately on application of 3–5% acetic acid and they may be found inside or beyond the TZ (Figs 4.2a and b).

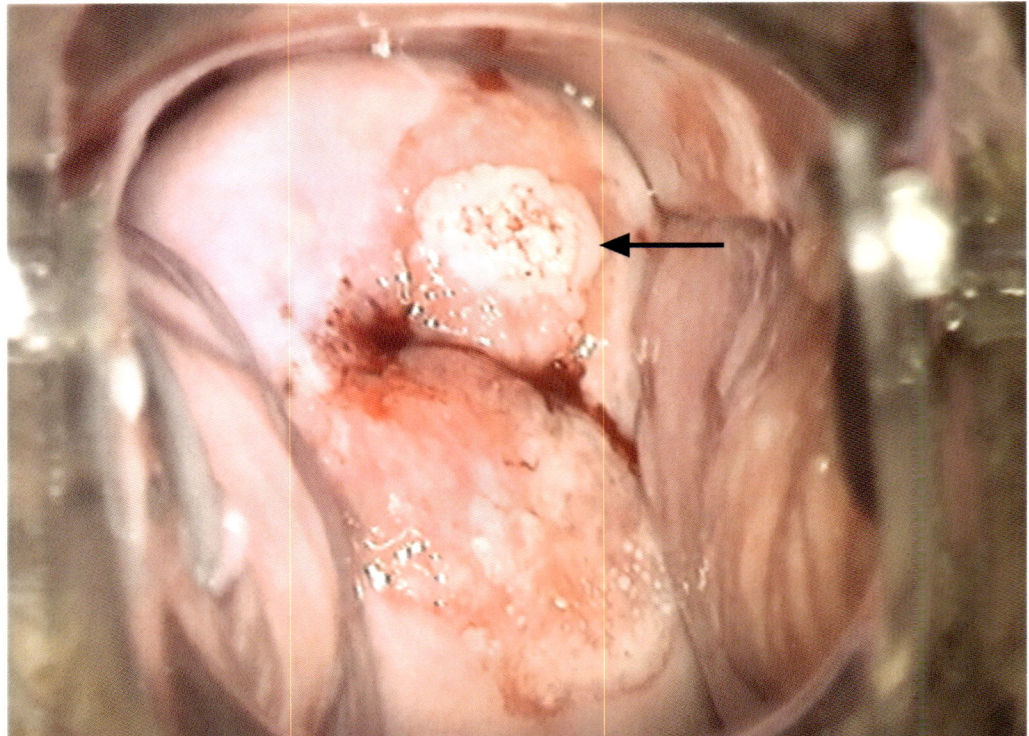

Fig. 4.2a: Exophytic condyloma

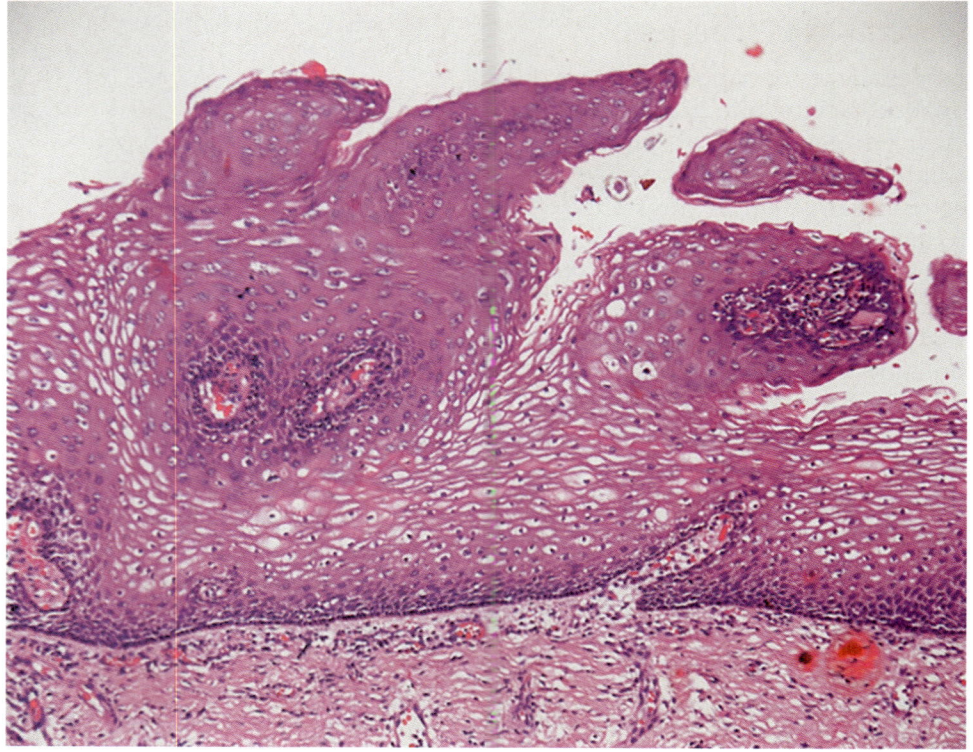

Fig. 4.2b: Histology of condyloma

Low-Grade Squamous Intraepithelial Lesion (LSIL)—CIN 1 (Figs 4.3a, b and 4.4a, b)

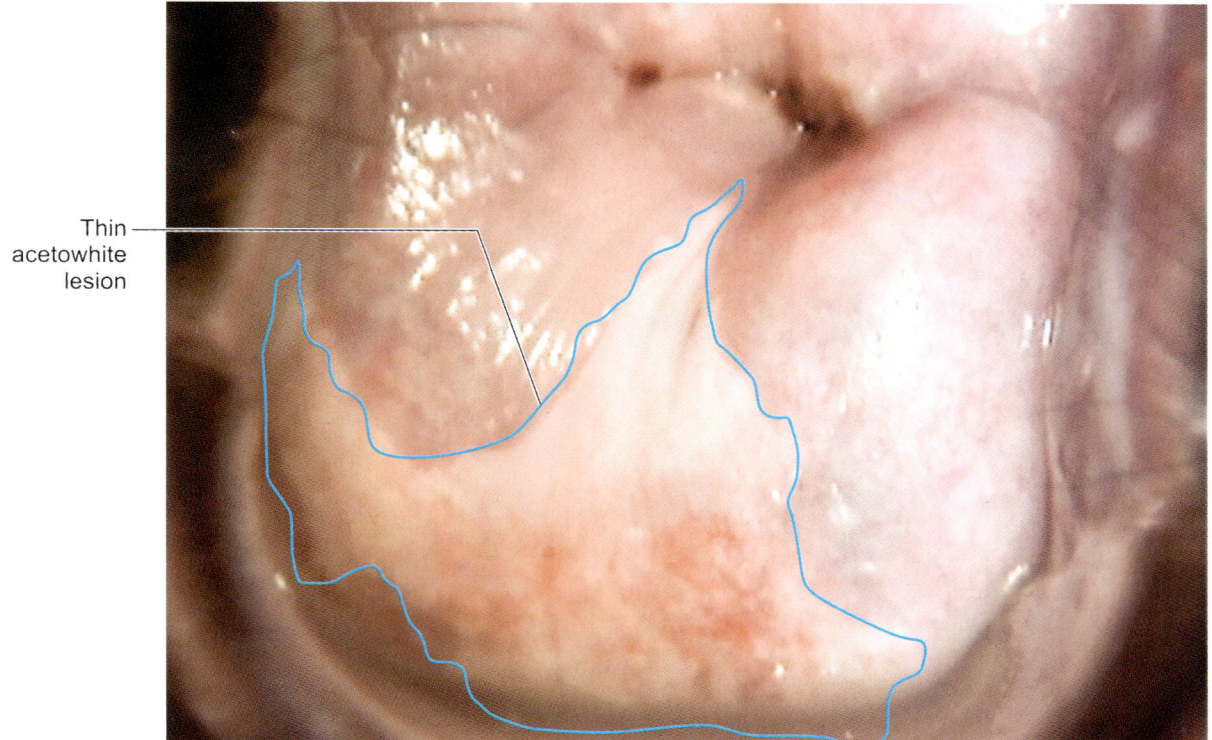

Thin acetowhite lesion

Fig. 4.3a

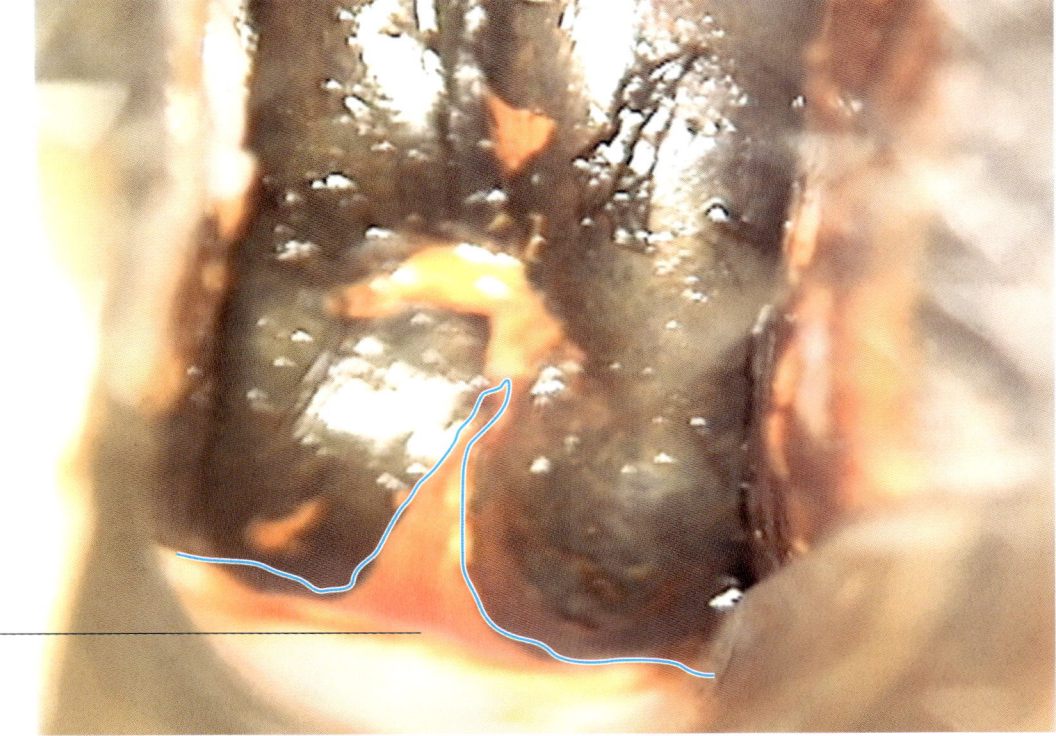

Lugol's iodine uptake negative with variegated uptake

Fig. 4.3b

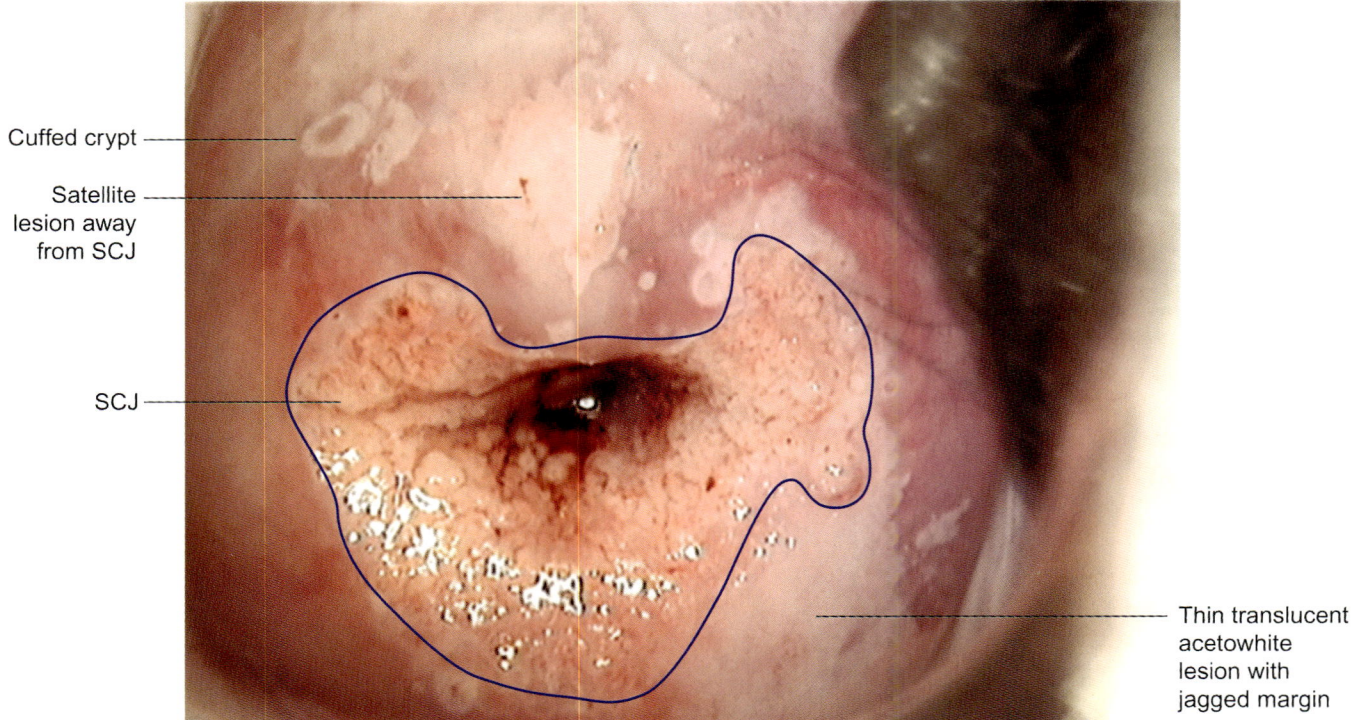

Cuffed crypt

Satellite lesion away from SCJ

SCJ

Thin translucent acetowhite lesion with jagged margin

Fig. 4.4a

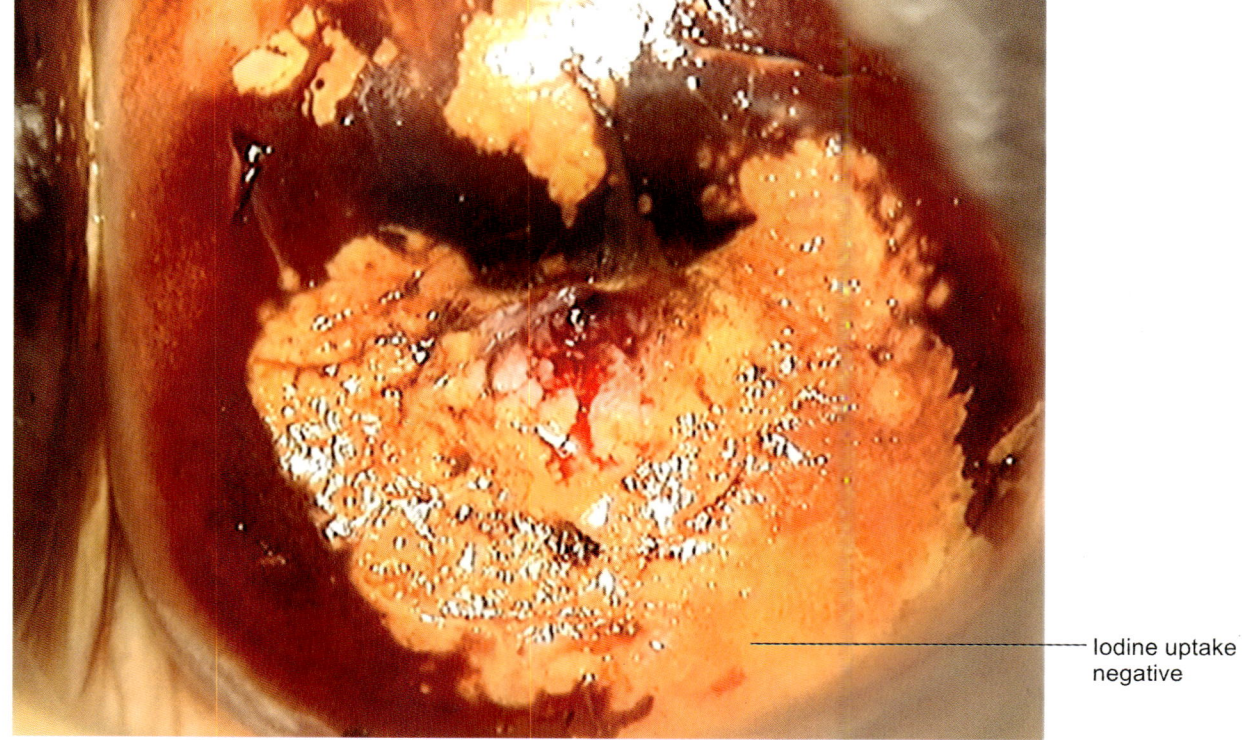

Iodine uptake negative

Fig. 4.4b

HIGH GRADE LESIONS (HSIL)

High grade lesions show thick, dense, opaque acetowhiteness arising from SCJ with well-demarcated, raised, rolled out margin, irregular undulating surface, and oyster egg white to chalky white, appearing rapidly after the application of acetic acid and persisting for long. The lesions show coarse punctations and coarse mosaic. In TZ 2/3, these lesions may extend into the endocervical canal (Fig. 4.5).

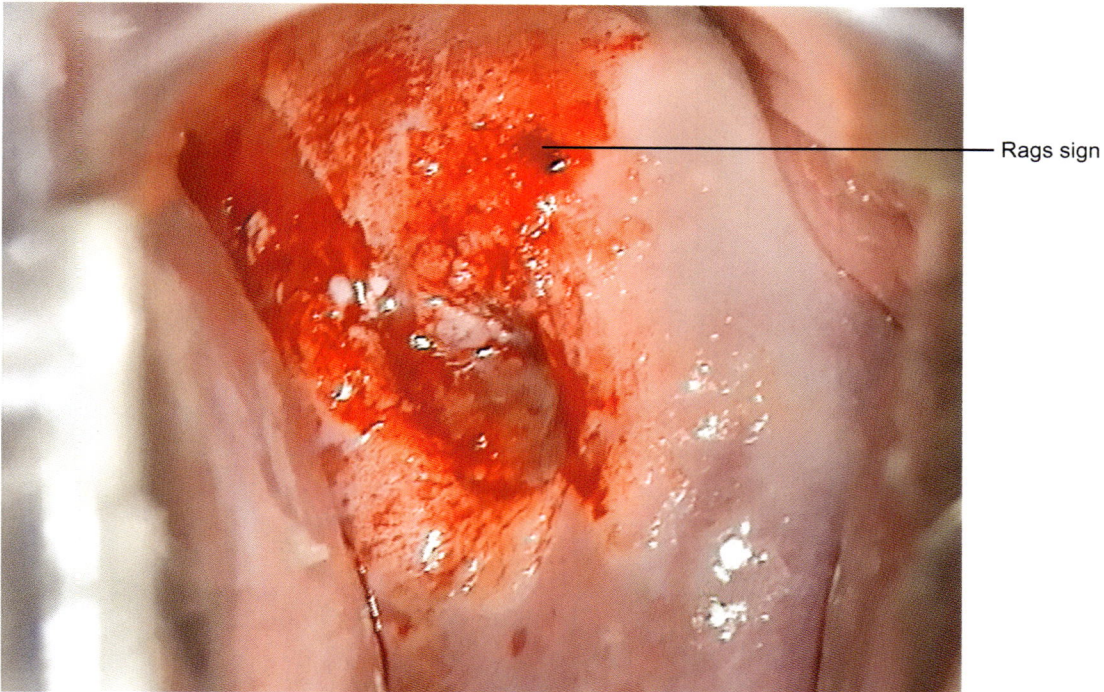

— Rags sign

Fig. 4.5: High grade lesion

HSIL lesions may peel off giving "Rags" appearance. Sometimes there are lesions within the lesions. The sharp demarcation between the thin and dense acetowhite areas that exists within the same lesion is known as "inner border sign" (Fig. 4.6).

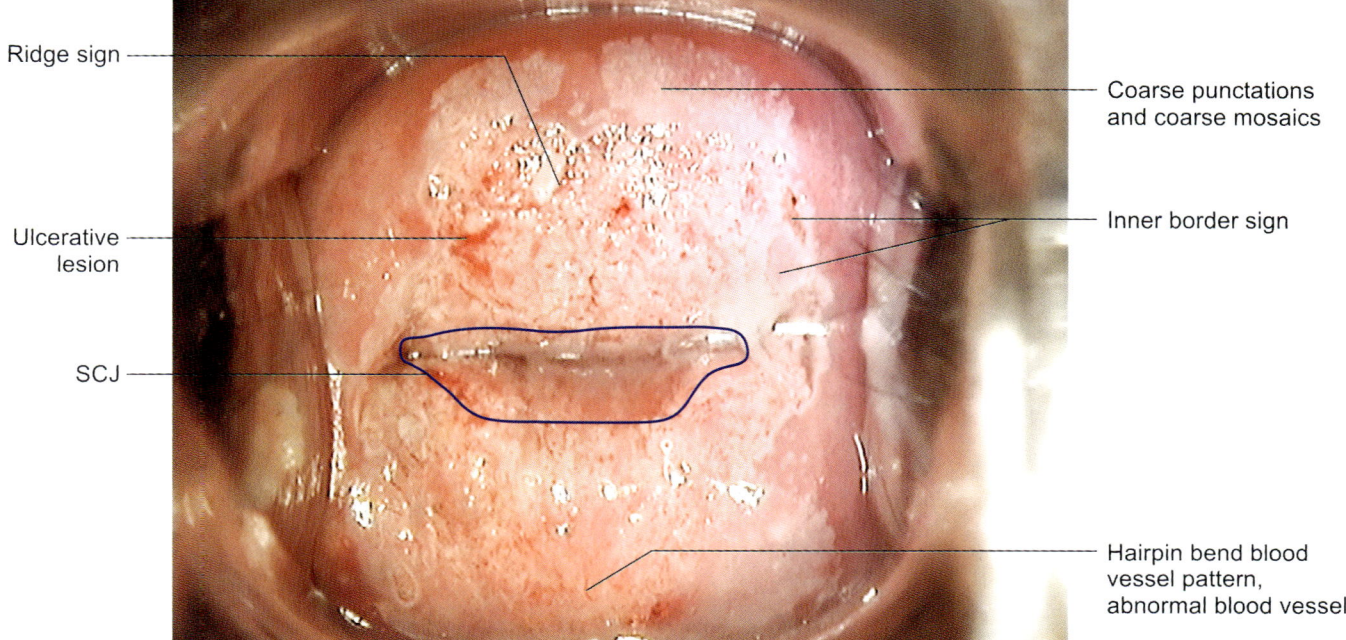

Ridge sign

Ulcerative lesion

SCJ

Coarse punctations and coarse mosaics

Inner border sign

Hairpin bend blood vessel pattern, abnormal blood vessel

Fig. 4.6: High grade lesion—CIN 3 with focal area of microinvasive lesions on LLETZ excision biopsy

CERVICAL INTRAEPITHELIAL NEOPLASIA GRADE 3 LESION (Figs 4.7a to c)

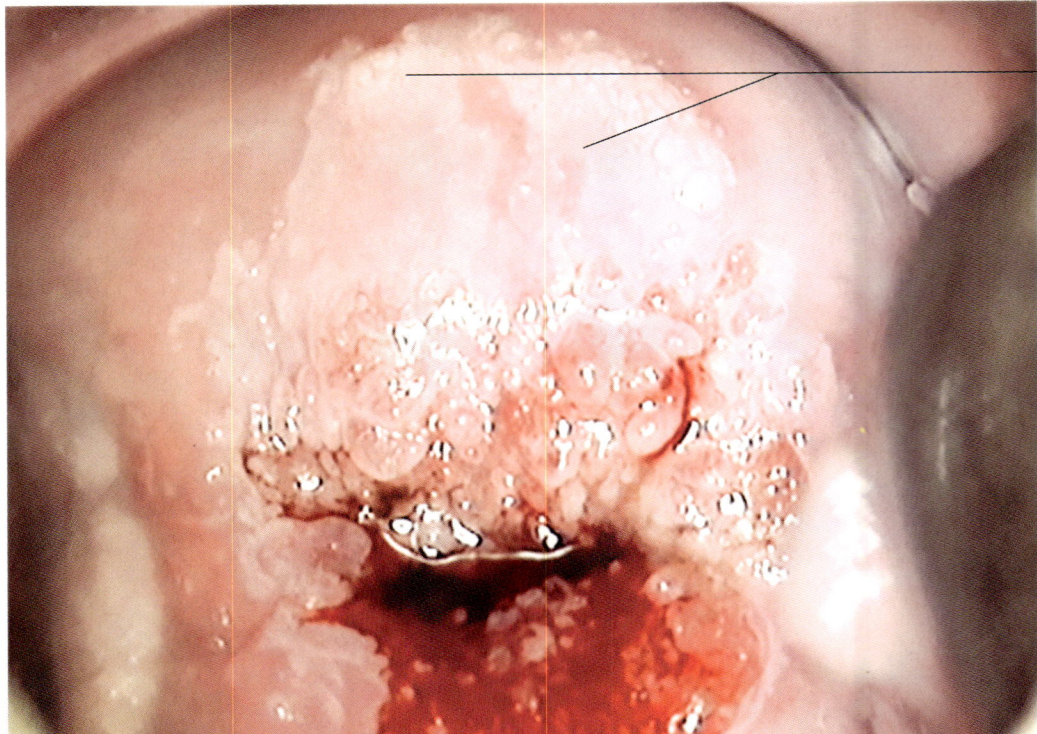

Dull opaque
acetowhite lesion
with sharp margin,
coarse mosaics

Fig. 4.7a

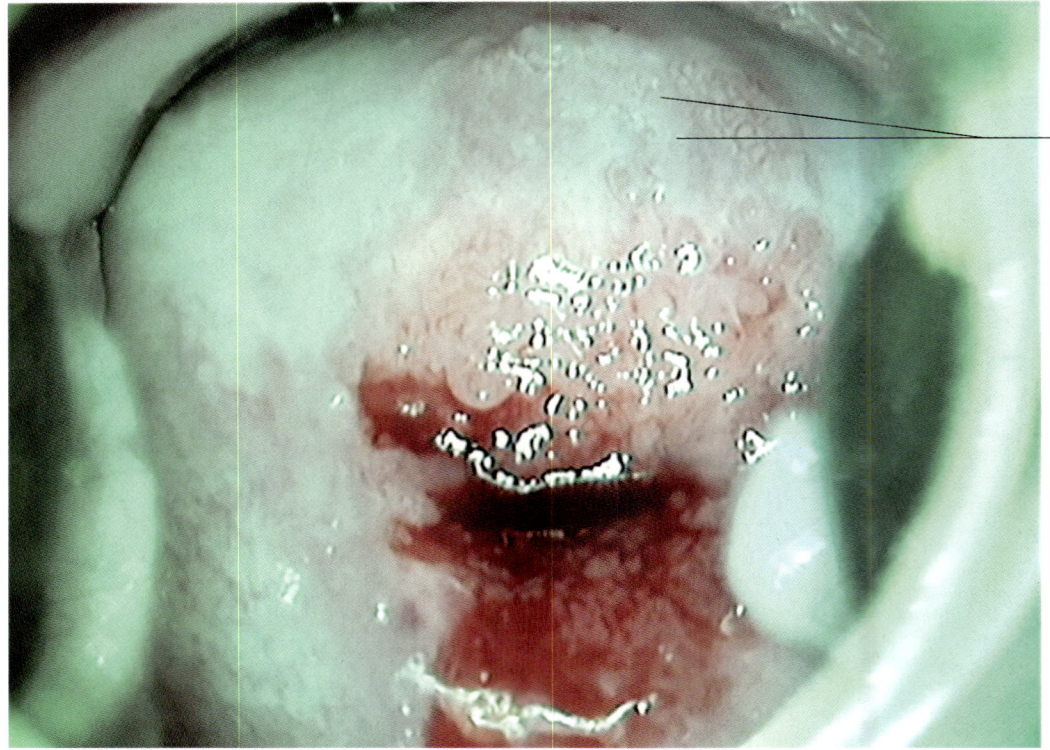

Abnormal blood
vessels, corkscrew
pattern

Fig. 4.7b

The rapidly dividing cells in high grade lesion do not accumulate glycogen in the cytoplasm thus turning yellow on iodine application.

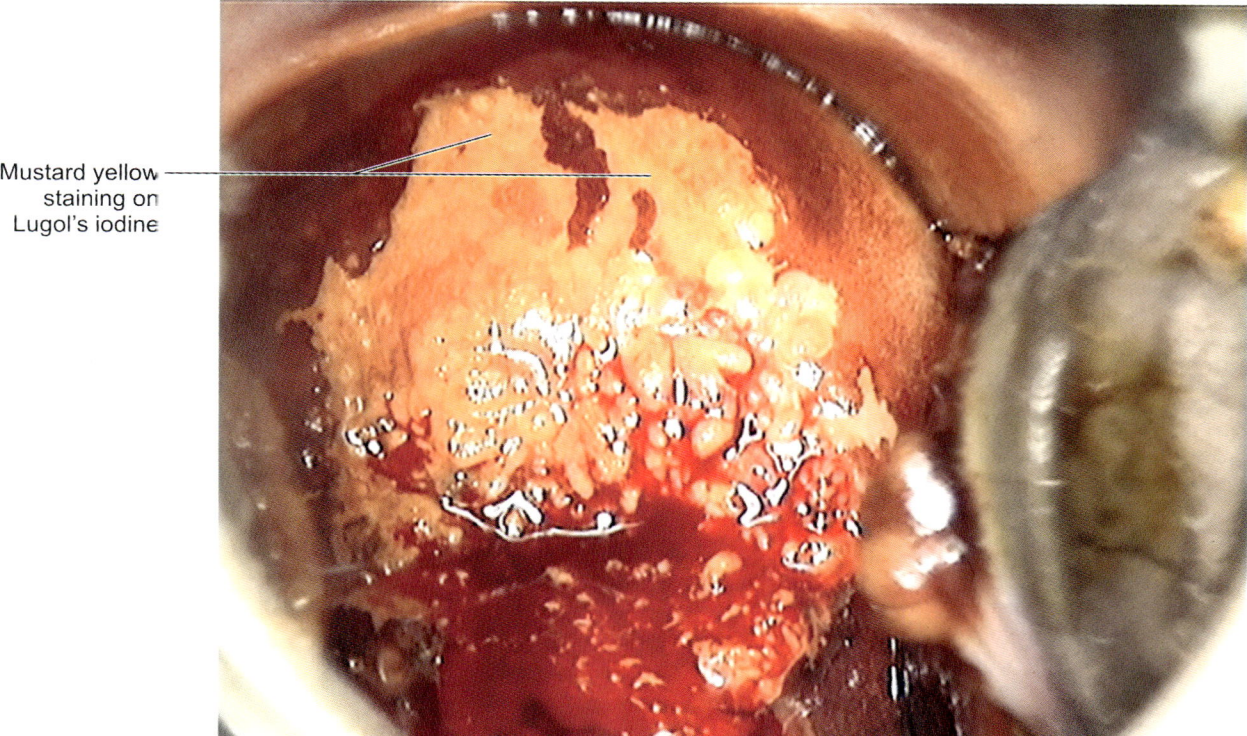

Mustard yellow staining on Lugol's iodine

Fig. 4.7c

MIXED LESION

Many a times, mixed lesions are noted in the cervix (Figs 4.8 a,b and 4.9 a,b)

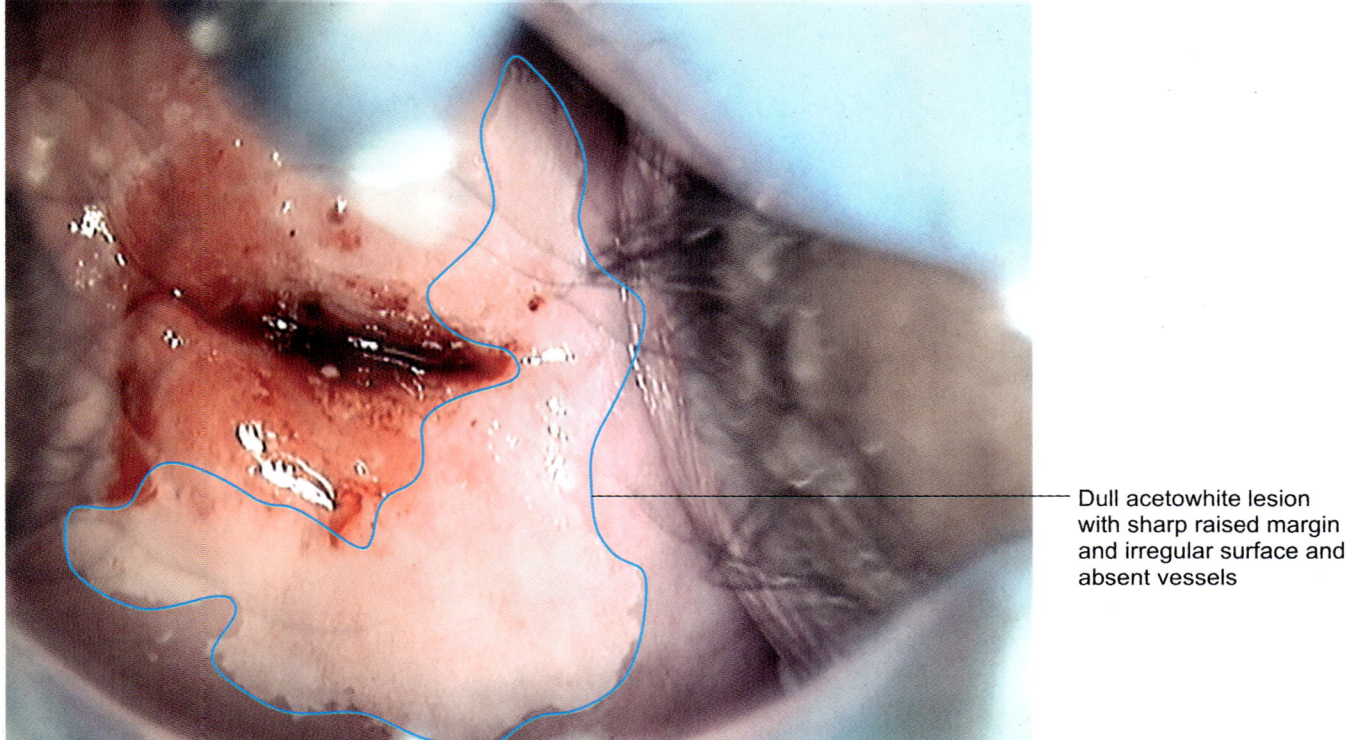

Dull acetowhite lesion with sharp raised margin and irregular surface and absent vessels

Fig. 4.8a: High grade CIN 2 lesions at the lower lip and CIN 3 at the upper lip

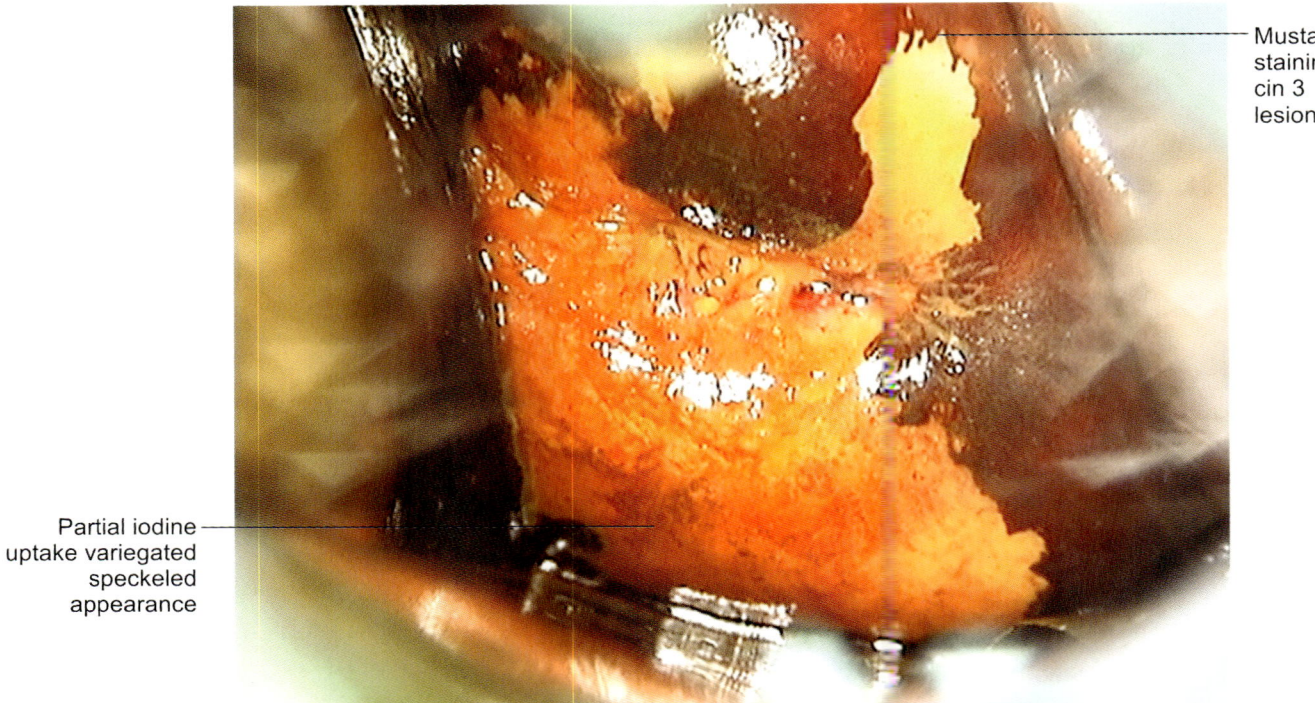

Mustard staining cin 3 lesion

Partial iodine uptake variegated speckeled appearance

Fig. 4.8b: High grade lesions with CIN 3 at the upper lip and CIN 2 at the lower lip

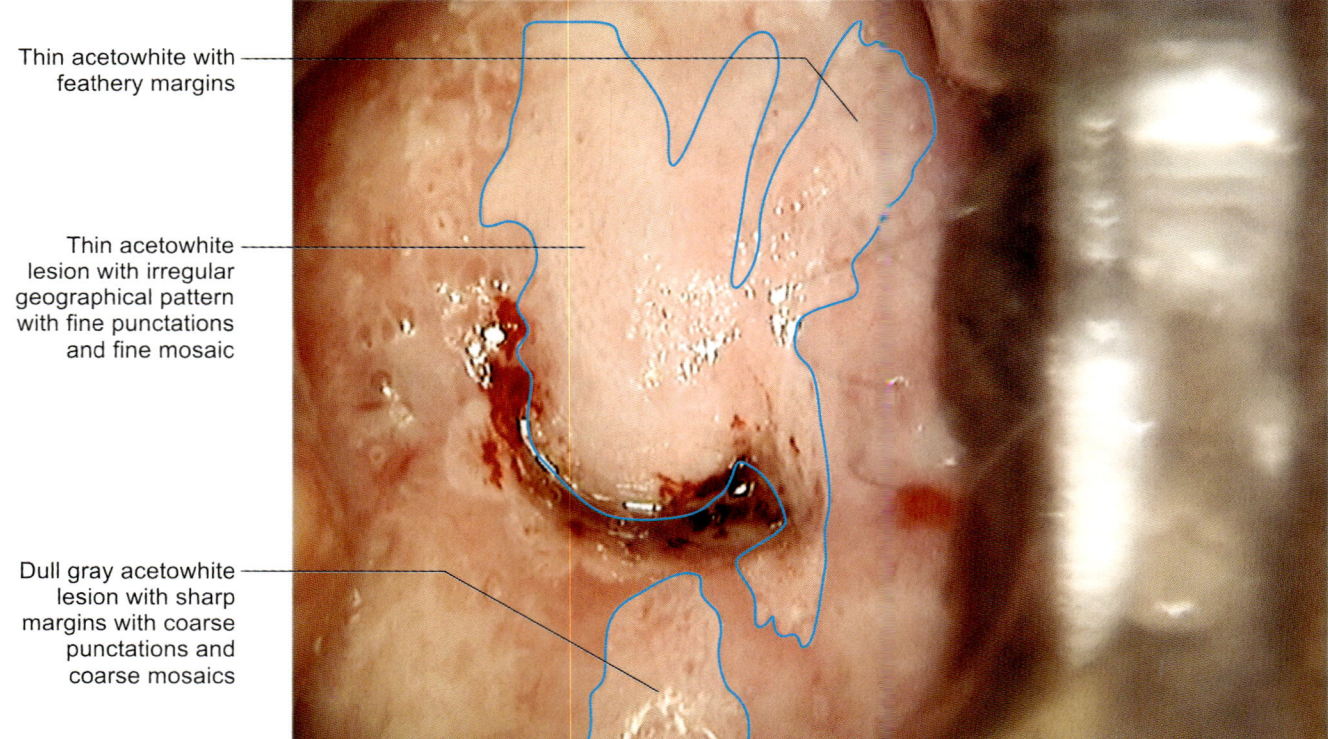

Thin acetowhite with feathery margins

Thin acetowhite lesion with irregular geographical pattern with fine punctations and fine mosaic

Dull gray acetowhite lesion with sharp margins with coarse punctations and coarse mosaics

Fig. 4.9a: CIN 1 lesions on upper lip with CIN 2 lesions on lower lip

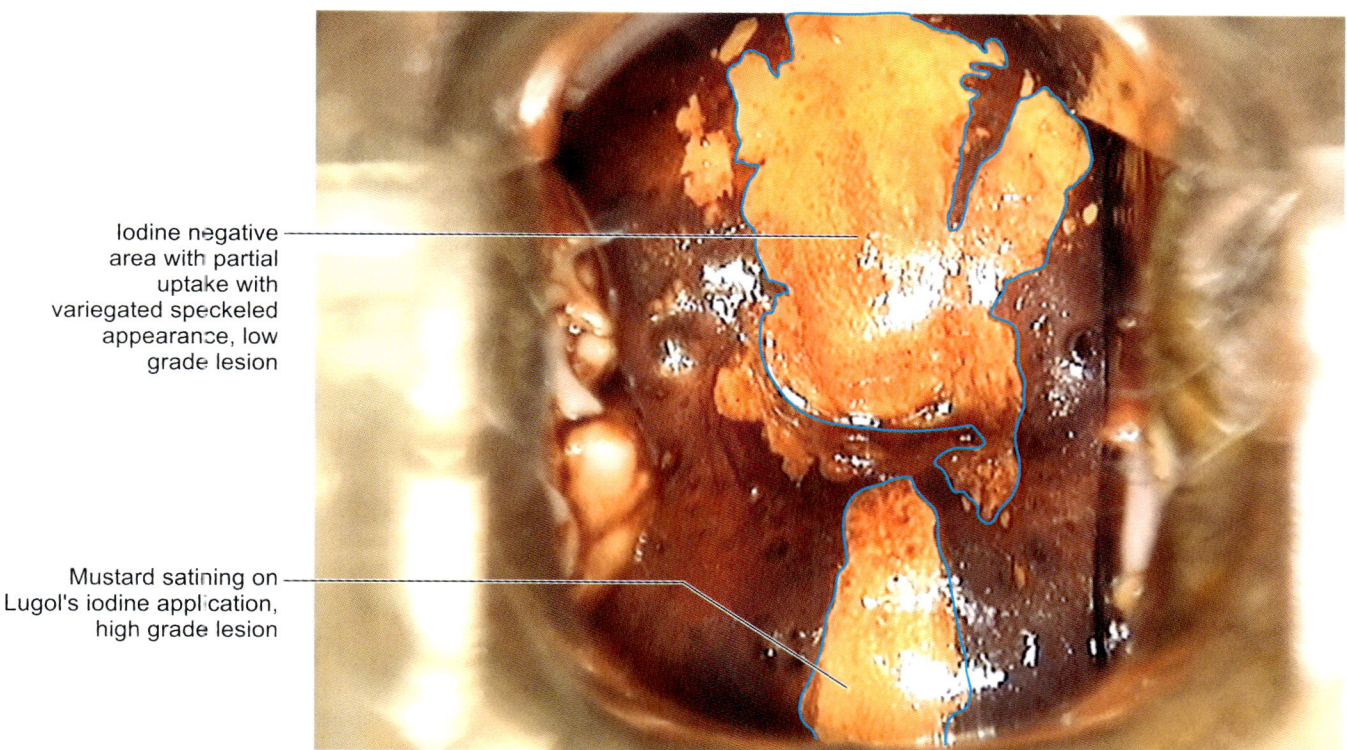

Iodine negative area with partial uptake with variegated speckeled appearance, low grade lesion

Mustard satining on Lugol's iodine application, high grade lesion

Fig. 4.9b

Ridge sign: High grade CIN 3 lesions can be characterized by dense opaque lesion having overhanging border resembling a ridge (Fig. 4.10).

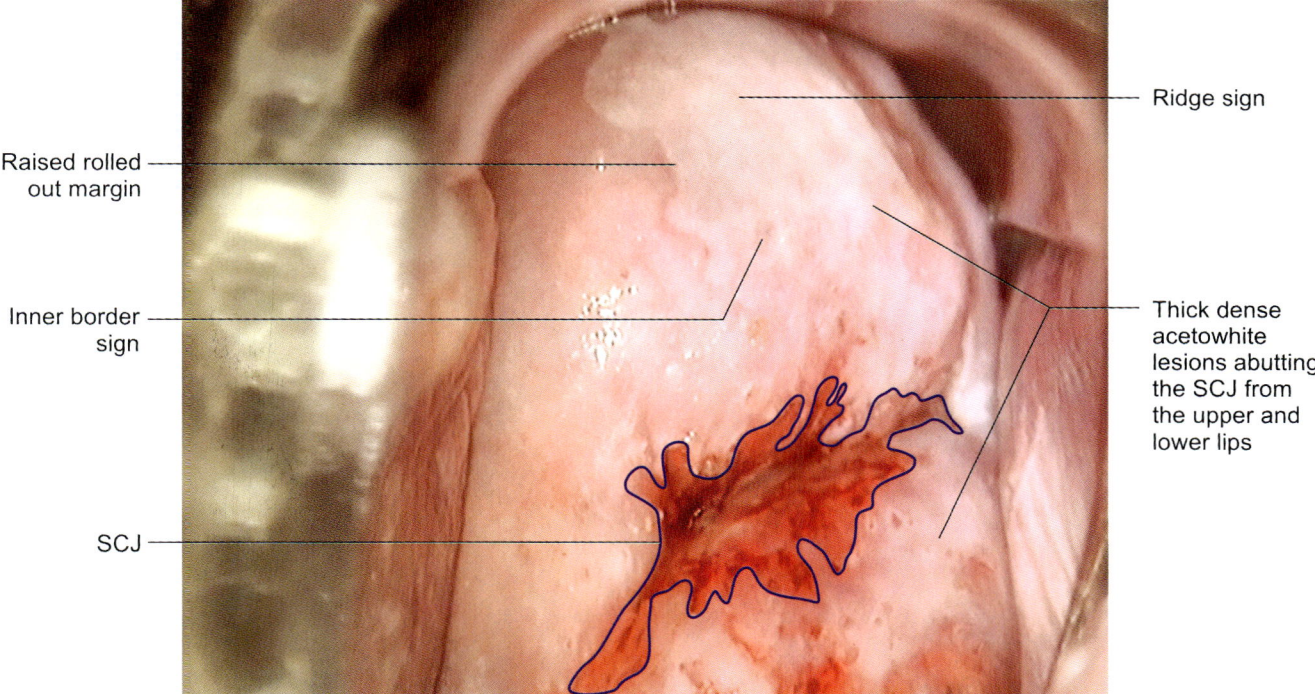

Raised rolled out margin

Inner border sign

SCJ

Ridge sign

Thick dense acetowhite lesions abutting the SCJ from the upper and lower lips

Fig. 4.10: High grade lesion on the upper and lower lips, dull gray acetowhite, rough surface with ridge sign, inner border sign

CIRCUMFERENTIAL LESION

Circumferential lesions usually cover all the 4 quadrants of the cervix (Figs 4.11, 4.12a–c and 4.13a, b).

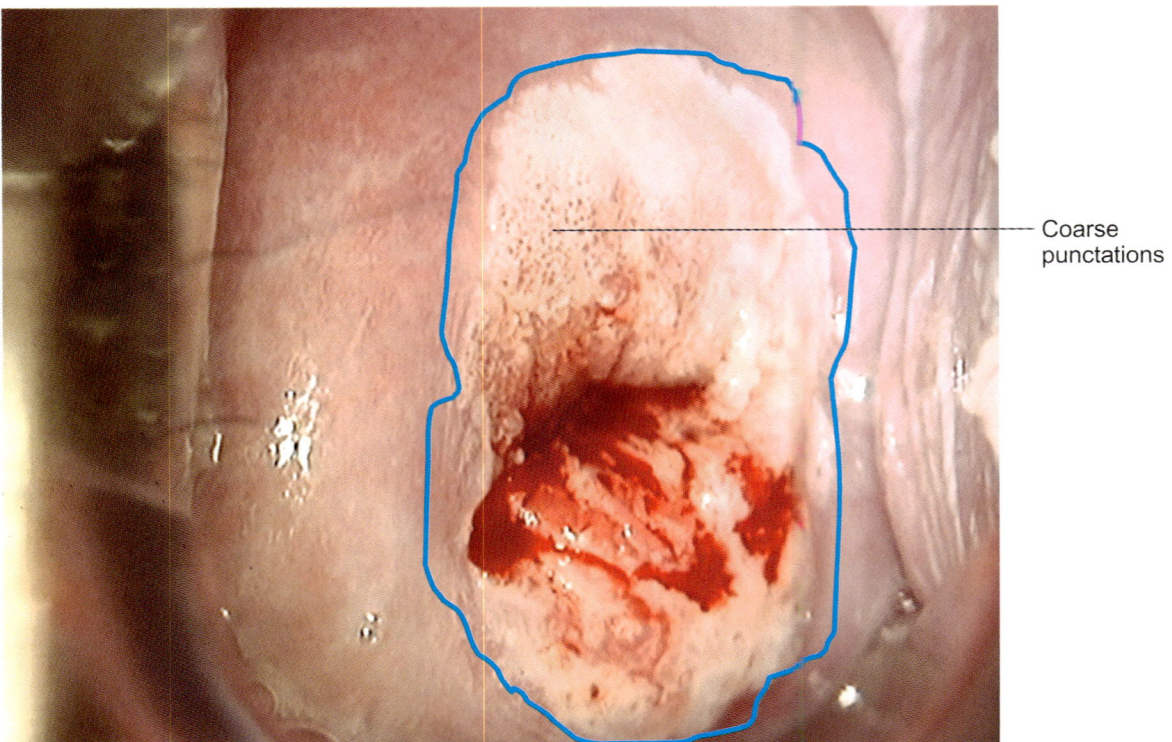

Coarse
punctations

Fig. 4.11: High grade circumferential lesion with rough surface, raised margins and coarse punctations

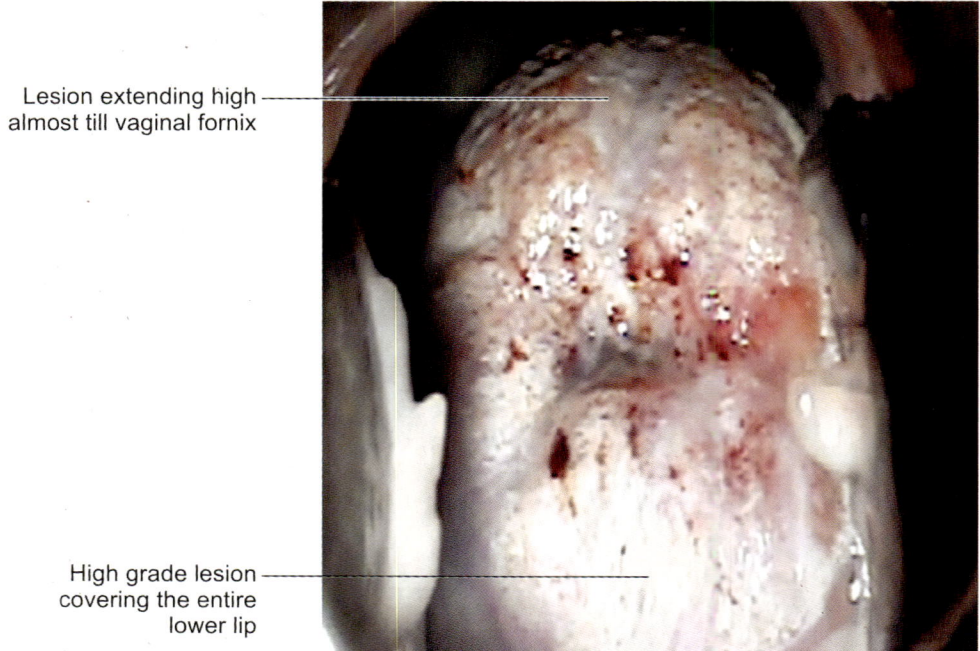

Lesion extending high
almost till vaginal fornix

High grade lesion
covering the entire
lower lip

Fig. 4.12a: Circumferential HSIL

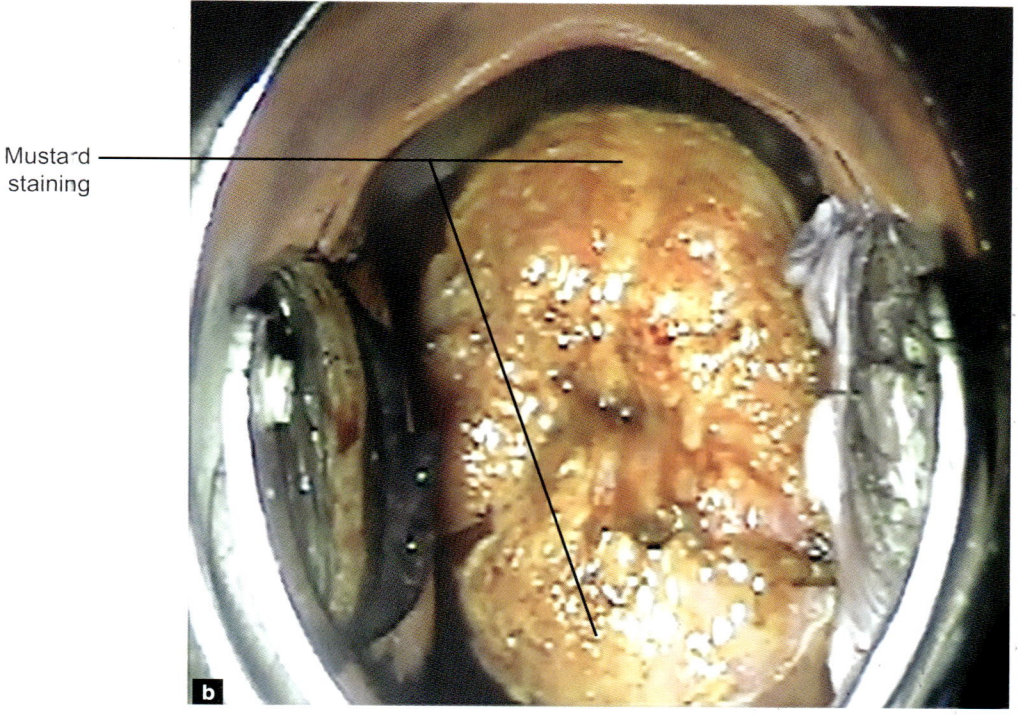

Mustard
staining

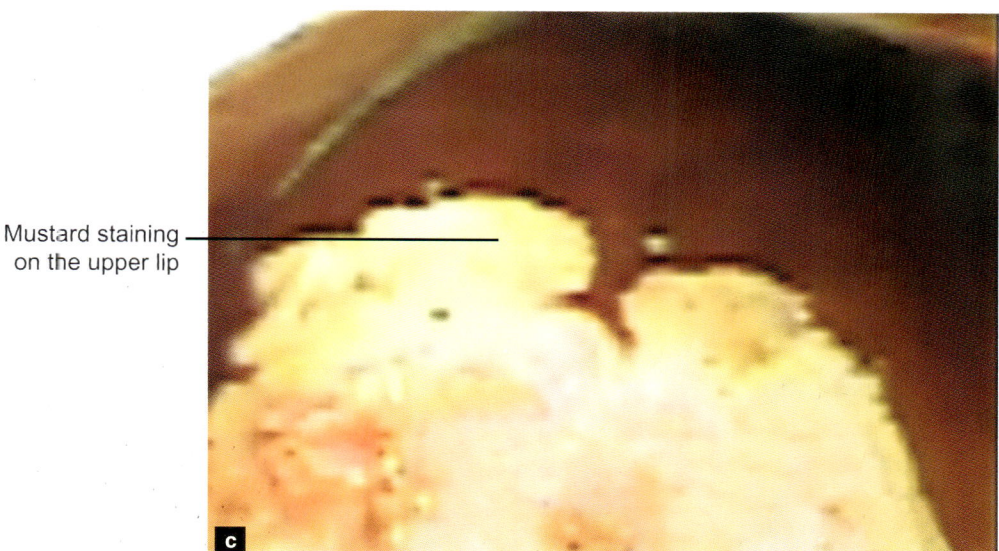

Mustard staining
on the upper lip

Figs 4.12b and c: On Lugol's iodine application

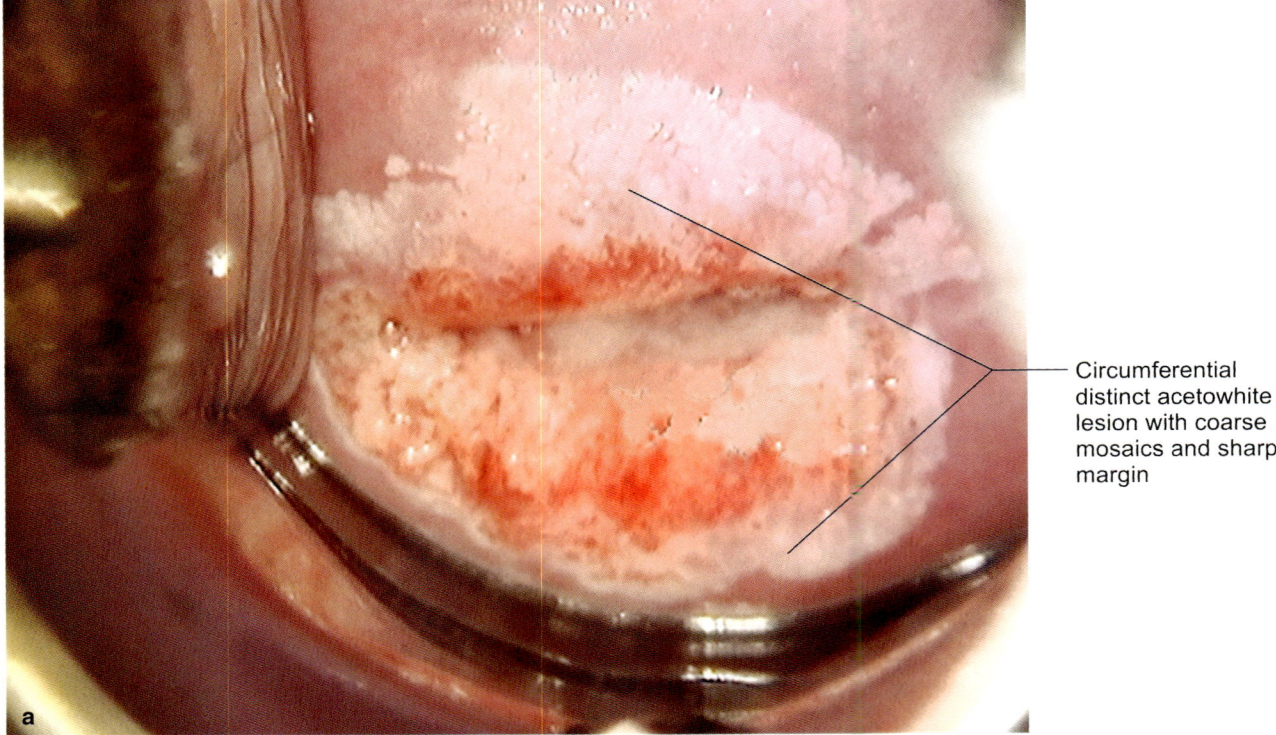

Circumferential
distinct acetowhite
lesion with coarse
mosaics and sharp
margin

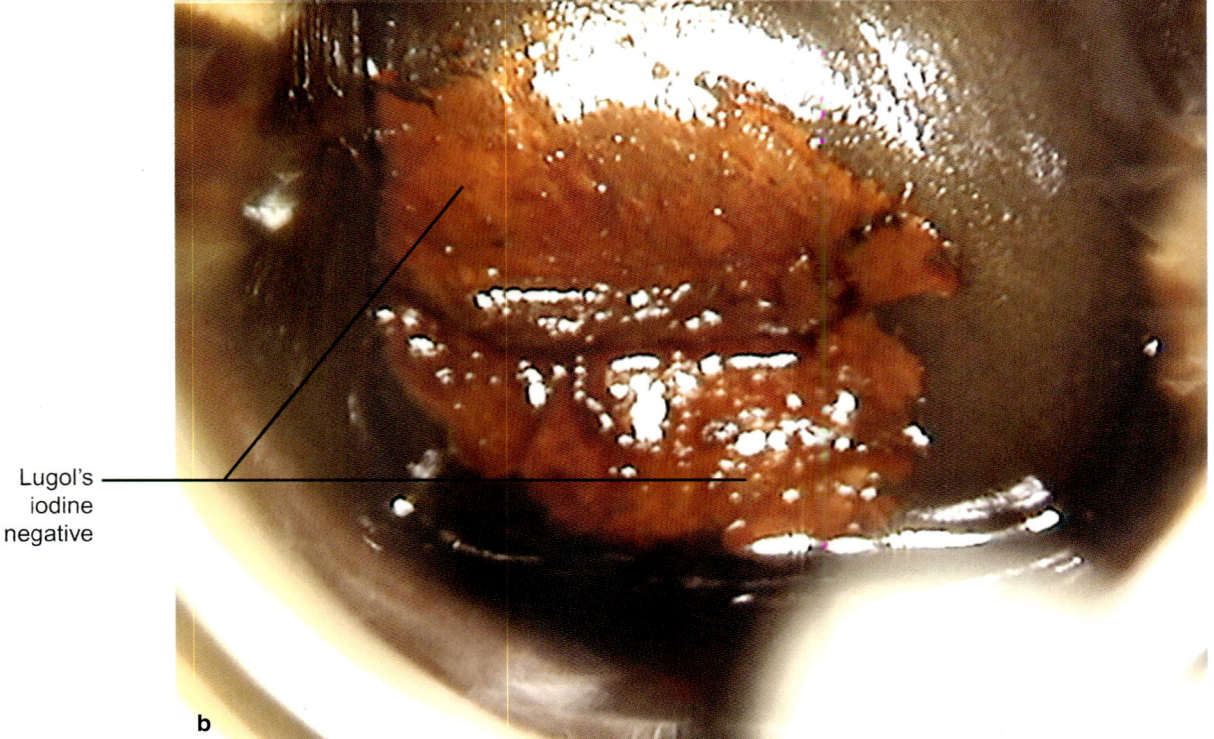

Lugol's
iodine
negative

Figs 4.13a and b: Circumferential lesion

PRECLINICAL INVASIVE CARCINOMA (Figs 4.14 and 4.15)

The prime responsibility of a colposcopist is to identify the preclinical invasive carcinoma. It is seen as rough, opaque, oyster egg white, raised acetowhite area with raised uneven surface. Breaking mosaics, atypical blood vessels are feature of microinvasice carcinoma. Atypical blood vessels have bizzare shape like waste thread, tendril, comma, corkscrew, etc.

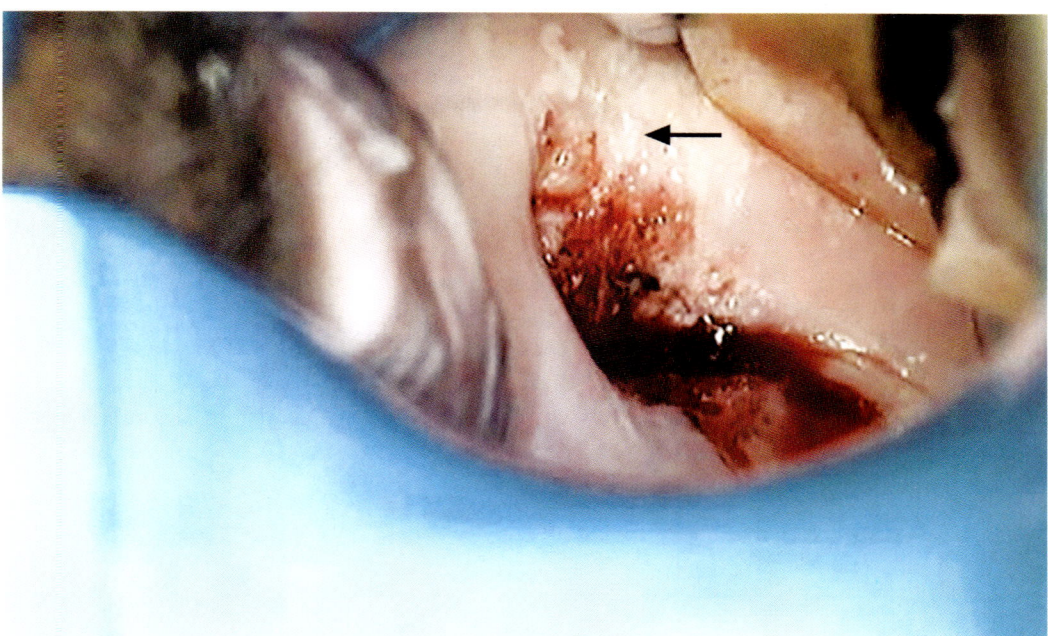

Fig. 4.14: Preclinical invasive carcinoma (arrow) on 5% acetic acid application—rough, oyster egg white, raised acetowhite area arising from SCJ with definite margins showing with margins. Coarse punctations and coarse mosaics, umbilications clearly noted on the lesions

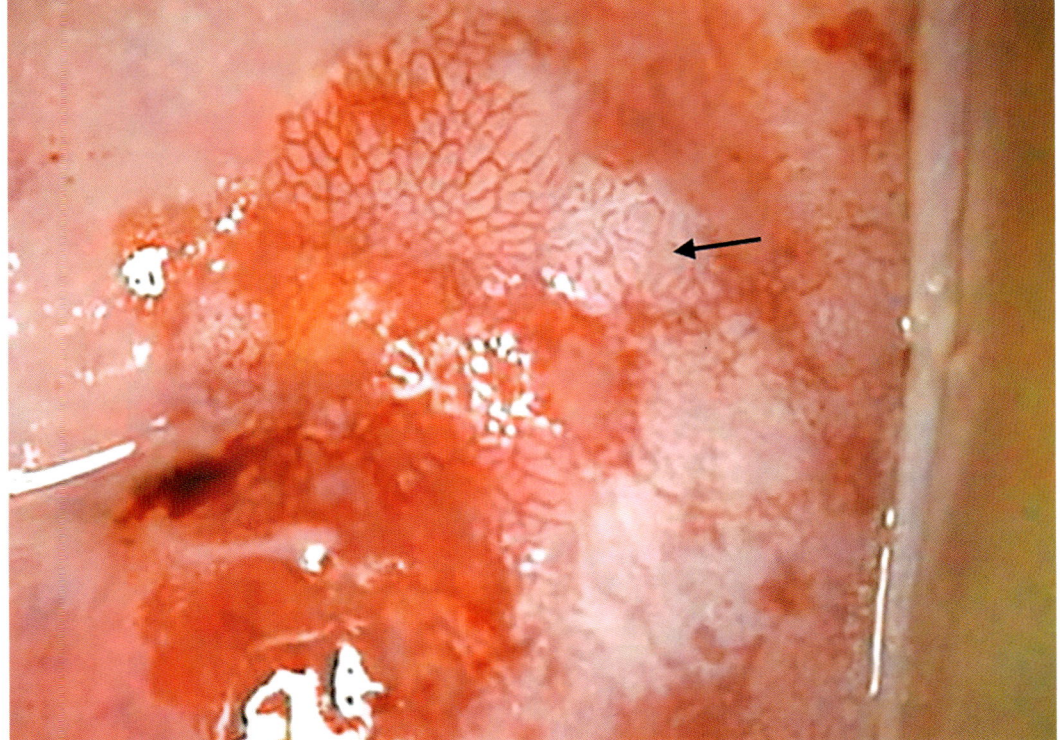

Fig. 4.15: Preclinical invasive carcinoma (arrow) on acetic acid: Dense, thick, rough, oyster egg acetowhite areas raised coarse mosaic

INVASIVE CARCINOMA (Figs 4.16a to c)

Invasive carcinomas on application of acetic acid appear thick, dense, opaque with rough, undulated surface, turning chalky white immediately and persisting for quite some time. They show lesion within lesion and have variegated appearance.

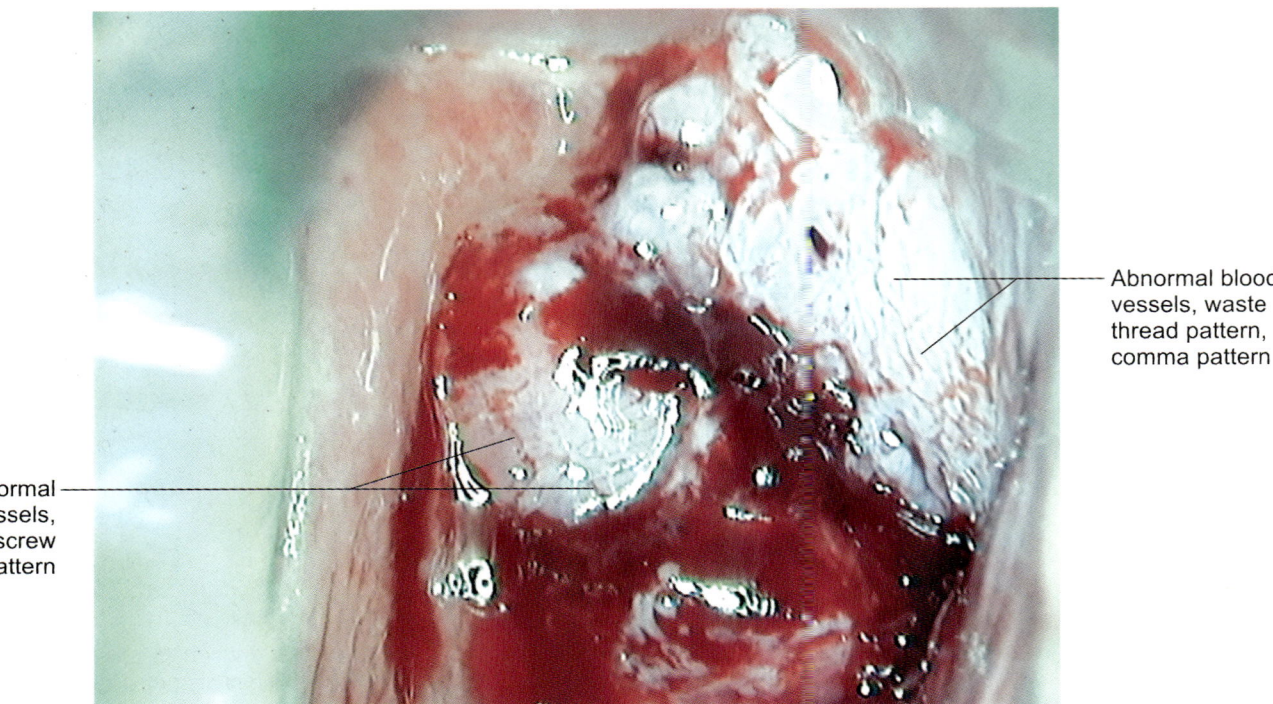

Abnormal blood vessels, corkscrew pattern

Abnormal blood vessels, waste thread pattern, comma pattern

Fig. 4.16a

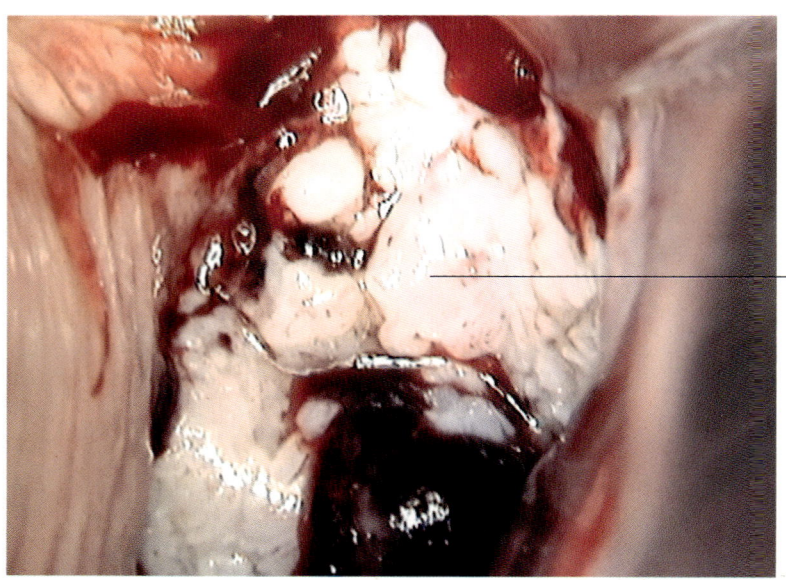

Chalky white elevated, dull, opaque lesions

Fig. 4.16b

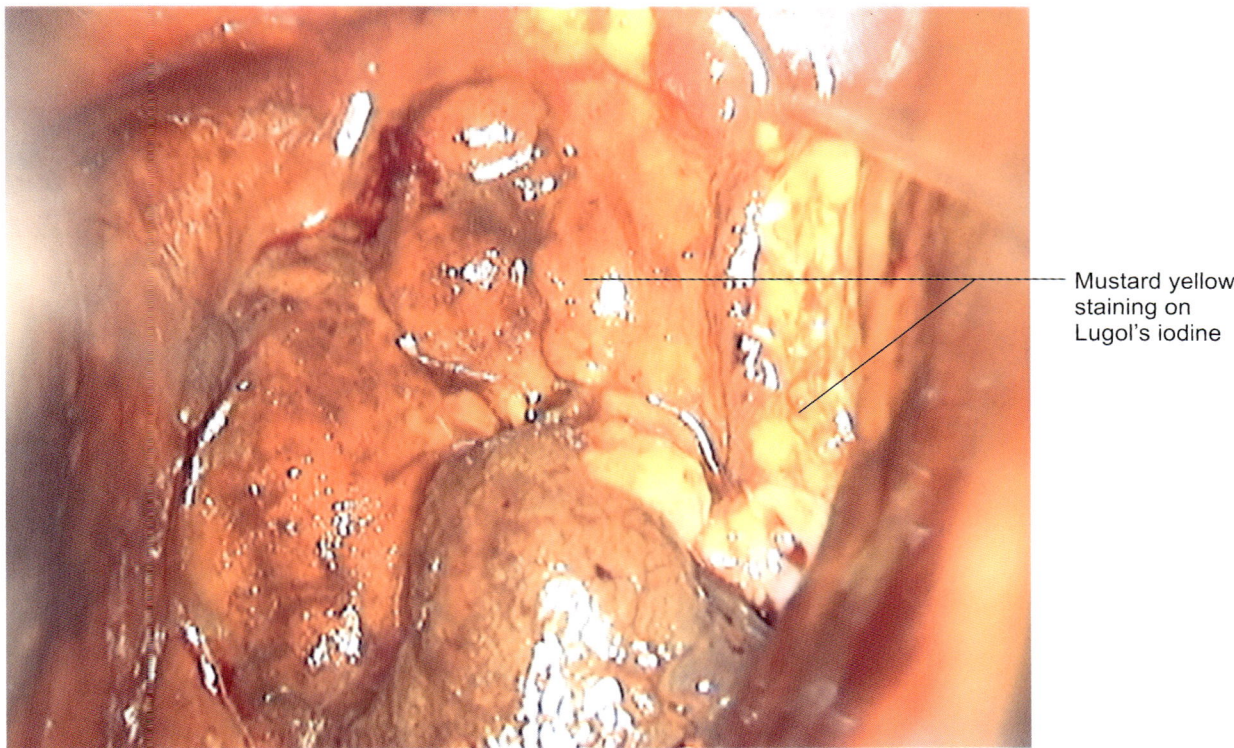

Mustard yellow
staining on
Lugol's iodine

Fig. 4.16c

ADENOCARCINOMA *IN SITU* (Figs 4.17a–c and 4.18a, b)

They are the precancerous lesions arising from the columnar epithelium usually found in the TZ area. The normal columnar epithelium is replaced by abnormal epithelium showing loss of polarity, altered size and shape with

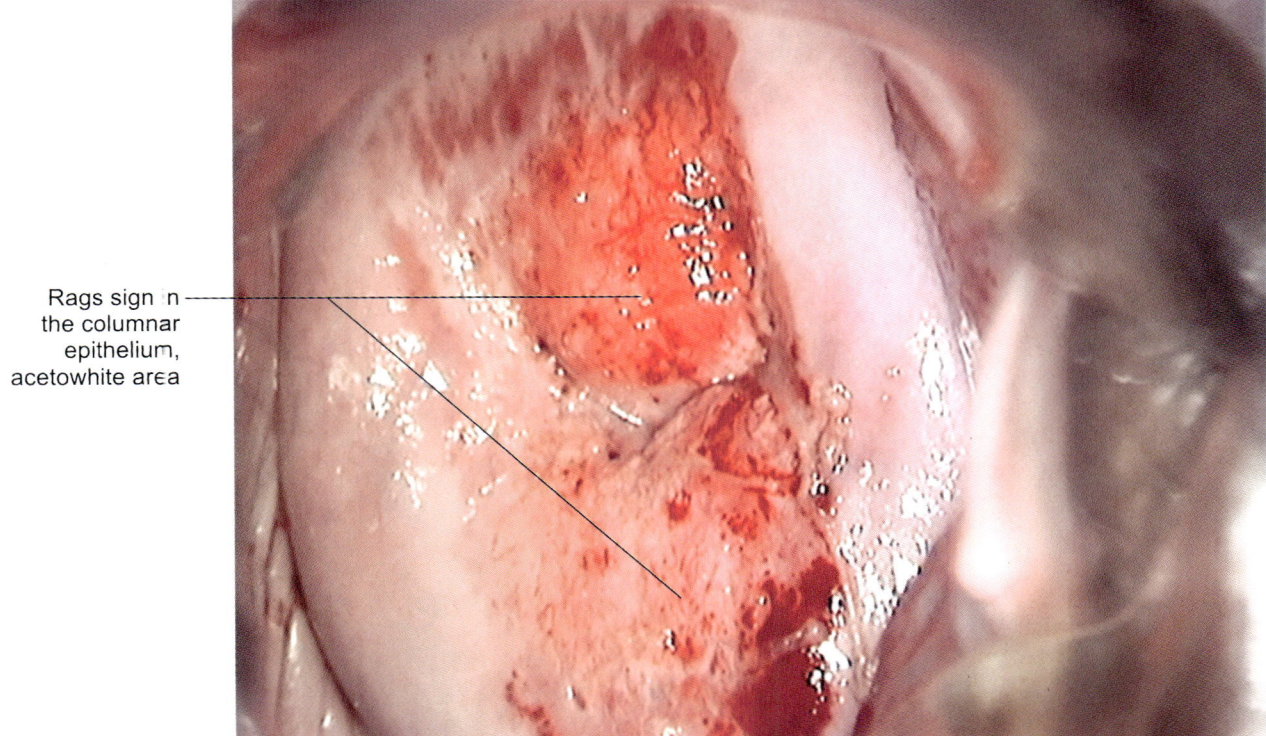

Rags sign in
the columnar
epithelium,
acetowhite area

Fig. 4.17a

nuclear pleomorphism, hyperchromasia, raised mitotic activity. Abnormal glands with intraluminar cellular projections are noted. Depending on the cell type, AIS is classified as:

- Endocervical
- Endometrioid
- Intestinal
- Mixed cell types.

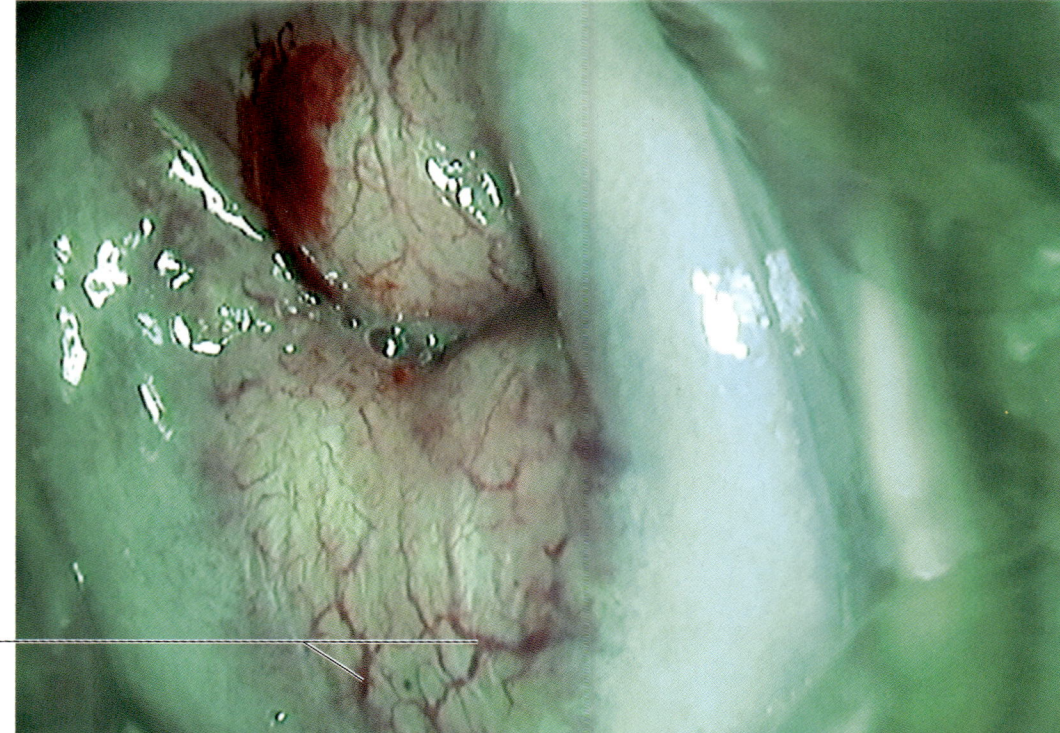

Abnormal dilated blood vessel pattern

Fig. 4.17b

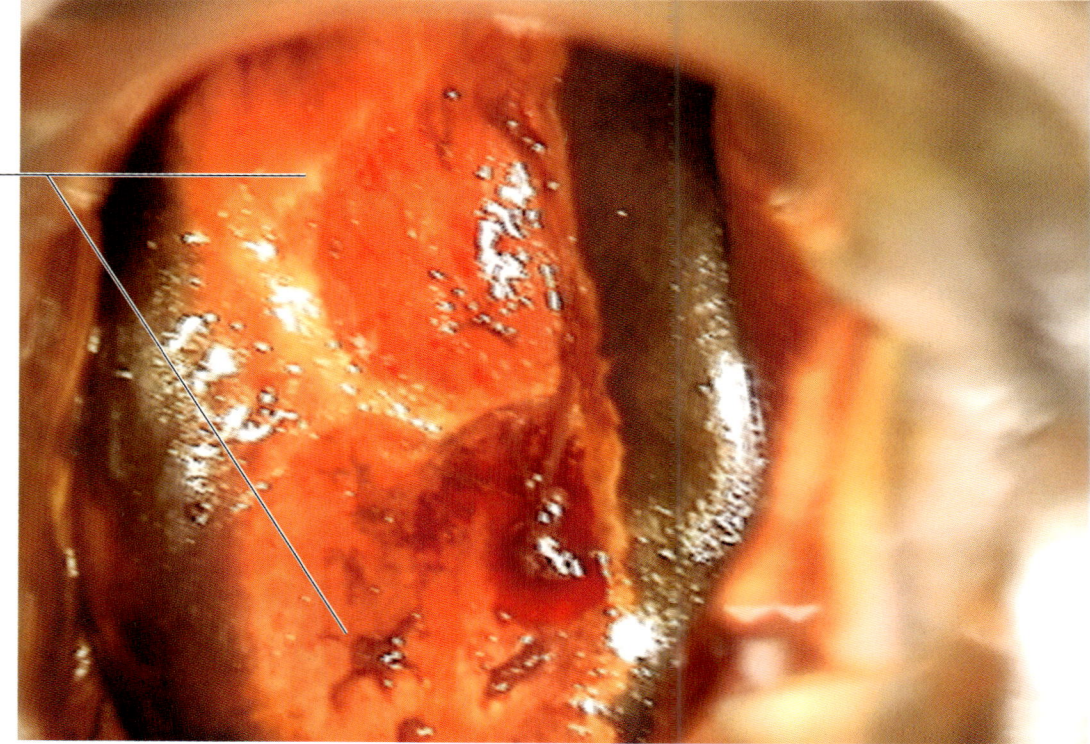

Mustard yellow staining on Lugol's iodine application

Fig. 4.17c

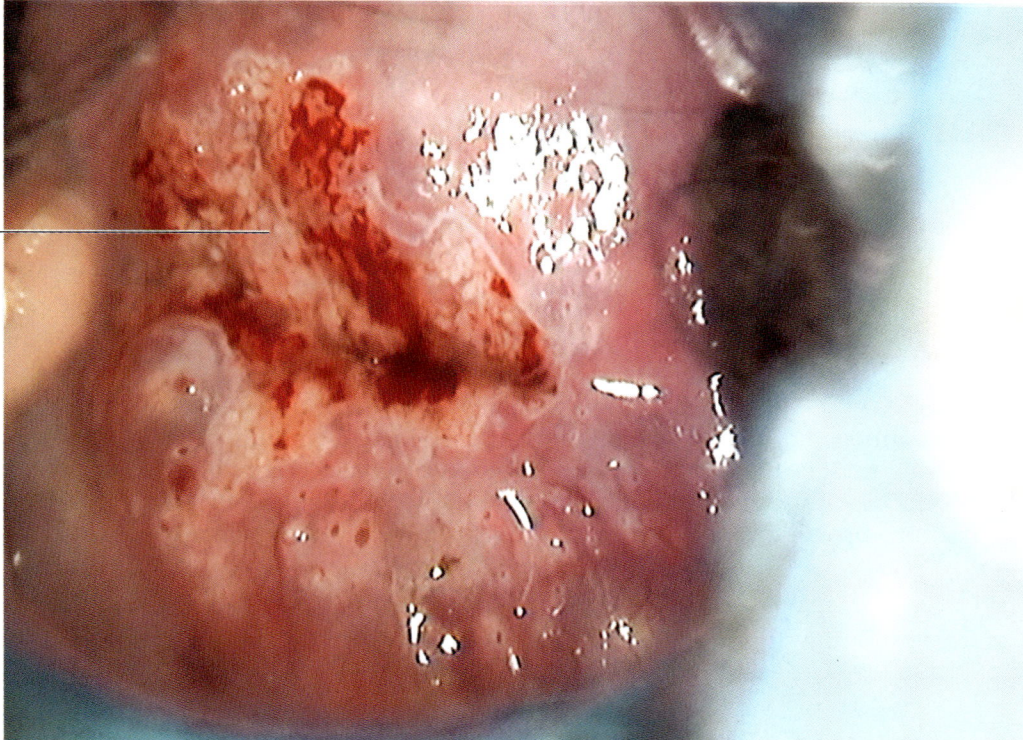

Adenocarcinoma *in situ* appearing dull, dense acetowhite on the columnar epithelium

Fig. 4.18a

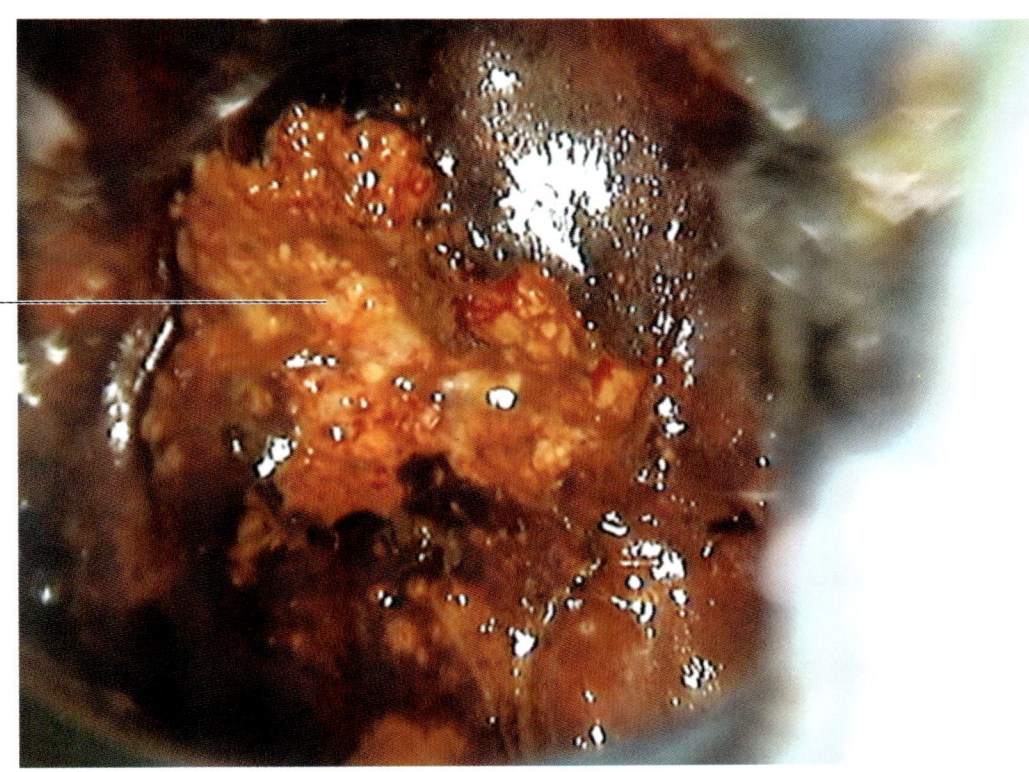

The lesion appears mustard yellow on Lugol's iodine

Fig. 4.18b

Vaginal Intraepithelial Neoplasia (VAIN)

VAIN is a condition that denotes premalignant histological findings in the vagina, which is characterized by dysplastic changes. It is a rare condition but colposcopist has to keep this in mind so as not to miss the diagnosis. While performing colposcopy, the vagina has to be smeared with acetic acid to note any acetowhite areas. These areas do not turn brown on Lugol's iodine application; whereas the normal vaginal mucosa turns dark brown.

CASE OF NECROTIC CERVICAL GROWTH EVALUATED FOR THE VAGINAL INVOLVEMENT (Figs 5.1a to e)

It is preferable to know the extent of vaginal involvement in the case to excise beyond that margins in radical surgery.

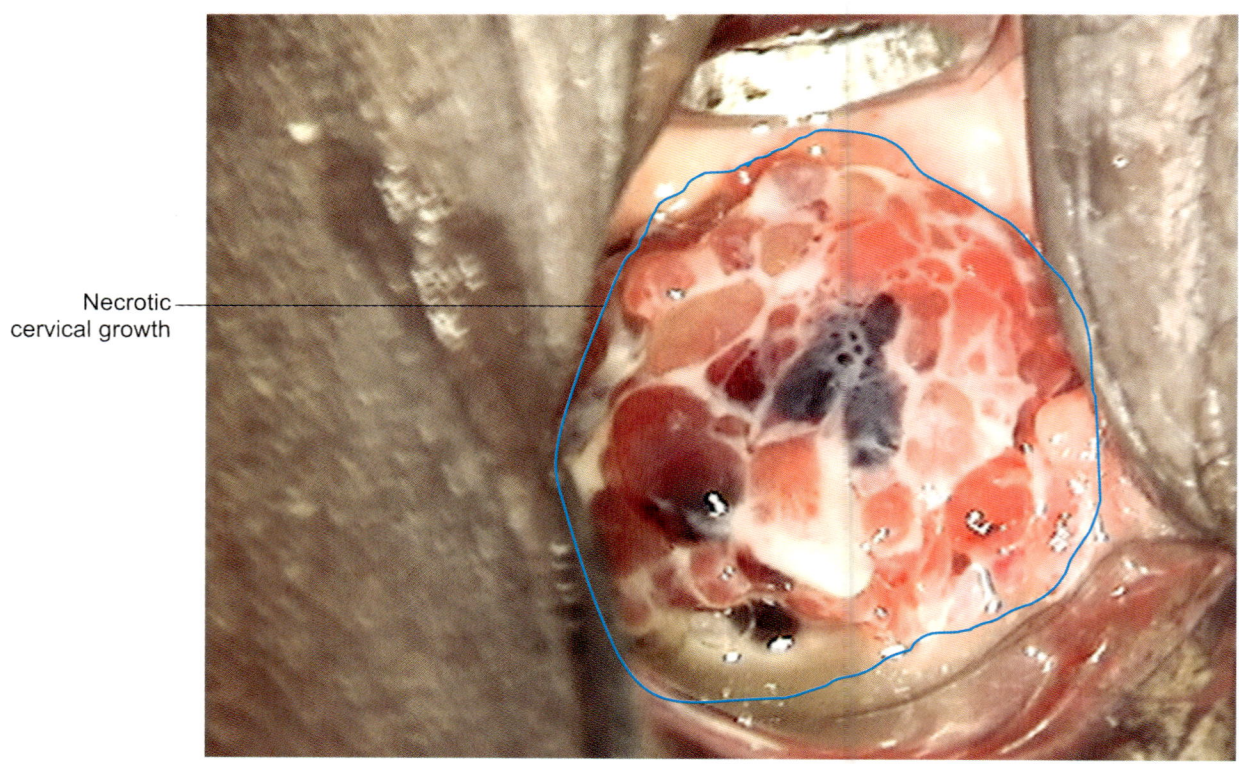

Necrotic cervical growth

Fig. 5.1a: Necrotic cancer growth flushed with the cervix

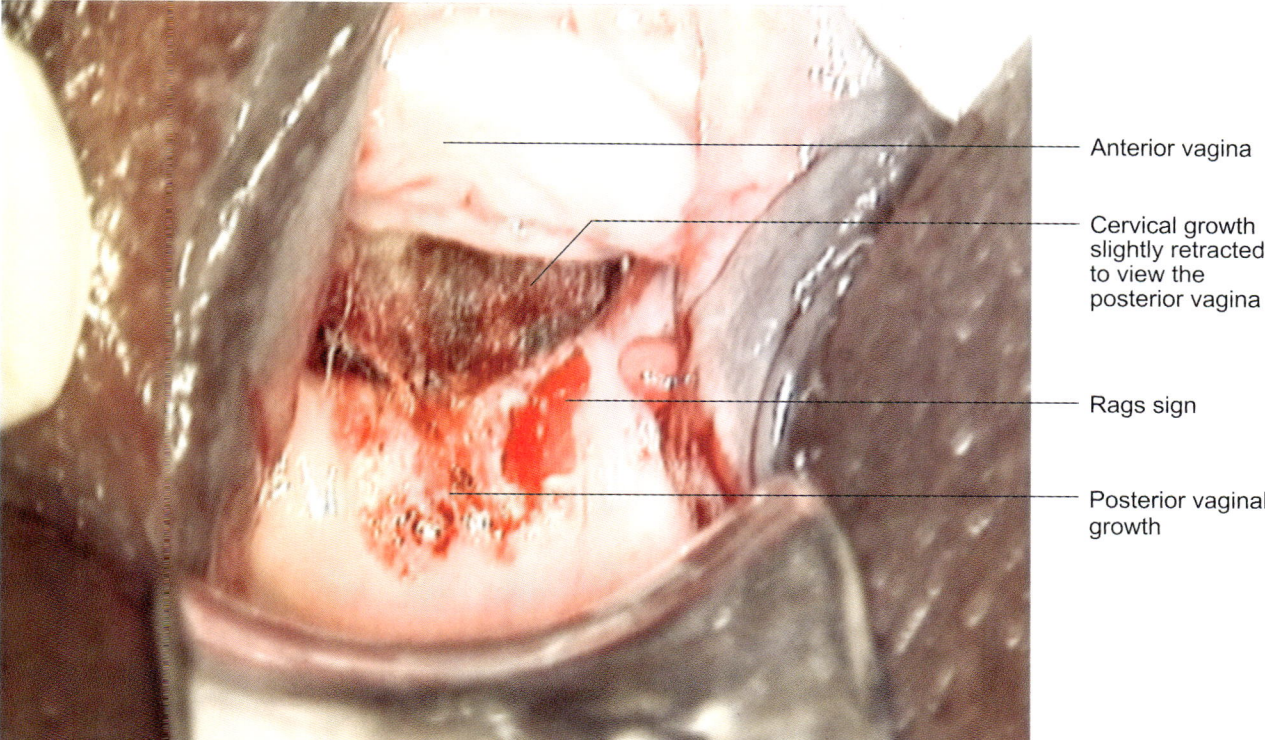

Anterior vagina

Cervical growth slightly retracted to view the posterior vagina

Rags sign

Posterior vaginal growth

Fig. 5.1b: Vaginal extension of invasive squamous cell cancer

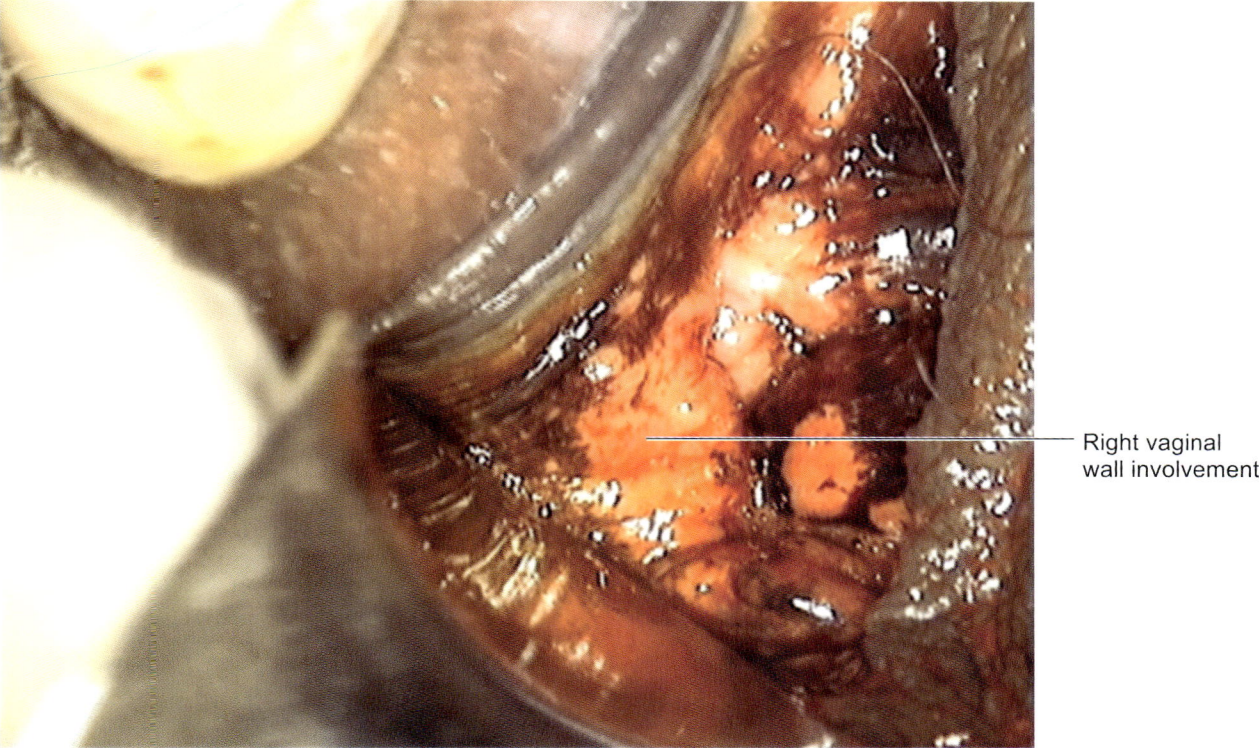

Right vaginal wall involvement

Fig. 5.1c: Demarcation of the extent of vaginal involvement in SCC

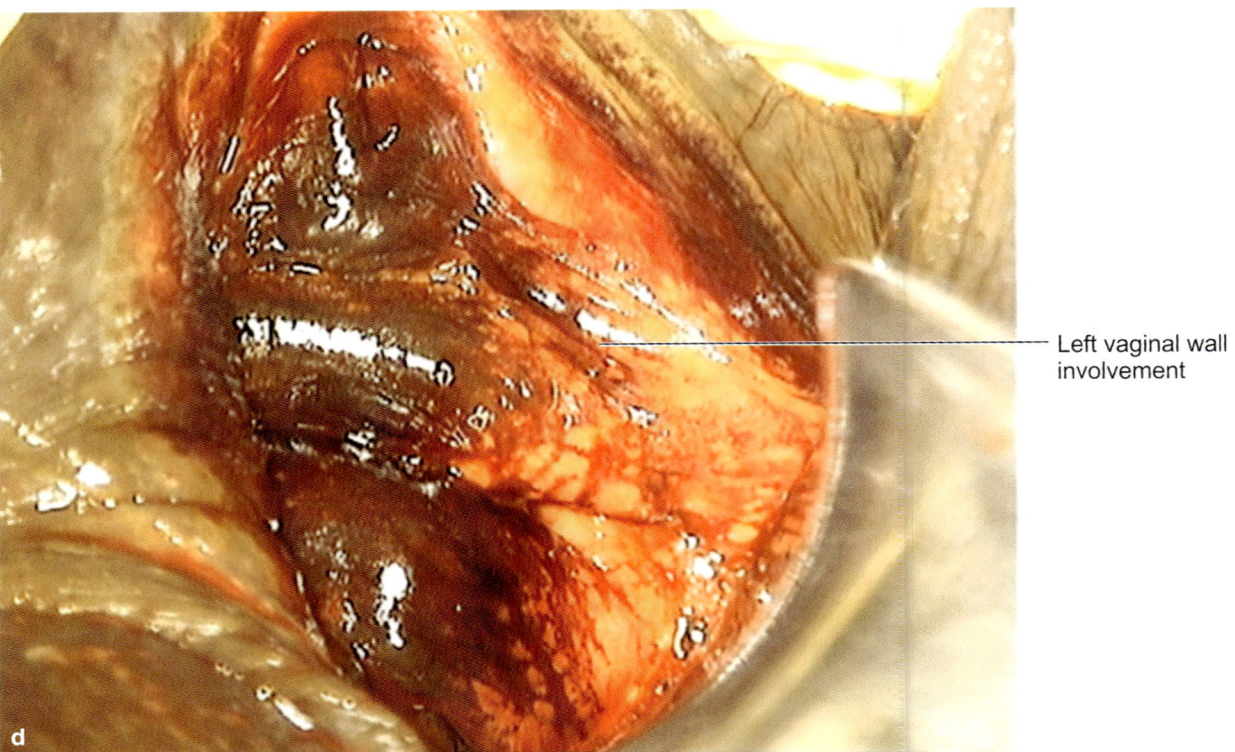

Left vaginal wall involvement

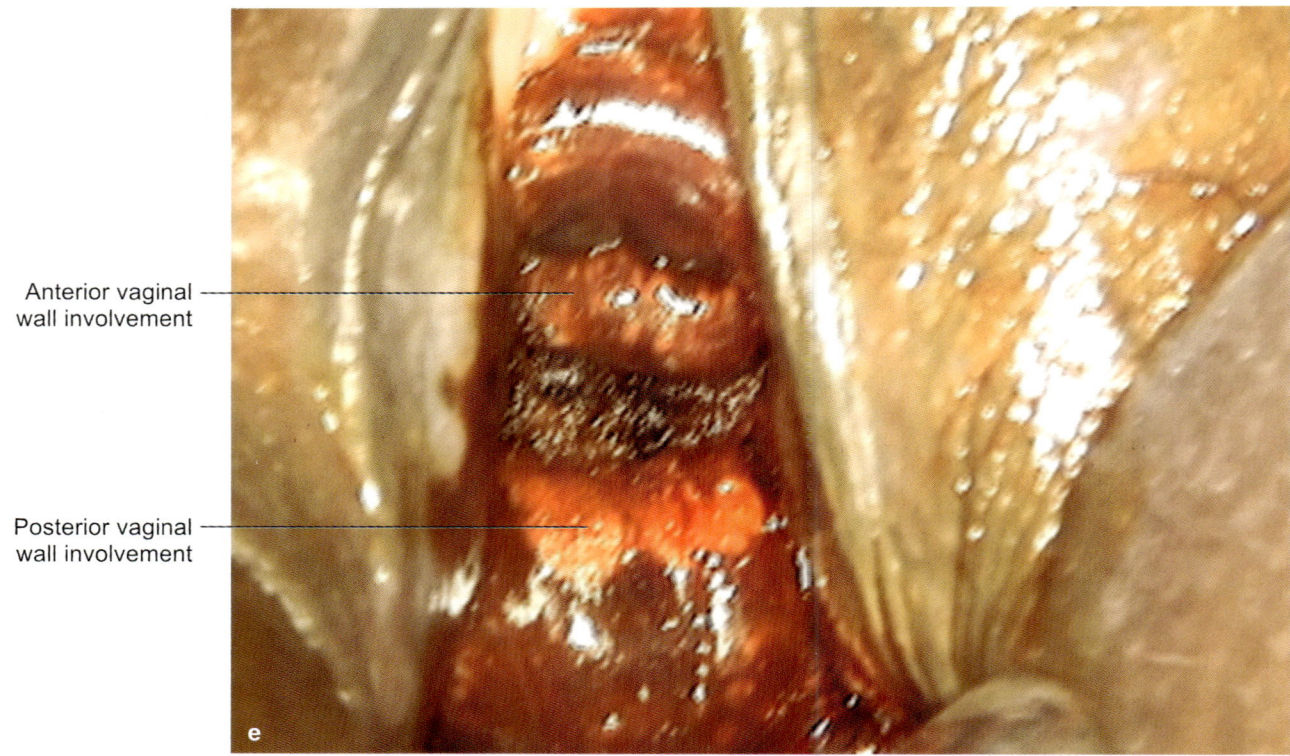

Anterior vaginal wall involvement

Posterior vaginal wall involvement

Figs 5.1d and e: Demarcation of the extent of vaginal involvement

VAULT COLPOSCOPY

Vault colposcopy is usually recommended for cases who have undergone hysterectomy for precancerous or cancerous lesions. Cytology is usually done along with colposcopy annually. If 3 consecutives annual check-up is negative, she can be put in 5 yearly surveillance protocol.

Healthy vault: On application of 5% acetic acid, there is no acetowhite area or discolouration of vault (Fig. 5.2).

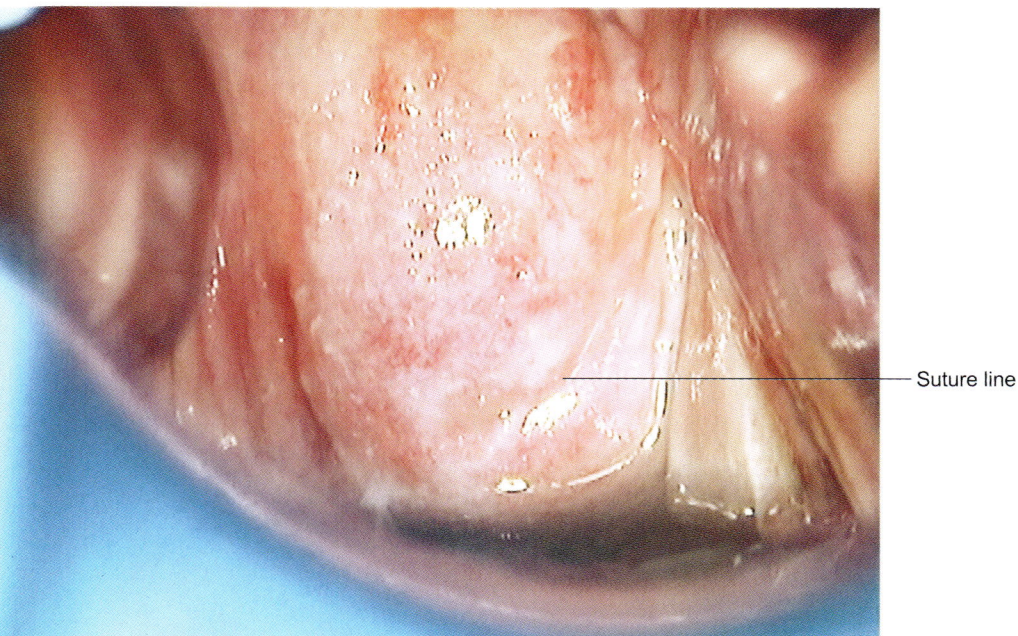

— Suture line

Fig. 5.2: Healthy vault

LEFT OUT CERVIX IN SUBTOTAL HYSTERECTOMY

Many a times, during obstetric hysterectomy, subtotal hysterectomy is performed leaving behind cervix. This is also encountered while performing hysterectomy in case of severe bladder adhesions, previous surgeries or endometriosis. In such cases, colposcopy examination reveals the left over cervical tissue (Fig. 5.3).

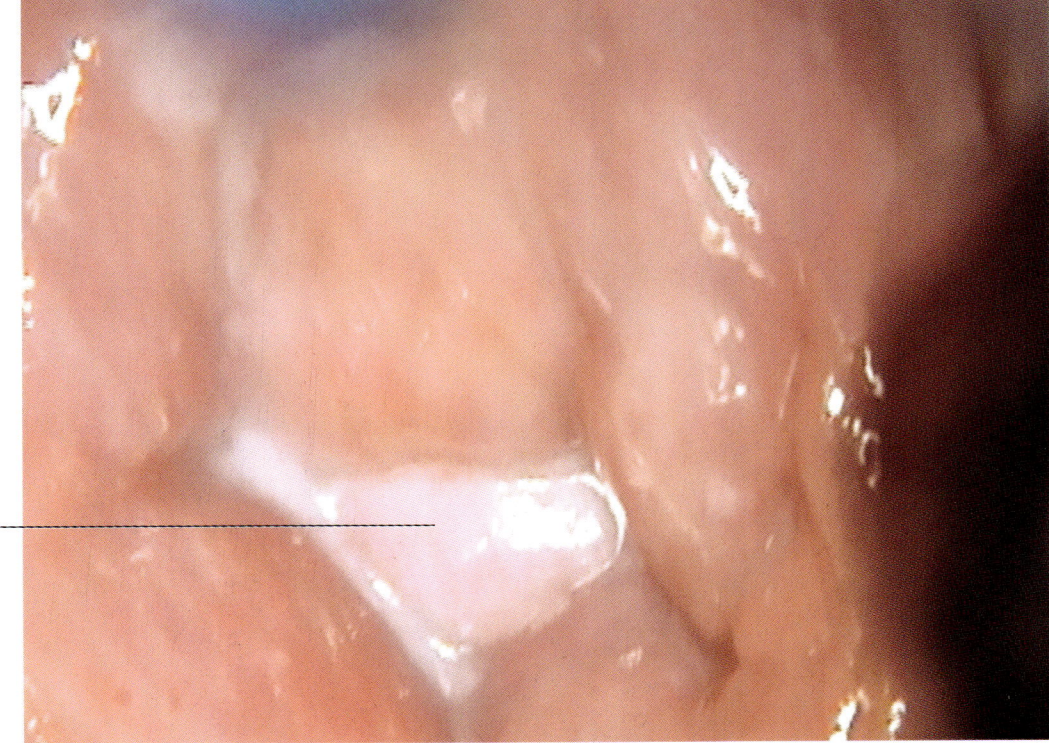

Left out cervix in subtotal hysterectomy

Fig. 5.3: Left out cervix in subtotal hysterectomy

Vault neoplasia (Fig. 5.4) is sometimes seen in case of SCC who have undergone radical hysterectomy.

The vault carcinomas are usually recurrent cervical cancers.

On application of 5% acetic acid on the vault, rough, dense acetohite lesions are noted, they can have rags sign (Fig. 5.5). On Lugol's application, the lesion appears mustard yellow (Fig. 5.6). In advance stage, vault carcinoma appears as growth on the vault, which bleeds on touch (Fig. 5.7).

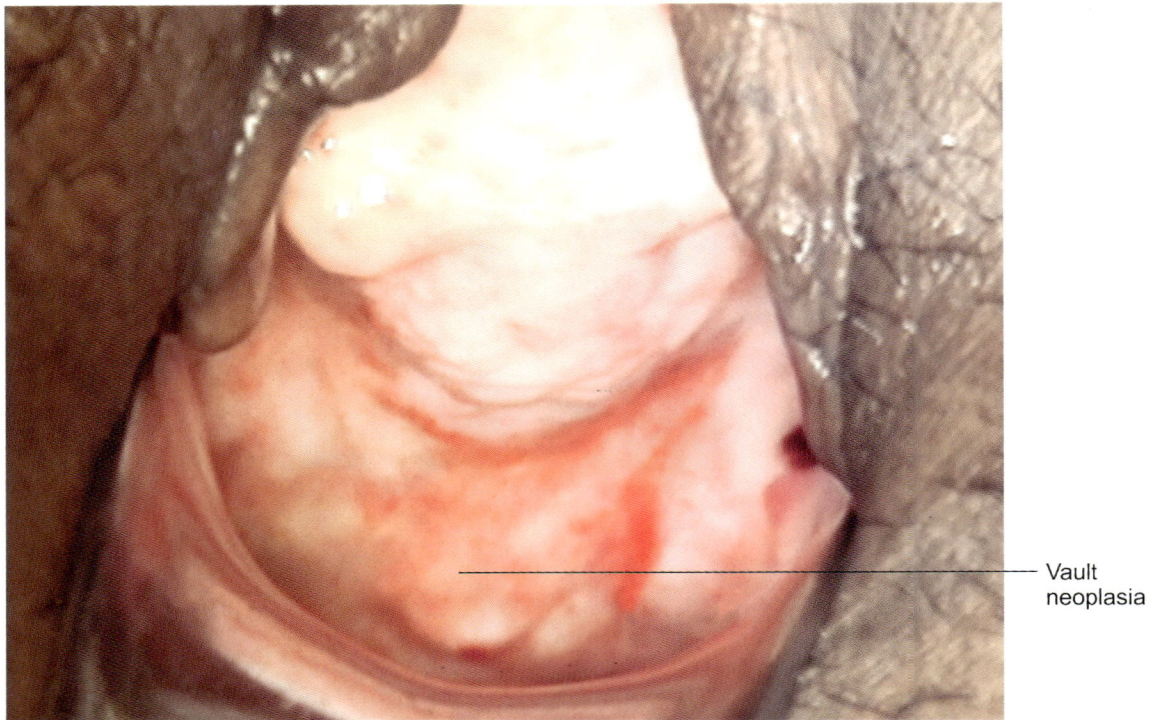

Vault neoplasia

Fig. 5.4: Vault carcinoma—post-radical hysterectomy done for SCC

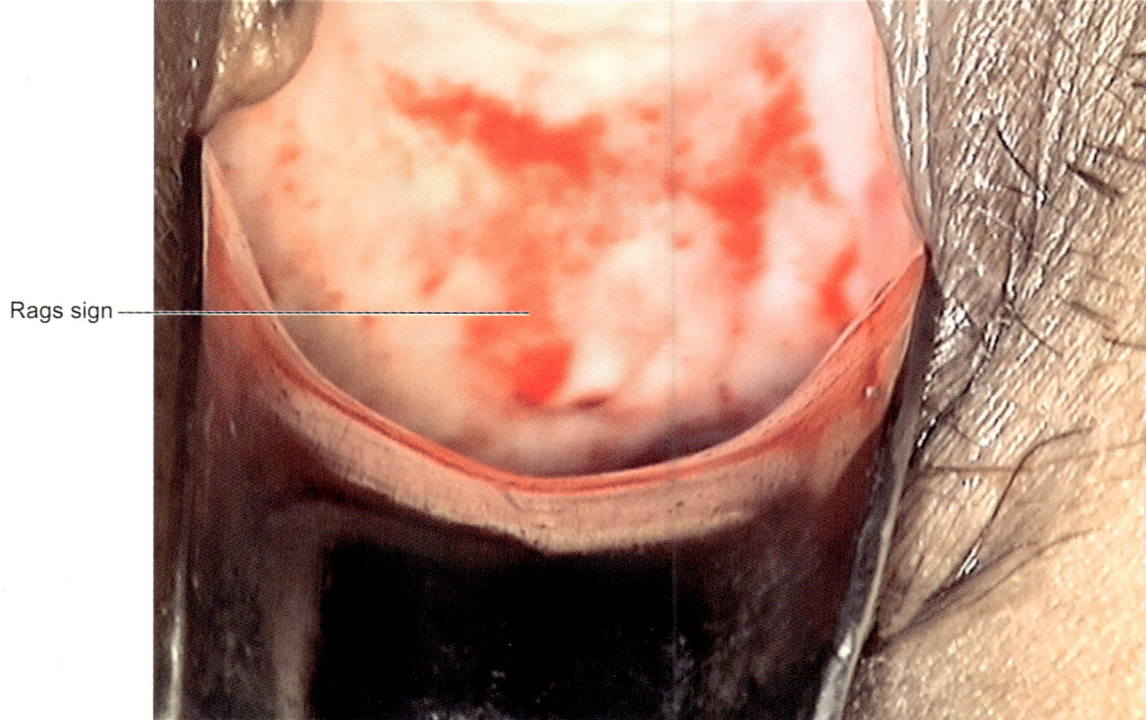

Rags sign

Fig. 5.5: Vault neoplasia on application of 5% acetic acid

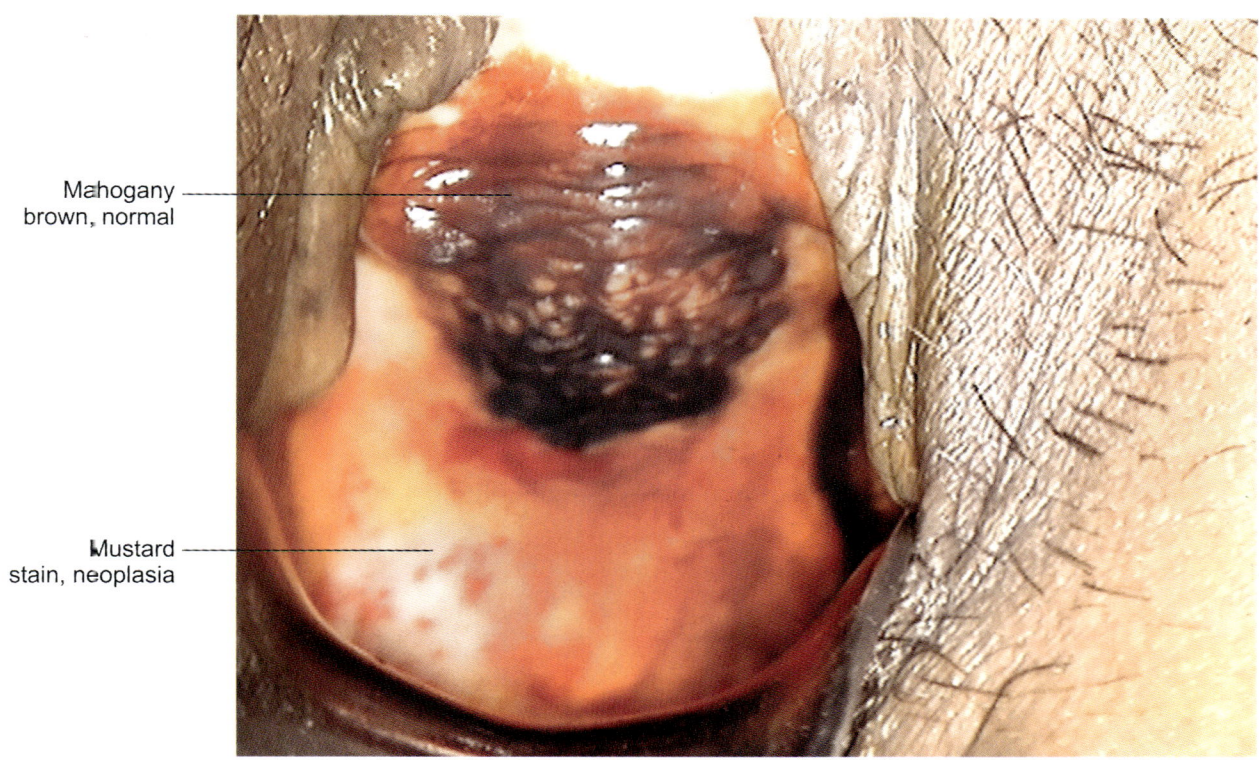

Mahogany brown, normal

Mustard stain, neoplasia

Fig. 5.6: Vault neoplasia—Lugol's iodine

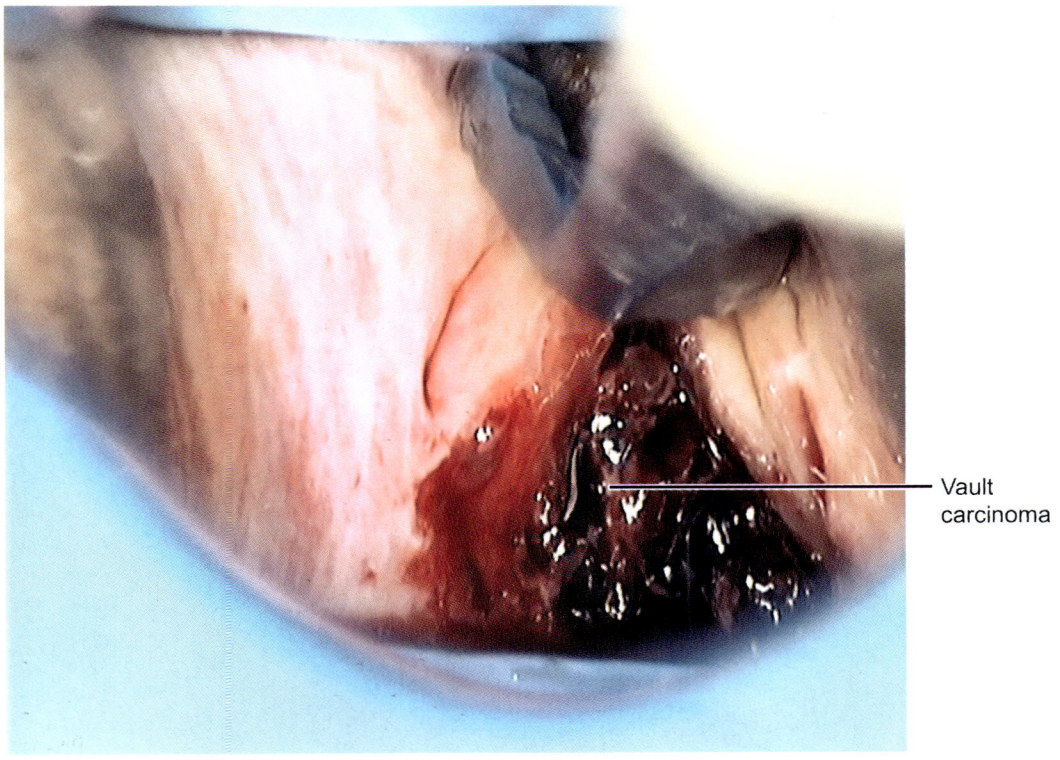

Vault carcinoma

Fig. 5.7: Vault carcinoma

Different Conditions of Cervix

1. ENDOCERVICAL POLYP (Figs 6.1 and 6.2)

A cervical polyp is an overgrowth and enlargement of single columnar epithelial papillae which appears as reddish mash protruding from the cervical os.

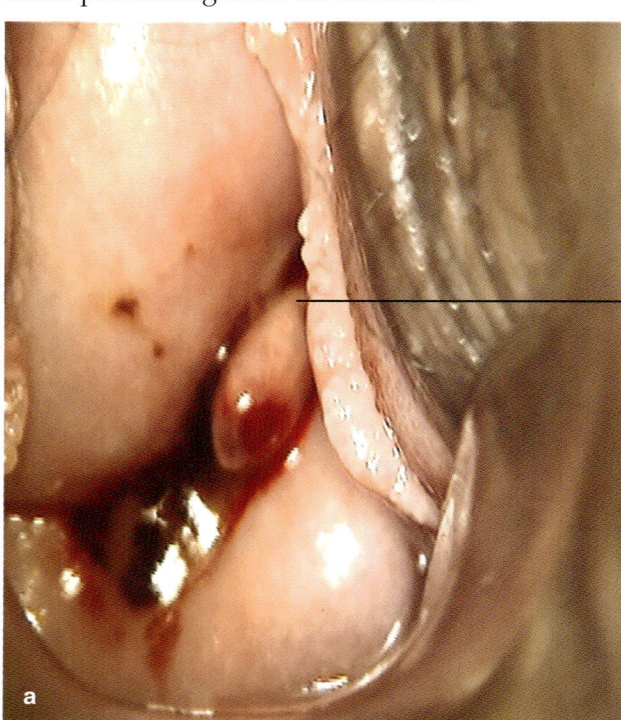

Cervical polyp, the stalk is seen very prominently in endocervical speculum examinations

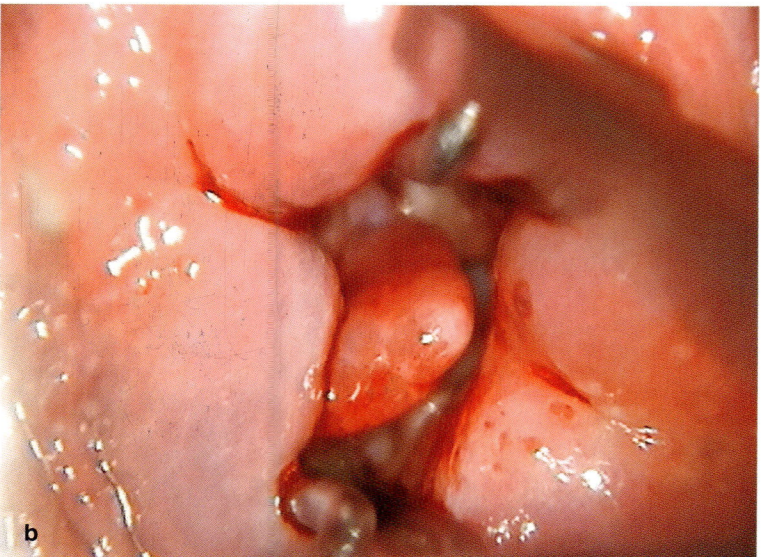

Figs 6.1a and b: Endocervical polyp

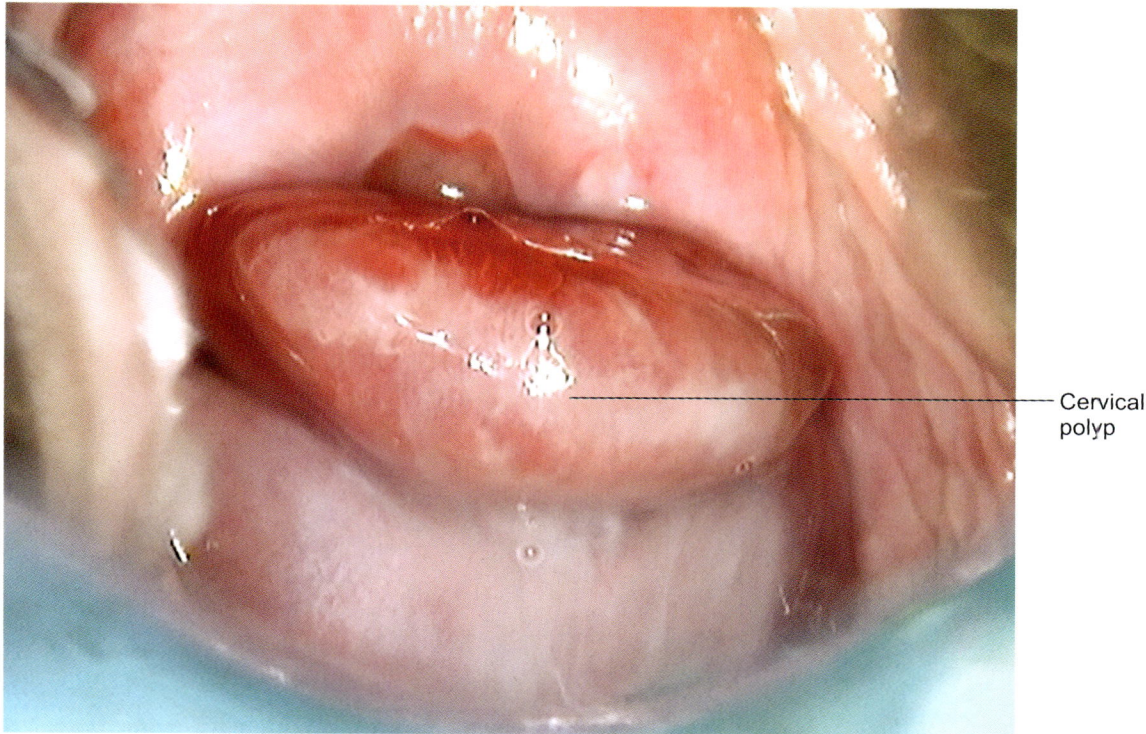

Cervical polyp

Fig. 6.2: Endocervical polyp

2. CERVICAL ENDOMETRIOSIS (Fig. 6.3a to c)

This is a rare entity found as cigar burn spots or blackish spots on the cervix, many a times ECC (endocervical curettage) specimen sent for HP reveals endometrial glands. Many a times, the endocervical cells are scanty. The features on HP suggest cervical endometriosis.

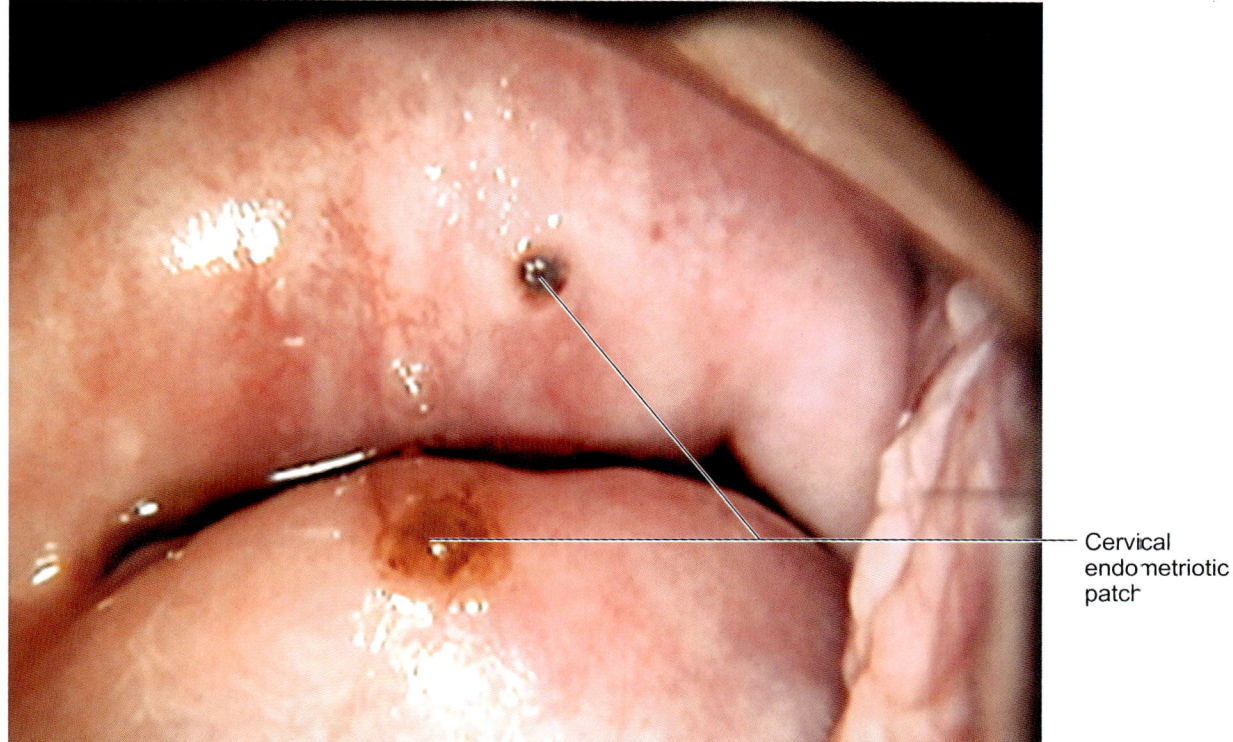

Cervical endometriotic patch

Fig. 6.3a: Cervical endometriosis had a case of post-coital bleeding

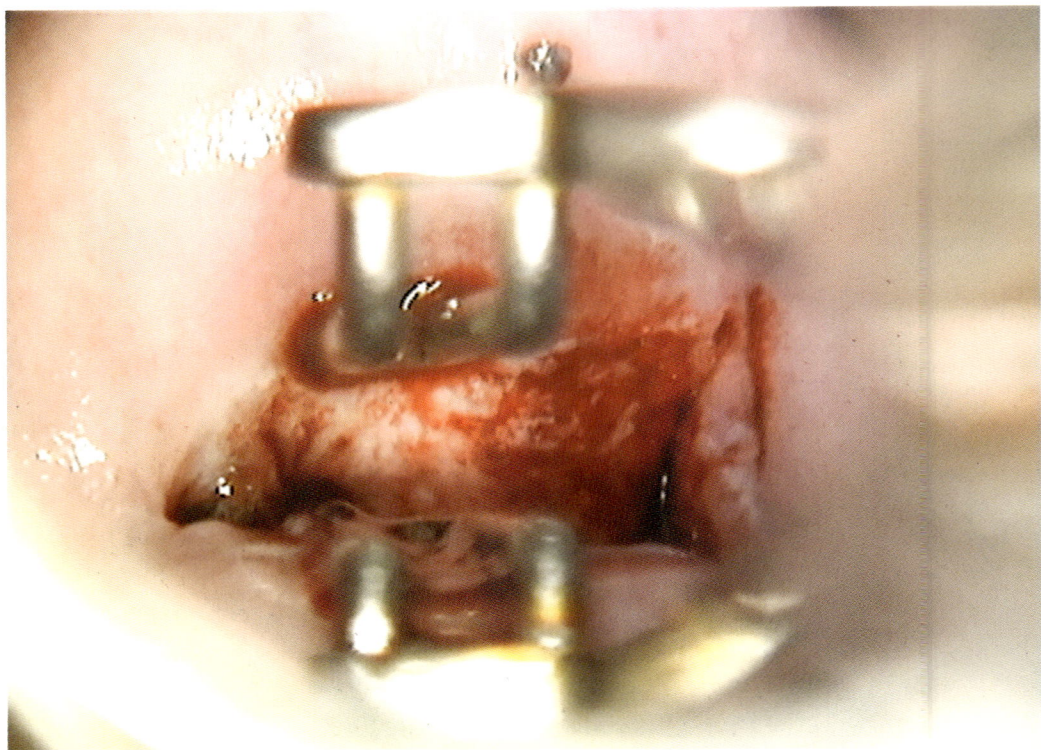

Fig. 6. 3b: Endocervical speculum examination of cervical endometriosis case, endocervical curettage HP-endometrial glands

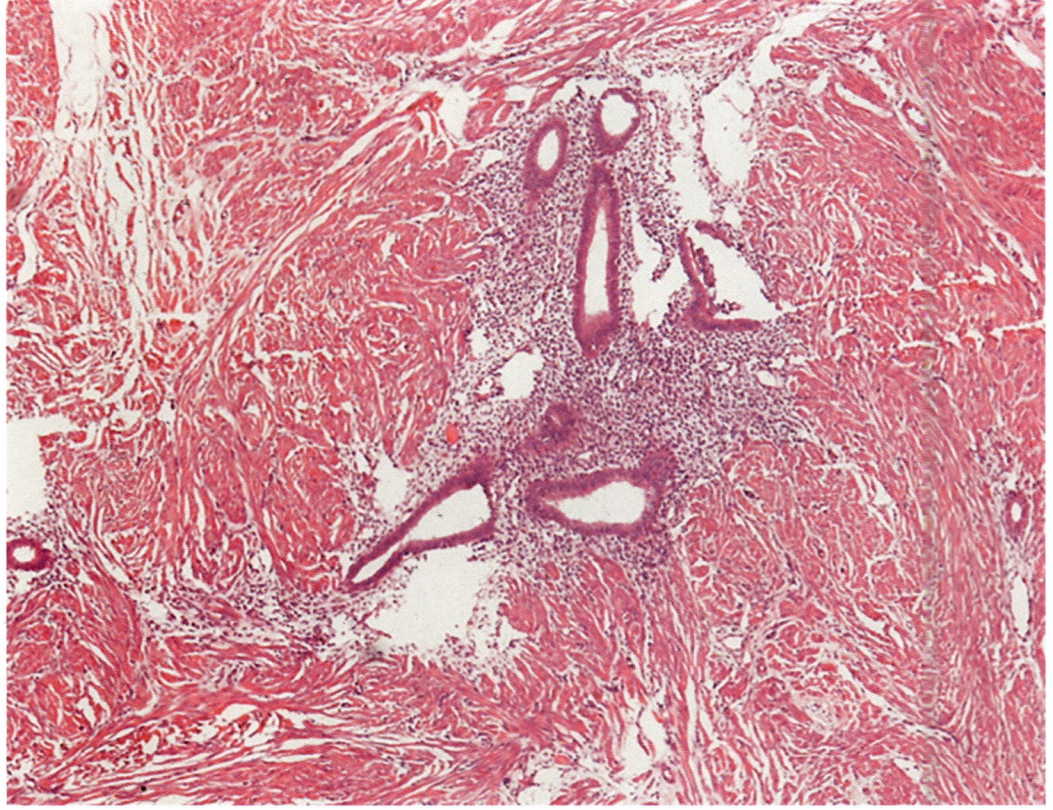

Fig. 6.3c: Histology of endometriosis

3. HYPERKERATOTIC PATCH (Fig. 6.4)

Hyperkeratotic patches are seen as white patch even without application of acetic acid due to high accumulation of keratin due to old trauma.

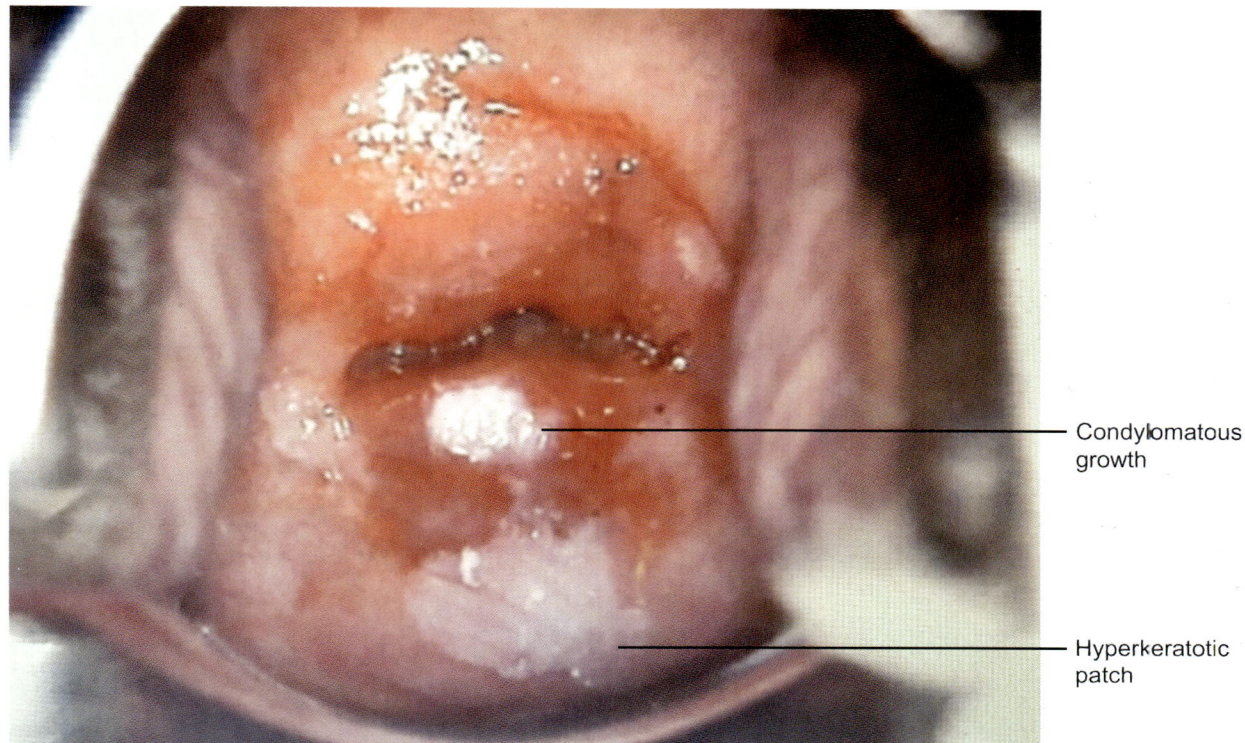

Condylomatous growth

Hyperkeratotic patch

Fig. 6.4: Hyperkeratotic patch

4. CERVICAL FIBROID

Tough fibroid growth from endocervix protruding from the cervical os (Figs 6.5a to d).

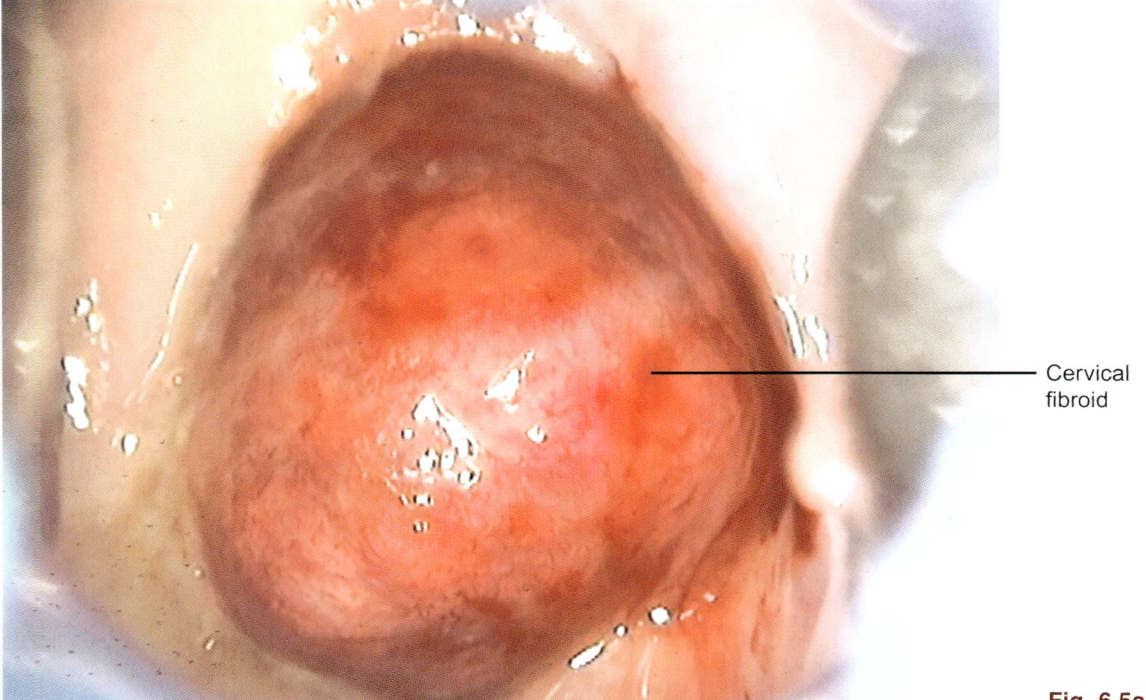

Cervical fibroid

Fig. 6.5a

Cervical fibroid removal can be performed during colposcopy examination, there is no need for GA/LA. This can be easily removed during the same sitting with ovum forceps/sponge holder forceps and given for HP.

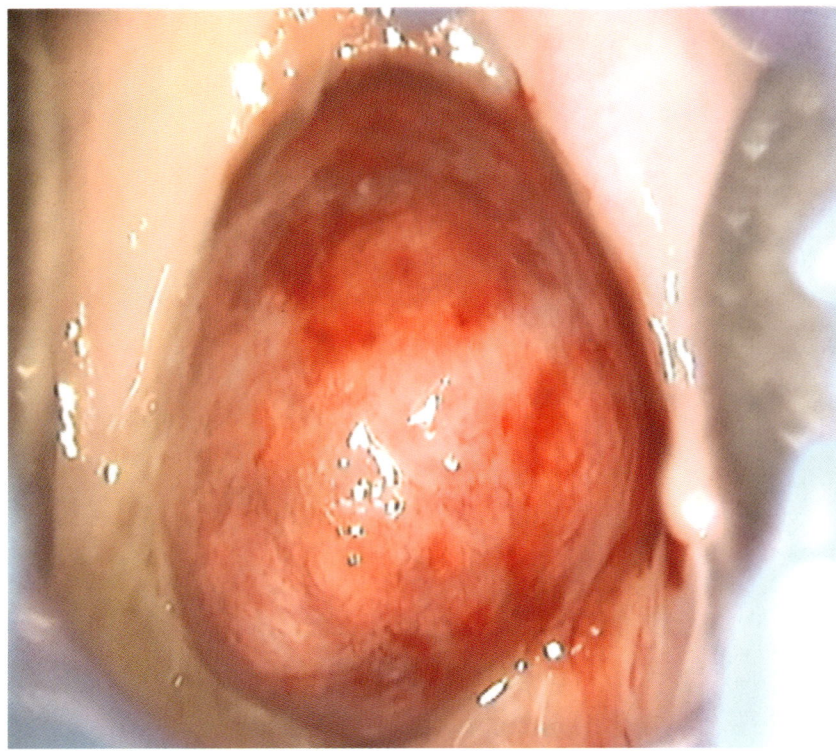

Fig. 6.5b

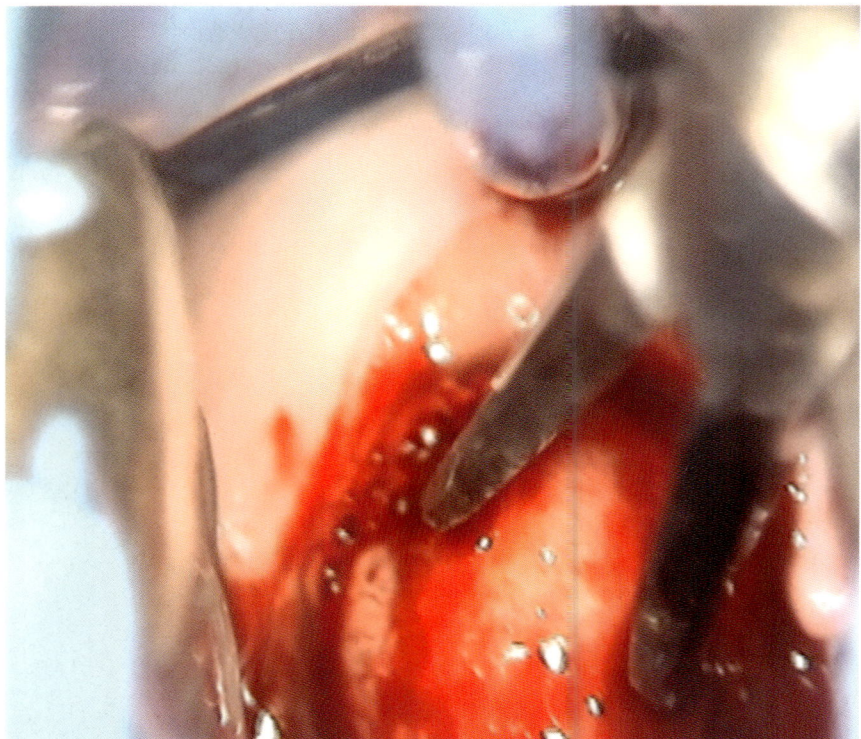

Fig. 6.5c

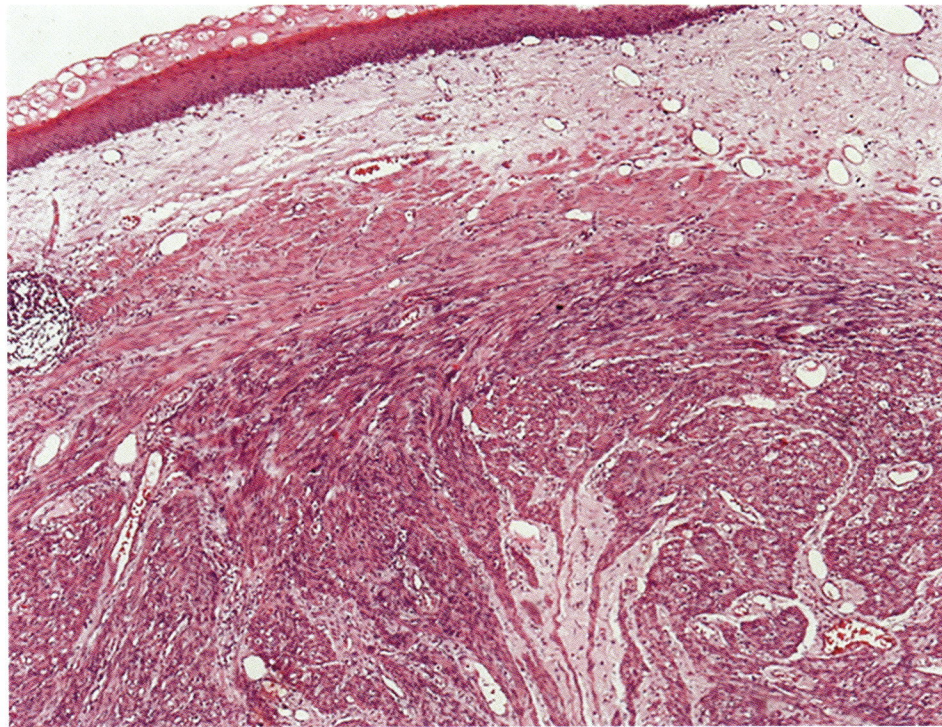

Fig. 6.5d

5. MENOPAUSAL AGE

The epithelium is thin, atrophic, lusterless. Application of acetic acid causes petechial hemorrhage (Fig. 6.6a). Due to lack of superficial stratified epithelium, Lugol's iodine uptake is negative (Fig. 6.6b).

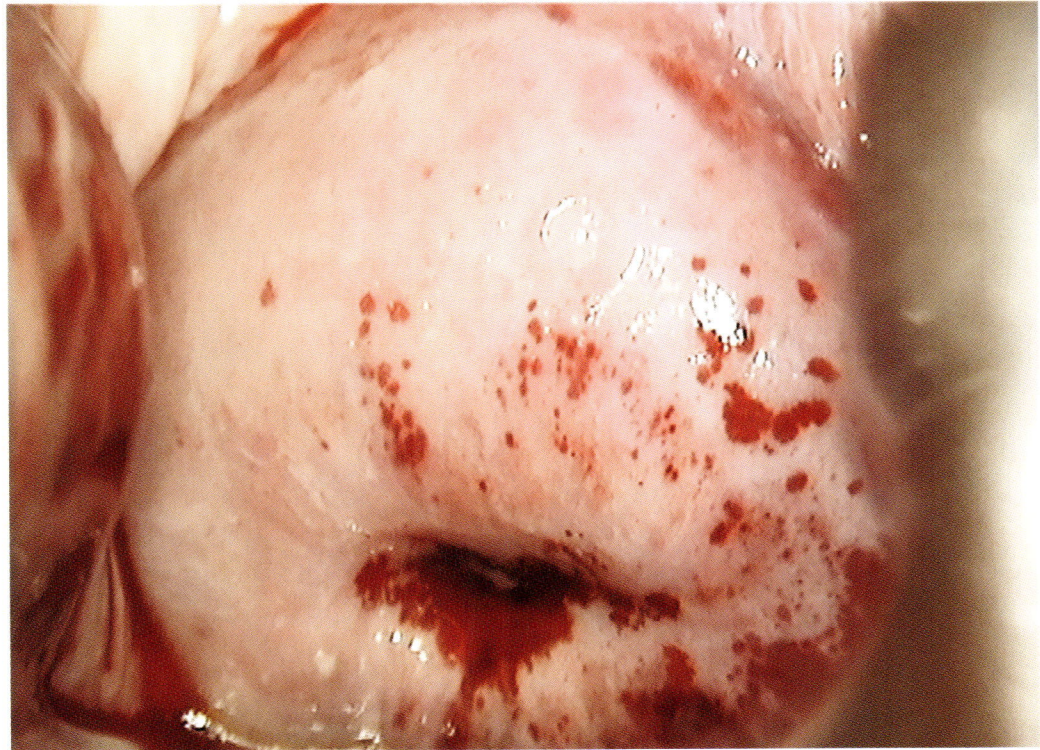

Fig. 6.6a

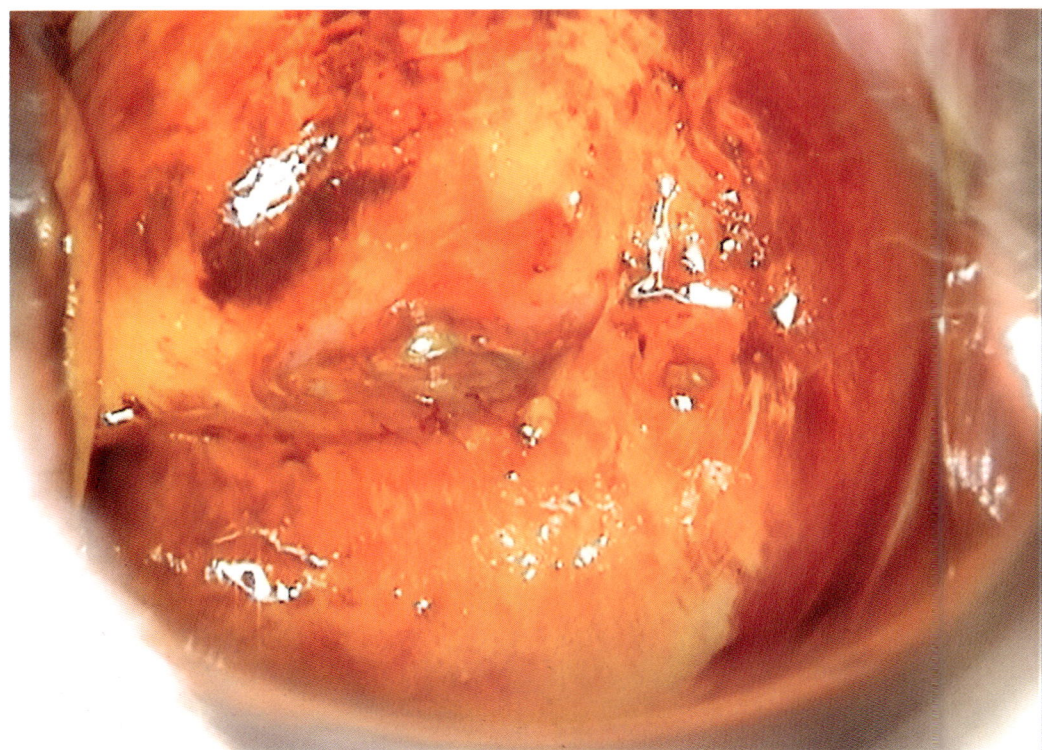

Fig. 6.6b

6. COLPOSCOPY IN CHALLENGING CASES LIKE MULLERIAN ANOMALIES (Figs 6.7a to d)

While routine examination, we may come across cases with mullerian anomalies like vaginal septum.

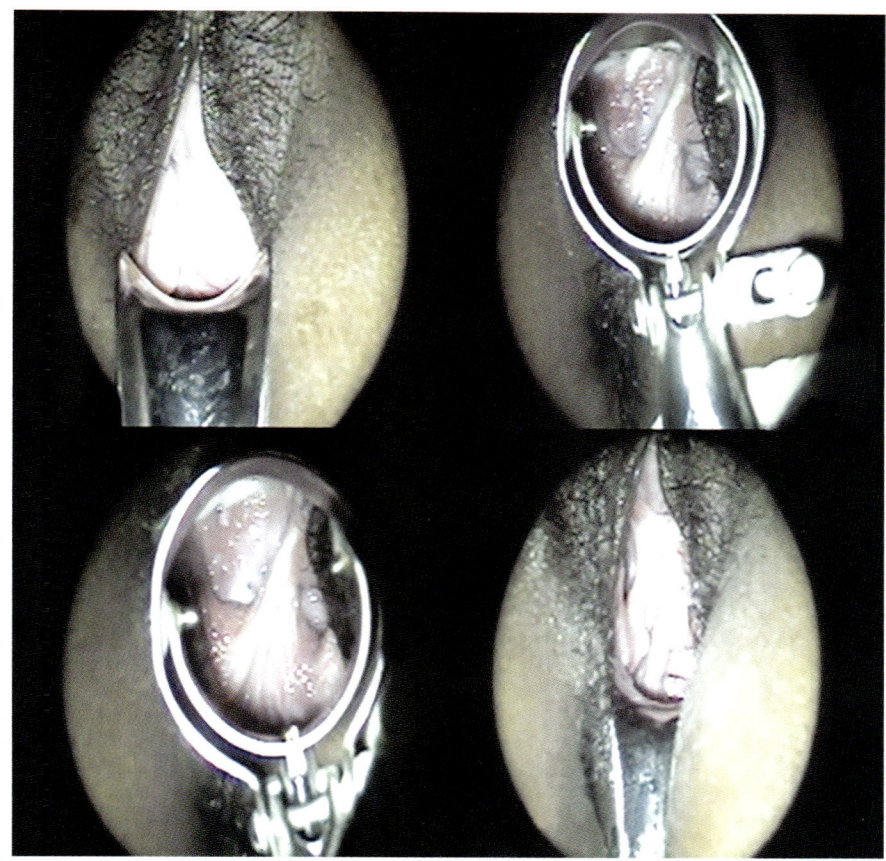

Fig. 6.7a: A complete vaginal septum

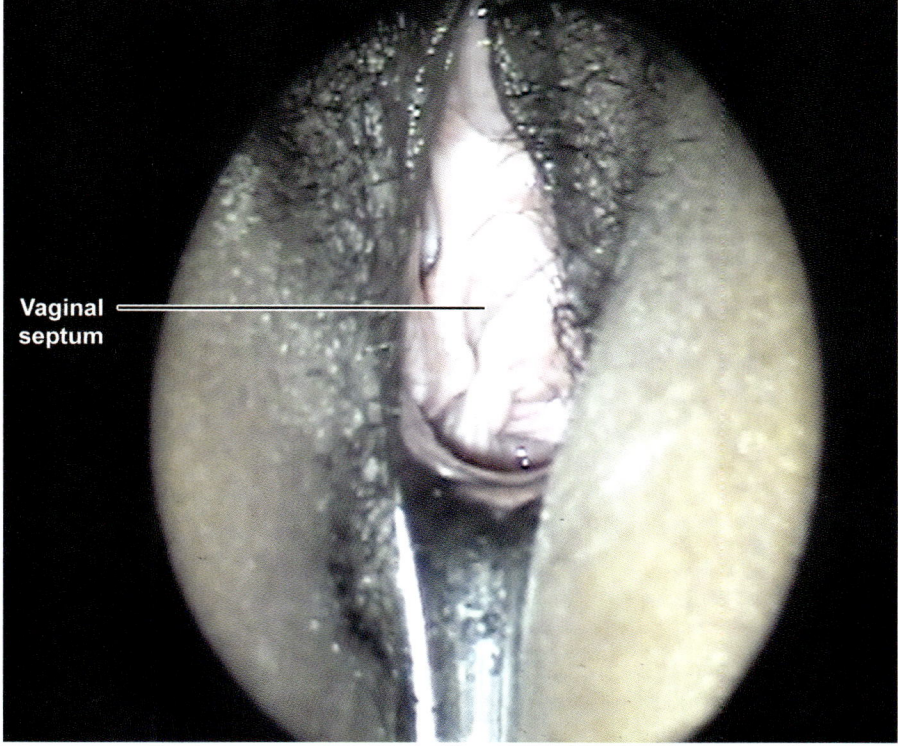

Vaginal septum

Fig. 6.7b: Complete vaginal septum noted during colposcopy examination

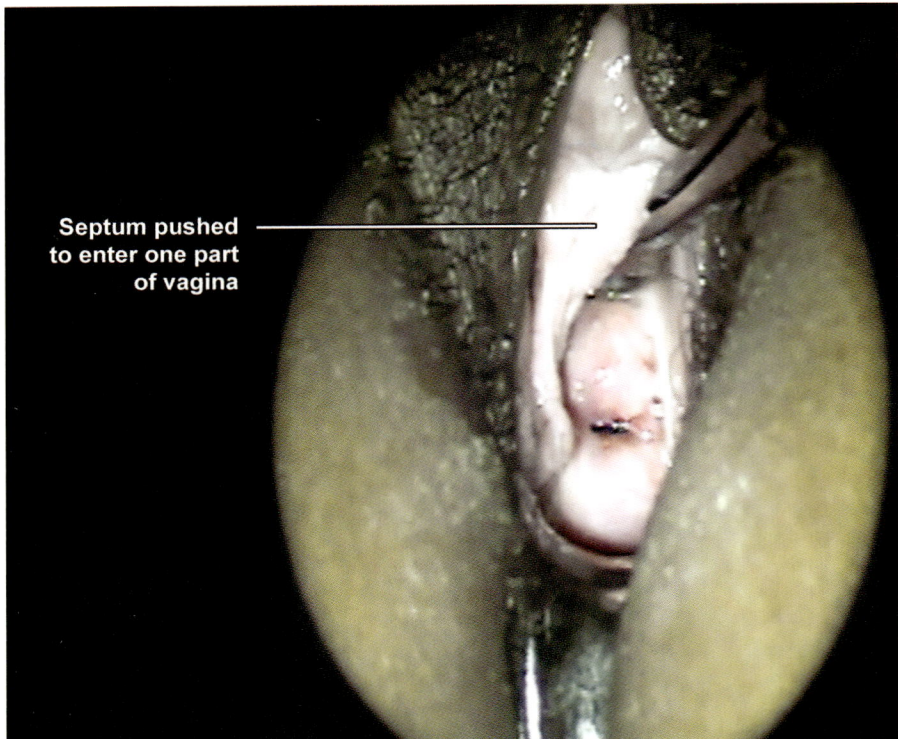

Septum pushed
to enter one part
of vagina

Fig. 6.7c: Cervix is located in one vaginal opening

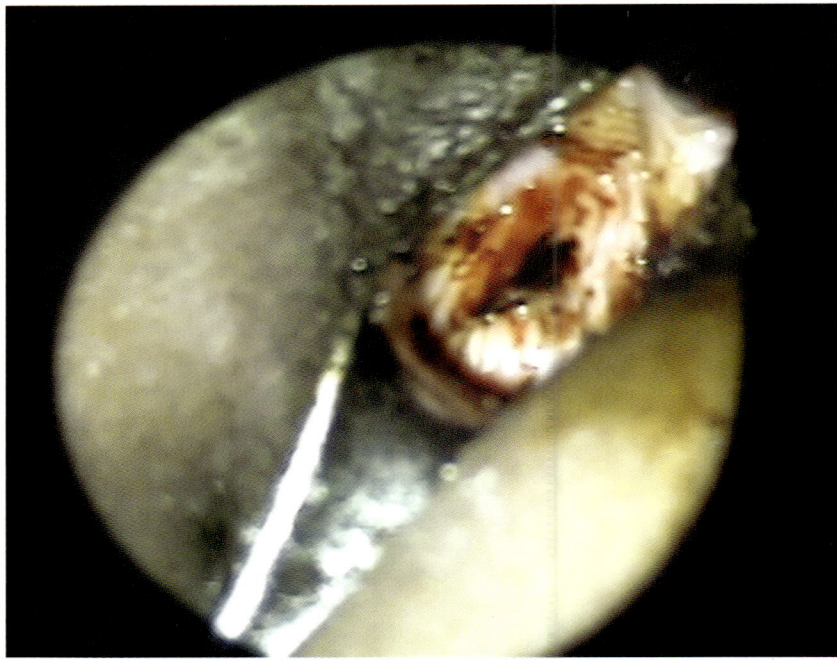

Fig. 6.7d: The second vaginal
opening is blind pouch

While performing colposcopy in such cases, one has to judiciously understand the anomaly. A through examination should be done to identify the cervix. In such cases, using of Sims vaginal speculum and anterior vaginal wall retractor is beneficial rather than Cusco's speculum.

Double cervical opening detected during colposcopy (Figs 6.7e to g).

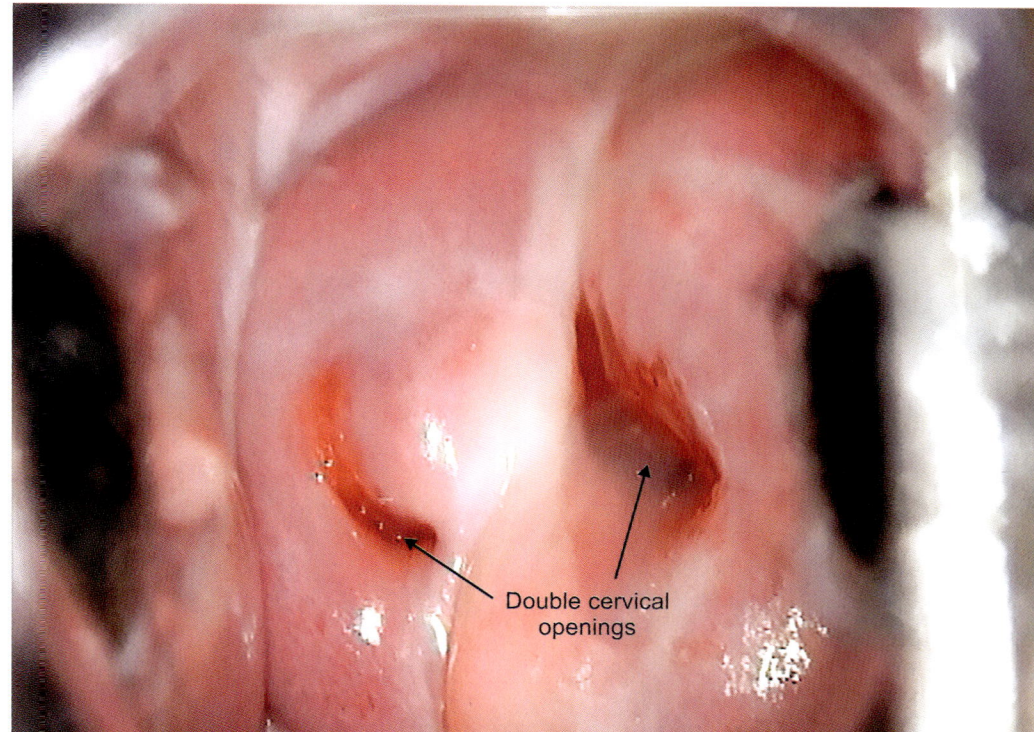

Double cervical openings

Fig. 6.7e

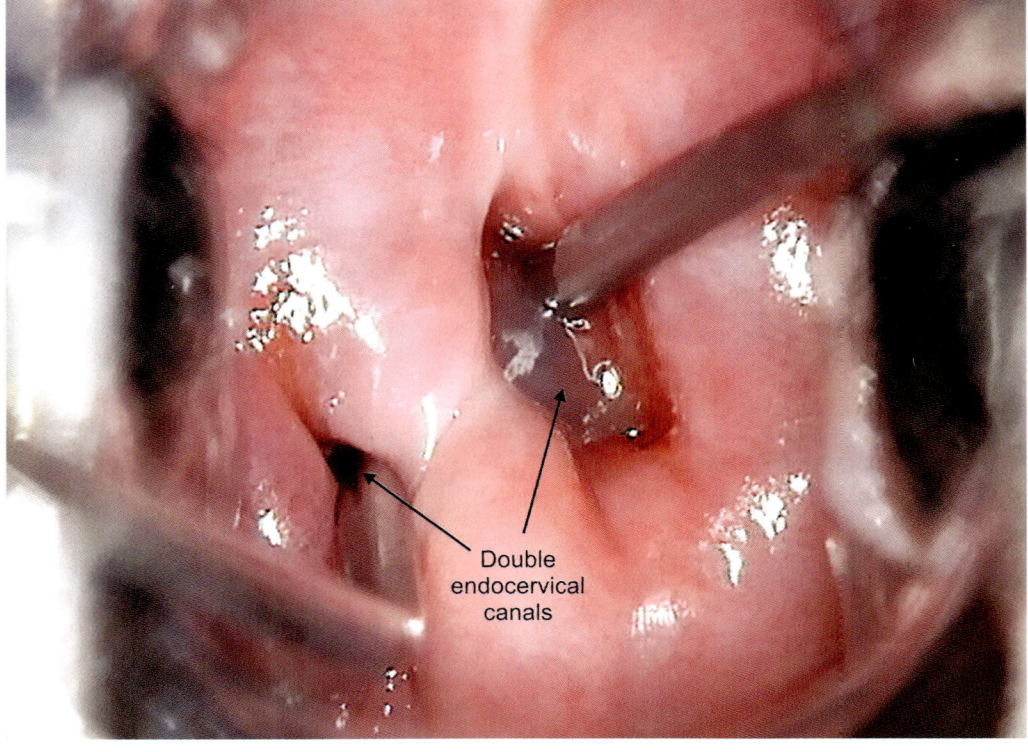

Double endocervical canals

Fig. 6.7f

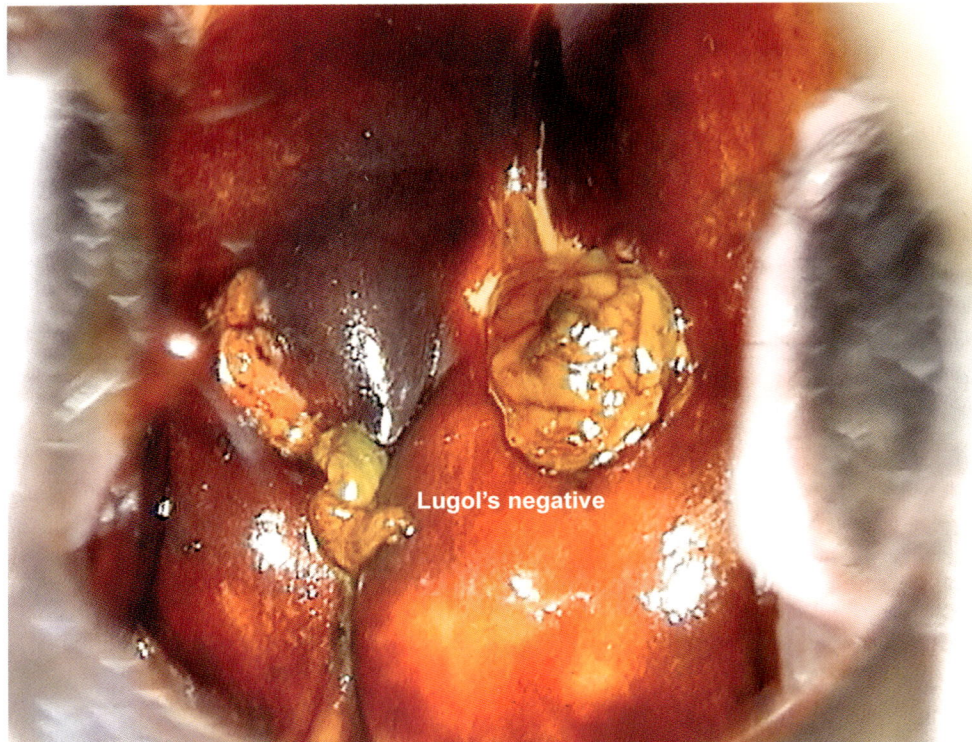

Lugol's negative

Fig. 6.7g

Real-time pelvis ultrasound report (TVS) of the case discussed above from Figs 6.7e to g
- Anatomically normal urinary bladder. Bicornuate uterus noted with two uterine cervix represents bicornuate bicollis uterus.
- Right uterine horn measuring 5.4 × 2.8 × 2.7 cm. No evidence of focal lesion. Myometrial echotexture is smooth and homogenous. The right horn endometrium is homogenous, measures 4 mm.
- Left uterine horn measuring 5.8 × 3.0 × 2.6 cm. No evidence of focal lesion. Myometrial echotexture is smooth and homogenous. The left horn endometrium is homogenous, measures 3.8 mm.
- Both the ovaries are well visualized and appear normal. No evdience of any ovarian or adnexal mass noted.
- The right ovary measures 2.8 × 2.2 cm. Dominant follicle of size 13 mm seen in right ovary.
- The left ovary measures 2.5 × 2.2 cm.
- Cervix appears unremarkable
- No e/o free fluid in pouch of Douglas.

Conclusion
- Bicornuate bicollis uterus. Suggest—MRI pelvis correlation to rule out longitudinal vaginal septum
- Normal ovaries and adnexa
- No other significant abnomrality is seen.

7. COLPOSCOPY IN PREGNANCY

Colposcopy is usually avoided during pregnancy. Pregnancy exaggerates the lesion. Hence it is advisable to do a repeat colposcopy during PNC 4th–6th month. Usually the lesion regresses. Cytology can be done in case of suspected conditions.

In this case, a high grade lesion was detected during 1st month of missing her period. On HP examination, it revealed CIN 2/1 lesion. Cytology showed NILM (Figs 6.8a and b).

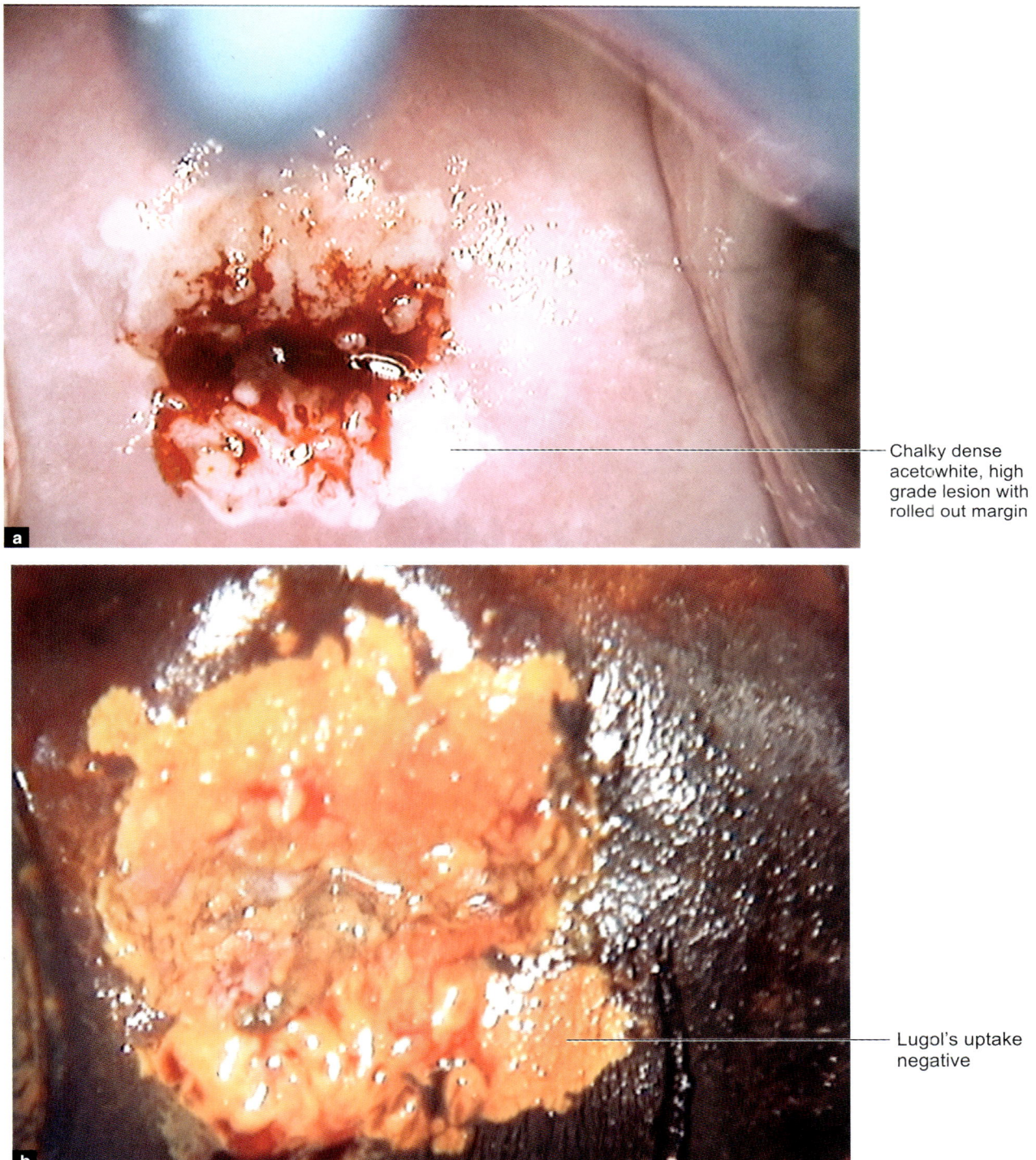

Chalky dense acetowhite, high grade lesion with rolled out margin

Lugol's uptake negative

Figs 6.8a and b: HSIL detected in pregnancy

Colposcopy was repeated again in this case at 4th month PNC. The lesion showed regression to LSIL. Pregnancy exaggerates the lesion due to high vascular state (Figs 6.9a and b)

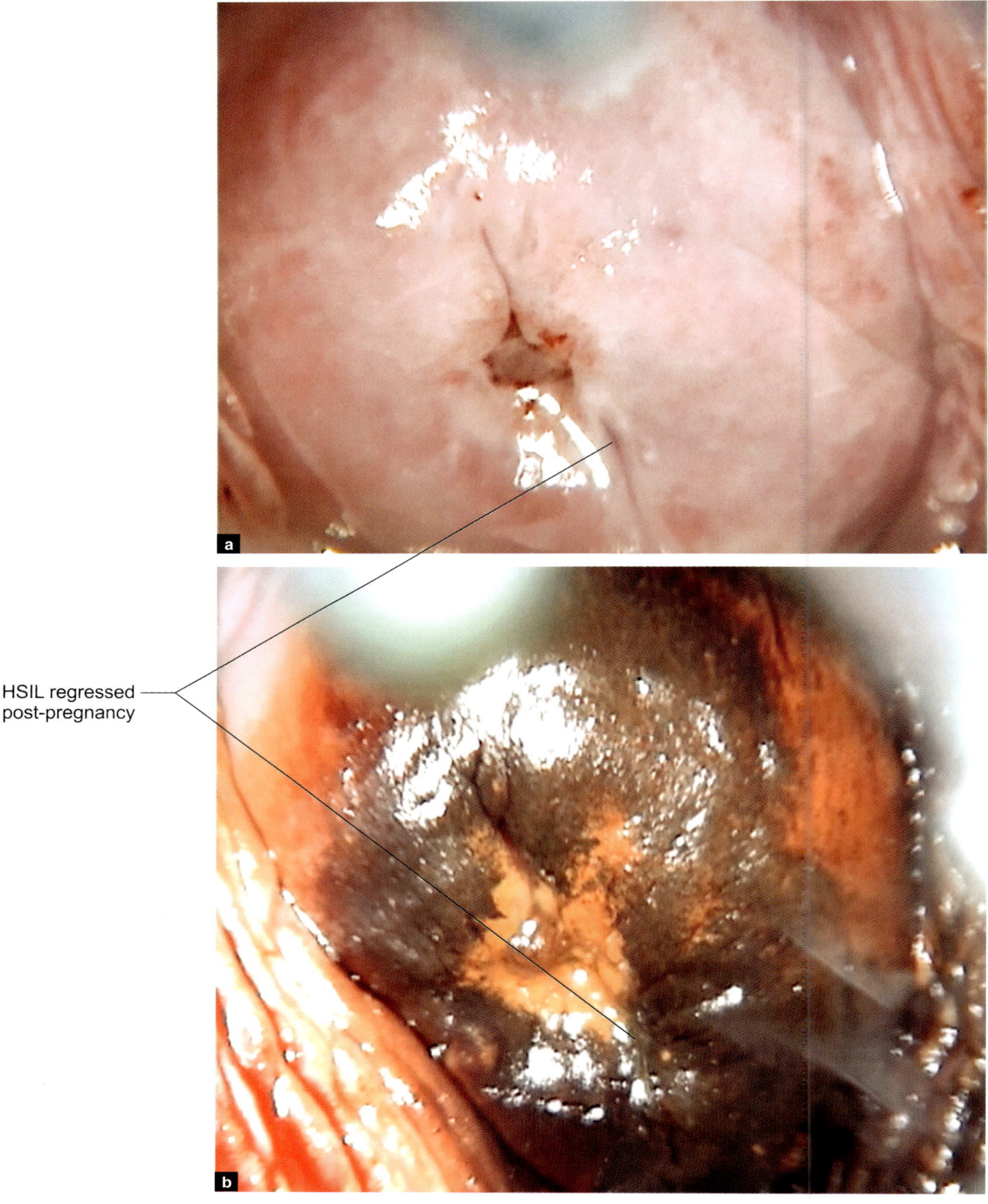

HSIL regressed post-pregnancy

Figs 6.9a and b: Post-pregnancy—LSIL

8. INFECTED NABOTHIAN CYSTS MIMICKING CERVICAL GROWTH

Rarely multiple nabothian cysts, which are long-standing and infected, appear as cervical growth. The tree branching blood vessel pattern on the nabothian cyst is very useful for identification. Manipulation of such lesion helps to resolve the condition (Figs 6.10a and b).

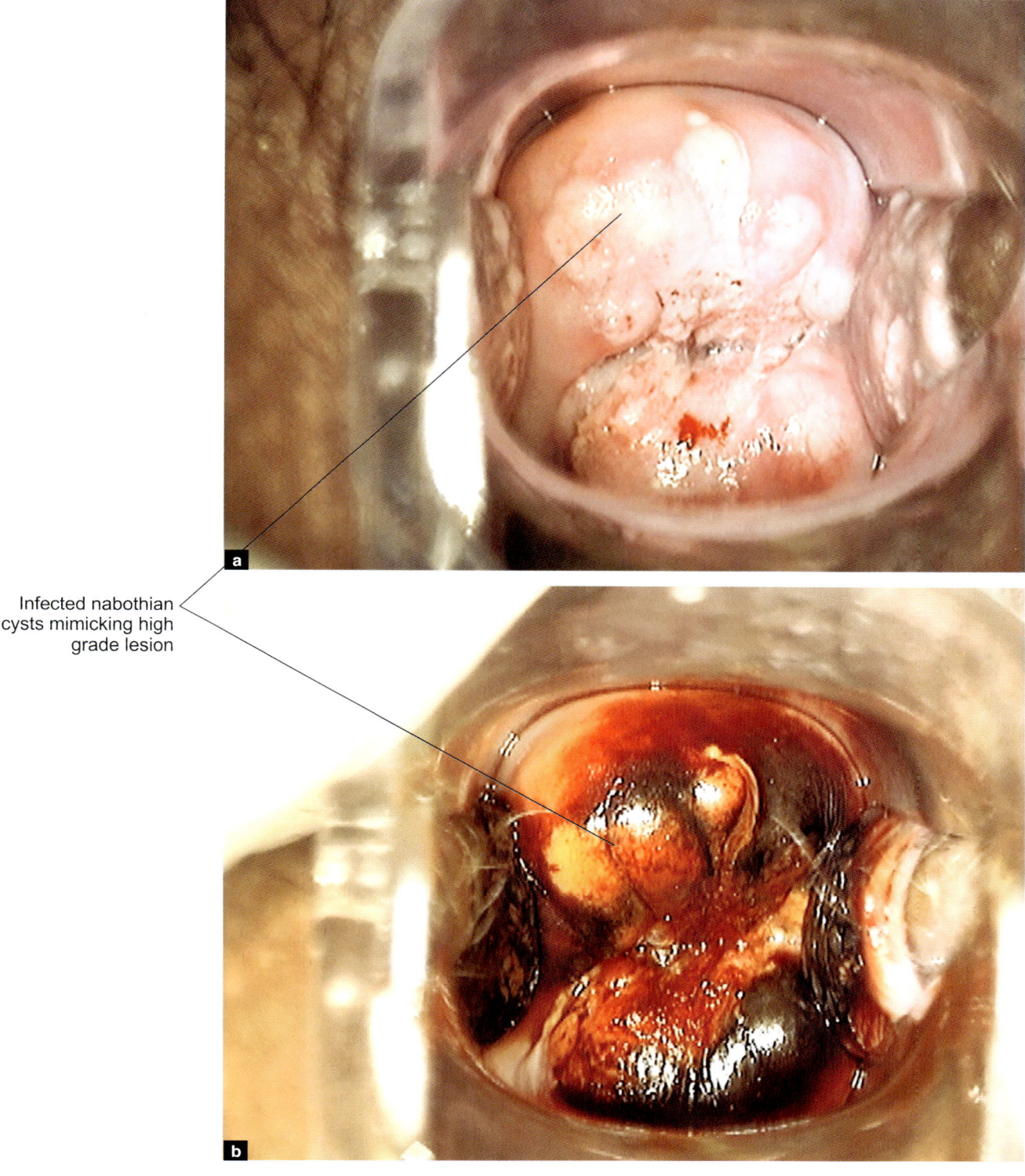

Infected nabothian cysts mimicking high grade lesion

Figs 6.10a and b: Nabothian cysts

9. HERPES SIMPLEX INFECTION (Figs 6.11a to d)

Herpes simplex type 1 is usually seen affecting oral mucosa,very commonly seen in oral sex practise. Herpes type 2 lesions are commoin in genital area.Very rare to find herpes simplex type 1 lesions in genital area. This is detected in scrape sent for multiplex PCR STI Panel detection (Figs 6.11a to d).

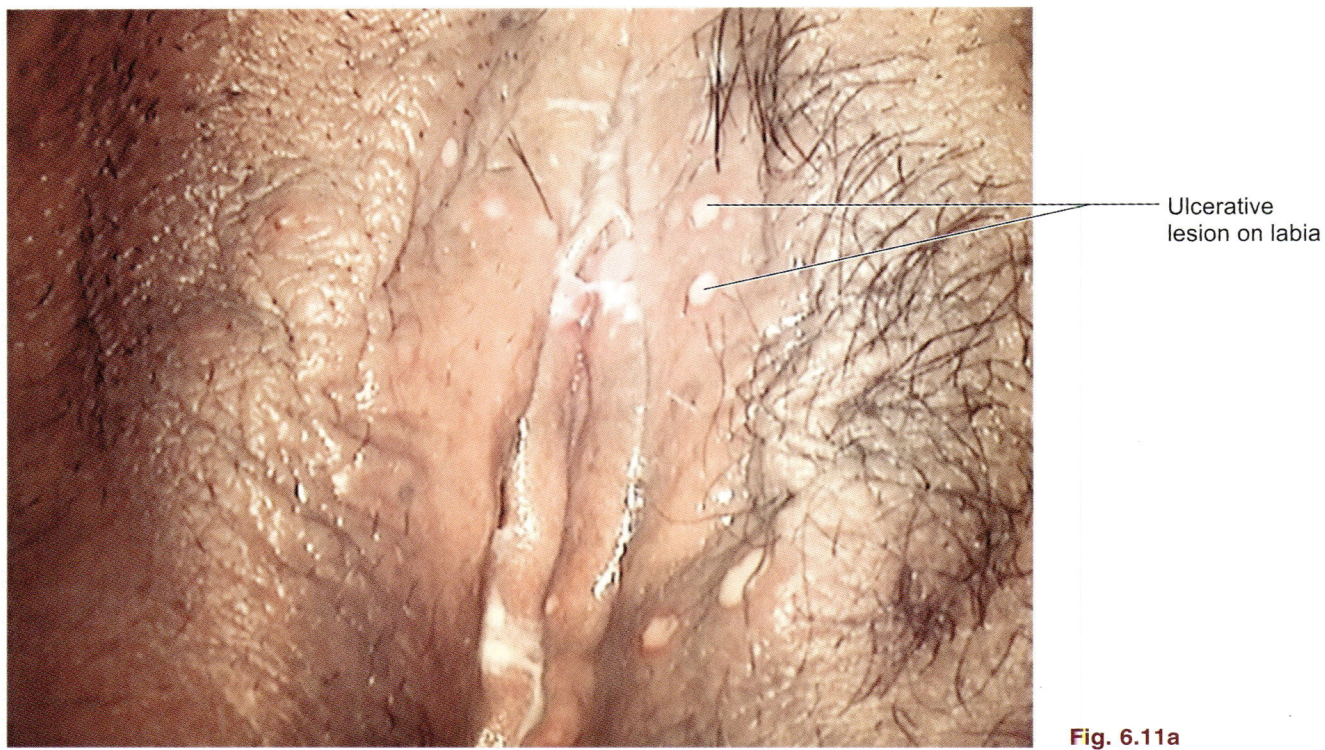

Ulcerative lesion on labia

Fig. 6.11a

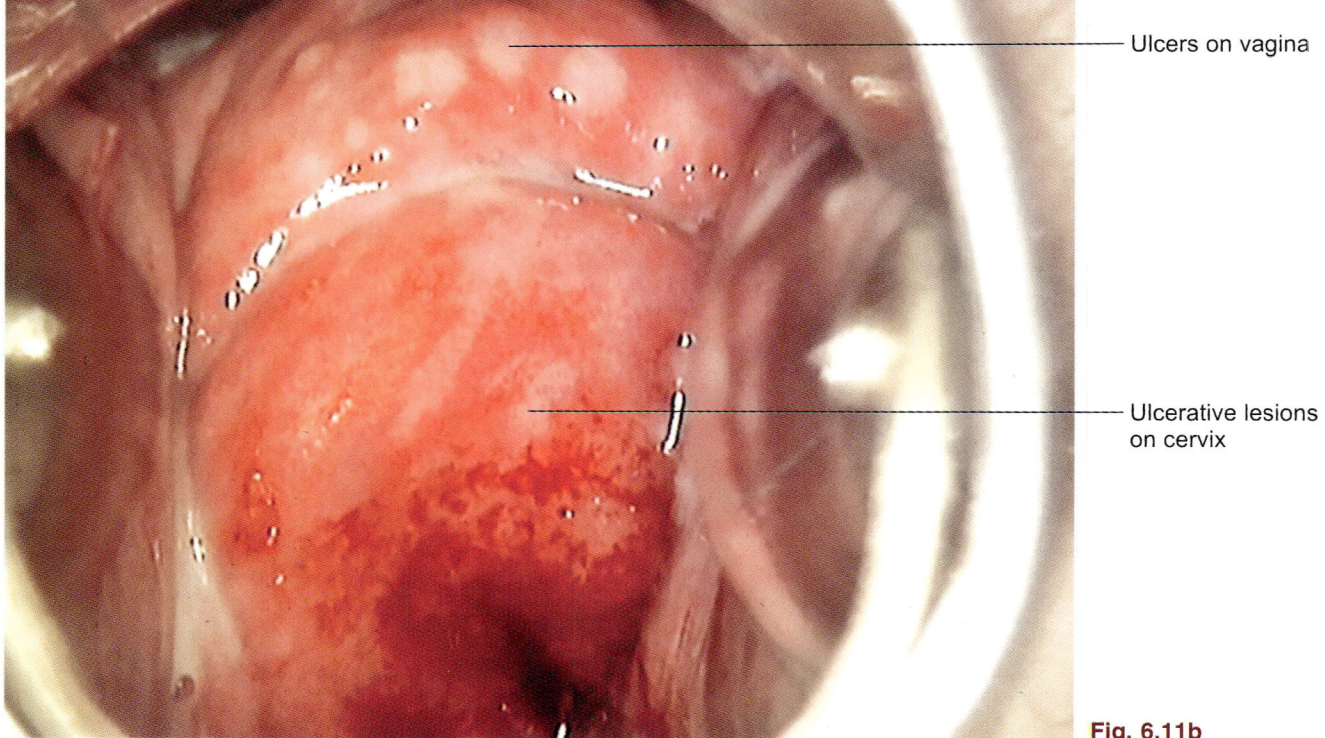

Ulcers on vagina

Ulcerative lesions on cervix

Fig. 6.11b

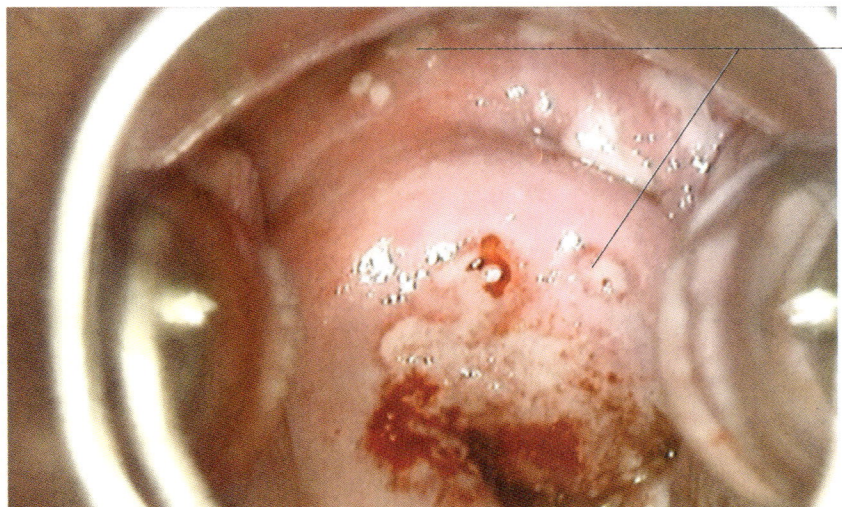

Ulcers have become prominent on 5% acetic acid

Fig. 6.11c

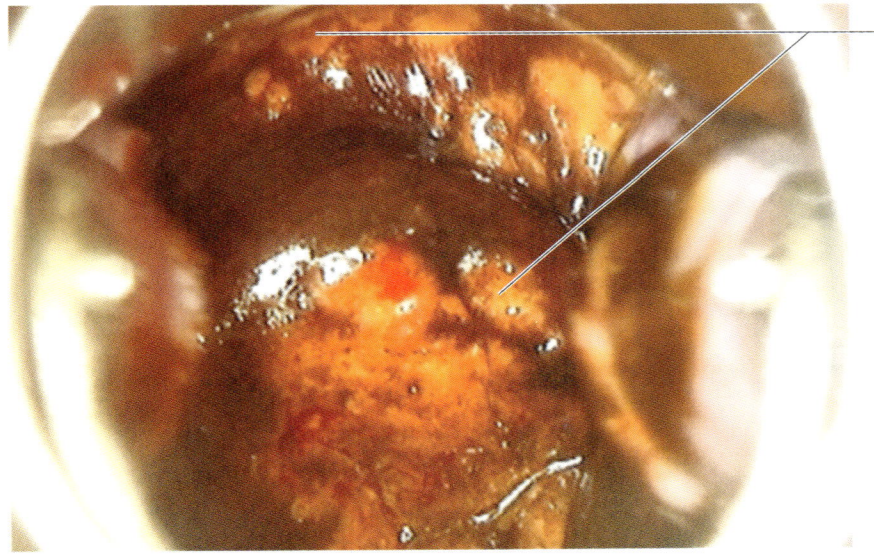

The lesions are Lugol's negative

Fig. 6.11d

Nomenclatures and Scoring System

INTRODUCTION

Scoring system is required for ease of reporting. There are various systems of reporting and nomenclatures, viz;

- IFCPC nomenclature
- Modified Reid scoring
- Swede scoring.

The elaborative explanation of various scoring systems is provided in author's *Textbook on Colposcopy in Practical Gynaecology*. This chapter explains Swede scoring system which is adopted by WHO/IARC and various organizations globally.

Strander *et al* from Sweden proposed a new scoring system in 2005.

The Swede scoring system includes lesion size as a variable in addition to the four original variables described in Reid's colposcopic index.

The Swede score			
Swede score	*0*	*1*	*2*
Acetowhite	Zero or transperent	Shady milky white neither transperent nor opaque	Distinct opaque white
Margins/surface	Diffuse	Sharp but irregular jagged, geographic satellites	Sharp, even difference in surface level, includes cuffing
Vessel	Fine regular	Absent	Coarse or atypical
Lession size	<5 mm	5–15 mm 2 quadrants	15 mm or 3 to 4 quadrants or undefined endocervically
Iodine staining	Brown	Fainty or patchy yellow	Distinct yellow
Total Score 10			

Total Swede Score 10

0, 1	Atypical HPV infection
2, 3, 4	CIN 1
5, 6, 7	CIN 2
8, 9, 10	CIN 3

UNDERSTANDING OF SWEDE SCORING WITH VARIOUS CASE DISCUSSIONS

1. 32-yr-old with C/O Irregular Menses

Colposcopy description: Adequate, SCJ visible, TZ 1, thin opaque milky white acetowhite lesions with sharp, jagged geographical pattern abutting from SCJ with fine punctations, with size less than 5 mm occupying one quadrant and patchy yellow on application of Lugol's iodine (Figs 7.1a to d).

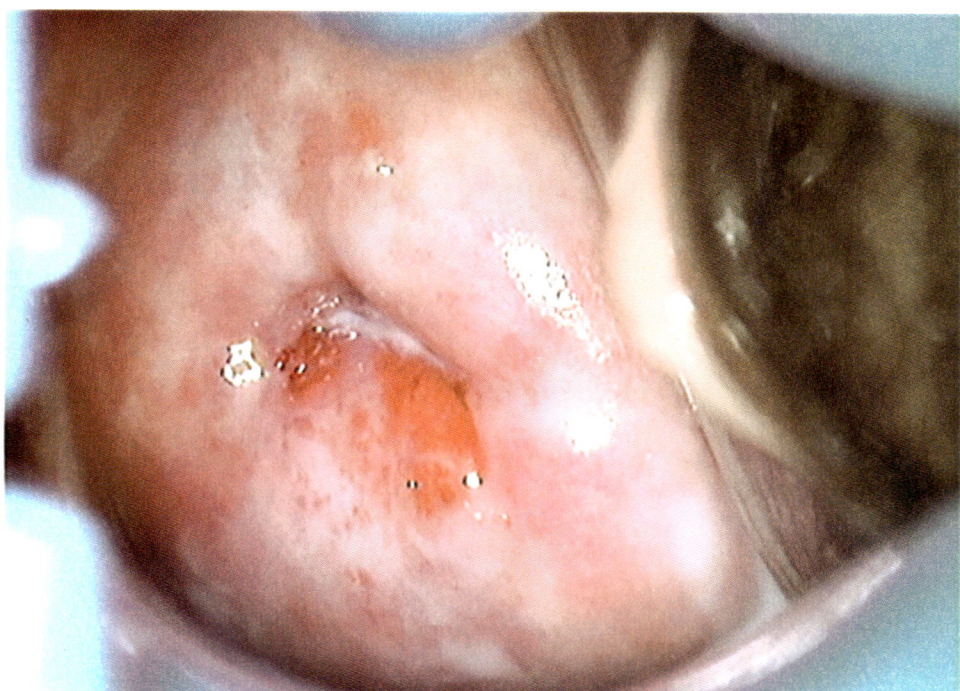

Fig. 7.1a: Normal saline

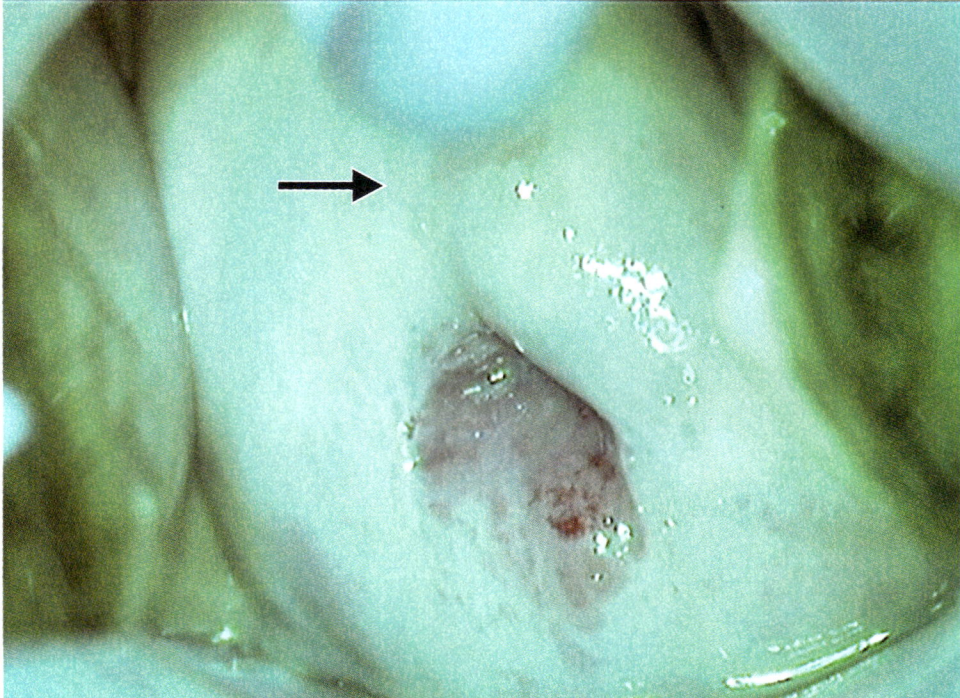

Fig. 7.1b: Green filter showing fine punctations

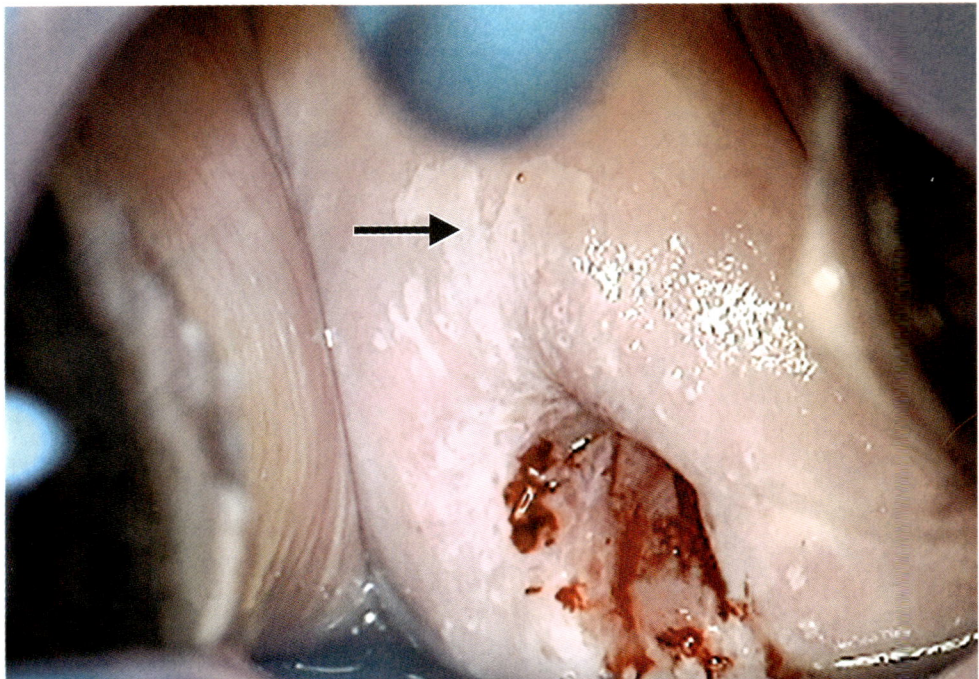

Fig. 7.1c: 5% acetic acid—thin opaque milky white lesion with sharp, jagged geographical pattern abutting from SCJ, having fine punctations and less than 5 mm, occupying one quadrant

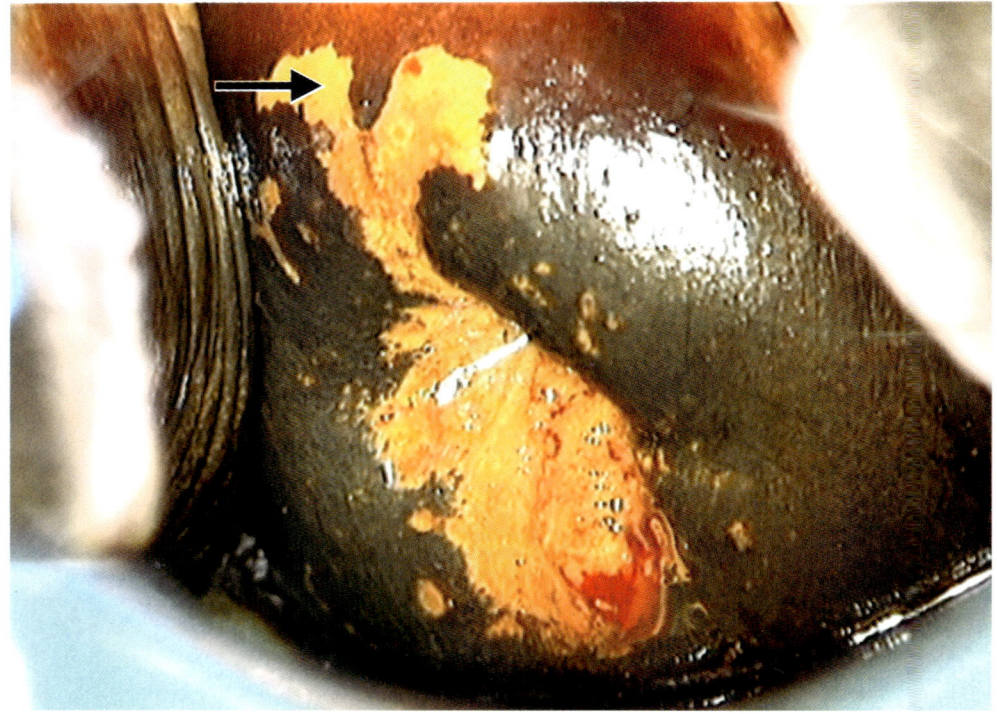

Fig. 7.1d: Lugol's iodine—variegated patchy yellow

Swede—1 + 1 + 0 + 0 + 1 = 3
CIN 1/LSIL
Cytology—Inflammatory smear
HP—Chronic cervicitis

2. 36-yr-old with White Discharge

Colposcopy description: Adequate, SCJ visible, TZ 1, thin milky white acetowhite lesions neither transparent nor opaque, abutting from SCJ within the TZ with jagged margins, having fine mosaics, occupying 2 quadrants and patchy yellow on Lugol's iodine application.

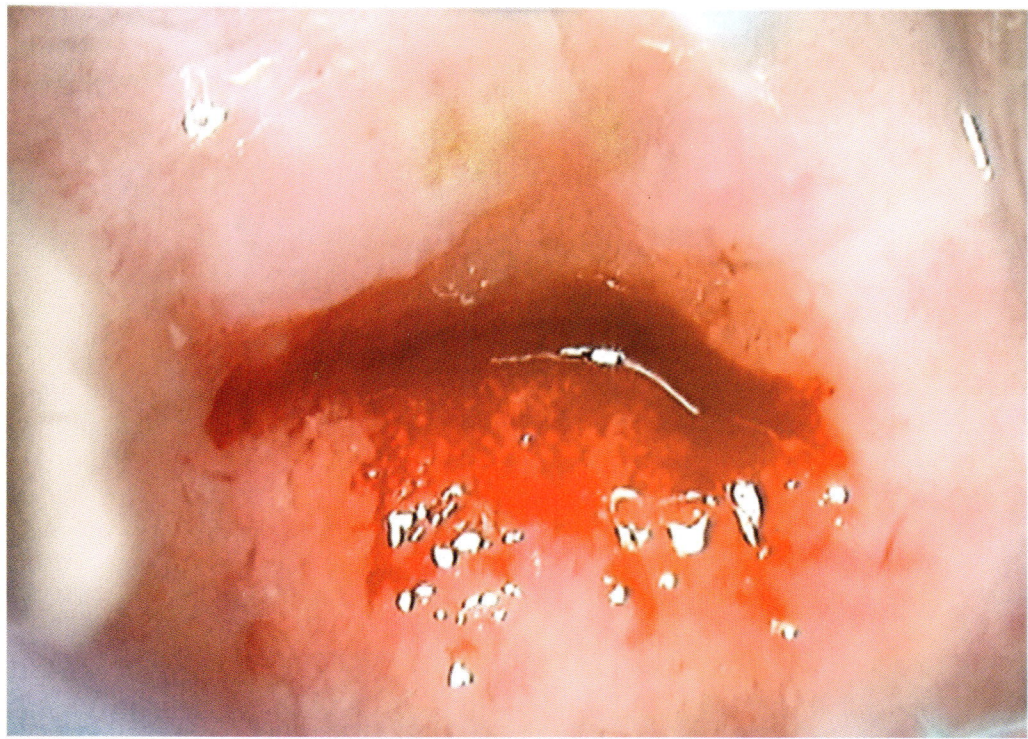

Fig. 7.2a: Normal saline

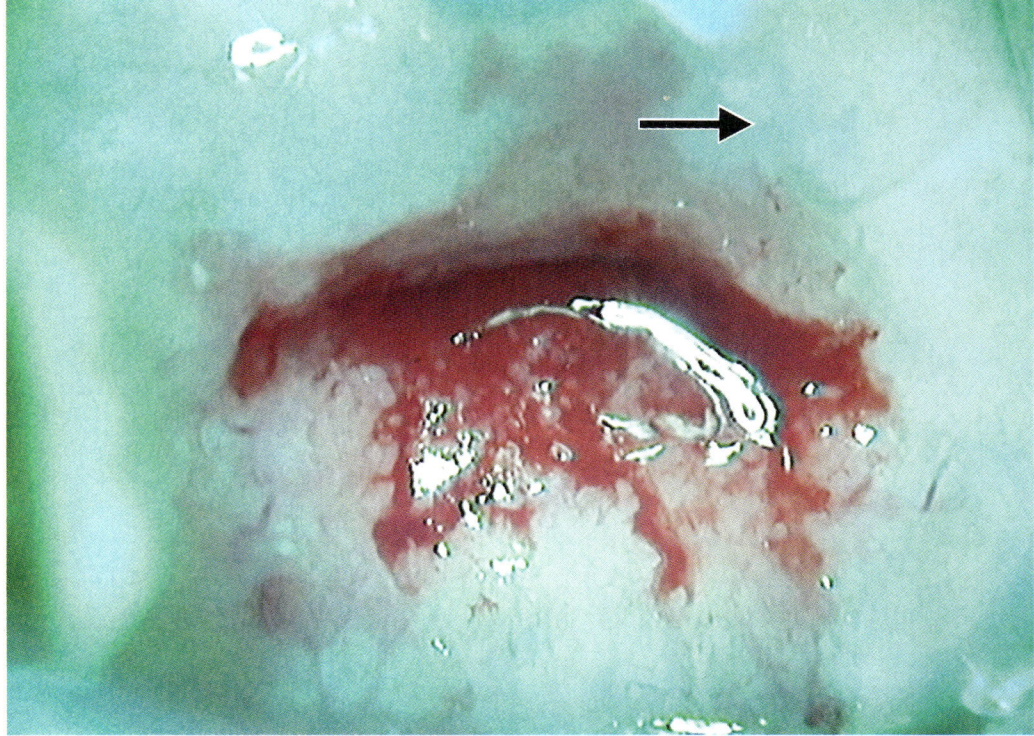

Fig. 7.2b: Green filter showing fine mosaics

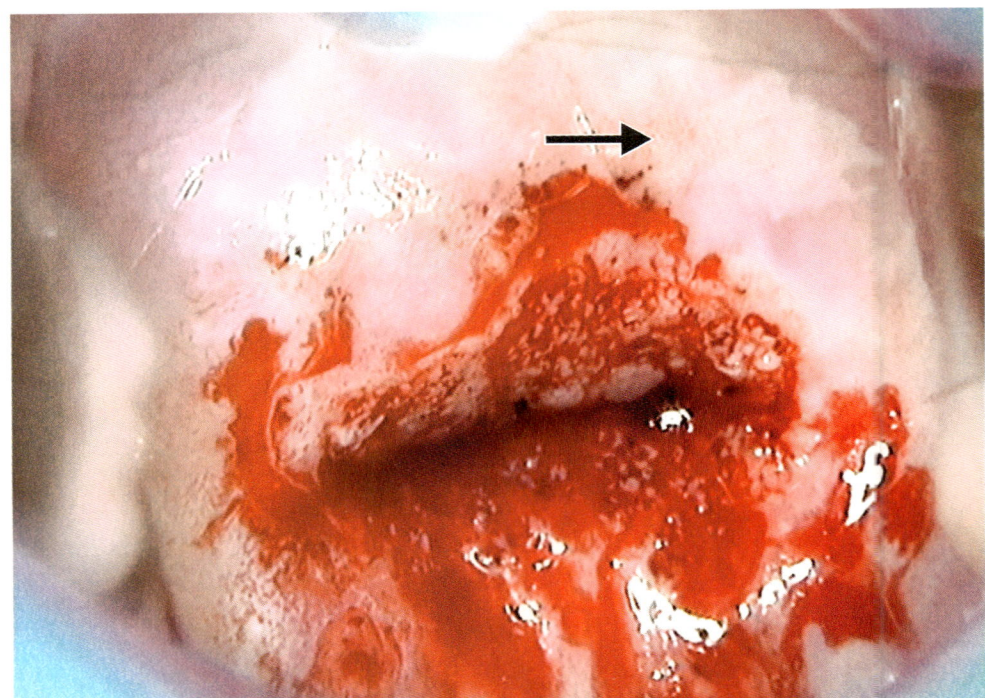

Fig. 7.2c: 5% acetic acid—thin milky white acetowhite lesions neither transparent nor opaque, abutting from SCJ within the TZ with jagged margins, having fine mosaics, occupying 2 quadrants

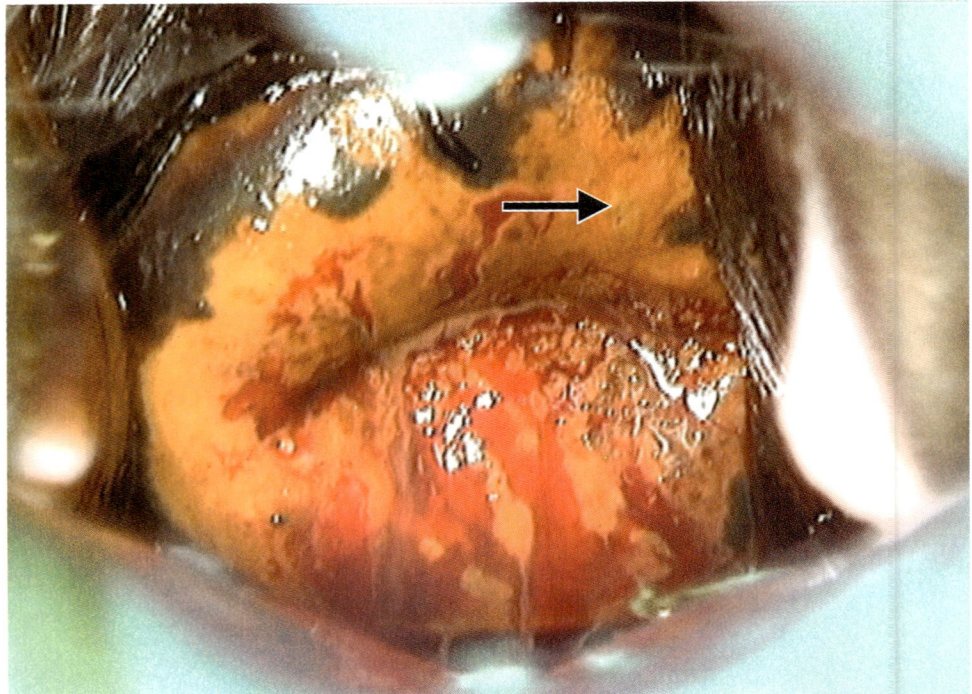

Fig. 7.2d: Lugol's iodine—variegated patchy yellow

Swede—1 + 1 + 0 + 1 + 1 = 4
CIN 1/LSIL
Cytology—CIN 1
HP—CIN 1

3. 32-yr-old with White Discharge

Colposcopy description: Adequate, SCJ visible, TZ 1, distinct opaque acetowhite lesion with sharp raised margin, coarse mosaics, abutting from SCJ, occupying 2 quadrants and patchy yellow on Lugol's iodine application.

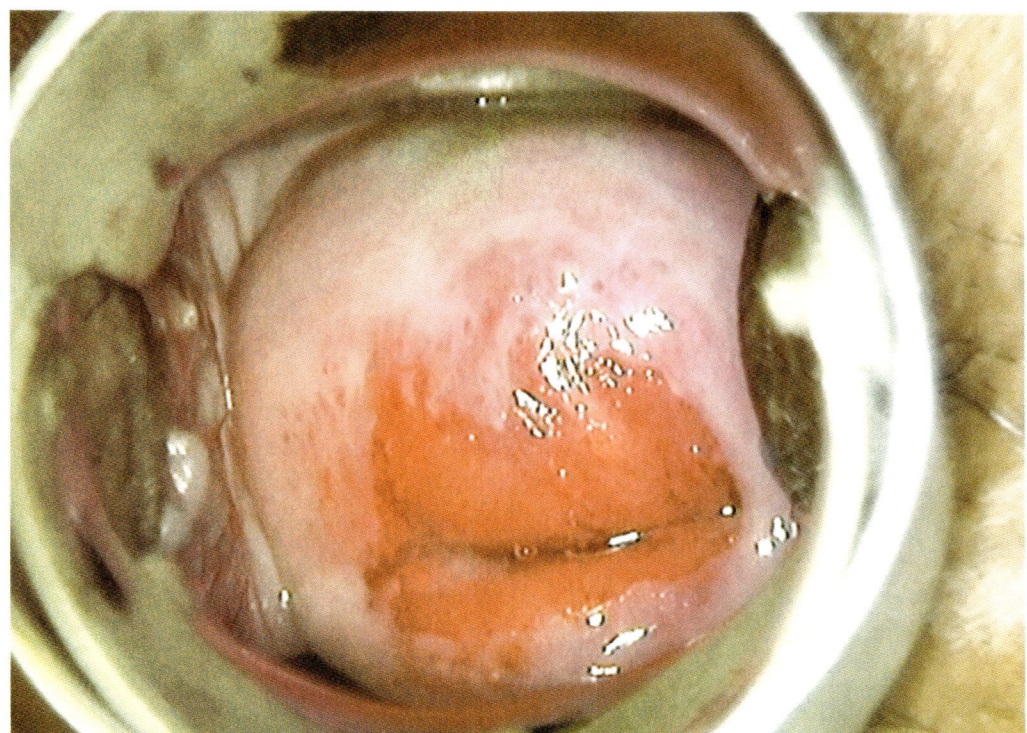

Fig. 7.3a: Normal saline

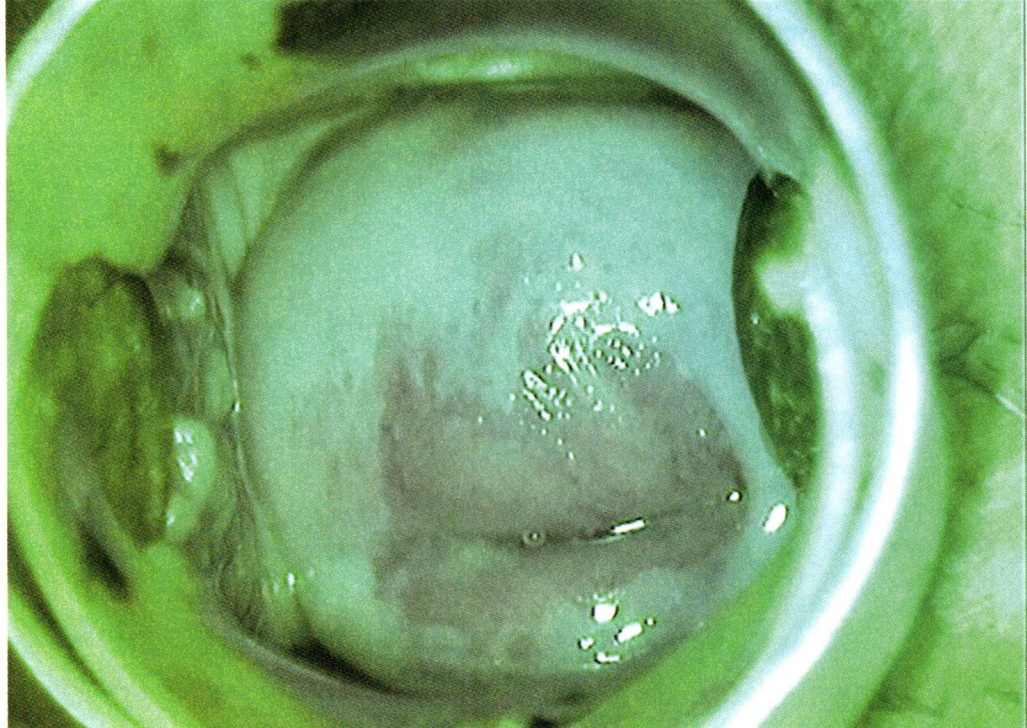

Fig. 7.3b: Green filter

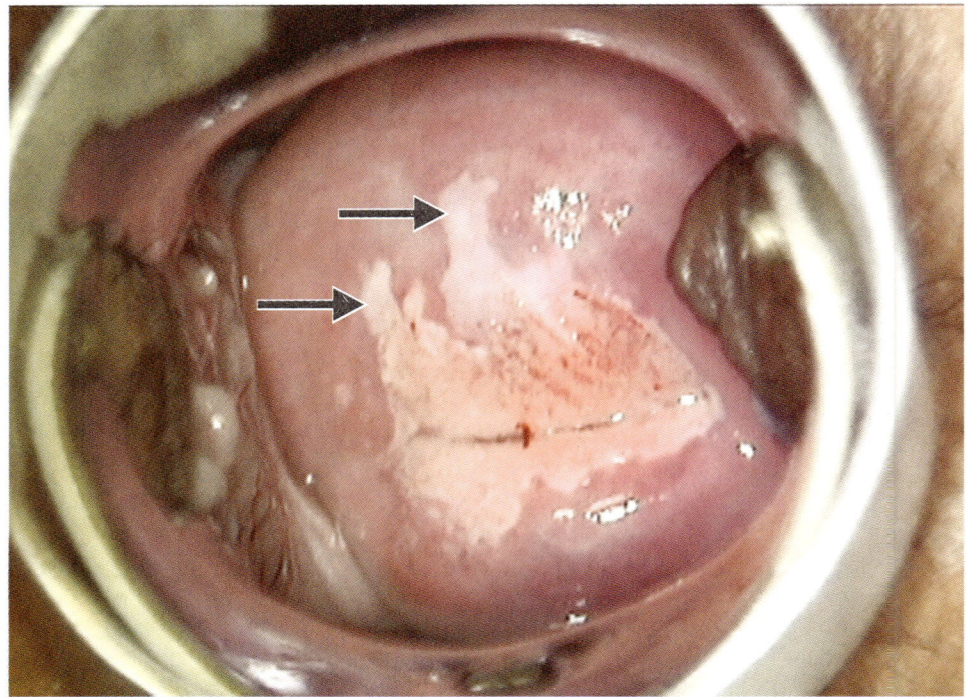

Fig. 7.3c: 5% acetic acid—distinct opaque acetowhite lesion with sharp raised margin, coarse mosaics, abutting from SCJ, occupying 2 quadrants

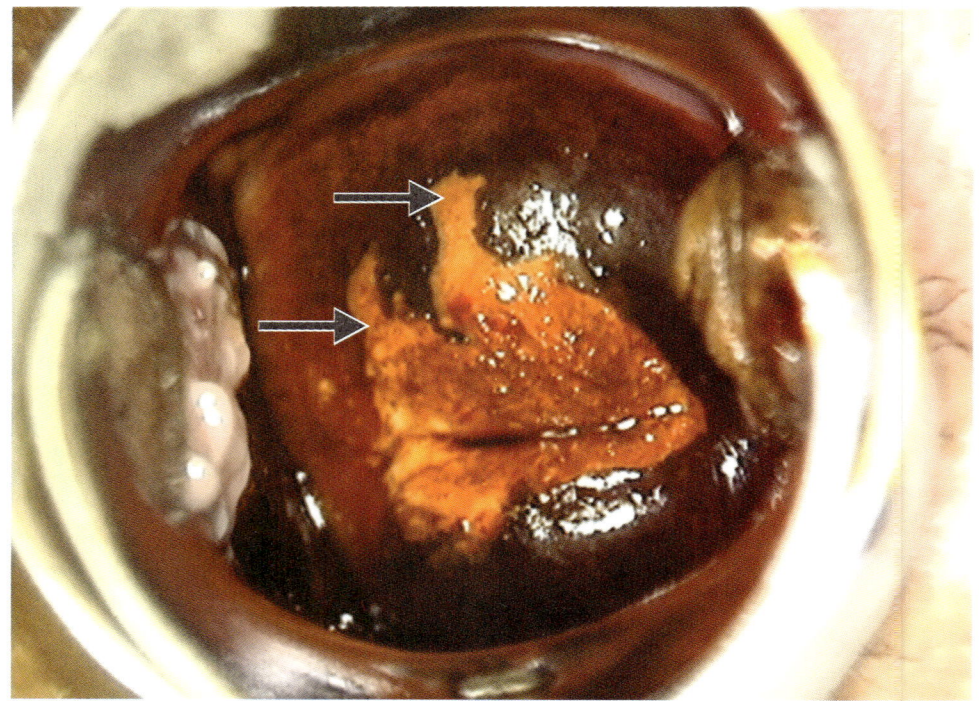

Fig. 7.3d: Lugol's iodine—variegated patchy yellow

Swede—2 + 2 + 2 + 1 + 1 = 8
CIN 3/HSIL
Cytology—CIN 2
HP—CIN 2

4. 42-yr-old with Repeated UTI and WD

Colposcopy description: Adequate, SCJ visible on the OS, TZ 2, distinct opaque acetowhite lesions with sharp margins, abutting from SCJ, having coarse mosaics and punctations, occupying 2 quadrants and variegated patchy yellow on Lugol's iodine application.

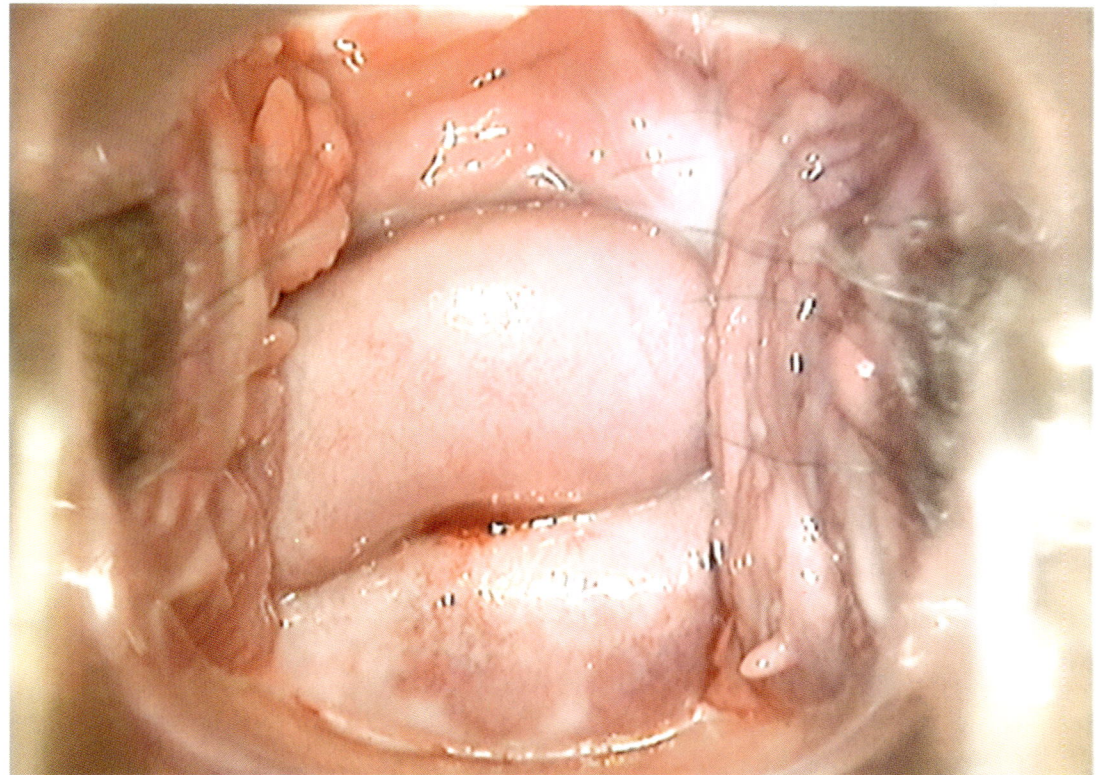

Fig. 7.4a: Normal saline

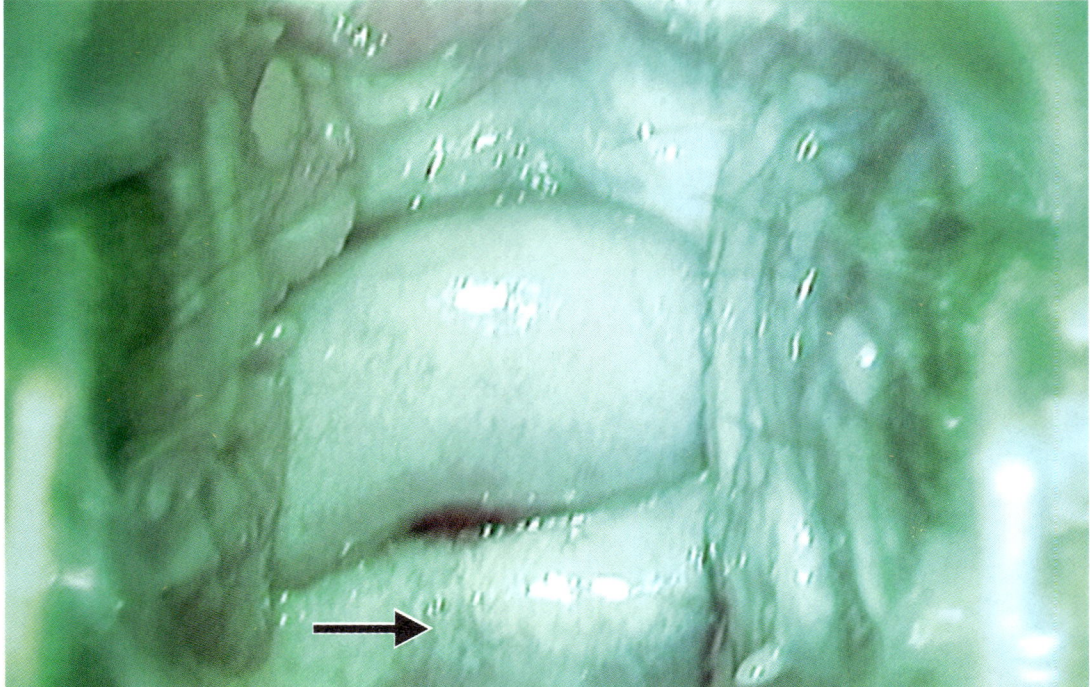

Fig. 7.4b: Green filter—coarse punctations

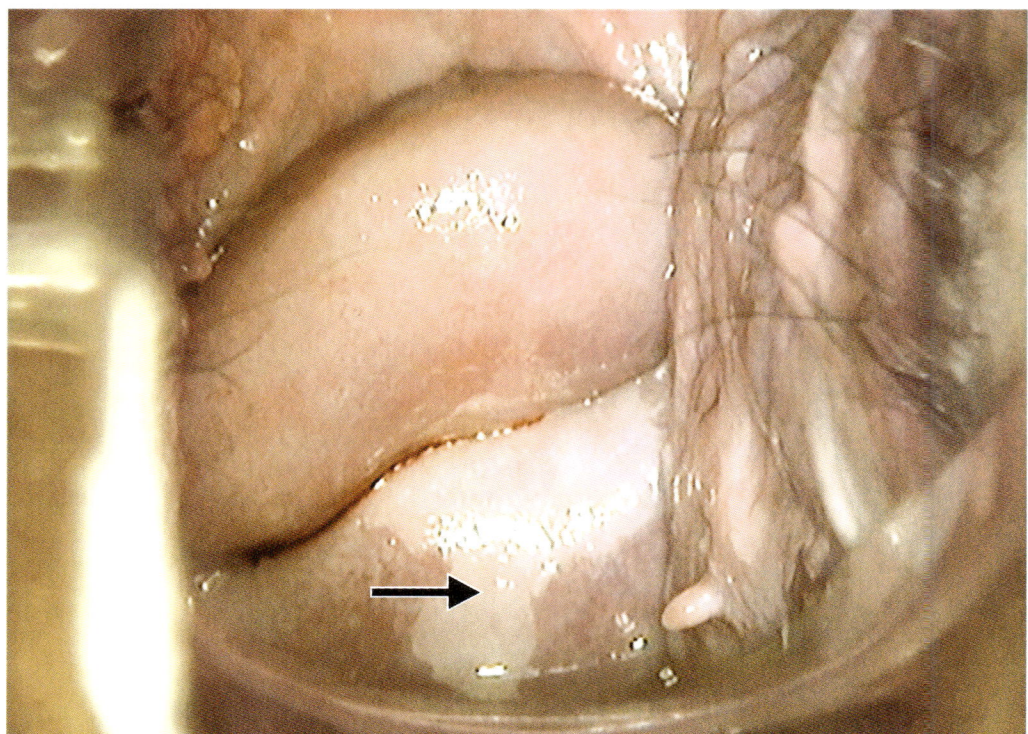

Fig. 7.4c: 5% acetic acid—distinct opaque acetowhite lesions with sharp margins, abutting from SCJ, having coarse mosaics and punctations, occupying 2 quadrants

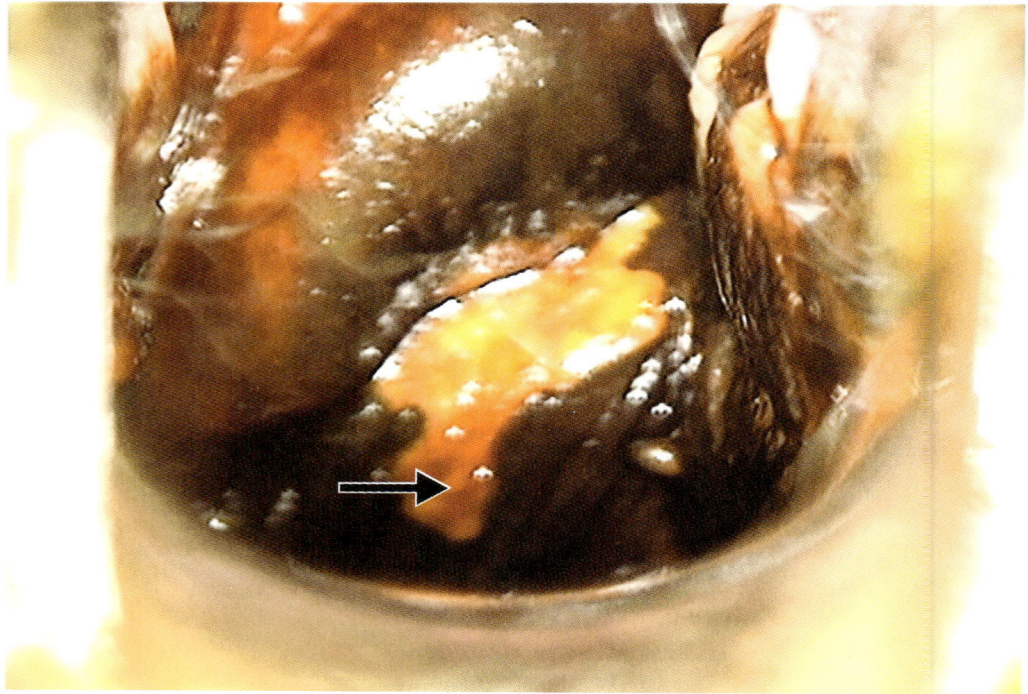

Fig. 7.4d: Lugol's iodine—variegated patchy yellow

Swede—2 + 2 + 2 + 1 + 1 = 8
CIN 3/HSIL
Cytology—ASC-H
HP—CIN 2

5. 36-yr-old with Repeated UTI

Cclposcopy description: Adequate, SCJ visible on the OS, TZ 2, distinct opaque acetowhite lesions with rolled out raised margins, abutting from SCJ, having coarse mosaics and punctations, occupying 2 quadrants and distinct yellow on Lugol's iodine application.

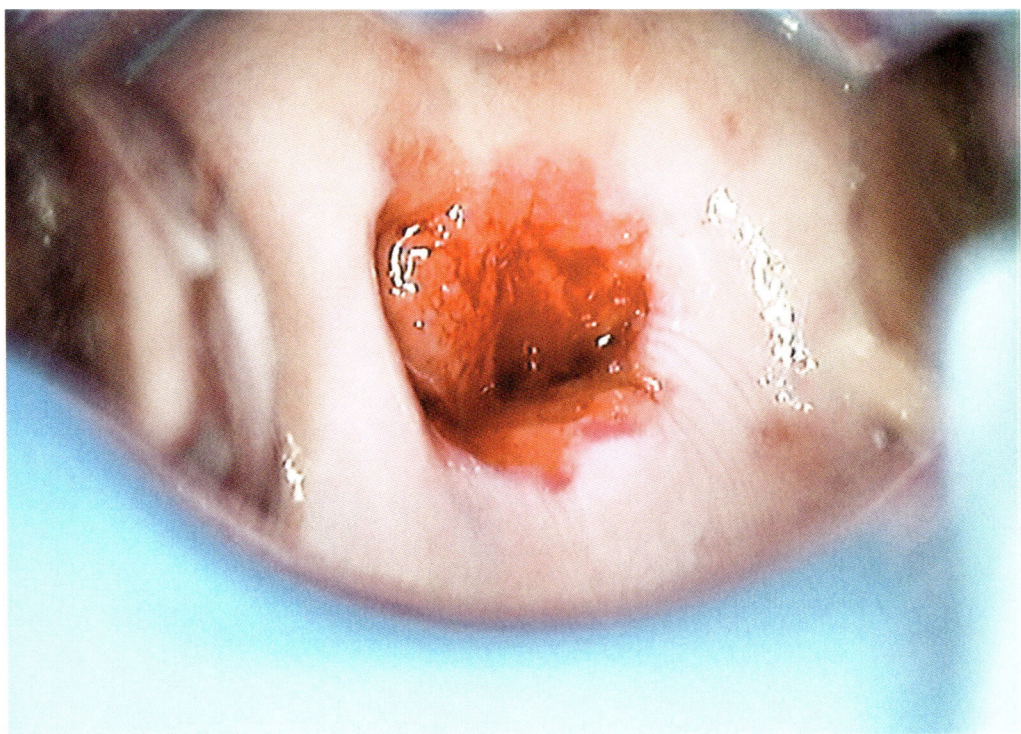

Fig. 7.5a: Normal saline

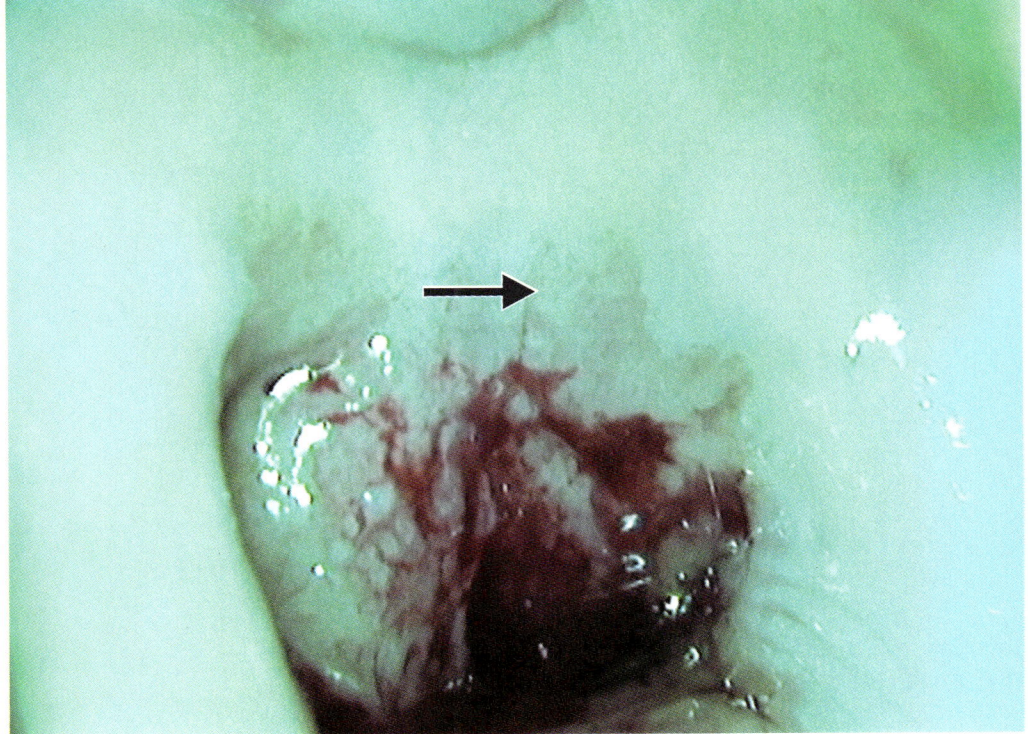

Fig. 7.5b: Green filter—coarse mosaics and punctations

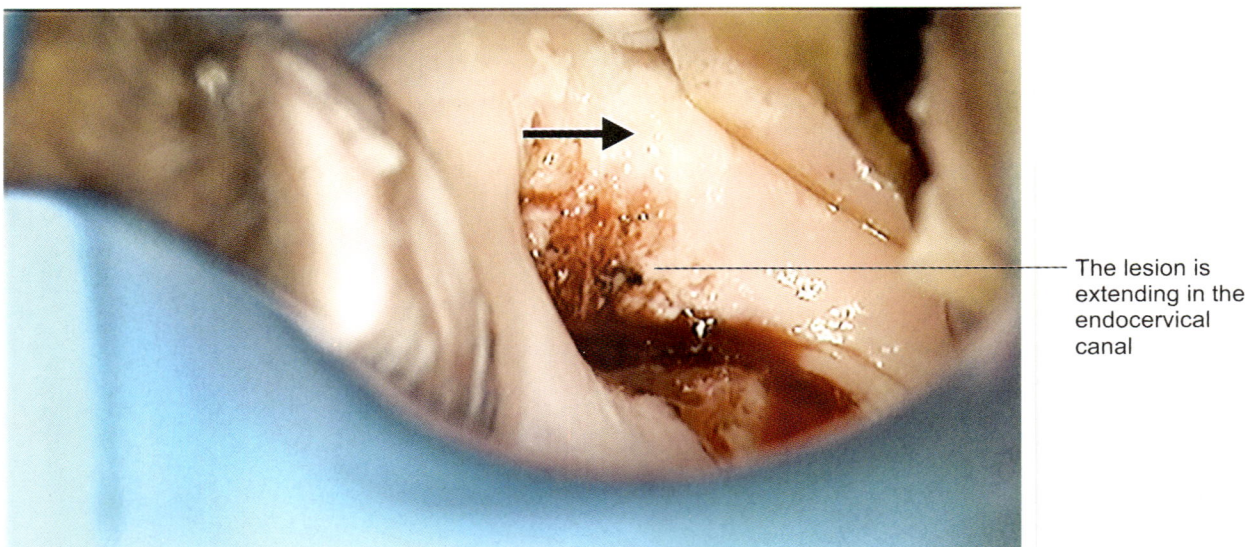

The lesion is extending in the endocervical canal

Fig. 7.5c: 5% acetic acid—distinct opaque acetowhite lesions with rolled out raised margins, abutting from SCJ, having coarse mosaics and punctations, occupying 2 quadrants

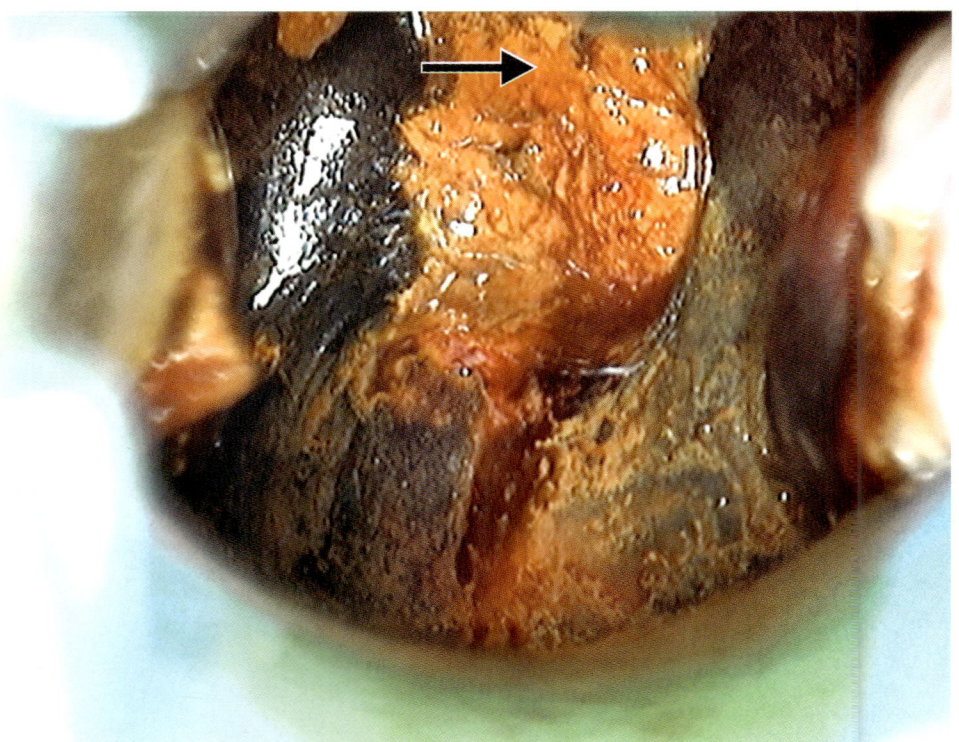

Fig. 7.5d: Lugol's iodine—distinct yellow

Swede—2 + 2 + 2 + 1 + 2 = 9
CIN 3/HSIL
Cytology—Atypical dysplasia
HP—Invasive SCC

6. 34-yr-old with Postcoital Bleeding

Colposcopy description: Adequate, SCJ visible, TZ 1, distinct opaque acetowhite lesions with raised margins, abutting from SCJ, having coarse mosaics and punctations, occupying 2 quadrants and variegated patchy yellow on Lugol's iodine application.

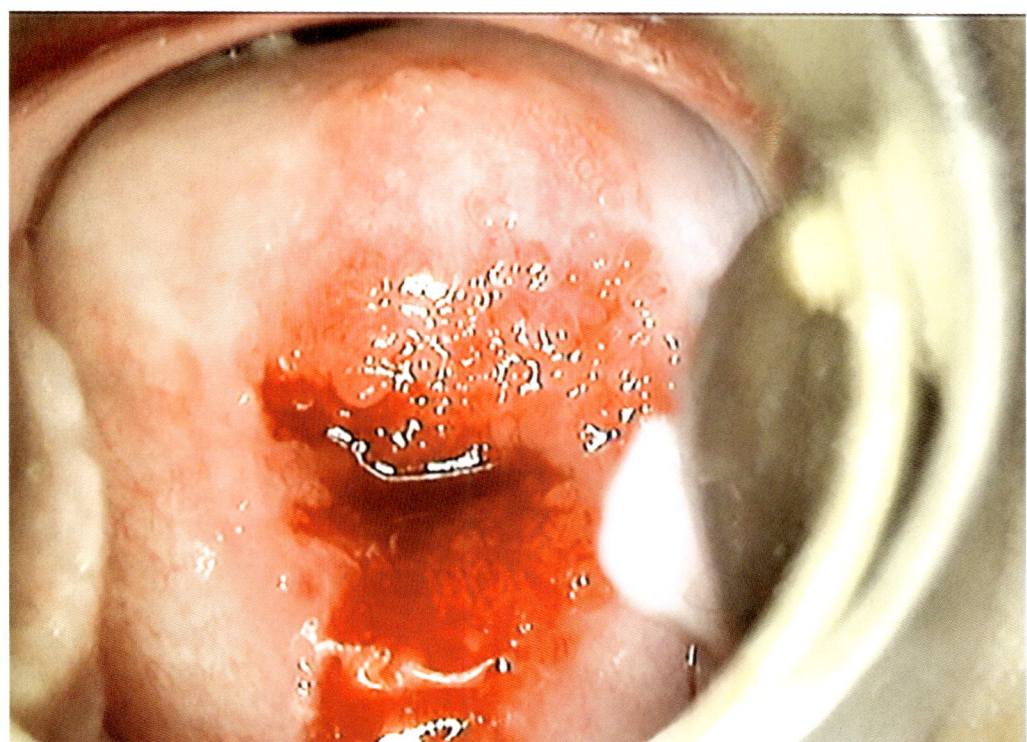

Fig. 7.6a: Normal saline

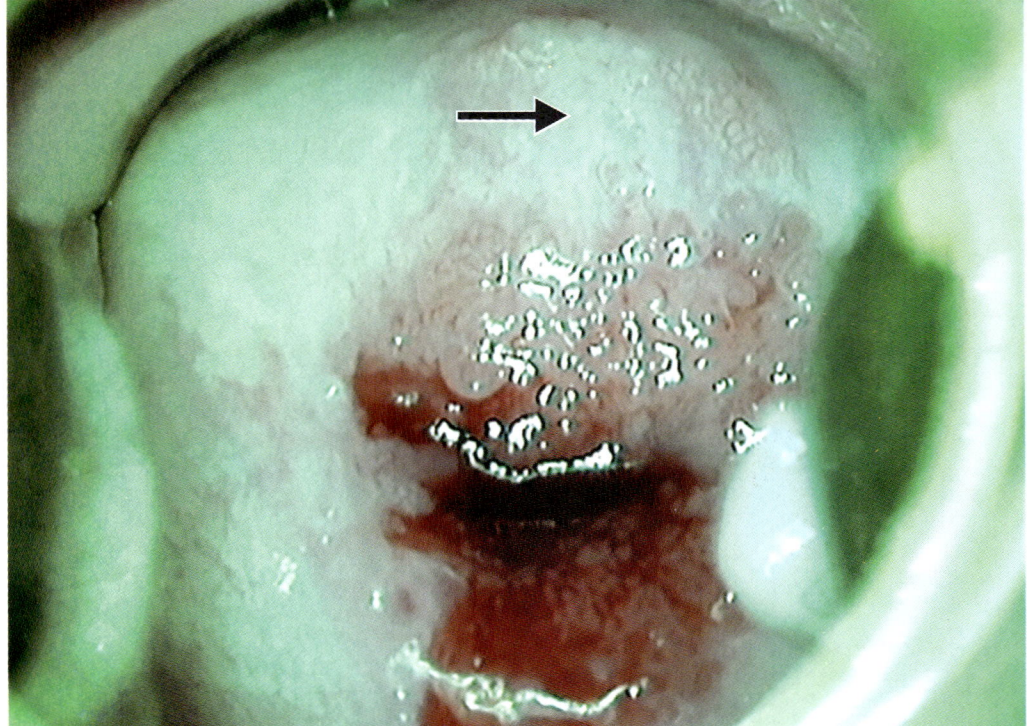

Fig. 7.6b: Green filter—coarse mosaics and punctations

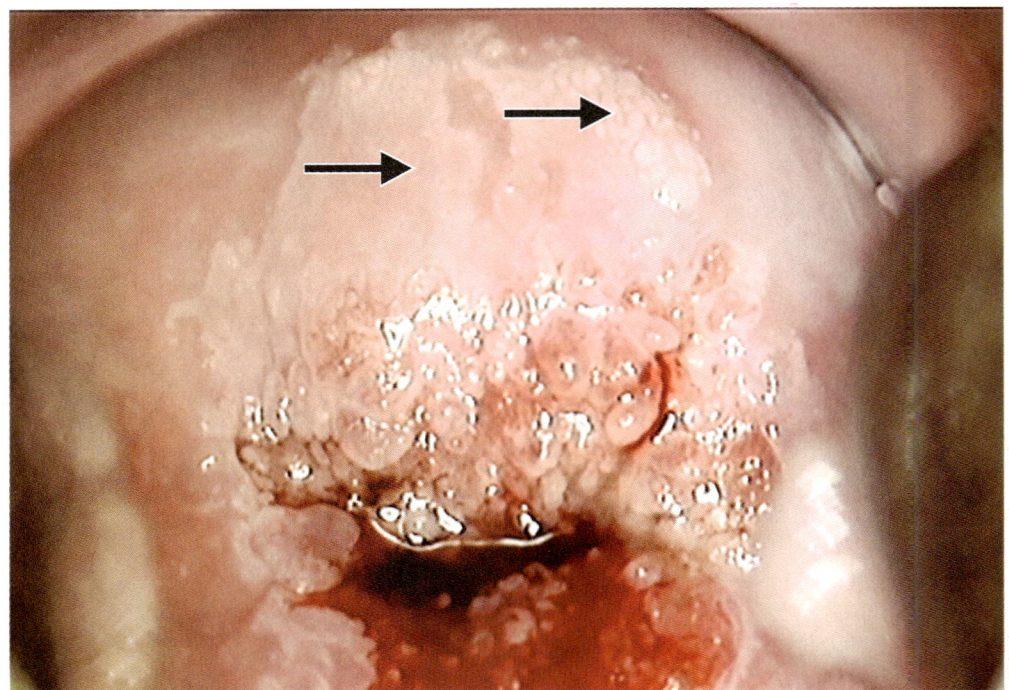

Fig. 7.6c: 5% acetic acid—distinct opaque acetowhite lesions with raised margins, abutting from SCJ, having coarse mosaics and punctations, occupying 2 quadrants

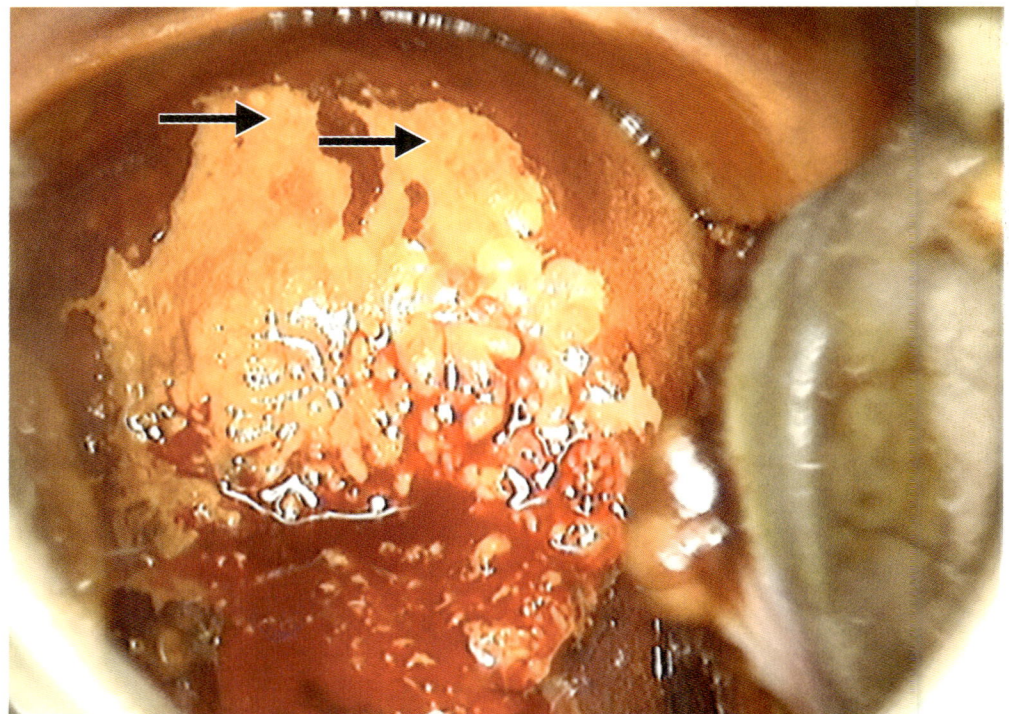

Fig. 7.6d: Lugol's iodine—variegated patchy yellow

Swede—2 + 2 + 2 + 1 + 1 = 8
CIN 3/HSIL
Cytology—CIN 3
HP—CIN 3

7. 26-yr-old with Recurrent UTI, WD

Colposcopy description: Adequate, SCJ visible, TZ 1, dense opaque circumferential lesion with jagged margin, abutting from SCJ within TZ, having coarse mosaics and coarse punctations, occupying all the 4 quadrants and variegated patchy yellow on Lugol's iodine application.

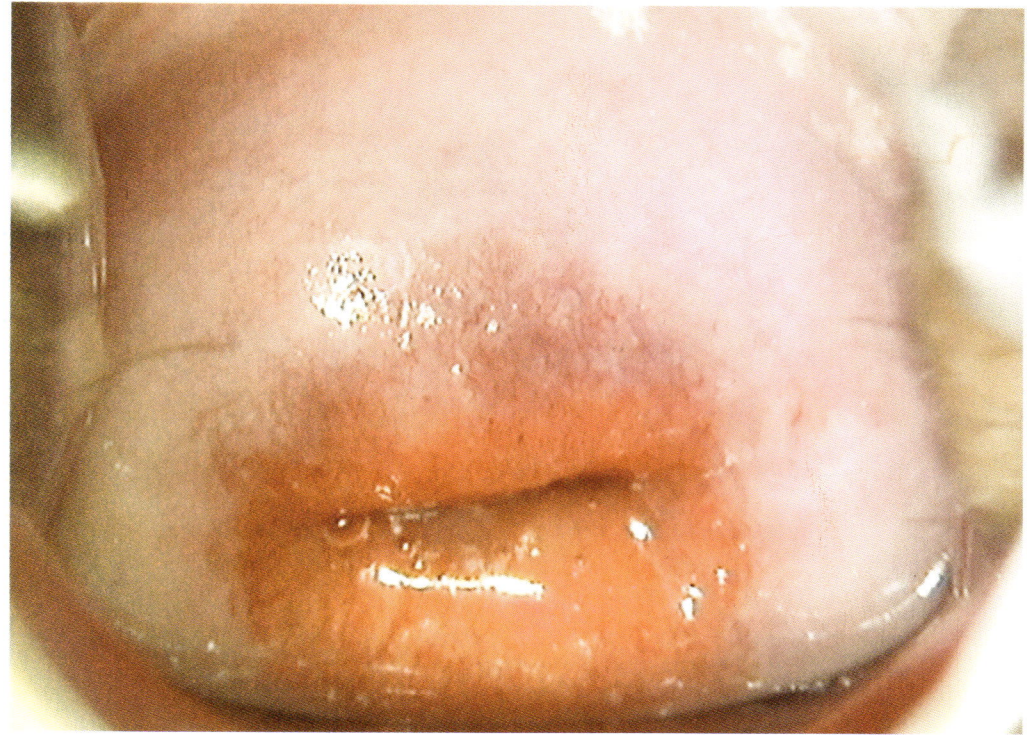

Fig. 7.7a: Normal saline

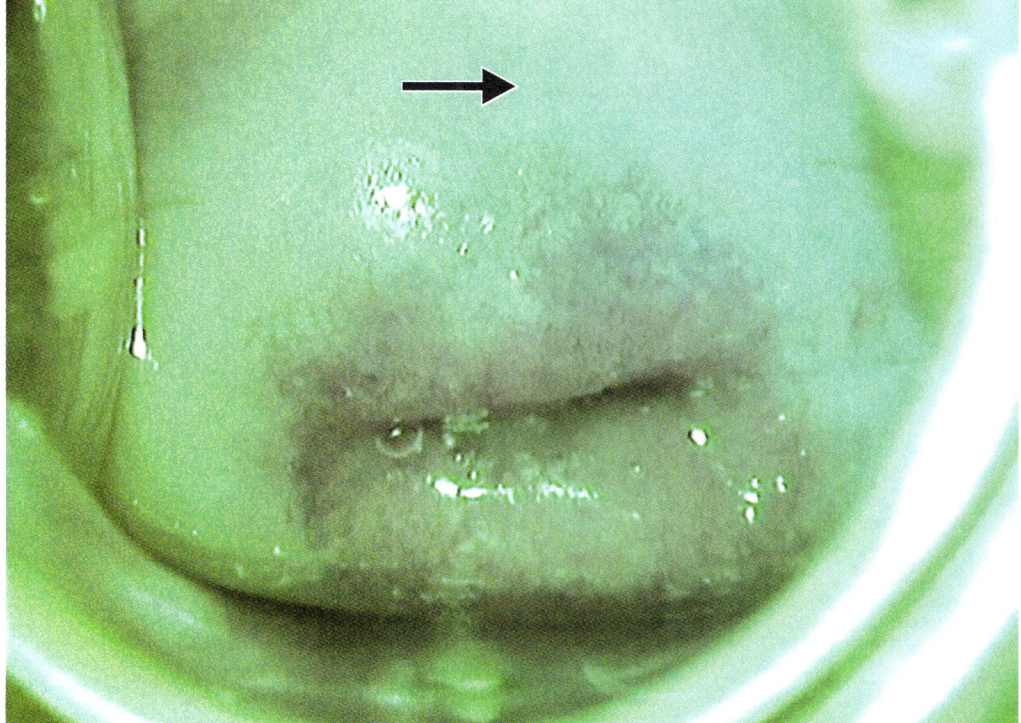

Fig. 7.7b: Green filter—abnormal blood vessels

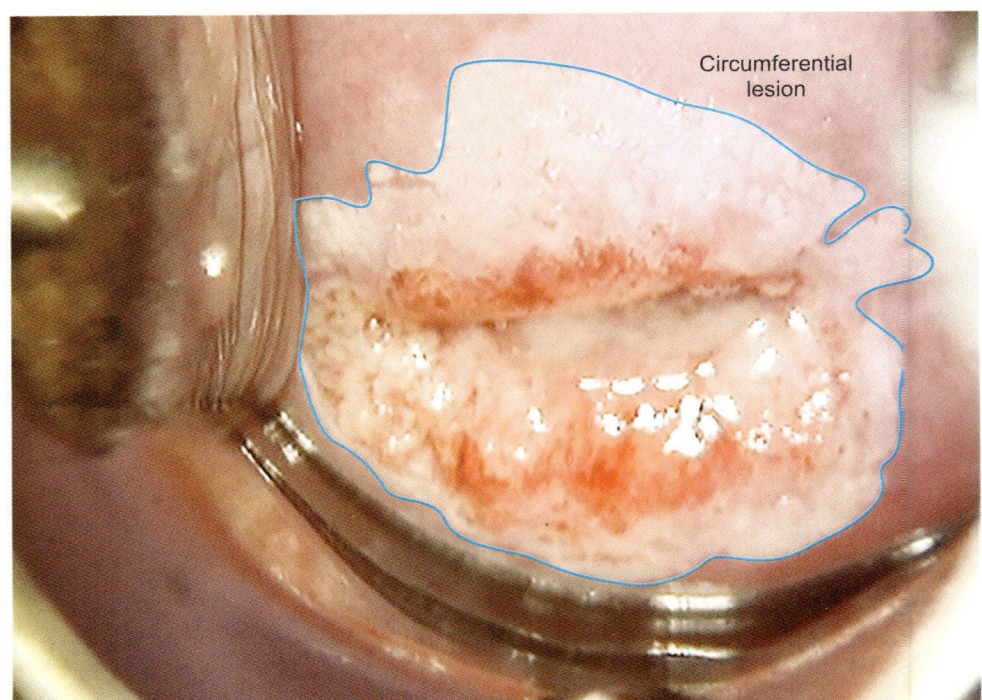

Circumferential lesion

Fig. 7.7c: 5% acetic acid—dense opaque circumferential lesion with jagged margin, abutting from SCJ within TZ, having coarse mosaics and coarse punctations, occupying all the 4 quadrants

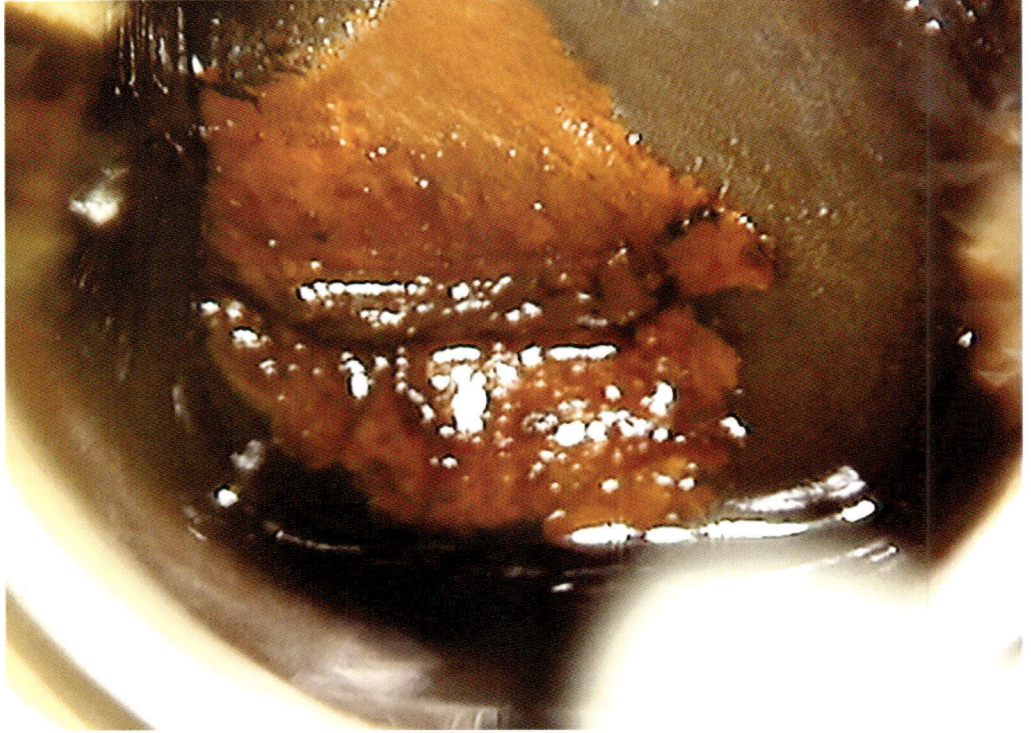

Fig. 7.7d: Lugol's iodine—variegated patchy yellow

Swede—2 + 1 + 2 + 2 + 1 = 8
CIN 3/HSIL
Cytology—ASC-H
HP—CIN 2

8. 41-yr-old with H/O Premenstrual Spotting and WD

Colposcopy description: Adequate, SCJ visible, TZ 1, distinct opaque acetowhite lesions with sharp raised margins, abutting from SCJ within the TZ with absent blood vessels, occupying 2 quadrants and variegated patchy yellow on Lugol's iodine application.

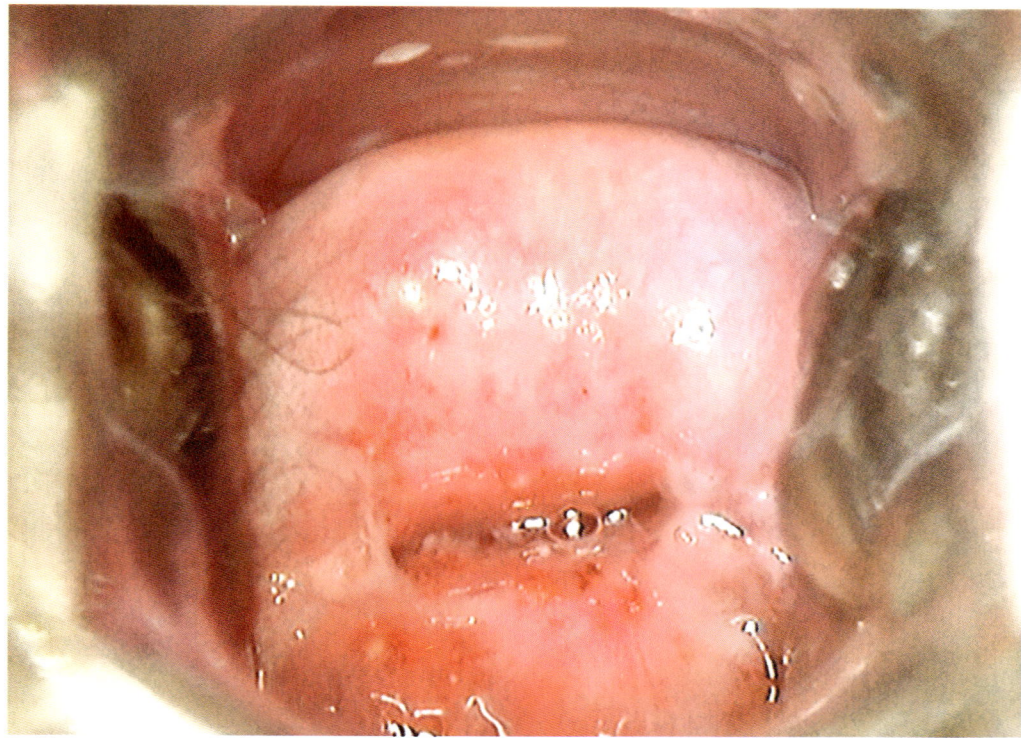

Fig. 7.8a: Normal saline

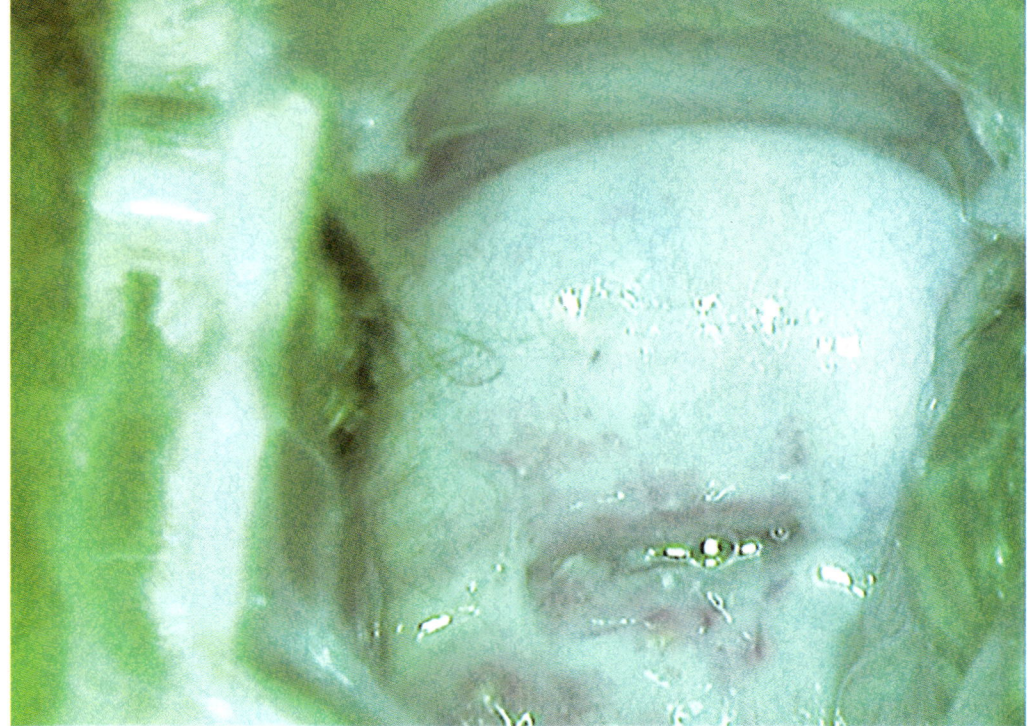

Fig. 7.8b: Green filter

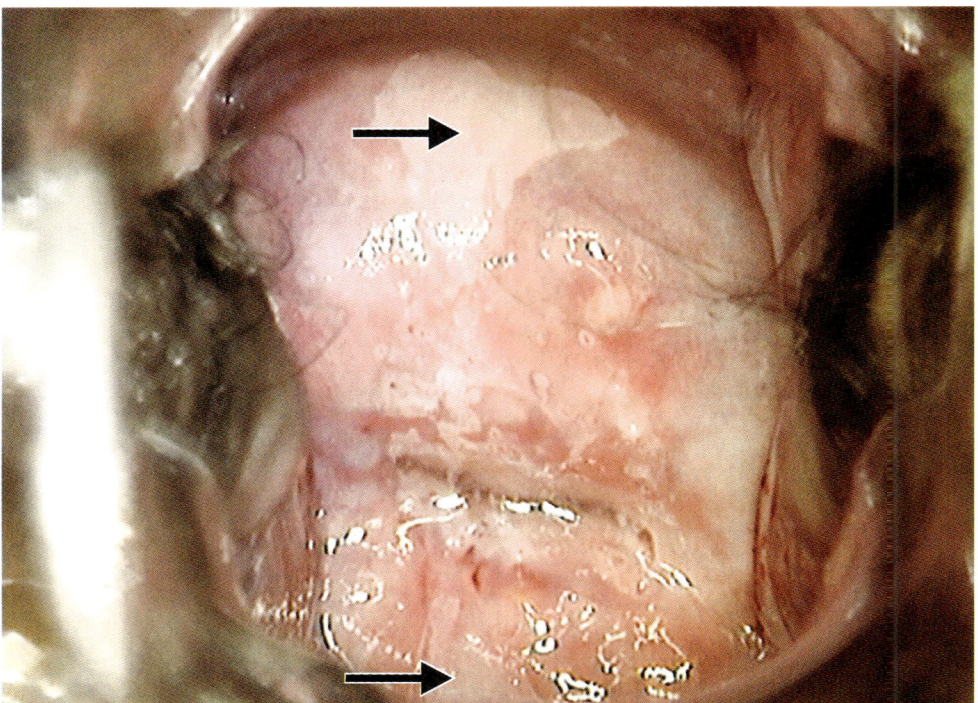

Fig. 7.8c: 5% acetic acid—distinct opaque acetowhite lesions with sharp raised margins, abutting from SCJ with absent blood vessels, occupying 2 quadrants

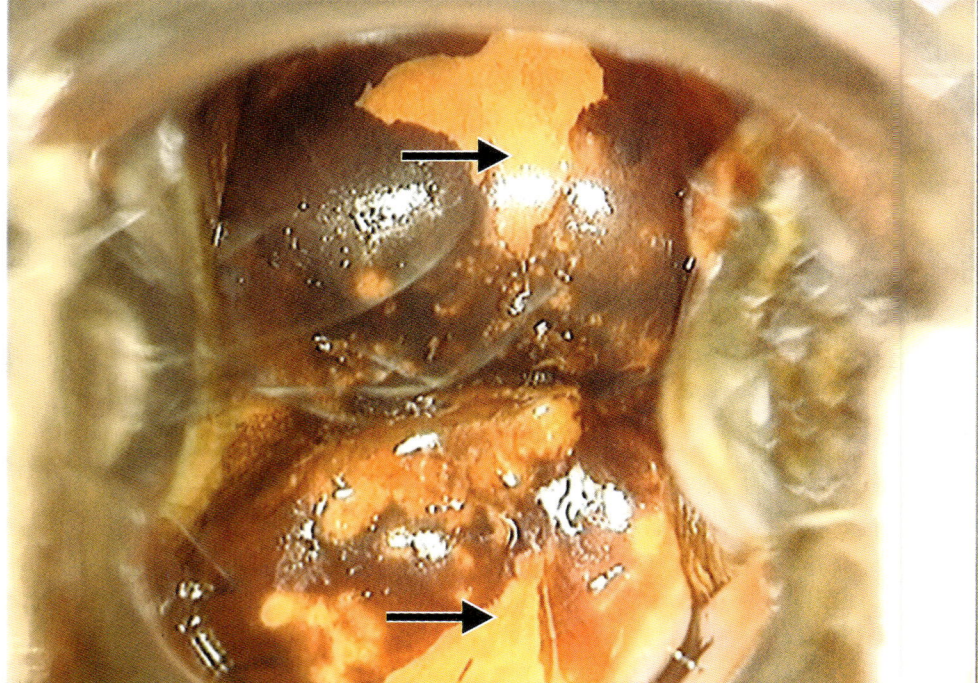

Fig. 7.8d: Lugol's iodine—variegated patchy yellow

Swede—2 + 2 + 1 + 1 + 1 = 7
CIN 2/HSIL
Cytology—CIN 1
HP—CIN 2

9. 35-yr-old with Postcoital Bleeding

Colposcopy description: Adequate, SCJ visible on the OS, TZ 2, thin milky acetowhite lesions with sharp margins, abutting from SCJ within the TZ, having coarse punctations and coarse mosaics, occupying 3–4 quadrants and variegated patchy yellow on Lugol's iodine application.

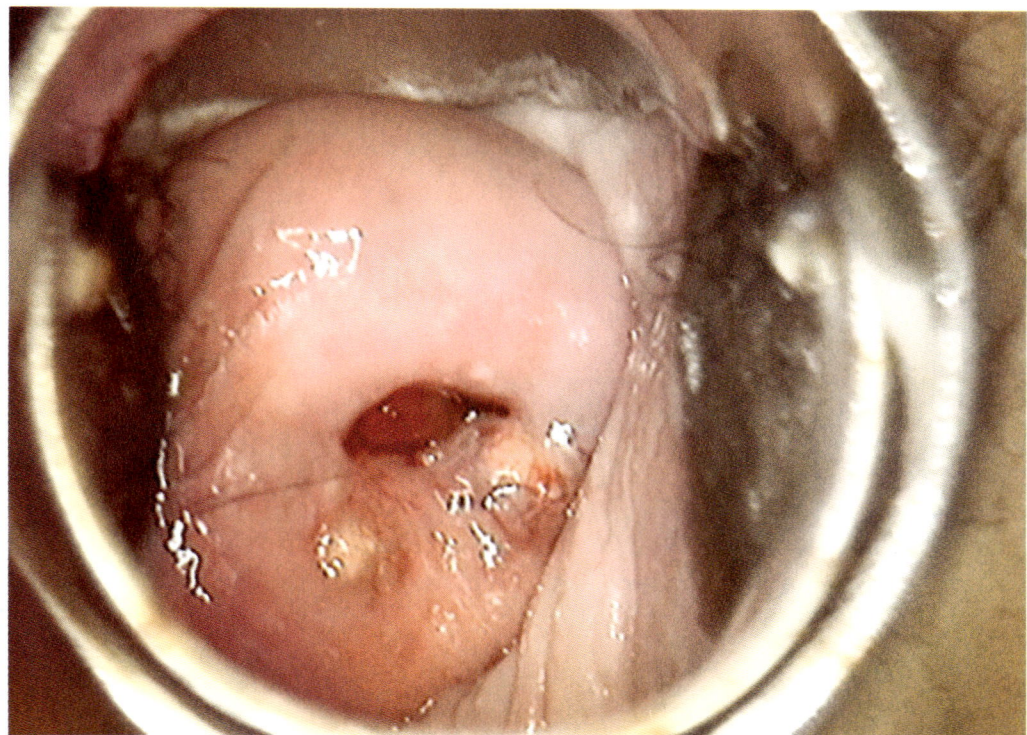

Fig. 7.9a: Normal saline

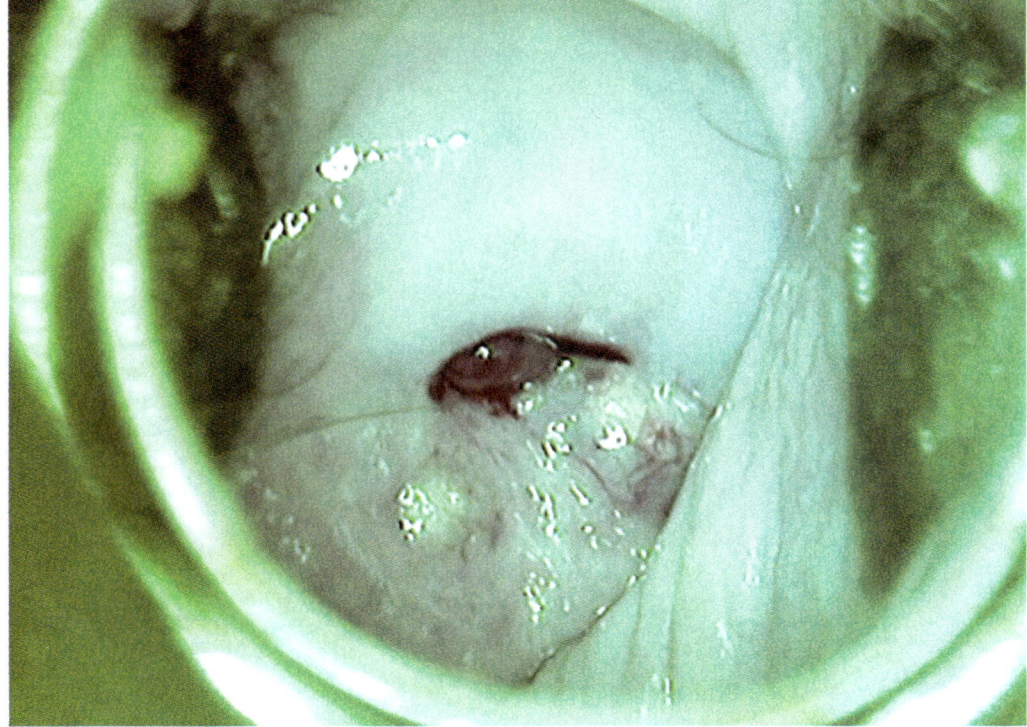

Fig. 7.9b: Green filter

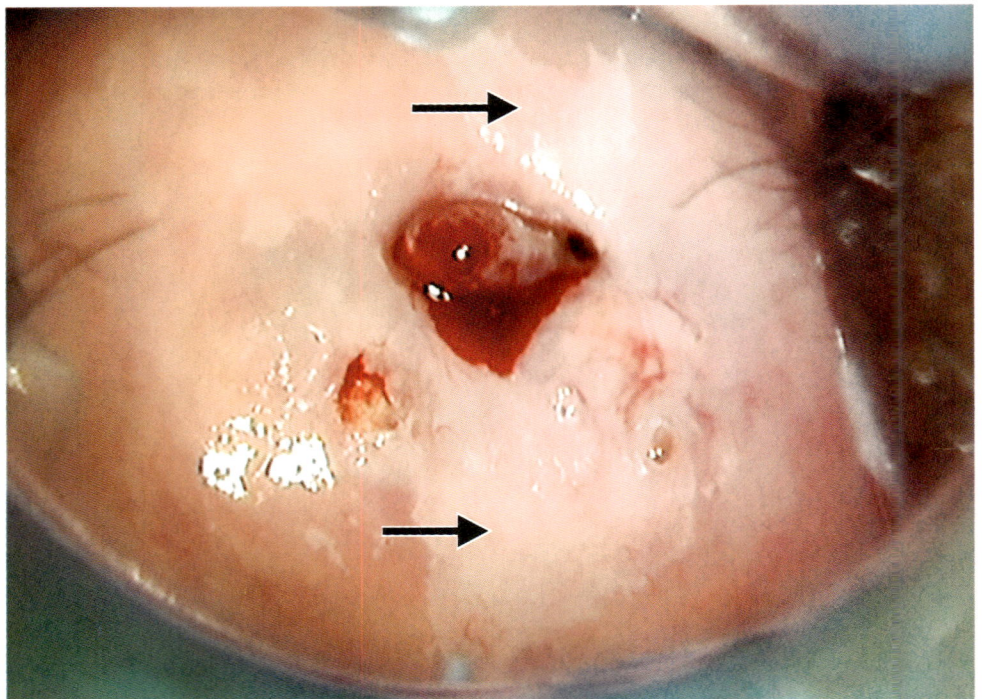

Fig. 7.9c: 5% acetic acid—thin milky acetowhite lesions with sharp margins, abutting from SCJ within the TZ, having coarse punctations and coarse mosaics, occupying 3–4 quadrants

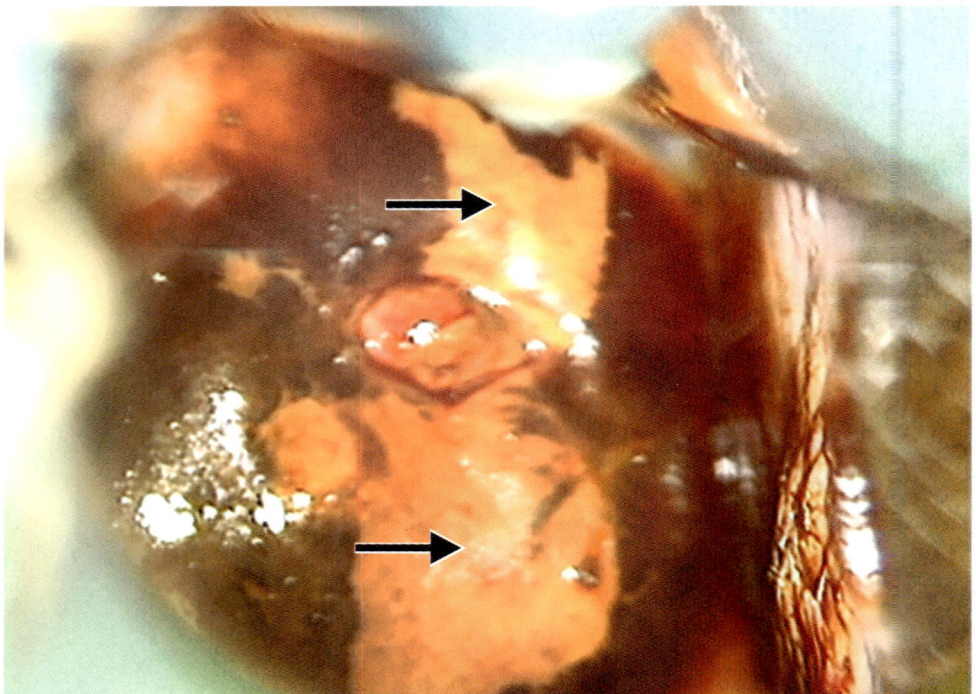

Fig. 7.9d: Lugol's iodine—variegated patchy yellow

Swede—1 + 2 + 2 + 2 + 1 = 8
CIN 3/HSIL
Cytology—Atypical dysplastic cells
HP—CIN 2

10. 43-yr-old with White Discharge

Colposcopy description: Adequate, SCJ visible, TZ 1, distinct opaque acetowhite lesions with raised rolled margins, abutting from SCJ within the TZ with coarse mosaics, occupying 2–3 quadrants and variegated patchy yellow on Lugol's iodine application.

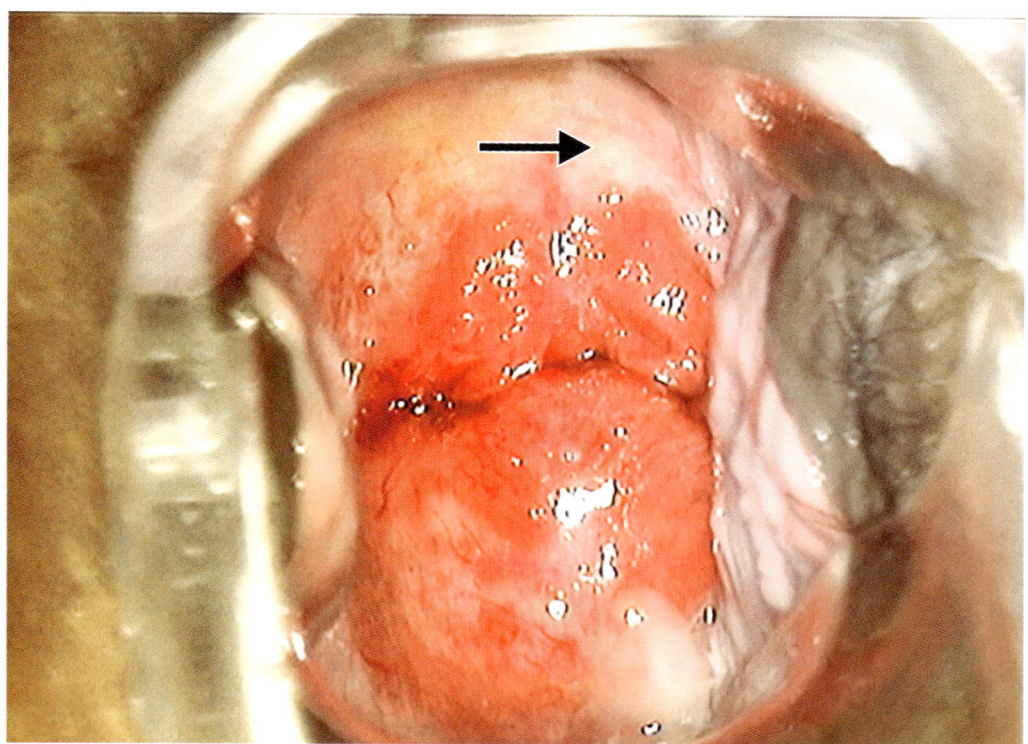

Fig. 7.10a: Normal saline

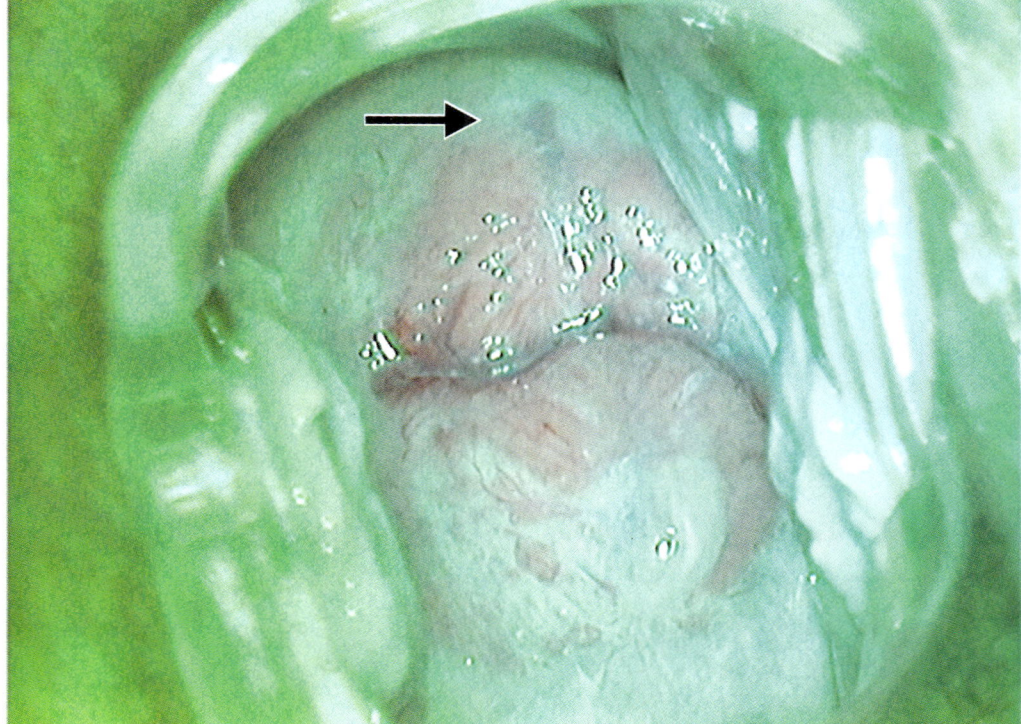

Fig. 7.10b: Green filter—coarse mosaics

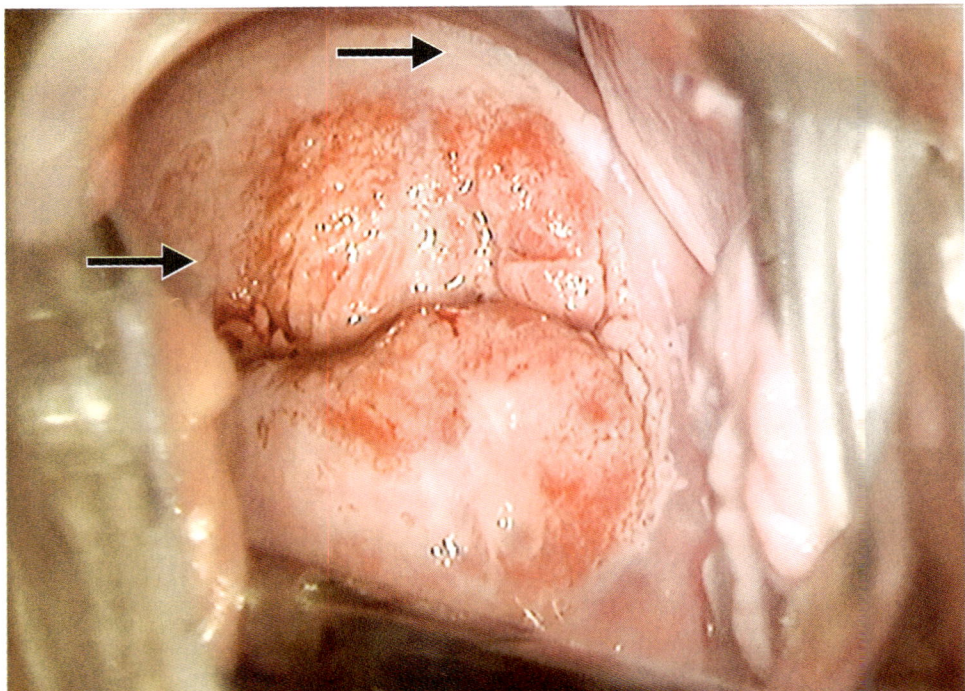

Fig. 7.10c: 5% acetic acid—distinct opaque acetowhite lesions with raised rolled margins, abutting from SCJ within the TZ with coarse mosaics, occupying 2–3 quadrants

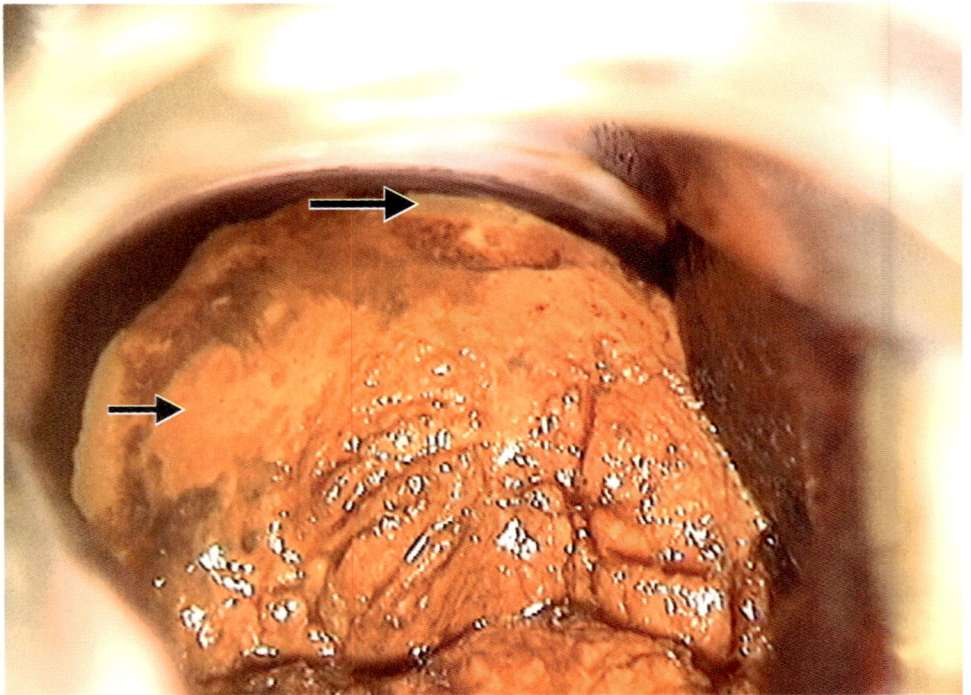

Fig. 7.10d: Lugol's iodine—variegated patchy yellow

Swede—2 + 2 + 2 + 2 + 1 = 9
CIN3/HSIL
Cytology—Inflammatory dysplasia
HP—CIN 2

11. 46-yr-old with Postcoital Bleeding

Colposcopy description: Inadequate due to bleeding, SCJ not visible, TZ 3, thick chalky white dense opaque acetowhite lesions with raised rolled margins, abutting from SCJ within the TZ with inner border sign, ridge sign, abnormal blood vessels, occupying 3–4 quadrants and mustard yellow on Lugol's iodine application.

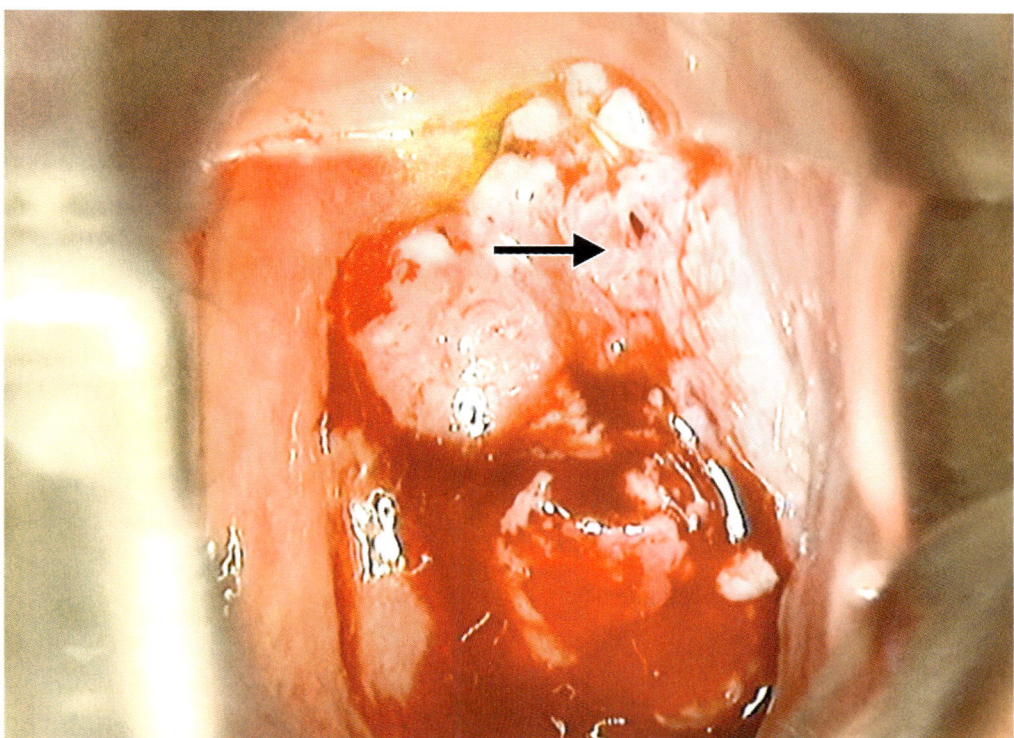

Fig. 7.11a: Normal saline—thick lesion visible

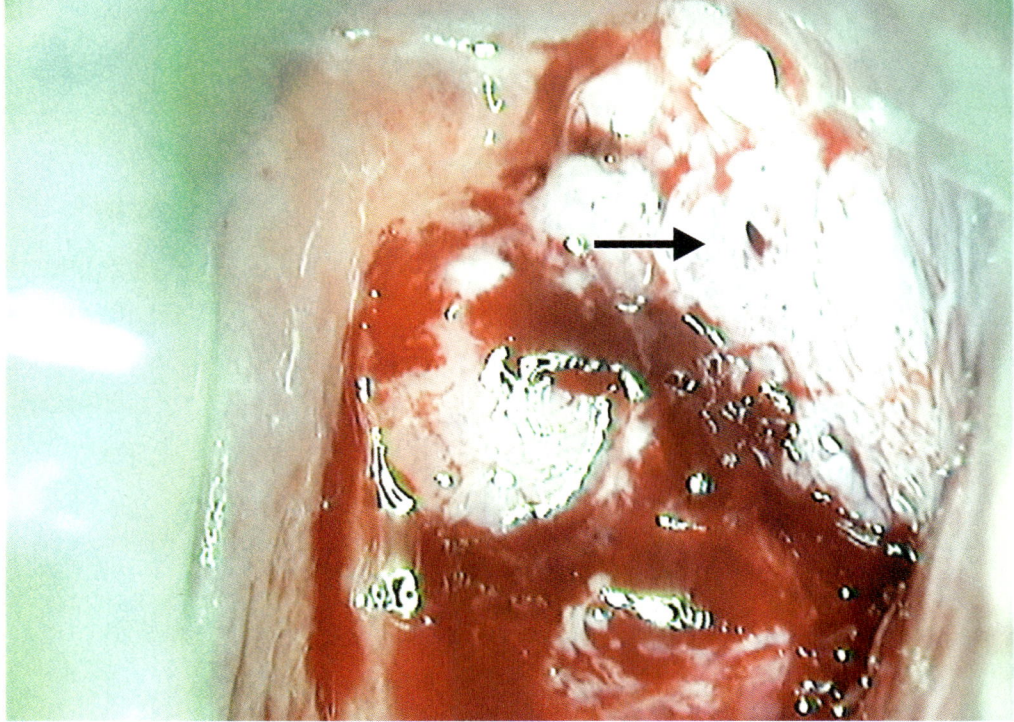

Fig. 7.11b: Green filter—abnormal blood vessels

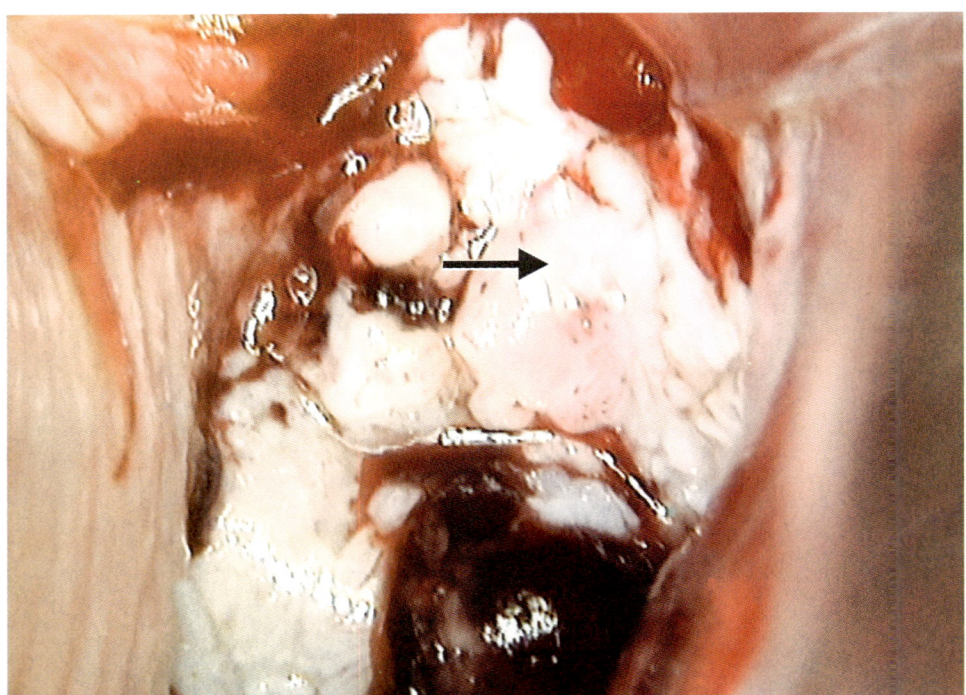

Fig. 7.11c: 5% acetic acid—thick chalky white dense opaque acetowhite lesions with raised rolled margins, abutting from SCJ within the TZ with inner border sign, ridge sign, abnormal blood vessels, occupying 3–4 quadrants

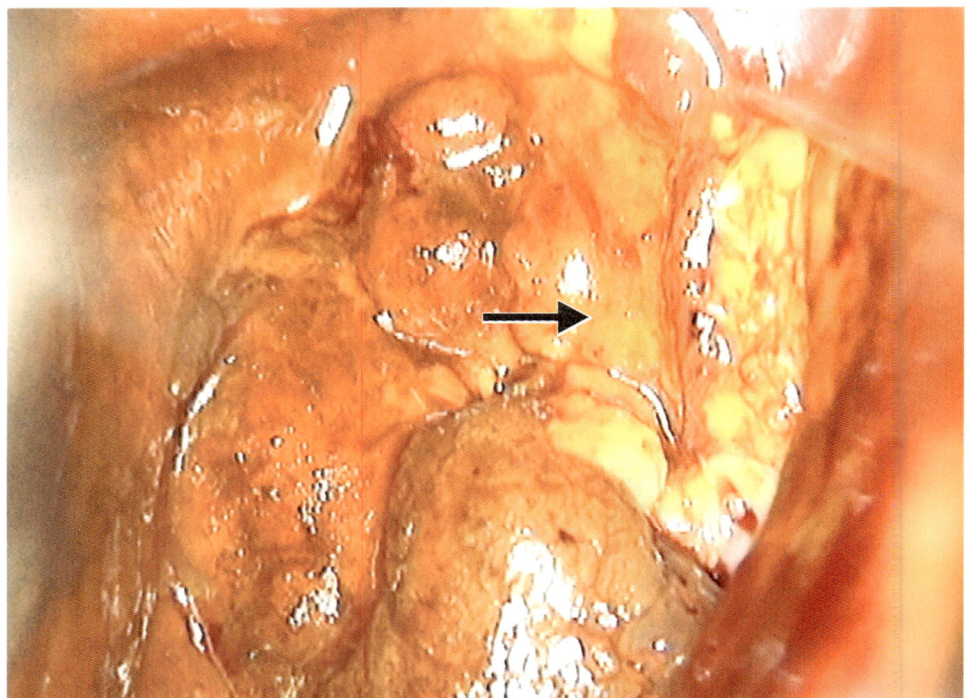

Fig. 7.11d: Lugol's iodine—mustard yellow

Swede—2 + 2 + 2 + 2 + 2 = 10
HSIL
Cytology—Squamous cell CA (SCC)
HP—SCC

Procedures and Therapies

CERVICAL PUNCH BIOPSY

We should use dedicated biopsy forceps for this purpose (Fig. 8.1).

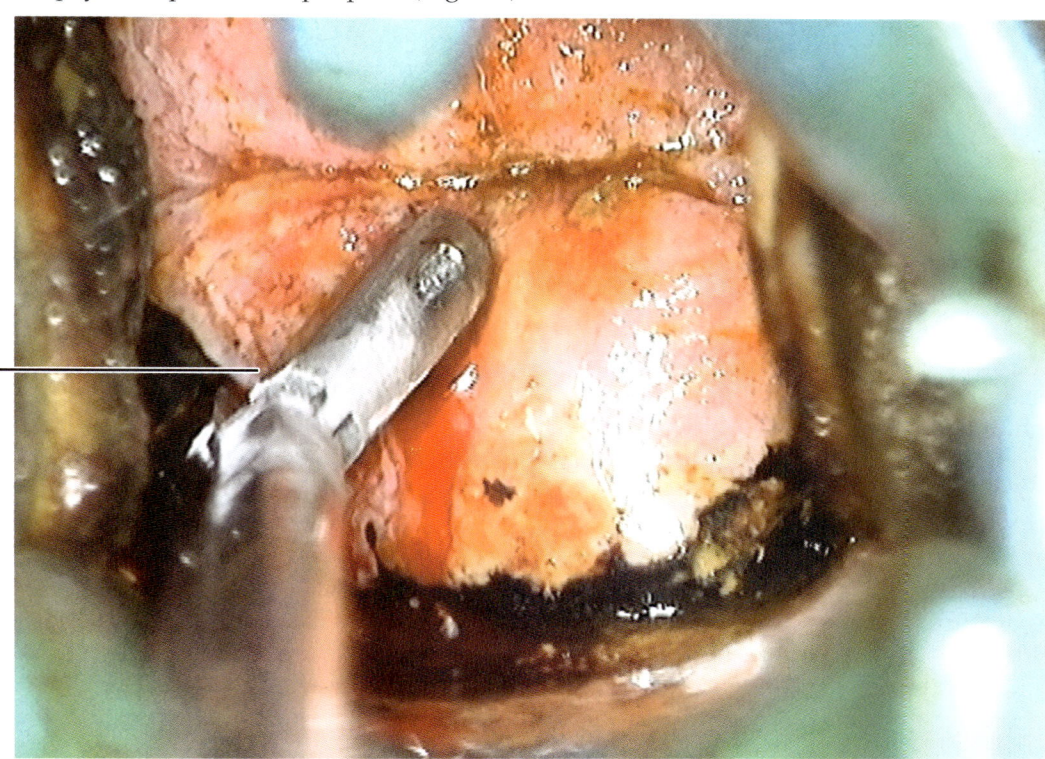

The punch biopsy should include SCJ with adequate tissue material which should not be fragmented

Fig. 8.1: Cervical punch biopsy with Tischler forceps

Case Management

Introduction

- The treatment of CIN should read as the management of women with CIN.
- Should never be dictated by an individual test results, even histology.
- Should incorporate all the case characteristics.
- Is a balance of benefit vs harm.

How to Safely Treat HSIL?

Safely means reducing the risk of cervical cancer to almost zero, reducing the side effects of treatment to as low as possible.

- Pretreatment counselling: Need, risk, follow-up, monitoring by cytology/HPV/colposcopy. Assessment of all case characteristics: Age, parity, future fertility.

Types of Treatment

The two main OPD-based treatments are:

- Ablative therapy which includes cryotherapy, electrocauterization, cold coagulation, and laser ablation.
- Excisional therapy includes cone biopsy, loop electrosurgical excision procedure (LEEP), large loop excision of transformation zone (LLETZ).

Advantages of these OPD Procedures

1. OPD procedure
2. Can be performed in low resource settings.
3. Easy to learn
4. 95–97% cure rate
5. Affordable to the patients
6. Well tolerated by patients
7. Avoids unnecessary hysterectomy (except when it is extremely necessary)
8. Preserves the fertility by avoiding hysterectomies
9. Halts the progression to cancer.

Effectiveness of the Therapy

- Depends upon the depth of the lesion. A right therapy has to be selected to prevent the recurrence.
- Electrocauterization reaches up to 4–5 mm in depth.
- Cryotherapy reaches a depth of 5–7 mm.
- LEEP reaches a depth of 7–8 mm.
- A treatment that is effective to a depth of 6–7 mm is necessary to destroy high grade lesions.

A. CRYOTHERAPY

It is a most popular ablative procedure practiced widely. It is economical, with less of side effects and cost-effective. It gives excellent results in CIN 1 and CIN 2 lesions. It is quite a safe procedure and does not require much expertise.

Principle of Cryotherapy

During the therapy, a cryoball made of ice is created around the cryogun. The tip of the gun is usually made of silver or copper. The core temperature of the crater formed is –68°C using carbon dioxide gas and –89°C using nitrous oxide gas. The temperature at the periphery is –20°C. Cryonecrosis of the cells occurs at this very low temperature and the intracellular water gets crystallized. There is vascular stasis, dehydration and protein denaturation. A rapid freezing for 3 minutes followed by slow thawing approximately for 5 minutes, allowing the color of the epithelium to return to original pink color followed by rapid freezing for 3 minutes is carried out. This practice of rapid freezing, slow thawing followed by rapid freezing and thawing is essential for the cryonecrosis.

Criteria for the Patient Selection

- It can be used in 'screen and treat' program.
- The lesion should not extend into the cervical canal.
- Chronic cervicitis and the active infection are to be cured first.
- There should be no evidence of PID. If so, the PID has to be cured prior to the therapy.
- The extent of the lesion should be within two-thirds of the diameter of the cryoball.

Prerequisites: The gas cylinder to be used should be completely full.

Instruments

A cryogun, large-sized self-retaining Cusco's speculum, nitrous oxide or carbon dioxide cylinder with a pressure gauge (Fig. 8.2). The pressure gauge shows three color zones—yellow, green, and red. After attaching the pressure gauge to the cylinder, note the position of the indicator showing in the gauge. Green indicates that the pressure in the cylinder is full; yellow indicates a very low pressure in the cylinder and so the cylinder has to be changed; red

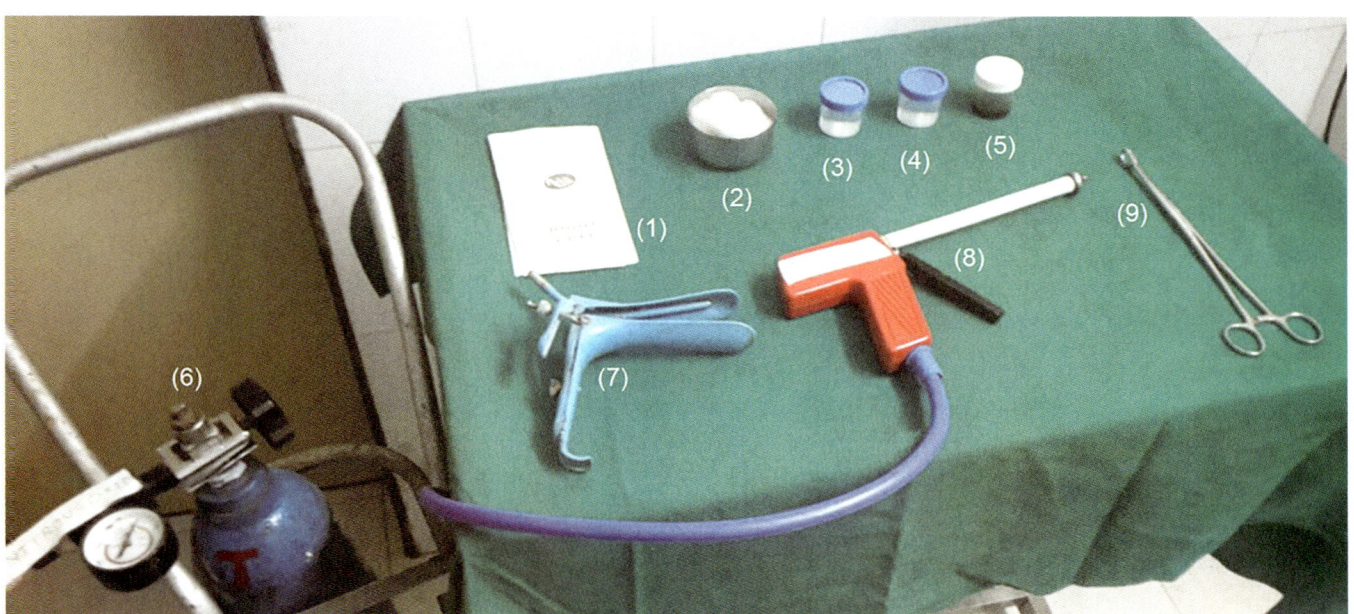

Fig. 8.2: Cryotherapy instruments: (1) Gloves, (2) cotton, (3) normal saline, (4) 5% acetic acid, (5) Lugol's iodine, (6) nitrous oxide, (7) Cusco's speculum, (8) cryogun for cryotherapy, and (9) sponge holder

indicates dangerously high pressure so some gas has to released before starting the procedure. Prior to starting of the procedure, the cryogun set has to be assembled, and the tubing of the cryogun along with the meter gauge has to be fixed to the gas cylinder.

Procedure

The filling of patient consent form is mandatory. After taking the consent and explaining the whole procedure to the patient in the language which she understands, the patient is given dorsal lithotomy position. An adequate size of self-retaining Cusco's speculum is inserted in the vagina. The cervical mucus is cleared with normal saline. With the application of 5% acetic acid, the lesion becomes more prominent. On application of Lugol's iodine, the margins of the lesion get delineated (Figs 8.3a to d). The cryoprobe with the cryogun is firmly held at the ectocervix with the center of the tip at the os. The vaginal wall should not come in contact with the cryoball. In case of lax vagina, use speculum covered with condoms. The timer is set and the handle of the cryogun is pressed to release the gas. The gas is released with a hissing sound. An ice ball is slowly formed on the tip of the cryogun, increasing in size and covering the lesion on the cervix. Release the handle after 3 minutes. By now the cryoprobe is stuck to the cervix along with the ice ball. Slow thawing is allowed till the cervix returned to original pink colour. During this time, the probe which was tightly adherent to the cervix gets released as the ice melts. Never pull the probe forcibly, if it is adhered to the cervix, to avoid injury to it.

After 5 minutes, the procedure is repeated again one more time. So we perform 3 minutes of rapid freeze and 5 minutes of slow thawing. A satisfactory freezing is achieved when the periphery of the cryoball covers the whole lesion adequately.

Cleaning of the cryogun: The cryogun probe is cleaned with running water and wiped with 60–90% ethyl alcohol or isopropyl alcohol and then kept dry.

Advice to the Patient after the Cryotherapy Procedure

The patient should be given verbal as well as written instructions that are to be followed after the procedure. They are as follows:
- There can be mild abdominal pain which subsides on its own or with mild analgesics.
- Mild raise of temperature is noticed. Patient can take one tablet of 500 mg of paracetamol, if temperature >100°C.
- There is usually no need of antibiotics.

- Watery discharge rarely blood stained can be there for about 21–30 days.
- Do not use any vaginal tampon or vaginal pessary.
- No sexual intercourse for 4 weeks.
- Report, if there is foul smelling discharge or excessive bleeding.
- To come for follow-up colposcopy examination after 3 months.

Healing of the Cervix

Healing usually takes place during the first 6 weeks of cryotherapy. Healing occurs by granulation tissue which appears during the first 2–3 weeks, followed by re-epithelialization of the surface. The wound heals completely within 6–8 weeks of the treatment. A repeat colposcopy is done by 6 months as a test of cure (Figs 8.4a and b).

Follow-up

The follow-up visits are at 3 months, 6 months and later 9–12 months. Then annually she is called once a year for 3 years. Once she is CIN negative during these three years, she is put in annual cytology screening program for 5 years. If three consecutive cytology reports are negative, then she need not come annually for screening. She is called once in 3–5 years till the age of 60 years.

Effectiveness of Cryotherapy

Cryotherapy is 95–97% effective with failure rate of only 3–5%. The treatment failure is manifested usually during the first year.

Reasons for Failure

- Faulty selection of patient for the cryotherapy. Remember the lesion size should be within two-thirds of the cryoball.
- The contact between the cryoprobe and the surface of the lesion on the cervix is inadequate.
- The channel of passage of gas in the cryoprobe could be blocked for some reason, thereby cryoball is inadequately formed.
- The cylinder is only partially full.
  The therapy is performed in haste without maintaining the principle of rapid freezing and slow thawing.
- Freezing done only once without repeating the process.
- Adenocarcinoma *in situ* (AIS) associated with CIN will not be benefited.

Management of Failure Cases

In case, if the patient come with the treatment failure, the colposcopy-guided biopsy should be repeated along with the endocervical curettage (ECC) histopathology to find out the cause of failure. Many a times, we find a few patches of CIN lesion which could not be covered in the cryoball and hence have been left out. In such cases, it is advisable to perform a repeat cryotherapy to tackle the lesion. As previously said, ensure that the cylinder is full and the procedure is performed correctly with 3 min freeze–5 min thaw–3 min freeze. Rarely we find a large lesion residues left over in spite of the previous treatment. In such cases, an alternative treatment modality is discussed and offered to the patient, which includes LEEP therapy, simple hysterectomy, if her family is complete and if she insists.

Complications and Long-Term Sequelae

- Excessive malodorous discharge—usually CIN cases are concurrent with pelvic inflammatory infection, bacterial vaginosis, and trichomoniasis. In such cases, the pathology of PID, cervicitis should be adequately treated prior to the treatment of CIN; otherwise there could be a flare up of PID.
- Both the sexual partners should be treated in the cases of reproductive tract infections, if any, or cervicitis, as the case may be. Use of condoms is highly recommended.
- Cervical stenosis occurs in less than 1% of women.

CASE 1

Case of HSIL treated with cryotherapy (Figs 8.3a to d)

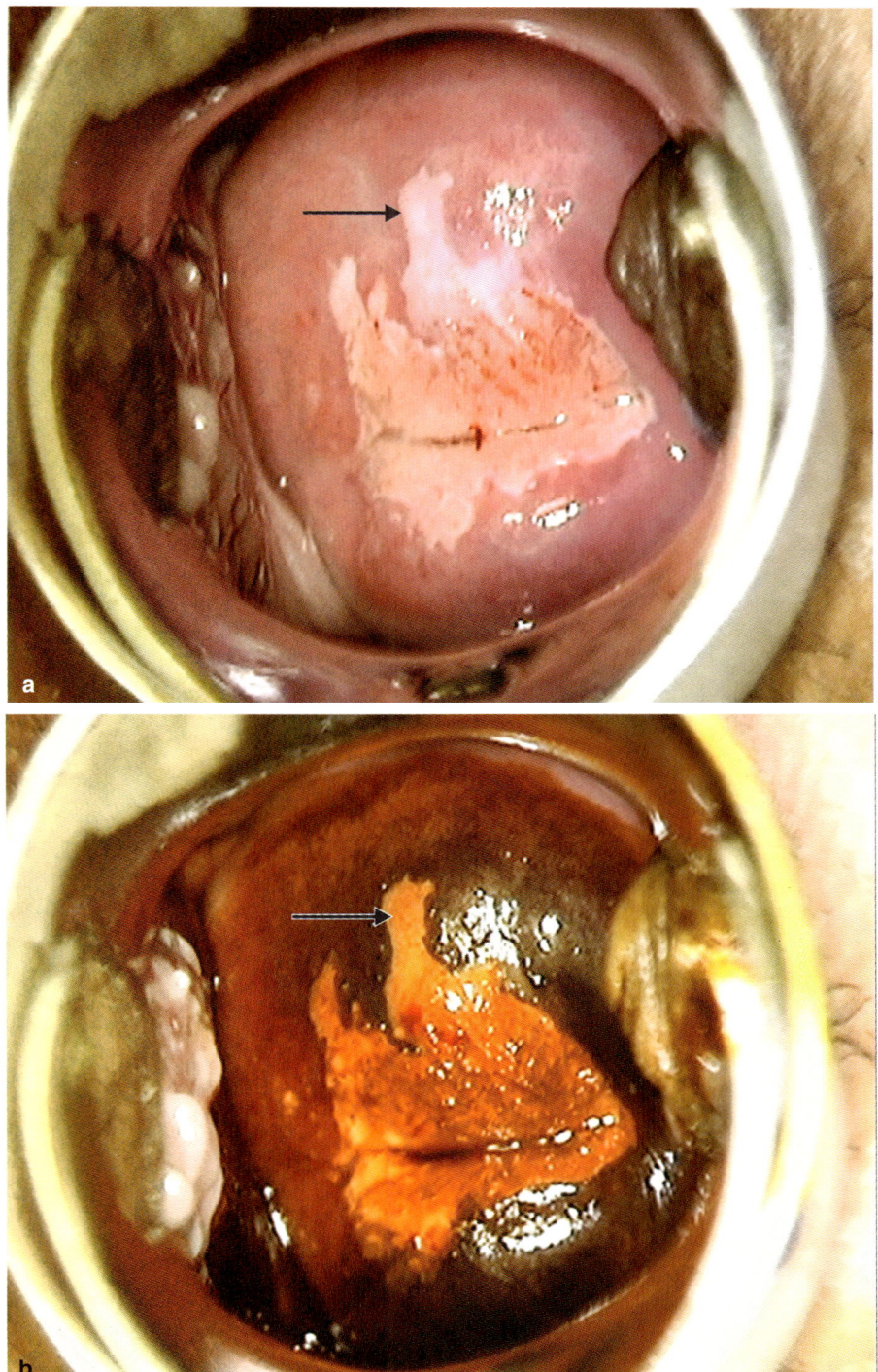

Figs 8.3a and b: A case of high grade lesion (CIN 2)

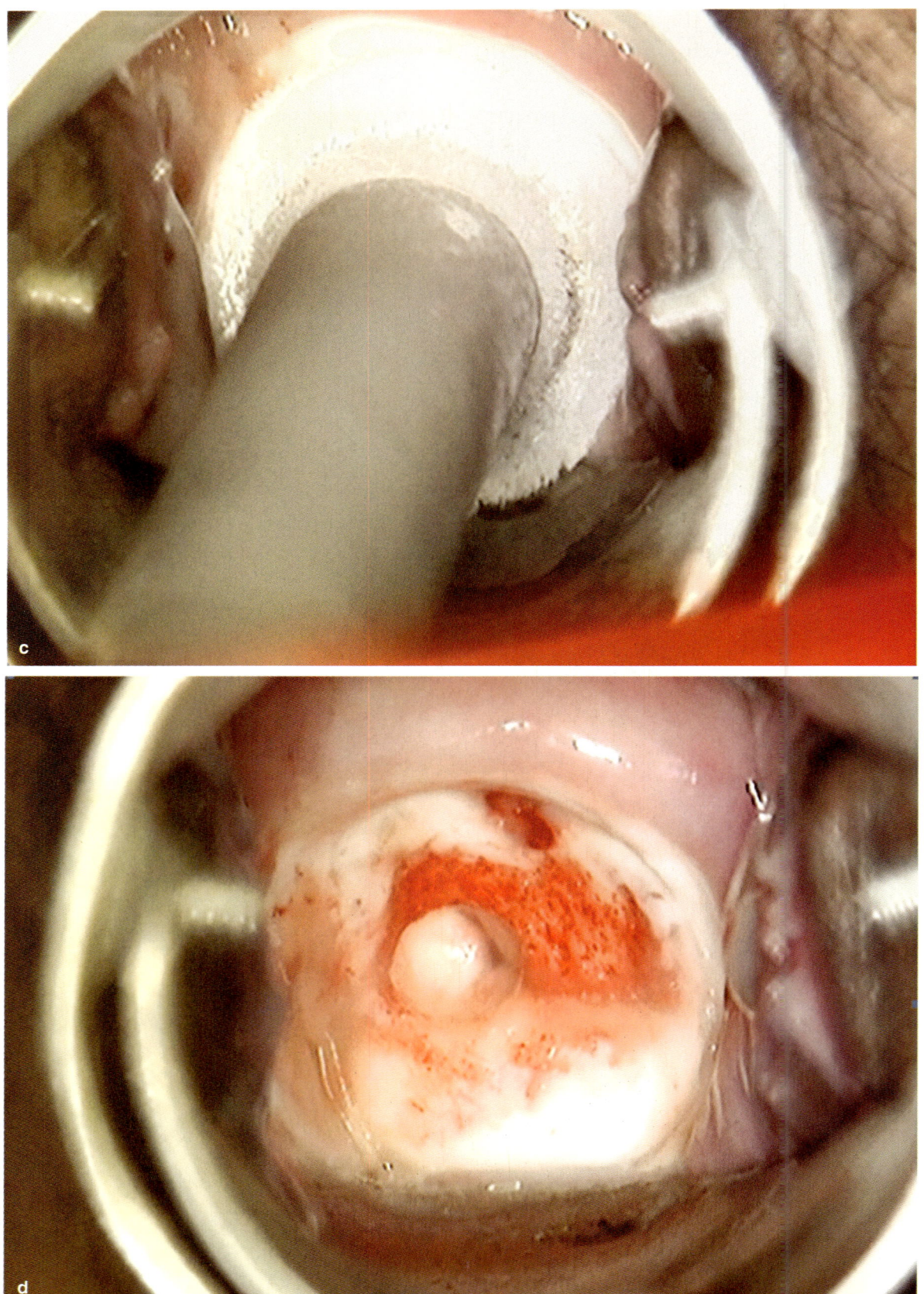

Figs 8.3c and d: Cryotherapy

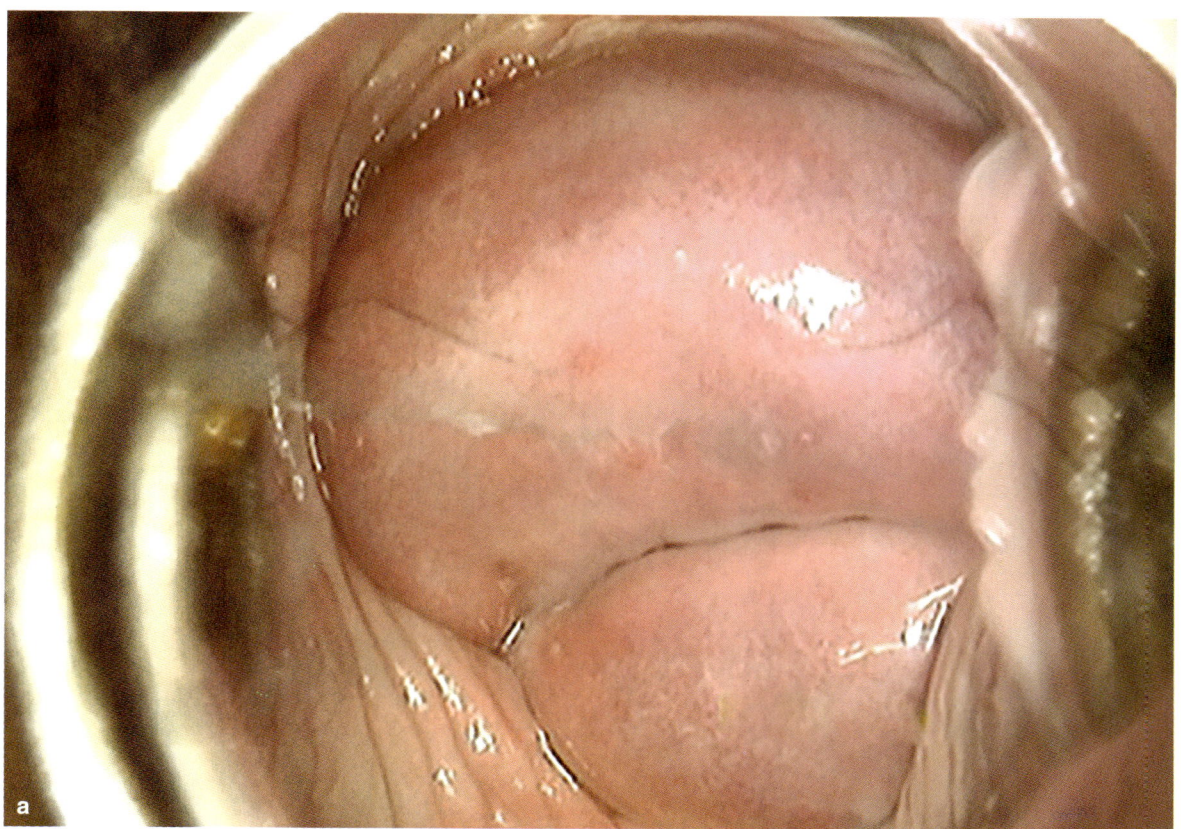

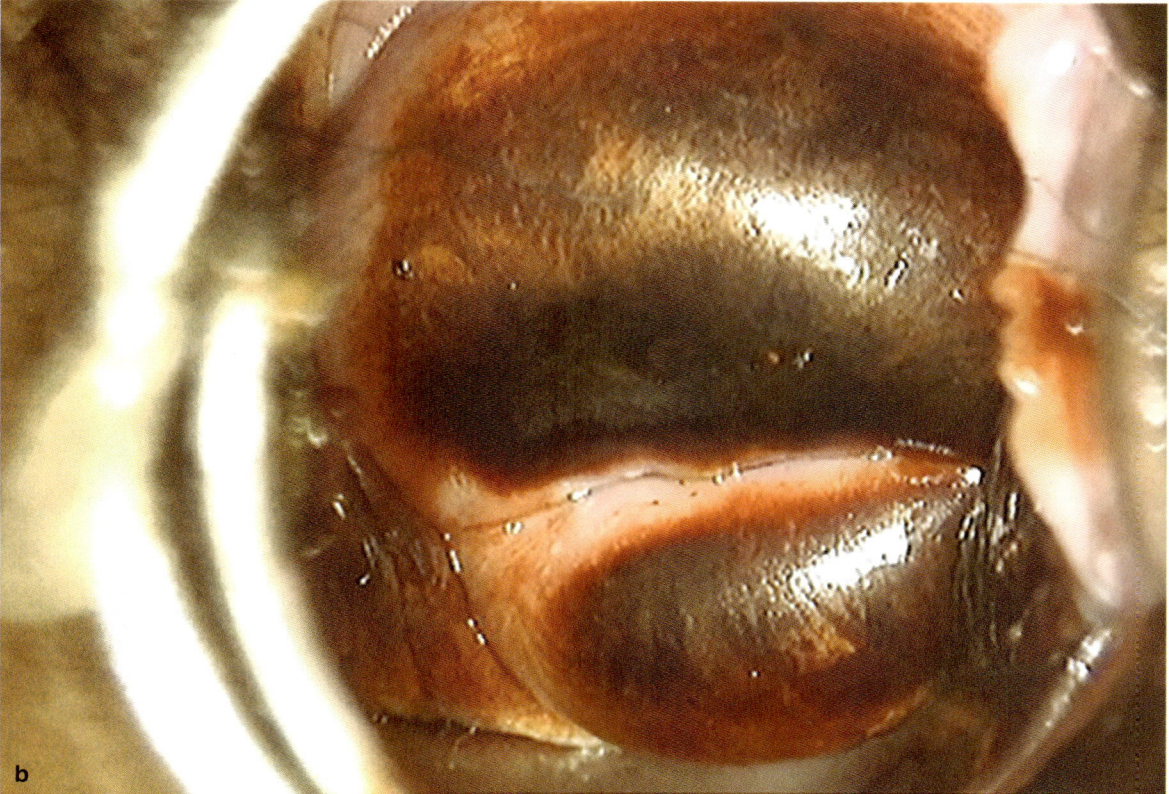

Figs 8.4a and b: Postcryotherapy—complete healing of the lesion (6 months later)

CASE 2

Case of LSIL treated with cryotherapy (Figs 8.5a to e)

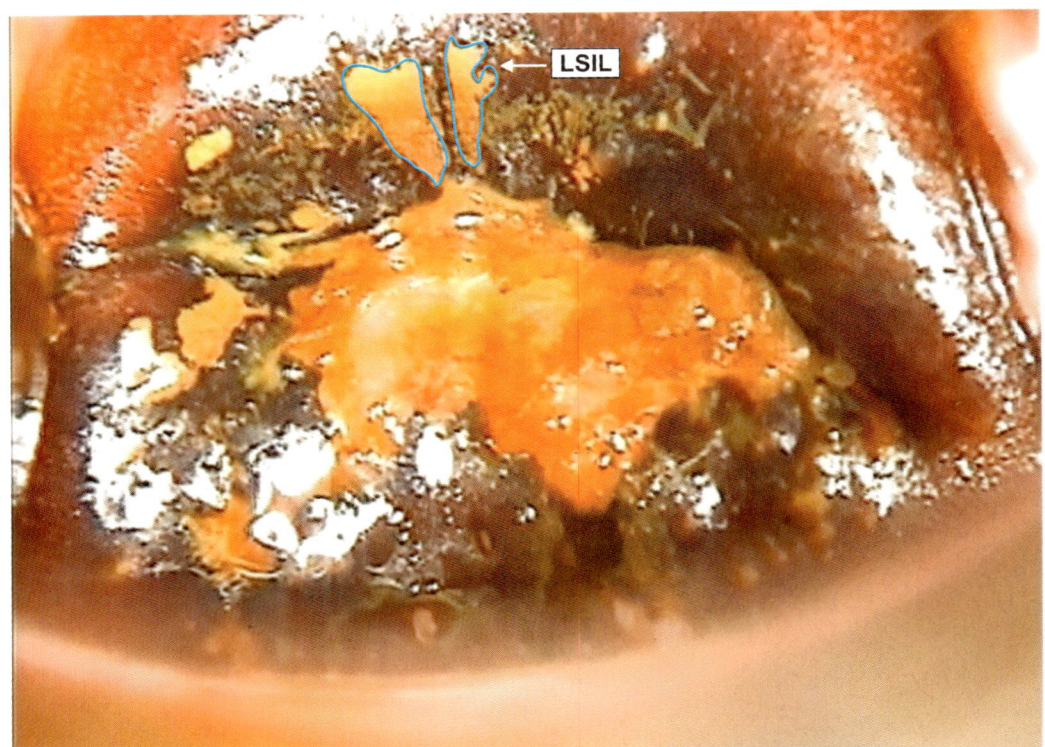

Fig. 8.5a: LSIL on colposcopy

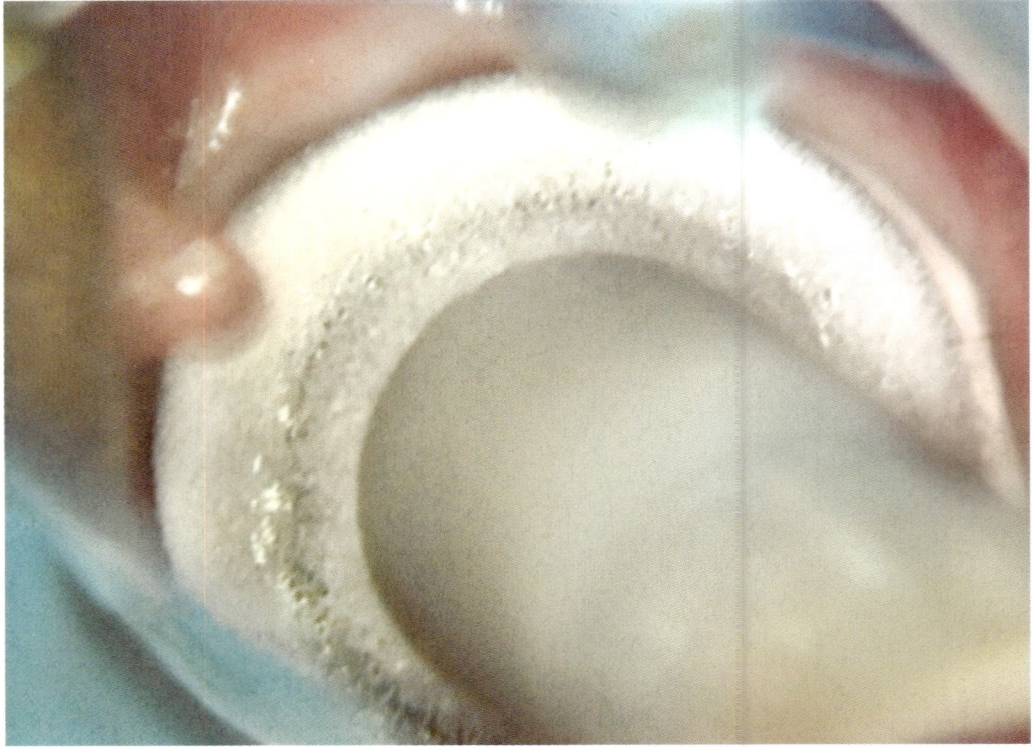

Fig. 8.5b: Cryotherapy with nitrous oxide

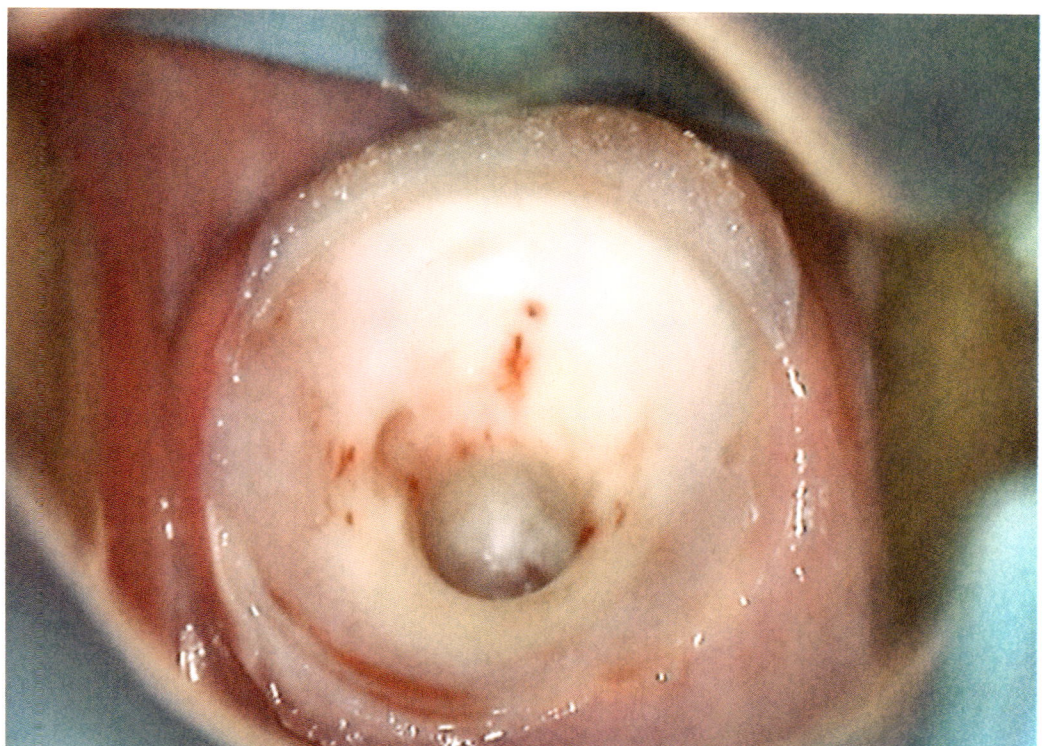

Fig. 8.5c: Post-cryotherapy

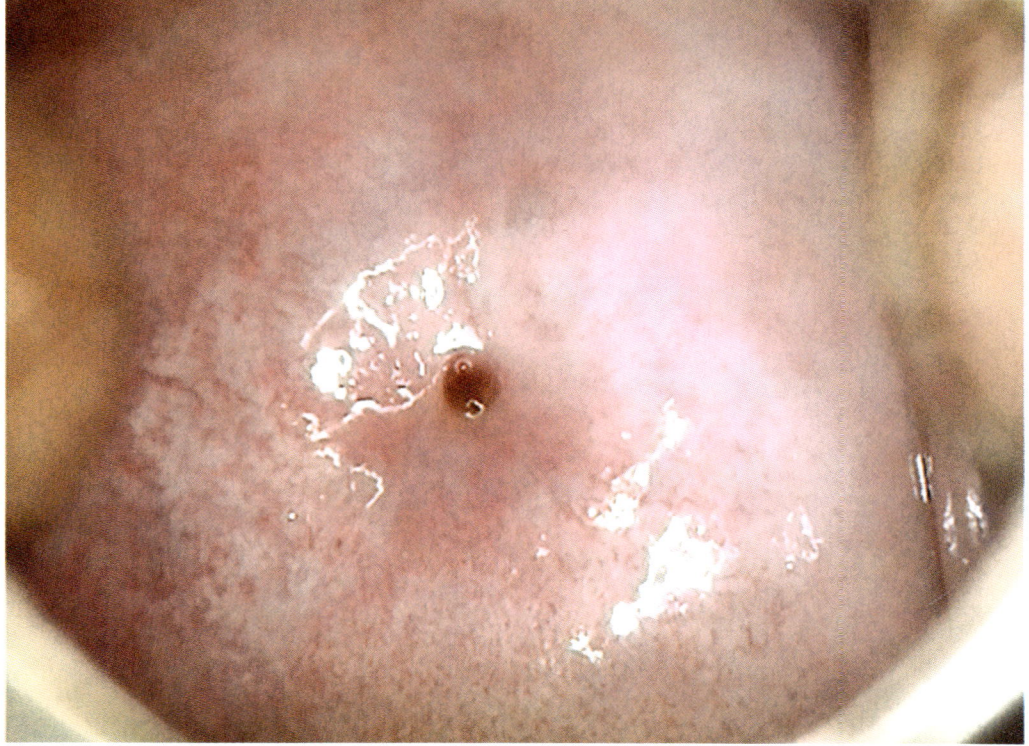

Fig. 8.5d: Post-cryotherapy follow-up after 6 months with 5% acetic acid

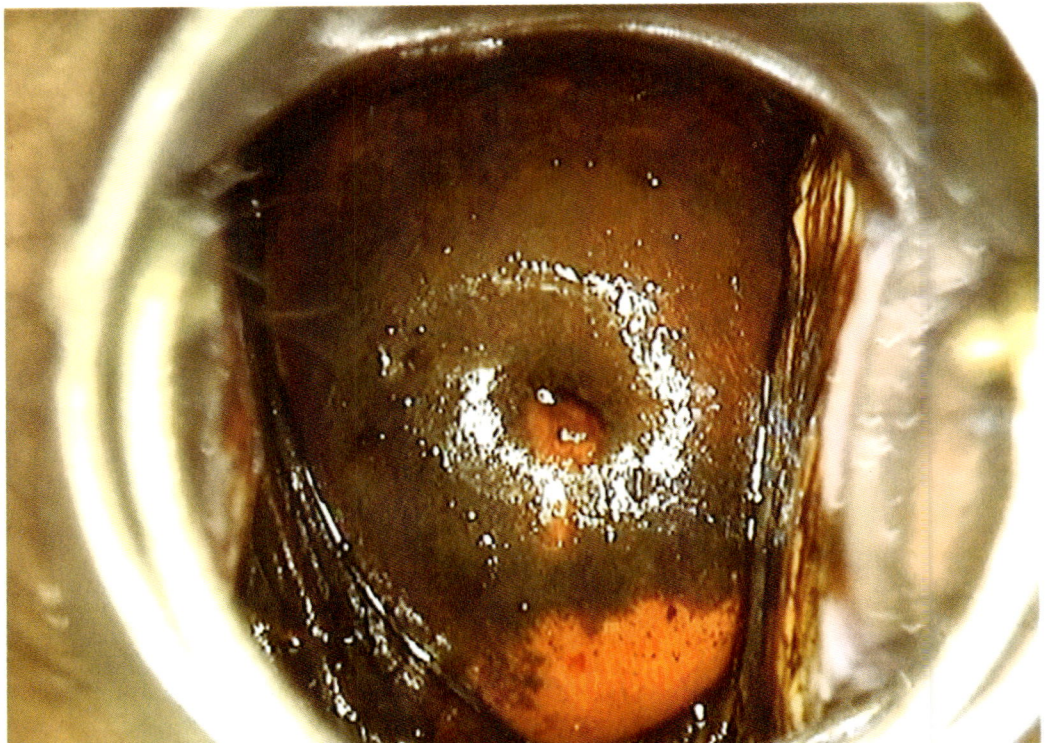

Fig. 8.5e: Post-cryotherapy follow-up after 6 months with Lugol's iodine

B. COLD COAGULATION OR THERMOCAUTERY

Introduction

It was introduced by Kurtz and Emm in 1966. It was originally used for cervical benign pathology and later from 1970 used in treatment of CIN.

Techniques

Cold coagulation is a misnomer as it is not cold. The probes are preheated to 120°C. The probe is applied in 40 sce pulses covering entire lesion in single or several applications. Local anesthesia is not required. It can be performed in see and treat approach.

Principle

It dessicates the intracellular water, denaturing the tissues, thus destroying the lesions.

Equipment (Figs 8.6a and b)

1. Portable operating unit with temperature control dial
2. Current models require main power supply
3. Detachable teflon-coated thermosound(s) probe

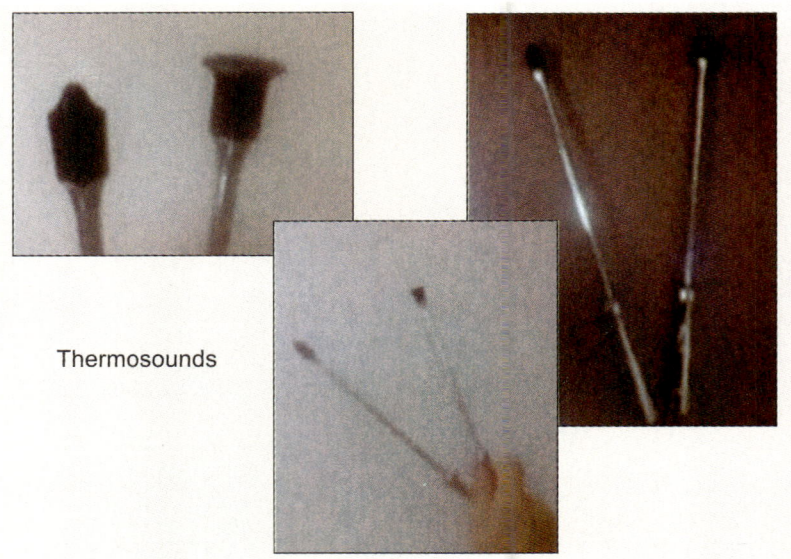

Thermosounds

Fig. 8.6a: Probes and thermosounds

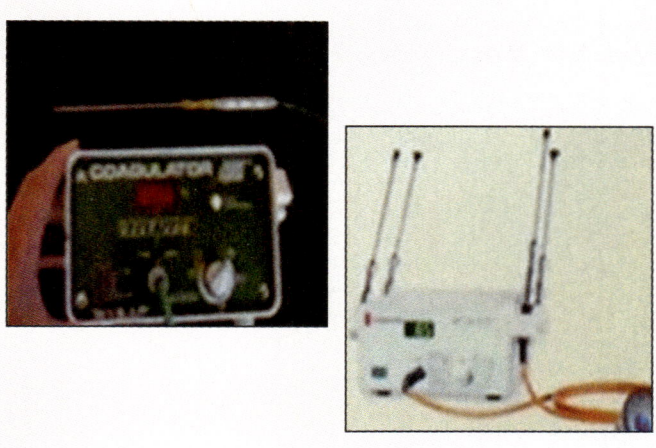

Fig. 8.6b: Portable operative unit

Advantages

- No refilling of gas.
- Operates on electricity, now battery operated is in experiment.
- Low learning curve.
- Can be used for see and treat.

Disadvantages

- Electricity recquired
- High cost (yet one time investment)
- No biopsy specimen

C. ELECTROCOAGULATION

Introduction

It is the usual treatment for ectropion and ectopy done with ball cautery. The whole exposed area of columnar epithelium is countered by ball cautery. The depth reached approximately 5 mm.

Principle

The subcolumnar reserve cells get stimulated to transform into metaplastic cells.

Advice

1. No sexual activity for 21 days.
2. Black discharge from vagina will be seen for a few weeks.

CASE 1

Electrocoagulation under Local Anesthesia (Figs 8.7a to d)

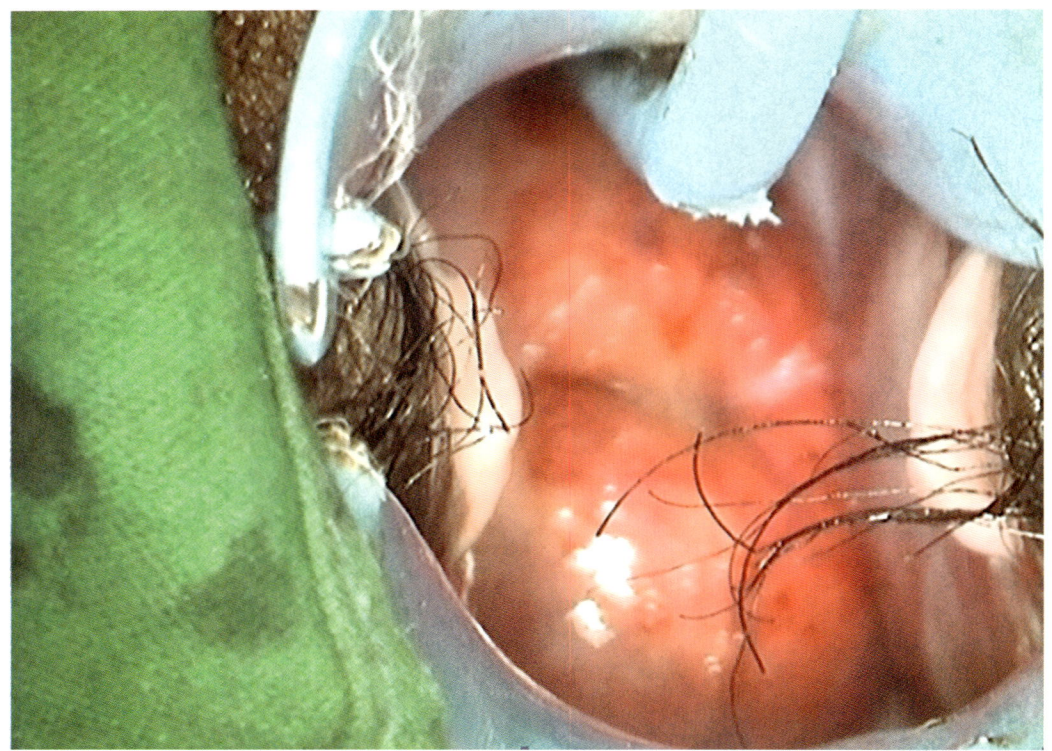

Fig. 8.7a: Case of ectropion

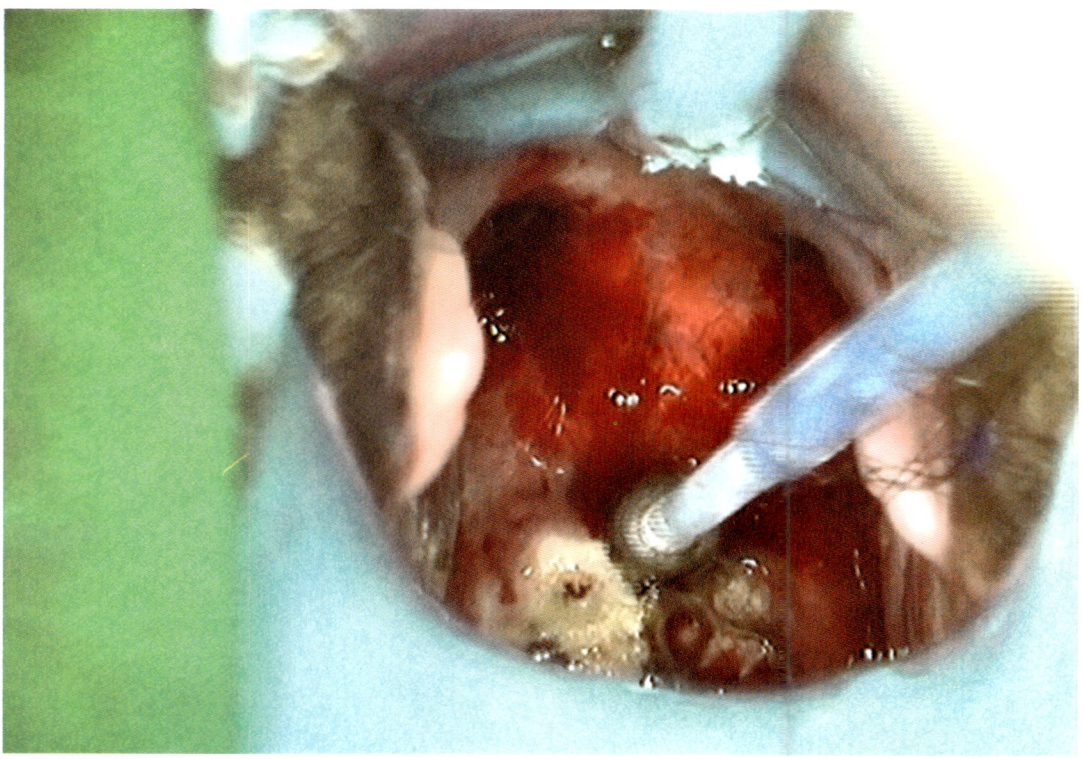

Fig. 8.7b: Cauterization with ball cautery

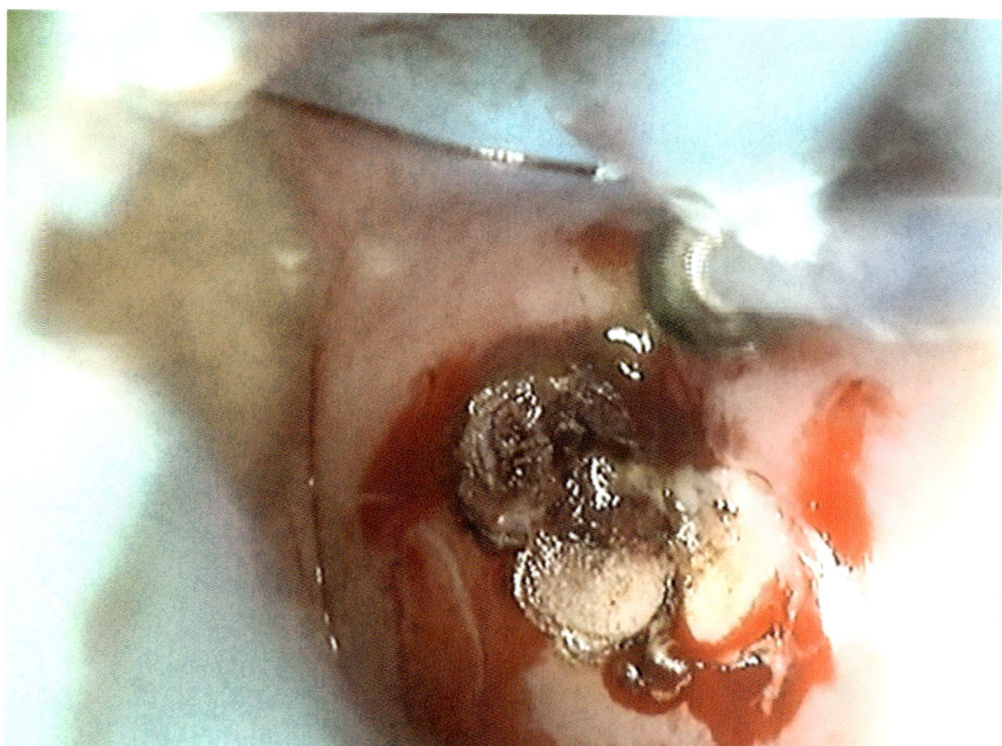

Fig. 8.7c: Ball cautery application covering whole of ectropion

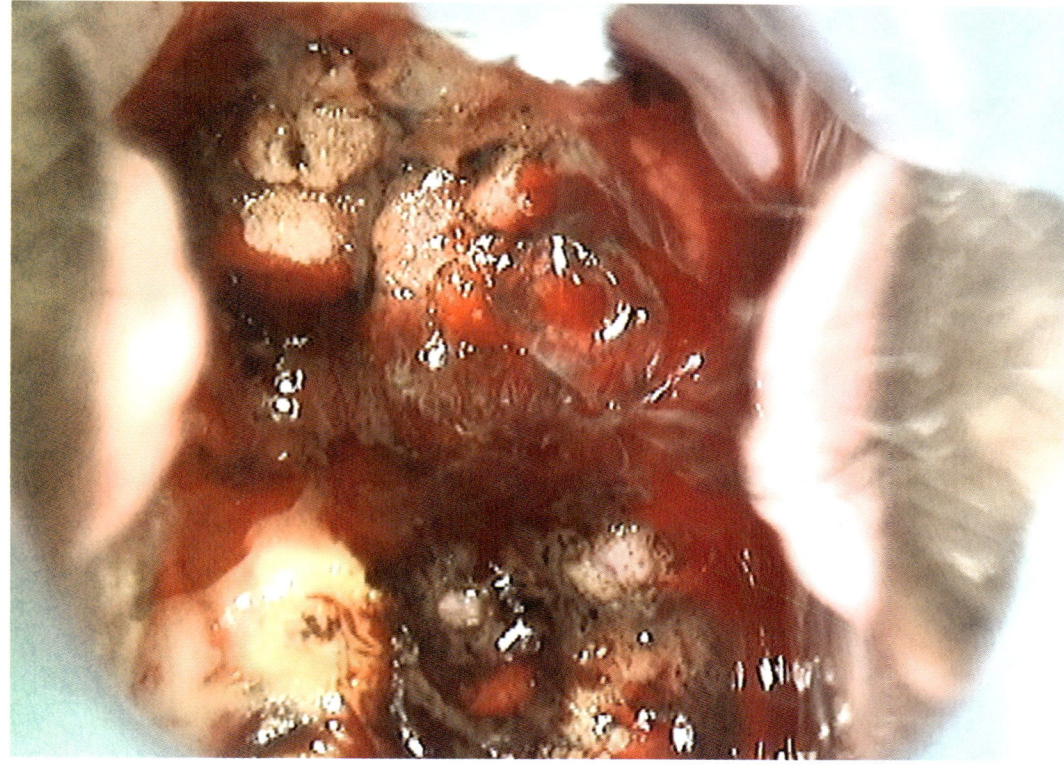

Fig. 8.7d: Complete ectropion cauterized with ball cautery

CASE 2

Case of Ectopy (treated with electrocautery—Figs 8.8a, b**)**

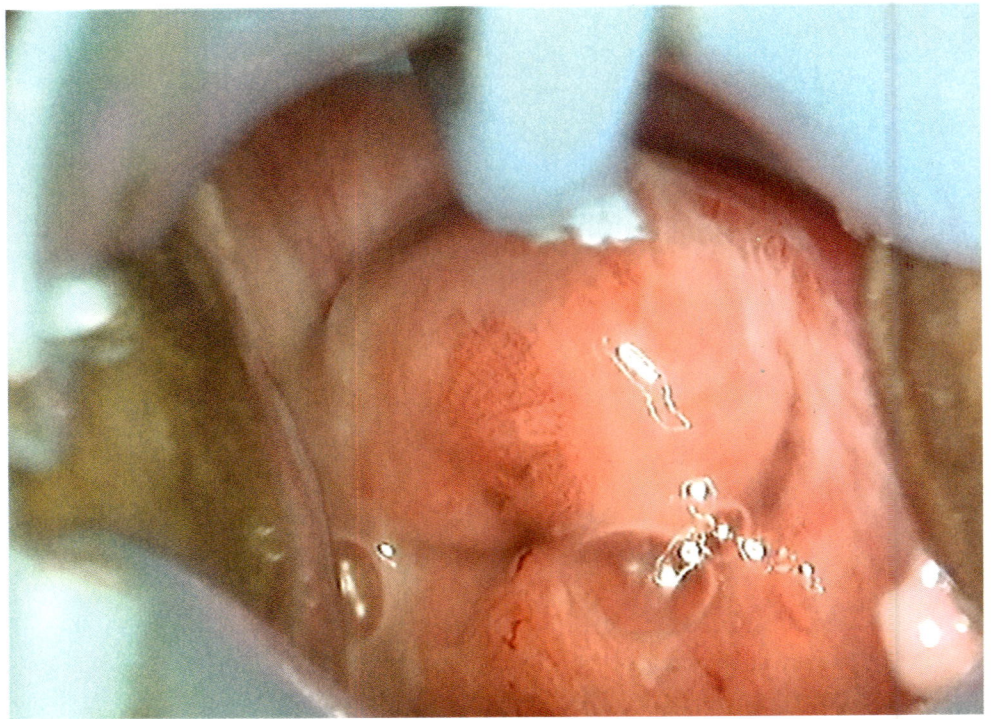

Fig. 8.8a: Case of ectopy

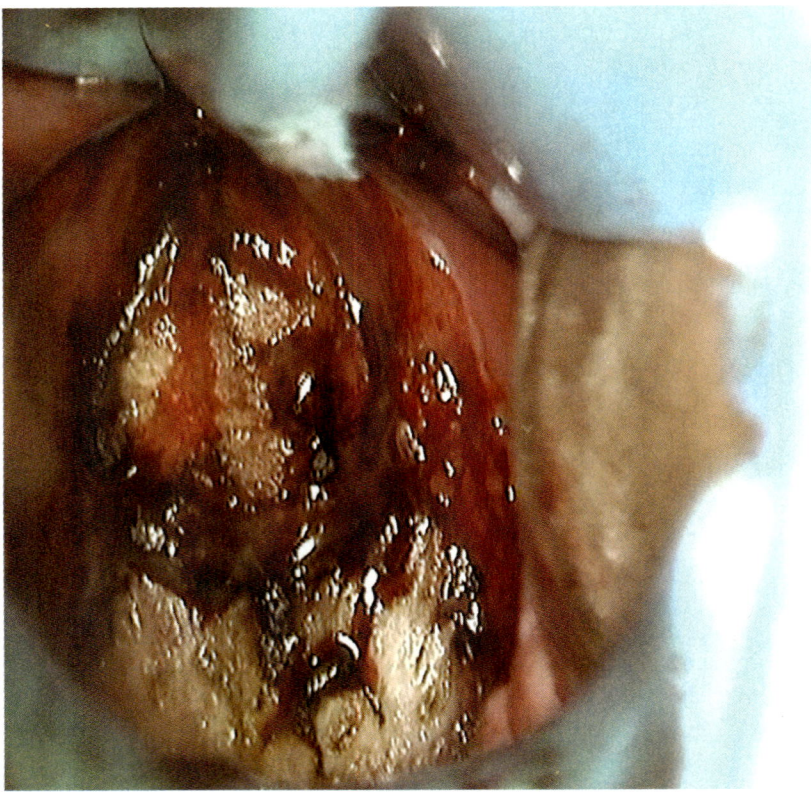

Fig. 8.8b: Treated by electrocautery using ball cautery

D. LOOP ELECTROSURGICAL EXCISION PROCEDURE (LEEP)

Large Loop Excision of Transformation Zone (LLETZ)

Introduction

The term LLETZ was coined by 'Rene Cartier' in early 1980s using a low voltage diathermy loop using thin wire under LA with blended diathermy. This term was coined to discriminate from small loop used by Ramey Kartey in Paris to take biopsy in early 1980s.

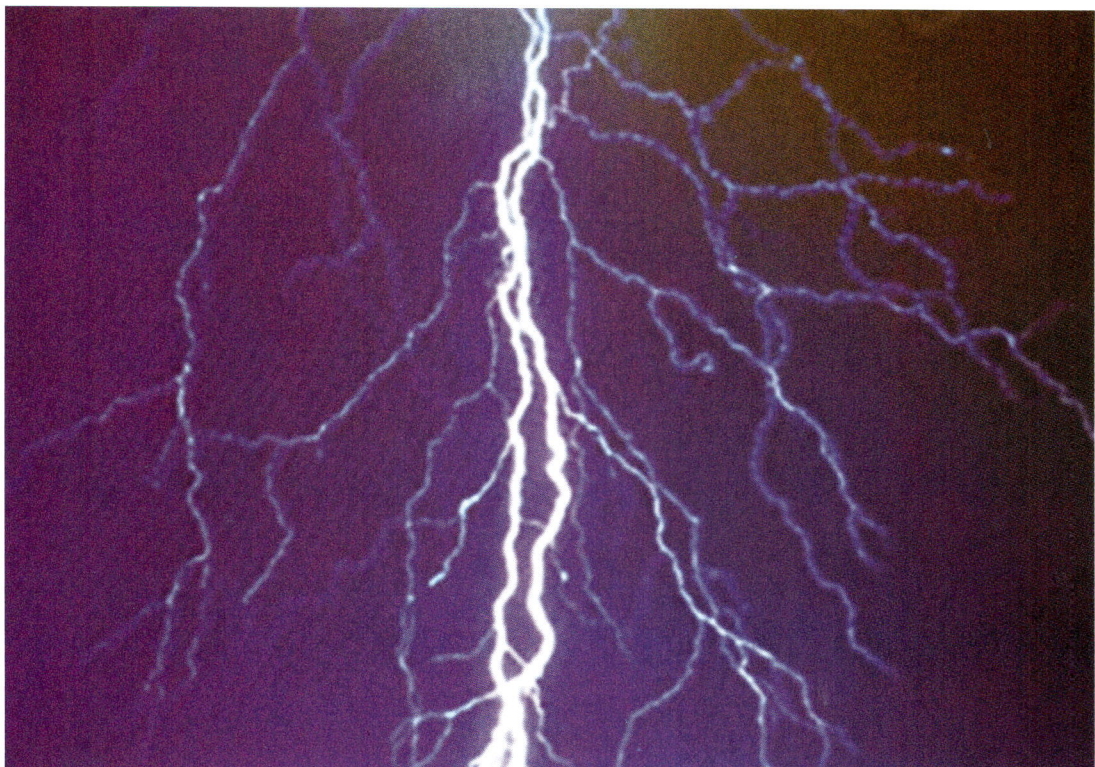

Fig. 8.9: High current

Principle

Based on discovery from Farday that the muscle does not contract by very high frequency alternating current (Fig. 8.9) greater than 100 kHz, it is possible to allow safe passage of electricity through controlled surface in the human body and to utilize the localised point of contact effect to achieve cutting, coagulation or combination blend of two. ESU operates to frequency above 300 KHz when contraction of muscle is overcome. The electrical energy used in electrosurgery is transformed into heat and light energy. The heat from a high voltage electrical arc between the operating electrode and the tissue has three effects on tissue depending on the power setting and the waveform of the current used—desiccation, cutting and fulguration. The tissue is cut by vaporizing tissue at 100°C or to coagulated by dehydrating tissue above 100°C. There are three types of coagulation–desiccation in which the active electrode touches the tissue; fulguration in which there is no contact between the active electrode withthe tissue, the electric current is sprayed with multiple sparks which flows between the electrode and the tissue; needle coagulation wherein a needle is inserted into the center of a lesion. The fulguration setting uses higher peak-to-peak voltage waveforms, coagulating the tissues with less current, and is, therefore, less harmful to the adjacent tissue. The waveform usually used is a blended waveform to control the bleeding during the procedure. Modern generators have the facility of blending both the coagulation current and the cutting current. Usually, the setting is made at 40 watts coagulation and 30 watts cutting to have a blended waveform. The settings can be adjusted accordingly. To complete the electrical circuit, a patient return electrode or dispersive plate should be placed in contact with patient's skin.

Fulguration vs desiccation

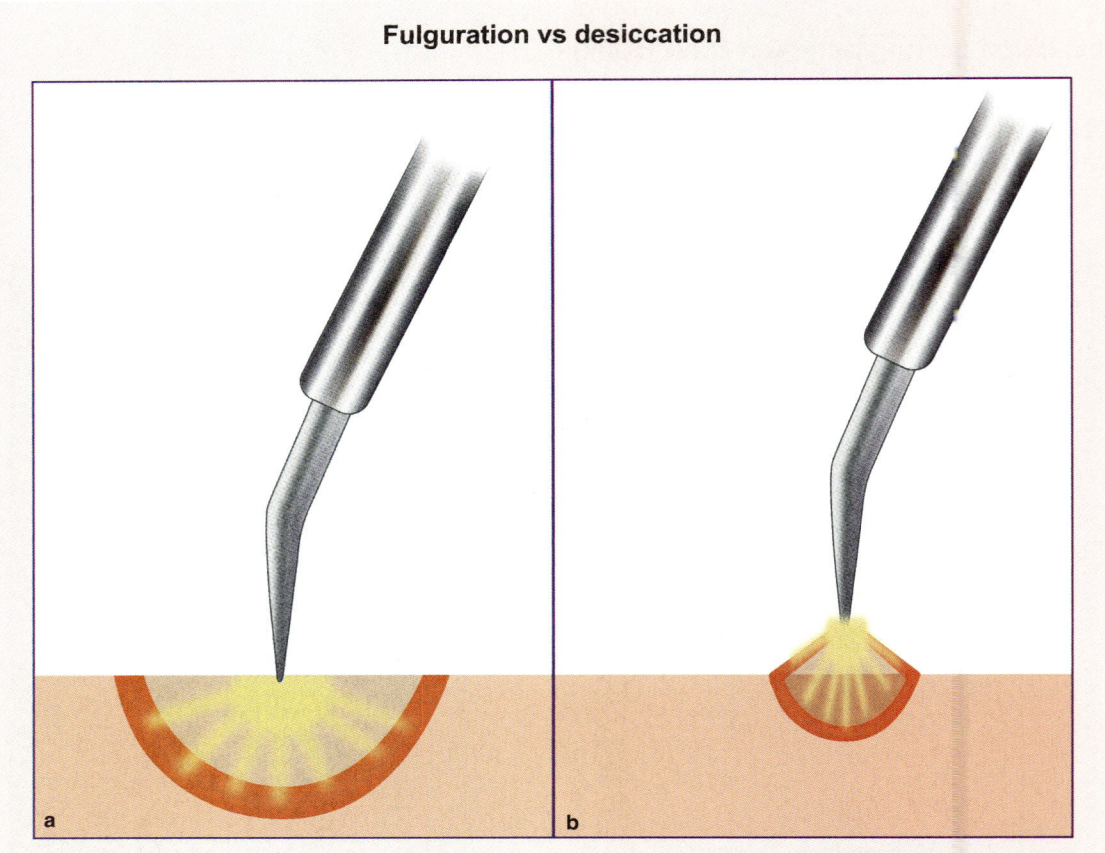

Figs 8.10a and b: a. Desiccation effect; **b.** Fulguration effect

Desiccation: There is full contact between the electrode and the tissue. ESU produces lower temperature but deeper diathermy effect, less coagulative and more damaging effect. This is usually useful in endometrial ablation (Fig. 8.10a).

Fulguration: The electricity passes through very small gap of tissue with relatively higher temperatures, used to achieve very less superficial tissue damage and sufficient cutting or coagulation effect (Fig. 8.10b).

How to achieve fulguration effect?
- Activate the electrode before contacting the tissue.
- Pass the loop slowly through the tissue whereby small stream window will occur between the loop and the tissue.
- Loop should not bend while passing the tissue or underneath the TZ.

Steps to be followed:
- Written informed consent should be taken.
- The procedure should be informed thoroughly to the patient. Also the alternative treatment modalities should be explained to the patient.
- In case of cervical atrophy in postmenopausal woman, topical application of estrogen is advisable before the procedure.
- *Instrument trolley* (Fig. 8.11): Insulated vaginal speculum or speculum covered by a condom, smoke evacuation tube, suction cannula, loop electrodes (Fig. 8.12), ball electrode, needle electrode, sponge holder, cotton balls, spinal needle no. 23 or 25, 5 cc syringe, 2% lignocaine, tooth forceps, cautery plate, Lugol's iodine, suture material, cautery handle, and monsel paste.
- Patient is made to lie on dorsal lithotomy position. Insulated vaginal speculum is inserted and the smoke evacuation tube is attached to the special operative speculum. The other end is attached to the suction machine.

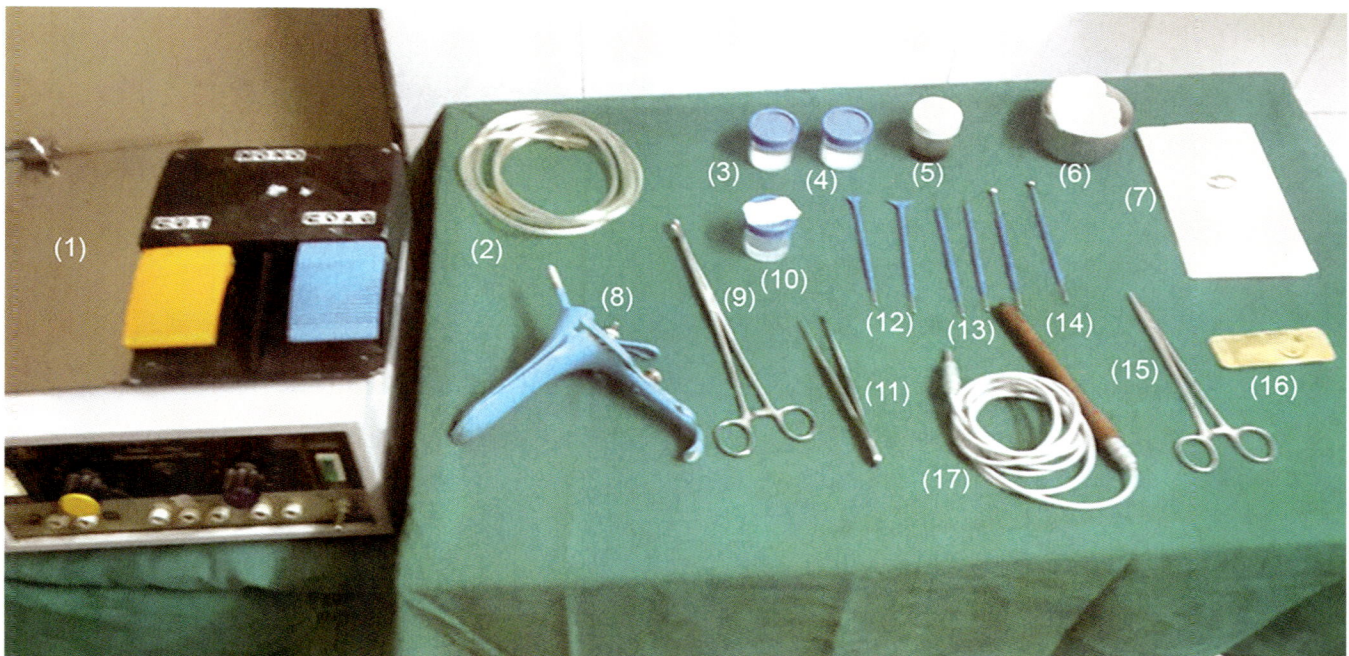

Fig. 8.11: Instrument trolley: (1) Cautery machine with foot pad, (2) smoke evacuation tube, (3) normal saline, (4) 5% acetic acid, (5) Lugol's iodine, (6) cotton balls, (7) gloves, (8) operative Cusco's speculum, (9) sponge holder, (10) specimen container, (11) tooth forceps, (12) LEEP's loops, (13) needle cautery, (14) ball cautery, (15) needle holder, (16) suture material, and (17) cautery handle

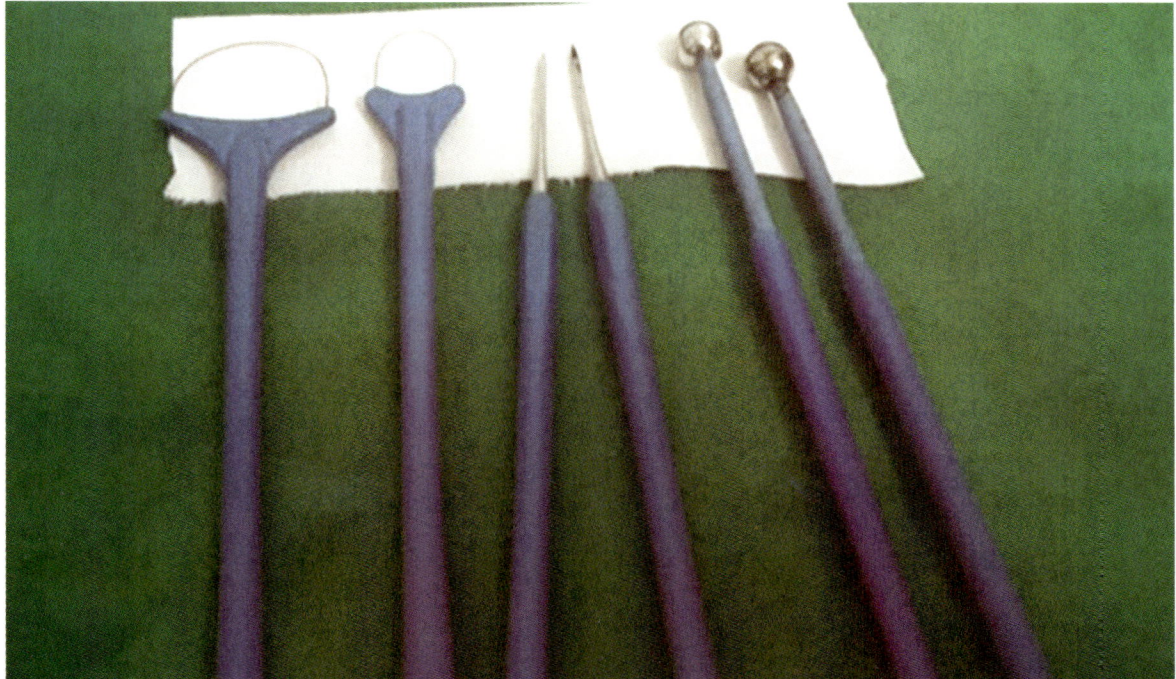

Fig. 8.12: Loop electrodes

The colposcopy procedure is repeated and the lesion is detected. Local anesthesia of 2% lignocaine is administered around the ectocervix using spinal needle. As the cervix is tough, there is some pressure to be applied for puncturing the tissue. Multiple sites are punctured to a depth of about 2 mm. Blanching of tissue is achieved while injecting the local anesthesia. To have a better field of vision, 1 drop of epinephrine can be added to the 10 ml of 2% lignocaine (to avoid epinephrine in case of high blood pressure). The smoke evacuation

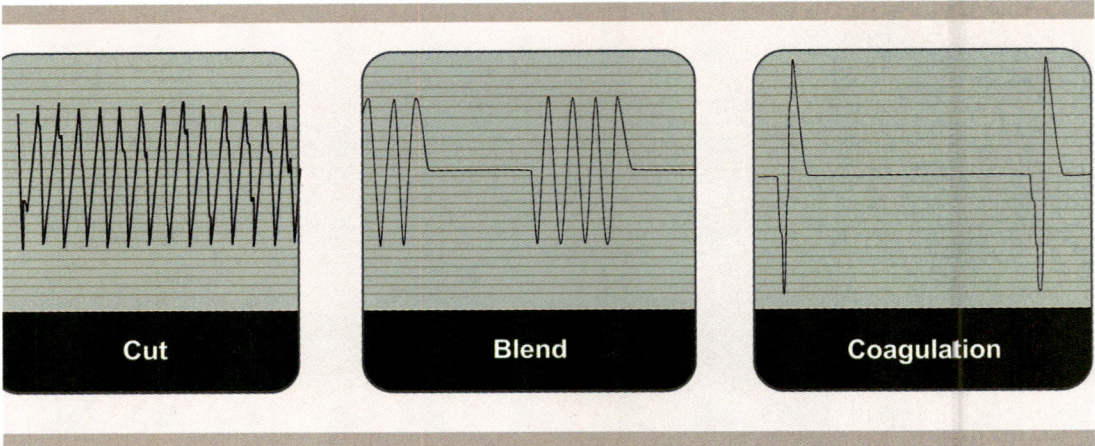

Fig. 8.13: Blended current

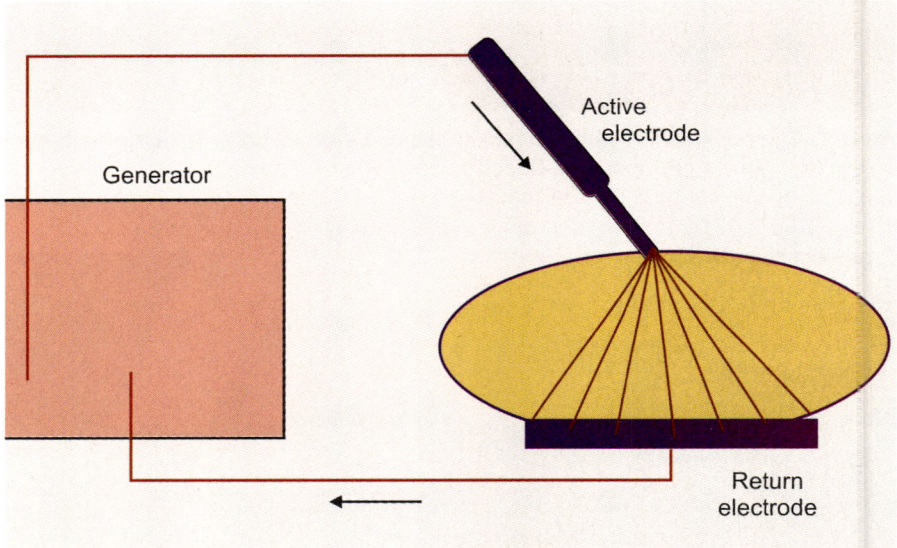

Fig. 8.14: Monopolar cautery

system is turned on. Just before the loop is placed on the cervix, the blended current is activated (Fig. 8.13), monopolar current is used (Fig. 8.14). The loop is placed on the tissue beyond the boundary of the lesion and simply cut through the cervical tissue without applying any pressure. The loop is guided parallel to the surface either horizontally or vertically with the handle perpendicular to the surface. Once the tissue is cut, the loop is withdrawn slowly and the dissected tissue is removed and sent for histopathology. The direction of movement can be from left-to-right; right-to-left; posterior-to-anterior (Fig. 8.15). But never from anterior-to-posterior as the excised tissue curls down and obscures the visual field. Once the tissue is removed, the surface is cauterized by ball cautery (Fig. 8.16). Minor bleeding is cauterized by needle cautery. Hemostasis is checked (Fig. 8.17). Intractable bleeding is tackled by taking a hemostatic stitch with late dissolving suture. Sometimes the lesion exceeds the width of the largest loop, in such cases multiple passes can be taken with different sizes of loop. The margins of the tissue removed should be lesion free on the HP report.

Instructions after the Procedure

- To avoid penetrative sexual contact for 4–6 weeks.
- Patient will have blackish brown discharge for 2–3 weeks.
- To report excessive bleeding or malodorous discharge.
- Follow-up at 3 months, 9–12 months, for test of cure (TOC Figs 8.18 a and b), and then yearly for 5 years.

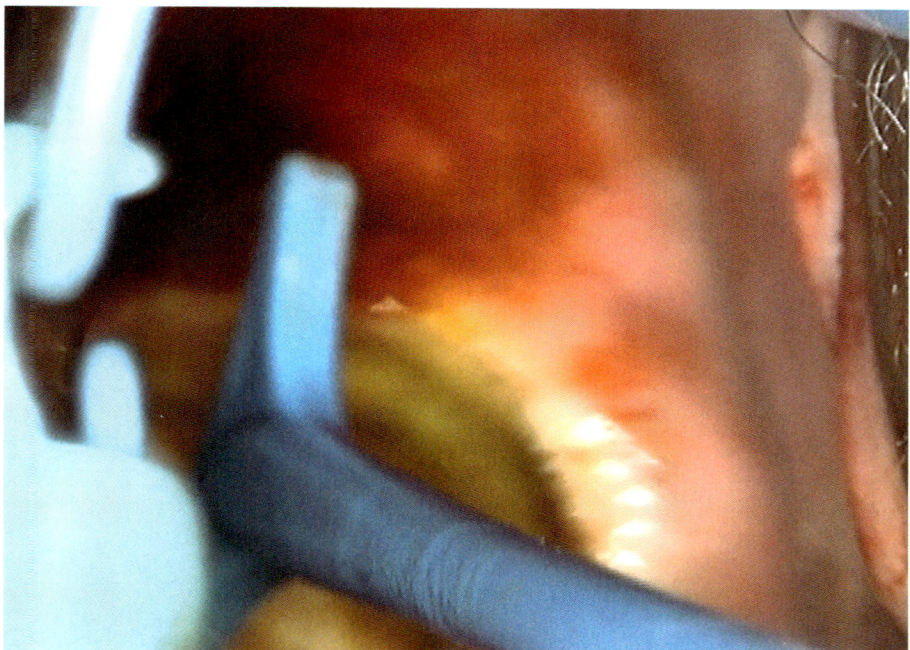

Fig. 8.15: Excision with loop electrode under LA

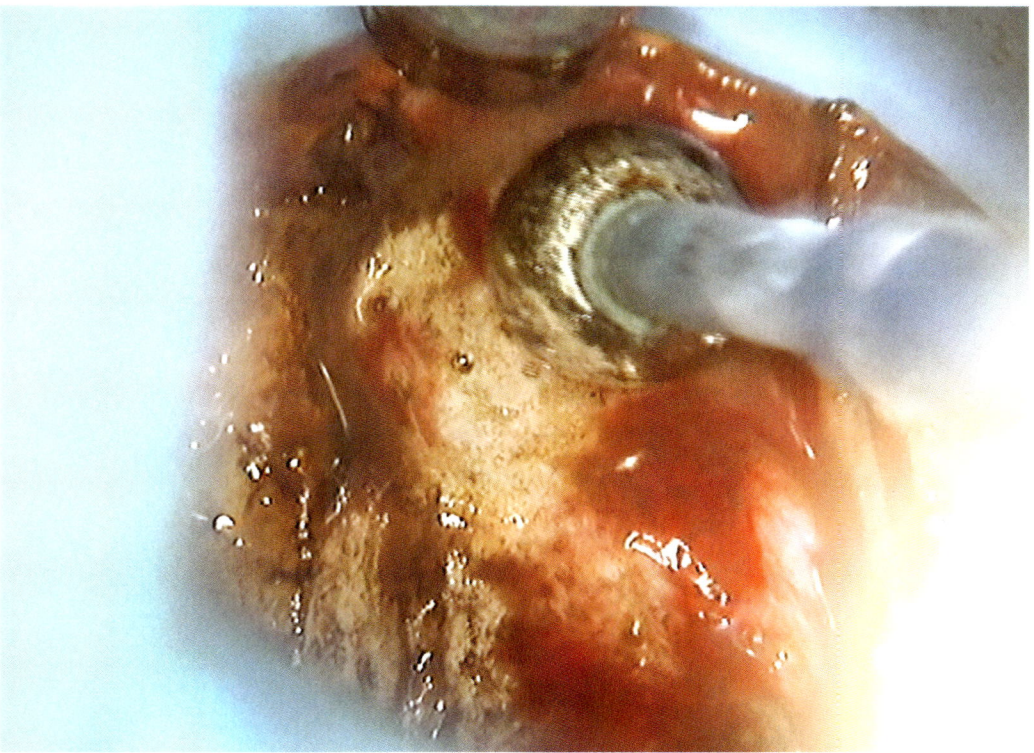

Fig. 8.16: Ball cautery used to achieve hemostasis

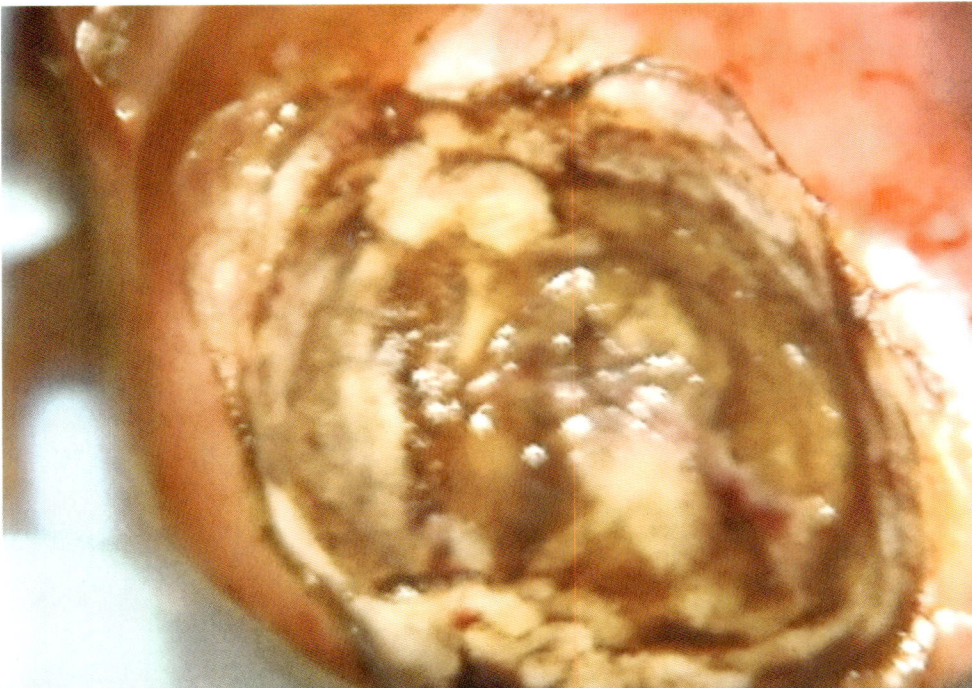

Fig. 8.17: Post-LEEP perfect hemostasis achieved

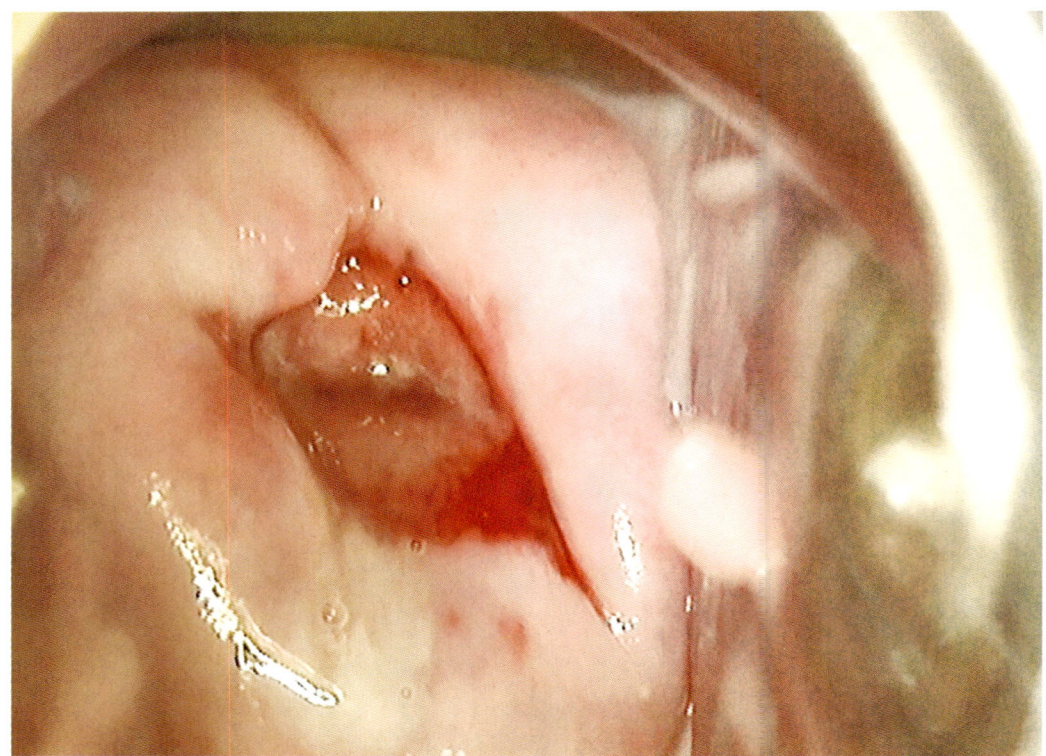

Fig. 8.18a: Post-LEEP follow-up after 6 months

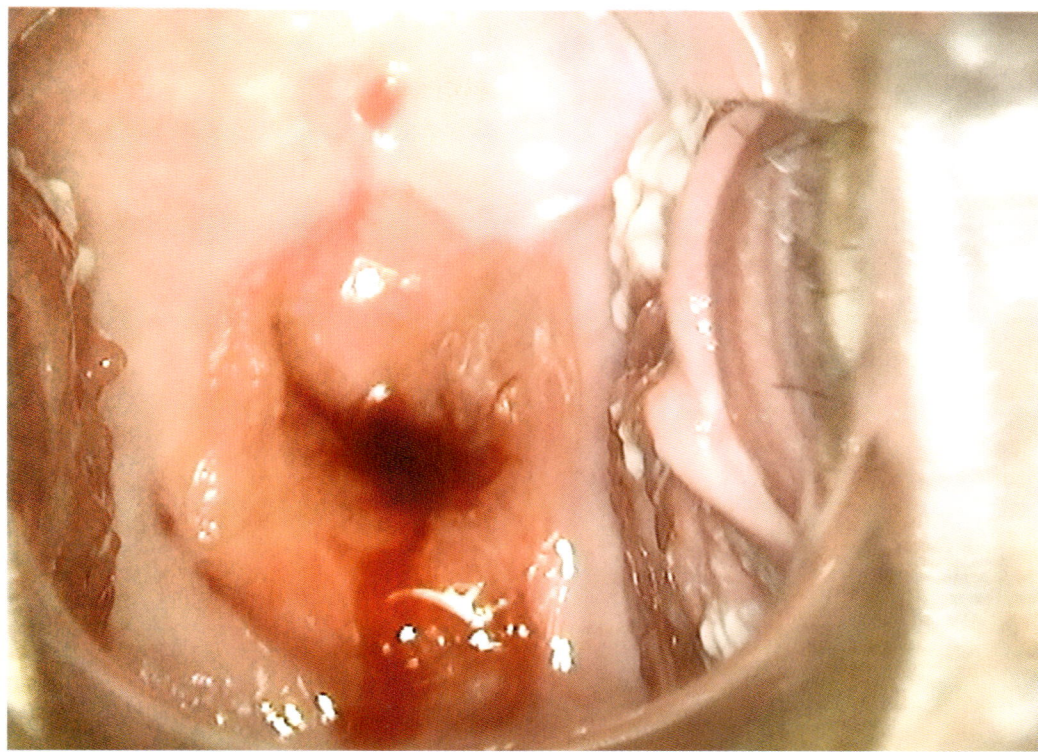

Fig. 8.18b: Follow-up post-LEEP after 1 year

Adverse Side Effects and Complications

- Excessive bleeding: Severe and moderate postoperative bleeding occurs in a few cases, which should be tackled immediately by fulguration or applying monsel paste or using a silver nitrate application stick. Rarely placement of suture is necessary.
- Postoperative infection.
- *Treatment failure:* This is seen in 10% of the cases. It is advisable and mandatory to biopsy all the persistent lesions to reporting of any preclinical invasive carcinoma. Persistent lesions can be treated with LEEP or cryotherapy.

Follow-up Post-Treatment

The valuation approach presented here is provided by the 2012 consensus guideliens of the American Society for Colposcopy and Cervical Pathology in collaboration with multiple professional societies and government organizations in the United States and Canada, including the American College of Obstetricians and Gynecologists, Society of Obstetricians and Gynaecologists of Canada, Society of Gynecologic Oncologists, American Cancer Society, Centers for Disease Control and Prevention, and the US Food and Drug Administration. The algorithms for the consensus guidelines can be found online.

After treatment with excision or ablation, women with cervical intraepithelial neoplasia (CIN) 2, 3 should be followed with:

- Human papillomavirus (HPV) cervical cytology cotesting at 12 and 24 months.
  - If both cotests are negative, cotesting should be repeated in three years. If cotesting is again negative, the patient may resume routine screening.
  - If there is abnormal cytology or a positive HPV test during follow-up, colposcopy with endocervical sampling should be performed.
- Routine screening is recommended for at least 20 years, even if screening continues beyond age 65 years.
- If CIN 2,3 is identified at the margins of an excisional procedure or postprocedure endocervical curettage (ECC), cytology and ECC at 4 to 6 months is preferred, but either repeat excision or hysterectomy may be performed.

Section II

Cytology

Understanding the Normal Cervix:
Histology and Cytology

Colposcopy requires a thorough understanding of the normal histology of the cervix. At a very basic level, the ectocervix is lined by stratified squamous epithelium. It is thick, due to multiple layers, and is opaque. At places, there are papillae which project upwards containing blood vessels. These are seen as red spots, when seen from above in colposcopy. Endocervix is lined by columnar epithelium which is unilayered and mucus secreting. Being single layered, it is translucent and hence underlying structures can be seen.

However, there are numerous other details of cervical histology which the colposcopist needs to understand—and the following section attempts to explain the details.

DEVELOPMENT

The endocervix is the site of the transformation zone—where the normal stratified squamous epithelium of the ectocervix abruptly changes to columnar mucus secreting epithelium of the endocervix.

During embryogenesis, the uterus, cervix and upper two-thirds of the vagina are of Mullerian duct origin. Hence, the original epithelial lining of the uterus, endocervix, ectocervix and vagina in the upper two-thirds of the organ is by cuboidal to columnar epithelium. The lower one-third of the vagina derived from the cloaca is lined by squamous epithelium derived from the ectoderm.

A wave of squamous metaplasia occurs later in embryogenesis, from below upwards. This transforms the columnar epithelium of the upper two-thirds of vagina and ectocervix into stratified squamous epithelium. This wave stops at the junction between endocervix and ectocervix. Hence, the endocervix continues to be lined by columnar epithelium which later differentiates to become mucin secreting in nature and also invaginates to form the endocervical glands.

The endocervical glands and surface lining are both similar, made up of tall columnar cells with basally located nuclei. The cytoplasm above the nucleus of each cell contains mucin. The glands are racemose in shape with the same type of mucinous epithelial lining as is present on the surface.

This is a process of normal embryological transformation and hence is not termed metaplasia. Metaplasia is defined as the process of transformation of one mature type of tissue into another mature type. Since the process is embryological, it is not metaplasia since the previous epithelium is not yet a mature type of tissue.

DEFECTS IN EMBRYOGENESIS

Defects in embryogenesis can occur either spontaneously or after administration of diethyl stilbesterol to the mother during pregnancy. In these situations, islands of columnar epithelium are left behind in the lining of the vagina where squamous transformation during embryogenesis fails to occur.

These islands can develop invaginations and cytoplasmic mucin production and form the lesion termed as vaginal adenosis.

HISTOLOGY OF NORMAL ECTOCERVIX

Normal squamous epithelium of vagina and cervix is a stratified and non-keratinized epithelium. It has a basement membrane, basal cells, parabasal cells which are small-sized cuboidal-shaped spinous cells, intermediate cells which are larger spinous cells above the parabasal cells, which have abundant cytoplasm configured flat over the surface plane, and superficial squamous cells which are even larger than the intermediate cells, again arranged flat over the surface plane and having increased cytokeratin intermediate filament in the cytoplasm. Parabasal and intermediate cells have a viable nucleus which is round with indistinct nuclear membrane and vesicular chromatin having a small inconspicuous nucleolus and a Barr body at the nuclear rim. The nucleus reduces in size as we go higher from the parabasal to the intermediate cells. Superficial cells have a pyknotic nucleus which is one-fourth the size of the intermediate cell nucleus.

Figure 9.1 shows normal ectocervical epithelium which is flat and is fully glycogenated, i.e. from secretory phase of the cycle. Parabasal cells do not have glycogen, intermediate cells have glycogen and superficial cells are few in number in this phase.

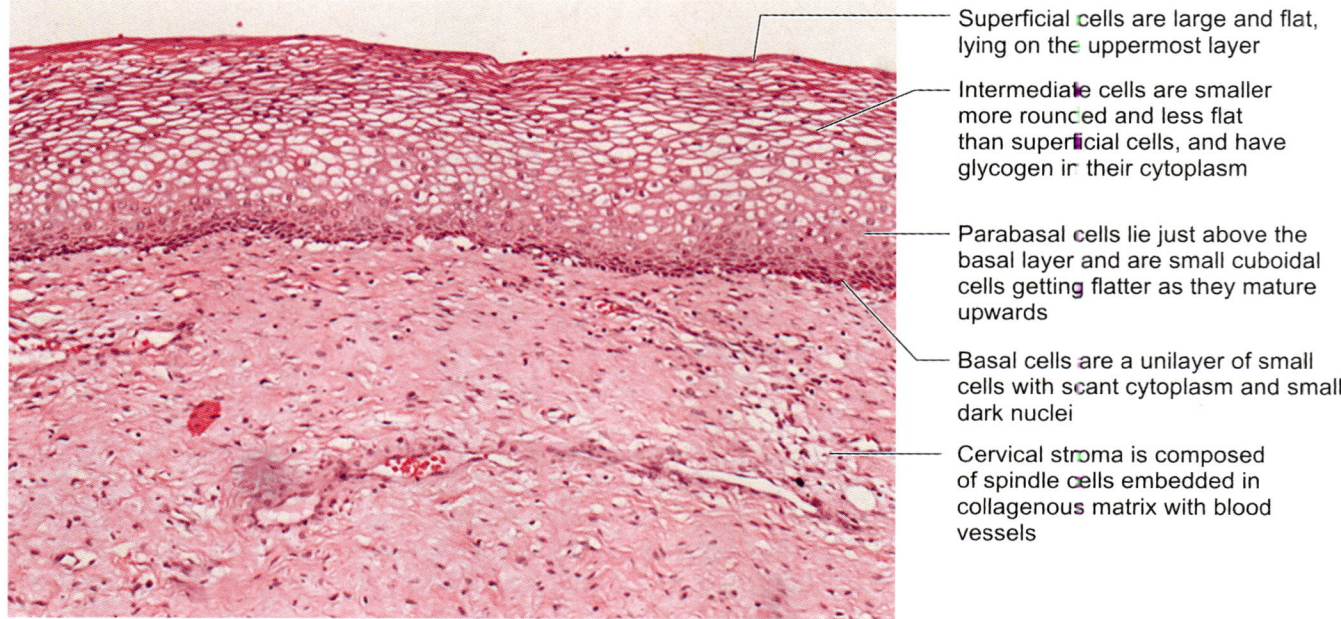

Superficial cells are large and flat, lying on the uppermost layer

Intermediate cells are smaller more rounded and less flat than superficial cells, and have glycogen in their cytoplasm

Parabasal cells lie just above the basal layer and are small cuboidal cells getting flatter as they mature upwards

Basal cells are a unilayer of small cells with scant cytoplasm and small dark nuclei

Cervical stroma is composed of spindle cells embedded in collagenous matrix with blood vessels

Fig. 9.1: Normal ectocervical epithelium

Figure 9.2 is of secretory phase showing glycogenated intermediate cells predominating. The basal cells and a small papilla are seen.

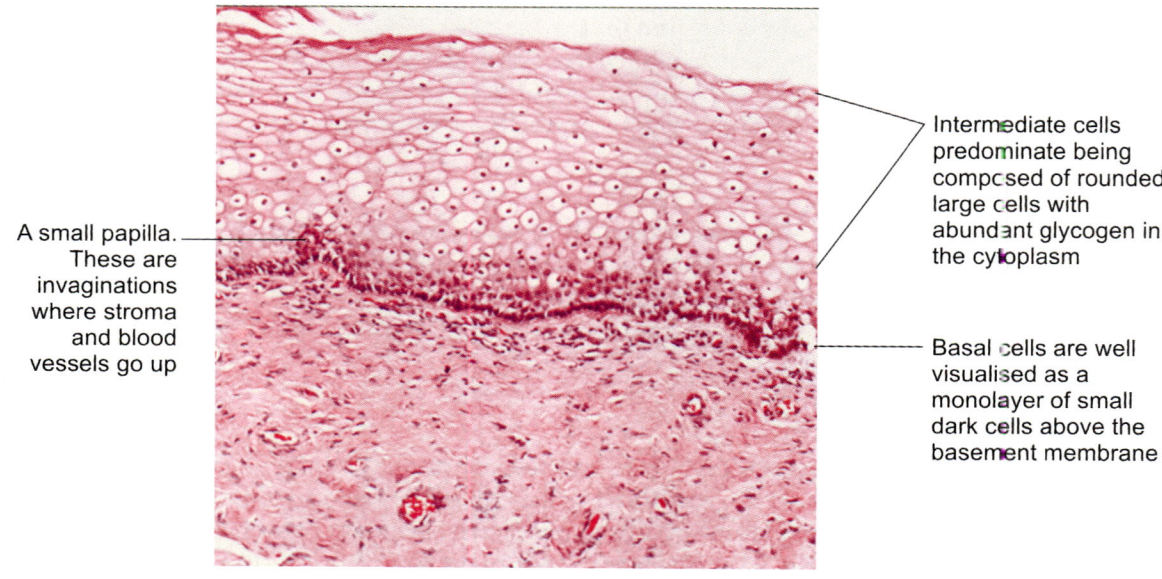

Intermediate cells predominate being composed of rounded large cells with abundant glycogen in the cytoplasm

A small papilla. These are invaginations where stroma and blood vessels go up

Basal cells are well visualised as a monolayer of small dark cells above the basement membrane

Fig. 9.2

Normal papillae (Figs 9.3 and 9.4) are invaginations where the blood vessels along with a sheath of stroma go up into the epithelium, so that all the layers of the epithelium can get oxygen and other nutrients by diffusion from the blood vessels. The overlying epithelium is thinner over these regions and hence can be seen on the surface as small spots of red due to the vessels.

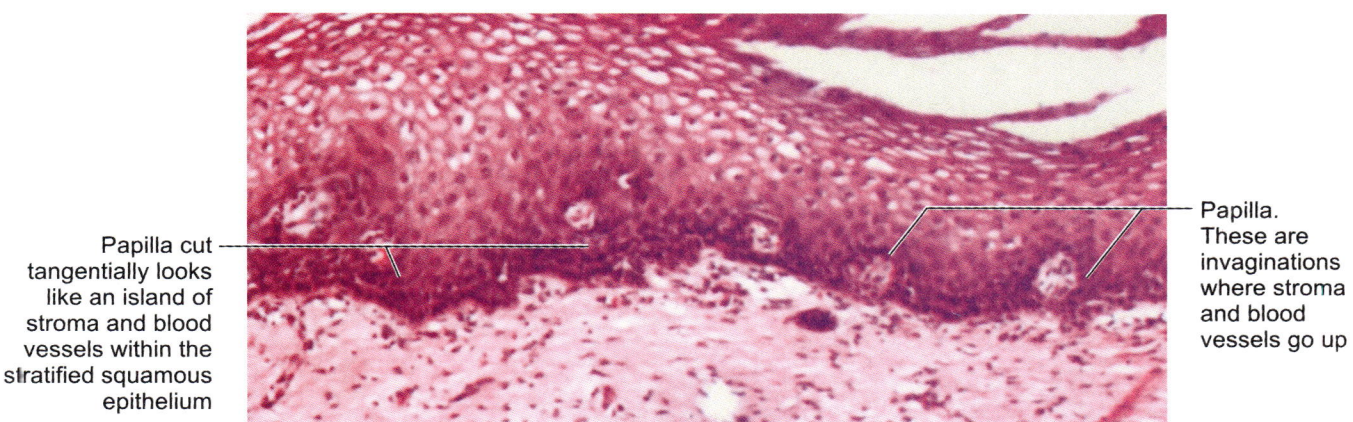

Papilla cut tangentially looks like an island of stroma and blood vessels within the stratified squamous epithelium

Papilla. These are invaginations where stroma and blood vessels go up

Fig. 9.3

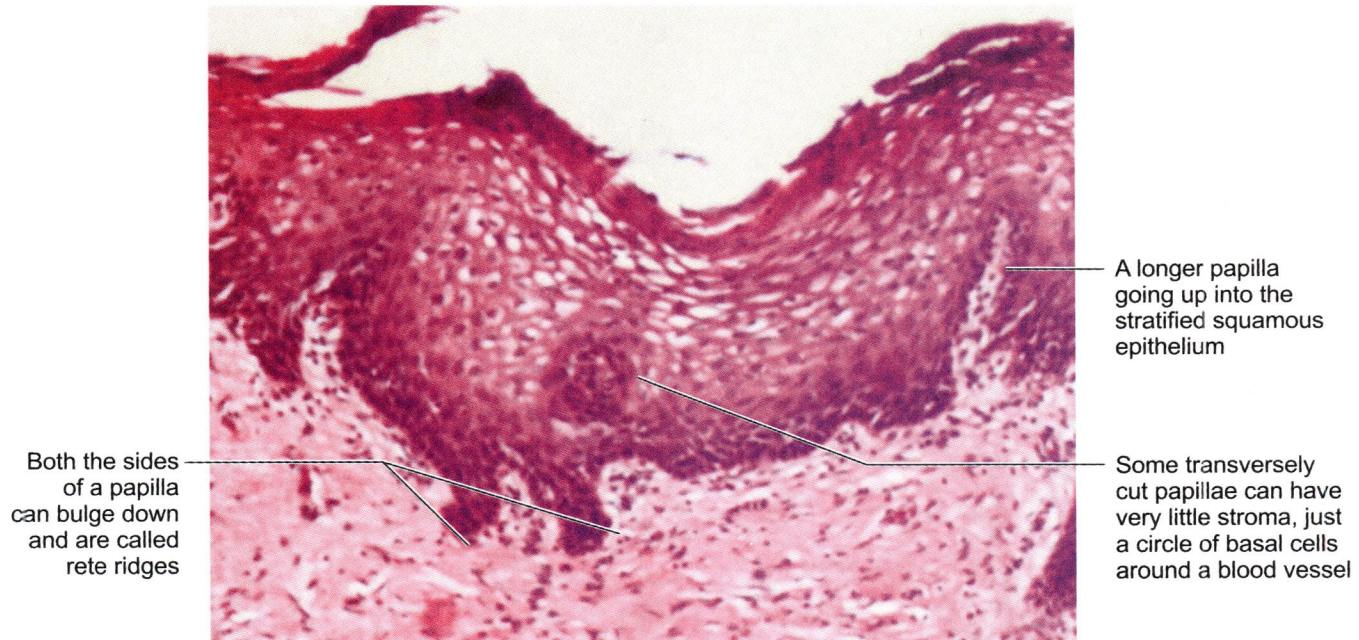

A longer papilla going up into the stratified squamous epithelium

Both the sides of a papilla can bulge down and are called rete ridges

Some transversely cut papillae can have very little stroma, just a circle of basal cells around a blood vessel

Fig. 9.4

CYTOLOGY OF CERVICAL SQUAMOUS CELLS (Figs 9.5 to 9.7)

Pap stain makes squamous cells either pink or green depending on its state of maturation. Cells with inactive cytoplasm stains pink with eosin. Cells with active cytoplasmic proteins stain green.

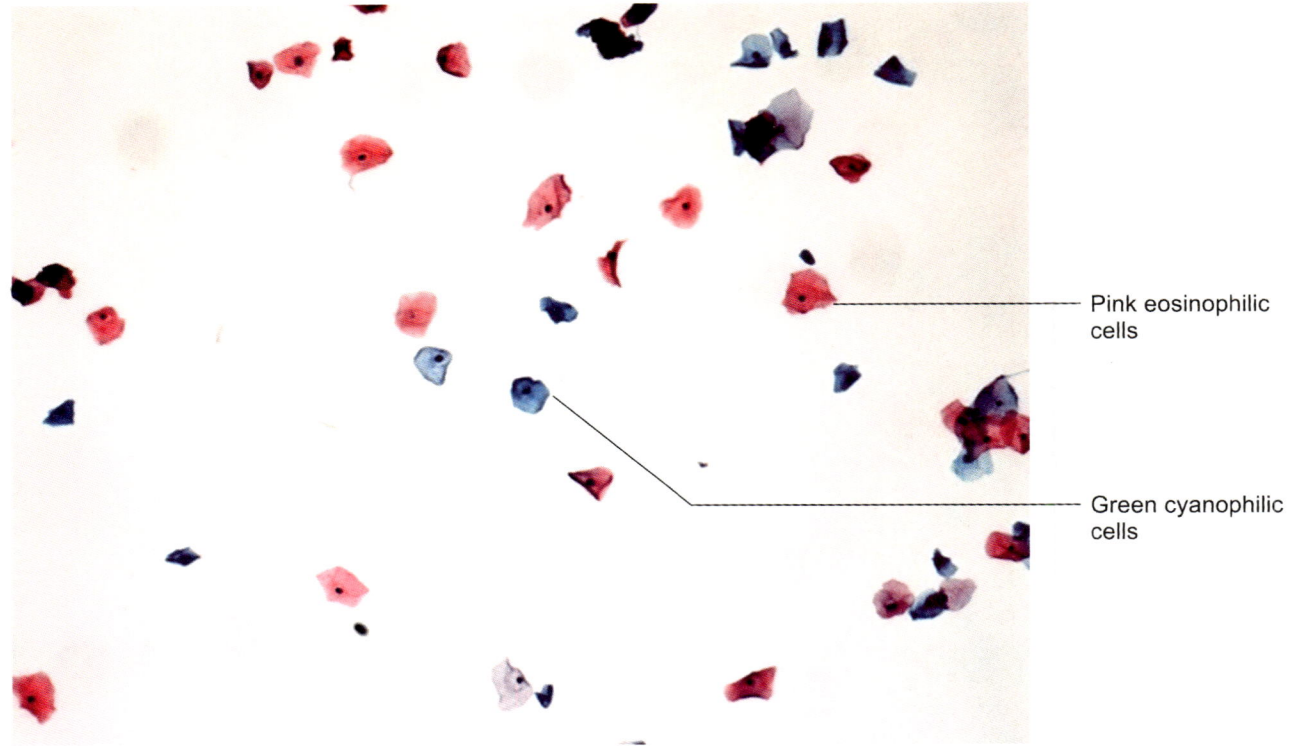

Pink eosinophilic cells

Green cyanophilic cells

Fig. 9.5

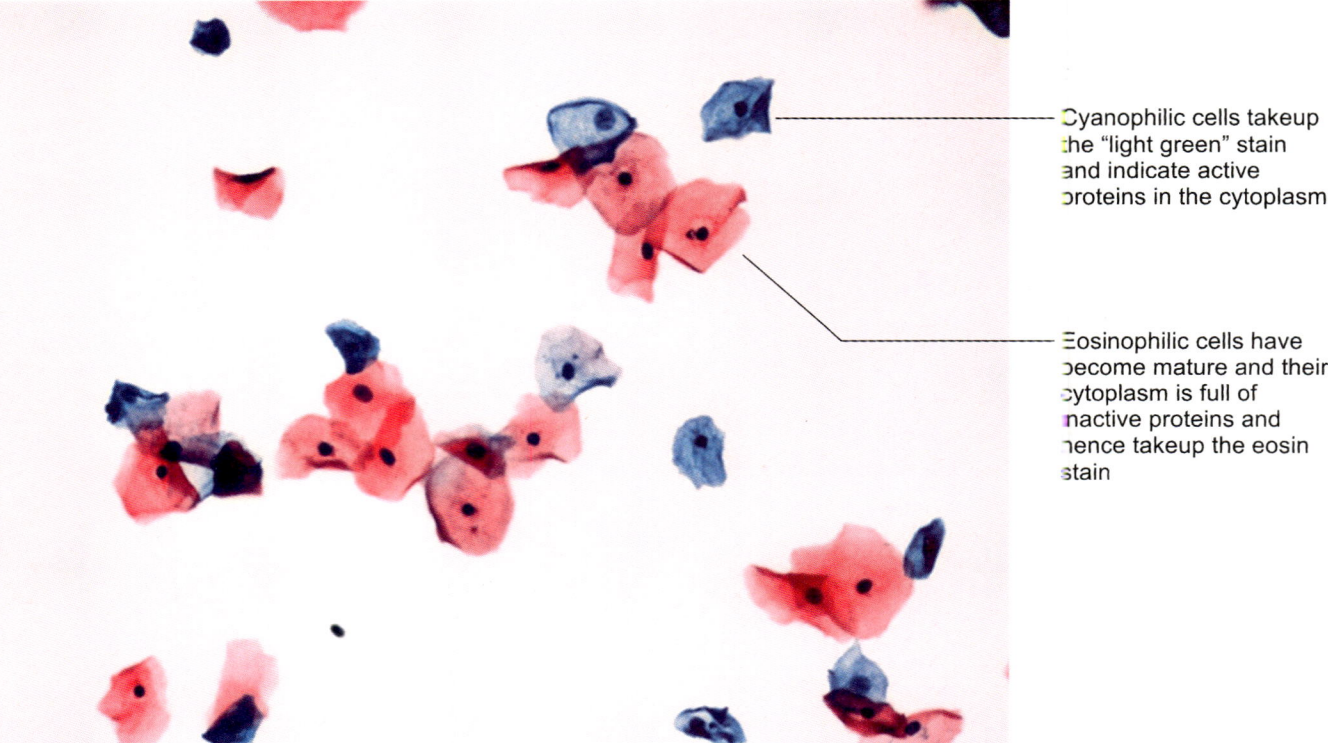

Cyanophilic cells takeup the "light green" stain and indicate active proteins in the cytoplasm

Eosinophilic cells have become mature and their cytoplasm is full of inactive proteins and hence takeup the eosin stain

Fig. 9.6

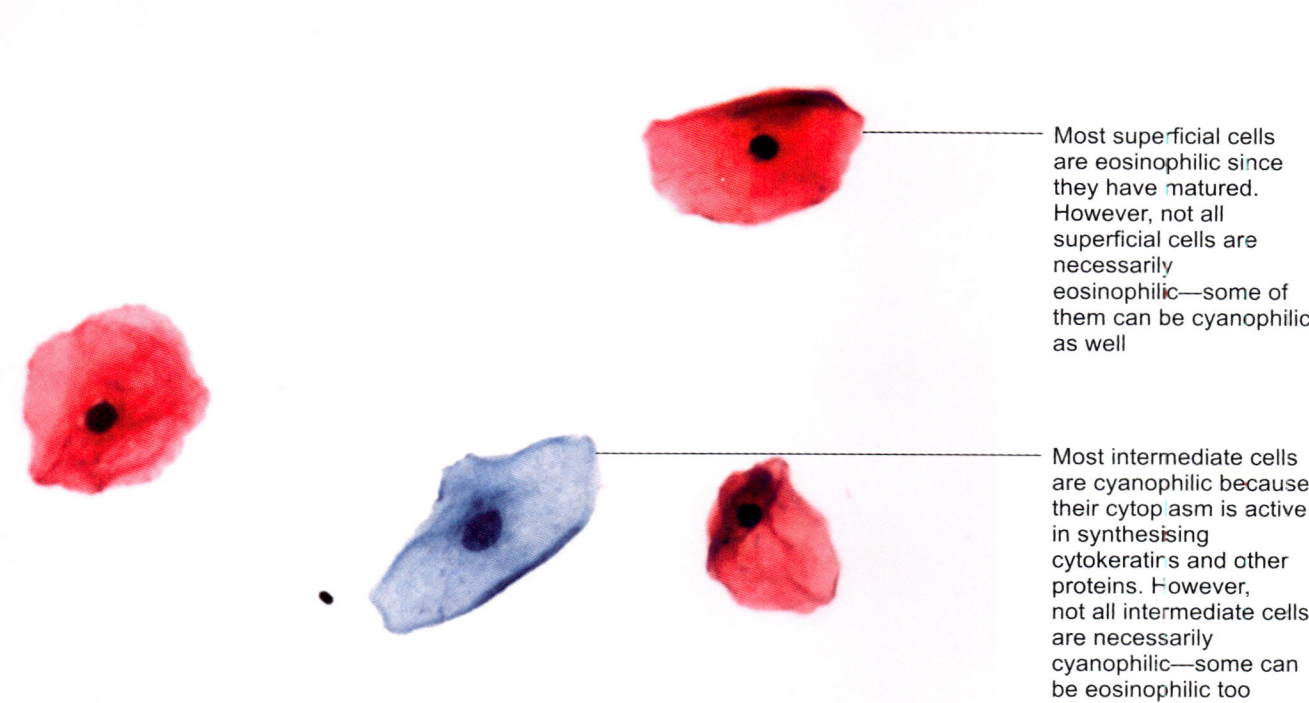

Most superficial cells are eosinophilic since they have matured. However, not all superficial cells are necessarily eosinophilic—some of them can be cyanophilic as well

Most intermediate cells are cyanophilic because their cytoplasm is active in synthesising cytokeratins and other proteins. However, not all intermediate cells are necessarily cyanophilic—some can be eosinophilic too

Fig. 9.7

SUPERFICIAL CELLS (Figs 9.8a and b)

The main distinction between a superfcial cell and an intermediate cell lies in the nature of their nucleus and not based upon the staining character of the cytoplasm.

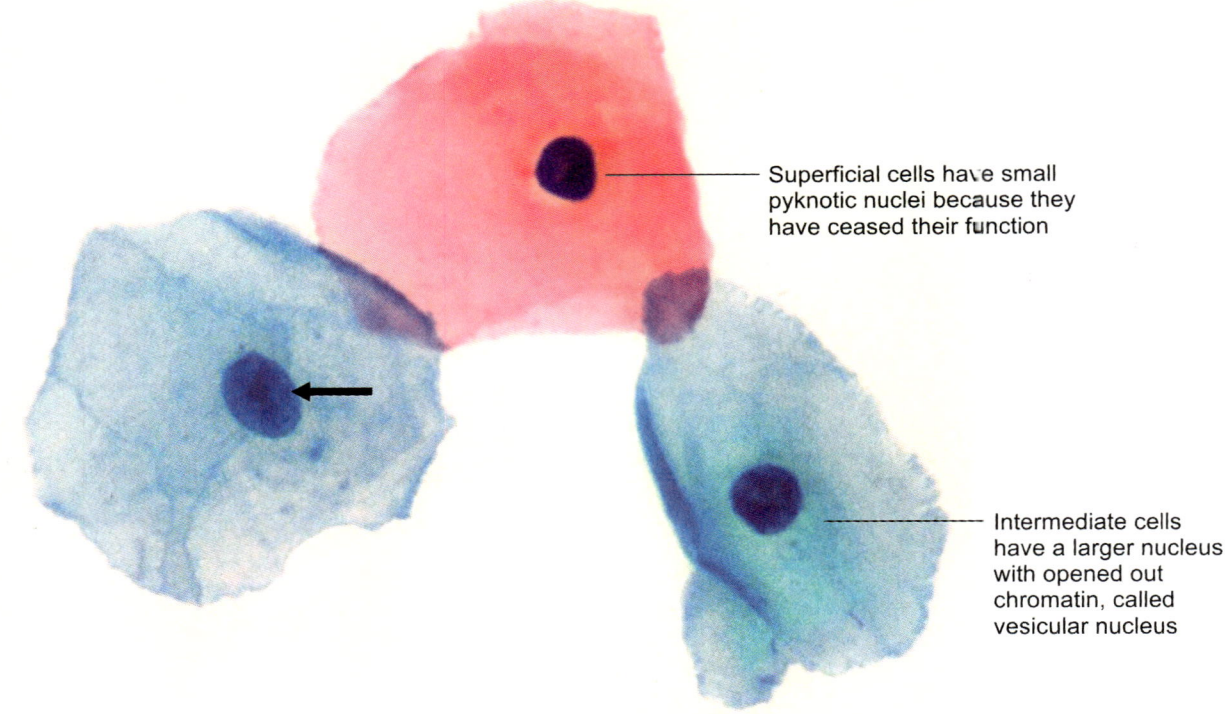

Superficial cells have small pyknotic nuclei because they have ceased their function

Intermediate cells have a larger nucleus with opened out chromatin, called vesicular nucleus

Fig. 9.8a

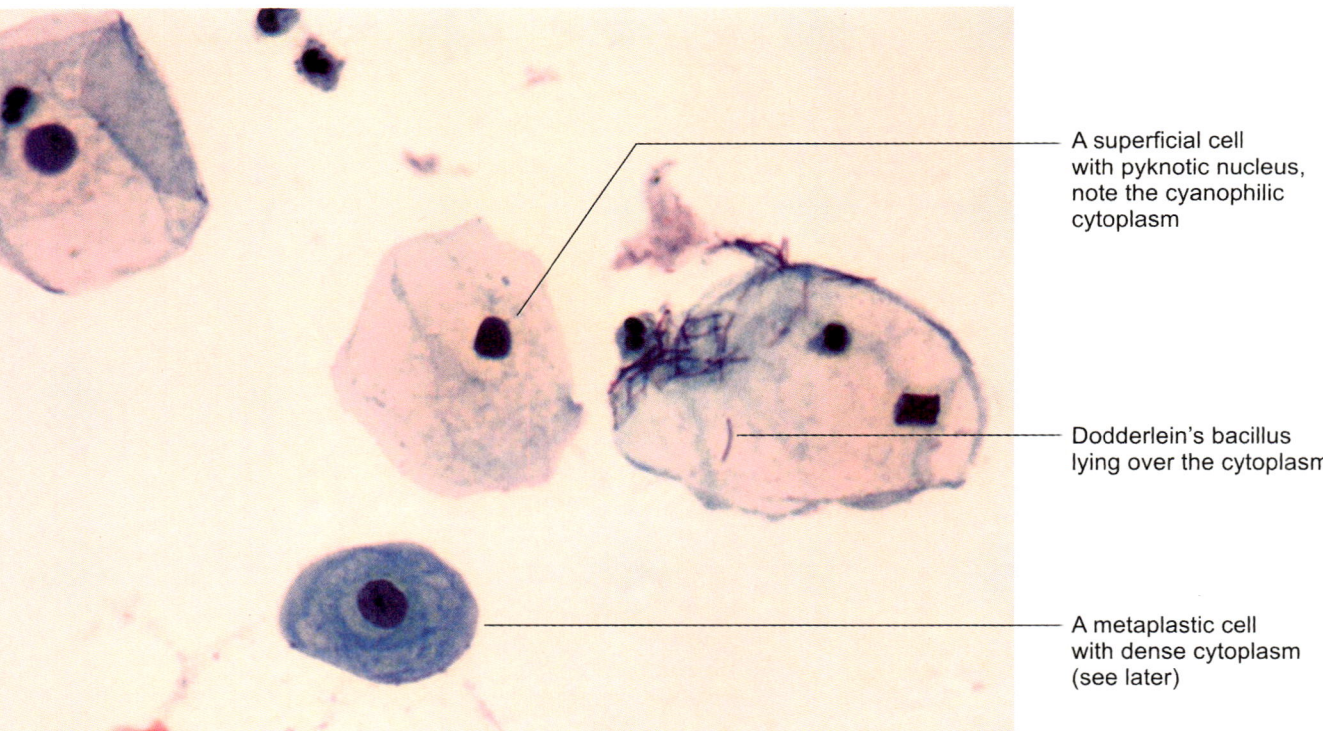

A superficial cell with pyknotic nucleus, note the cyanophilic cytoplasm

Dodderlein's bacillus lying over the cytoplasm

A metaplastic cell with dense cytoplasm (see later)

Fig. 9.8b

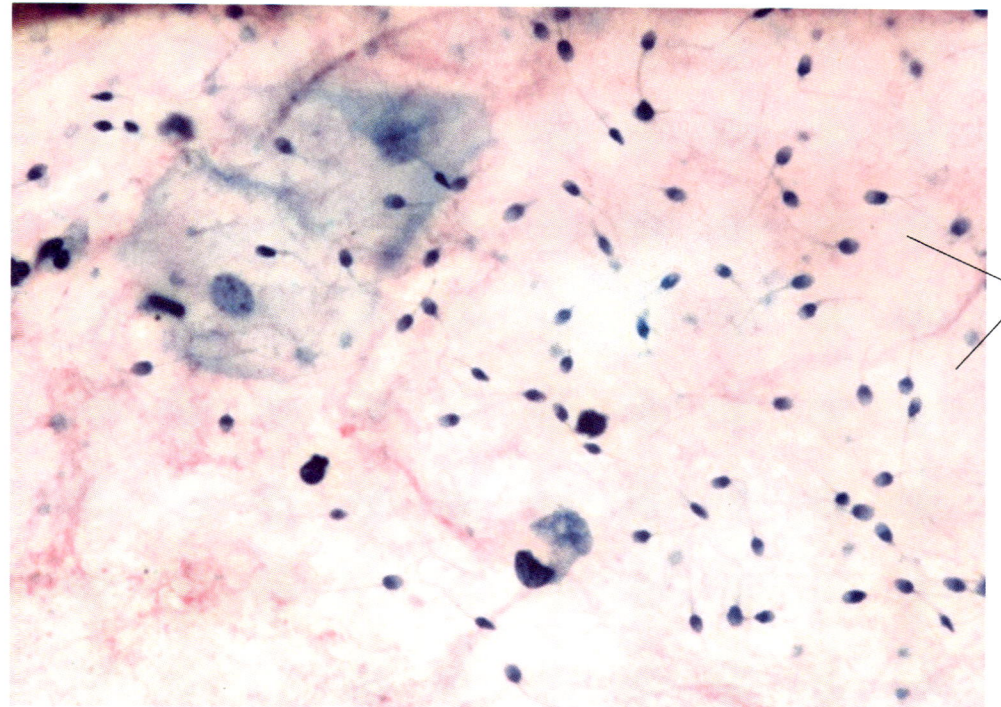

Sometimes one can see sperms (Fig 9.9) in the cervical smear due to coital activity prior to taking the smear. Note the head, cap neck and tail

Their presence is not supposed to be reported

Mild nuclear changes within normal limits can accompany such smears commonly

Fig. 9.9

INTERMEDIATE CELLS (Figs 9.10 and 9.11)

Keratohyaline granules are formed as a part of keratinization of cytoplasm. Normal squamous epithelium of cervix is not keratinised but still keratohyaline granules are frequent and must not be mistaken for parakeratosis seen in LSIL.

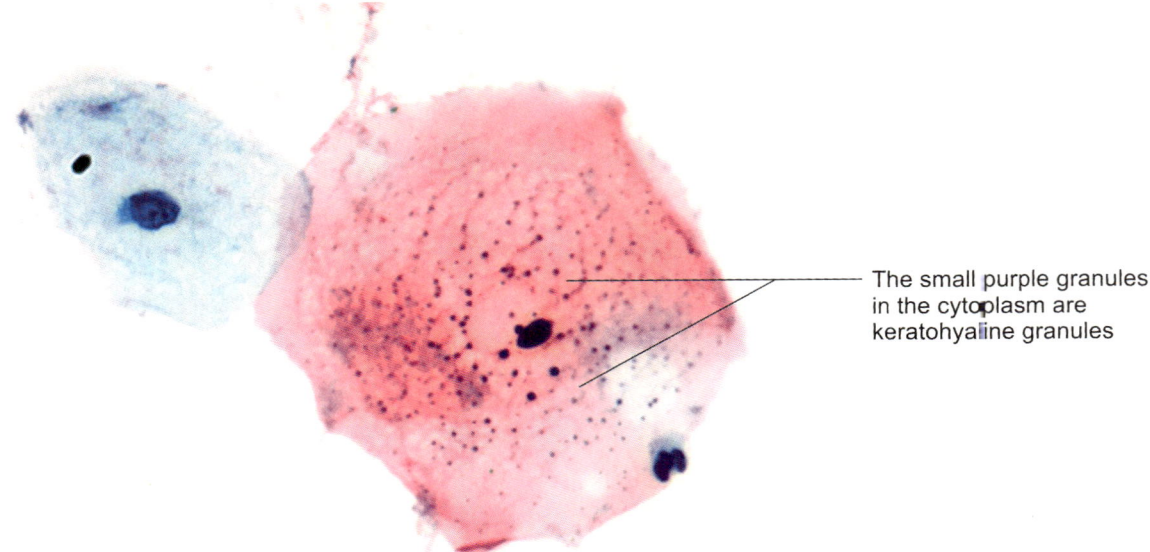

The small purple granules in the cytoplasm are keratohyaline granules

Fig. 9.10

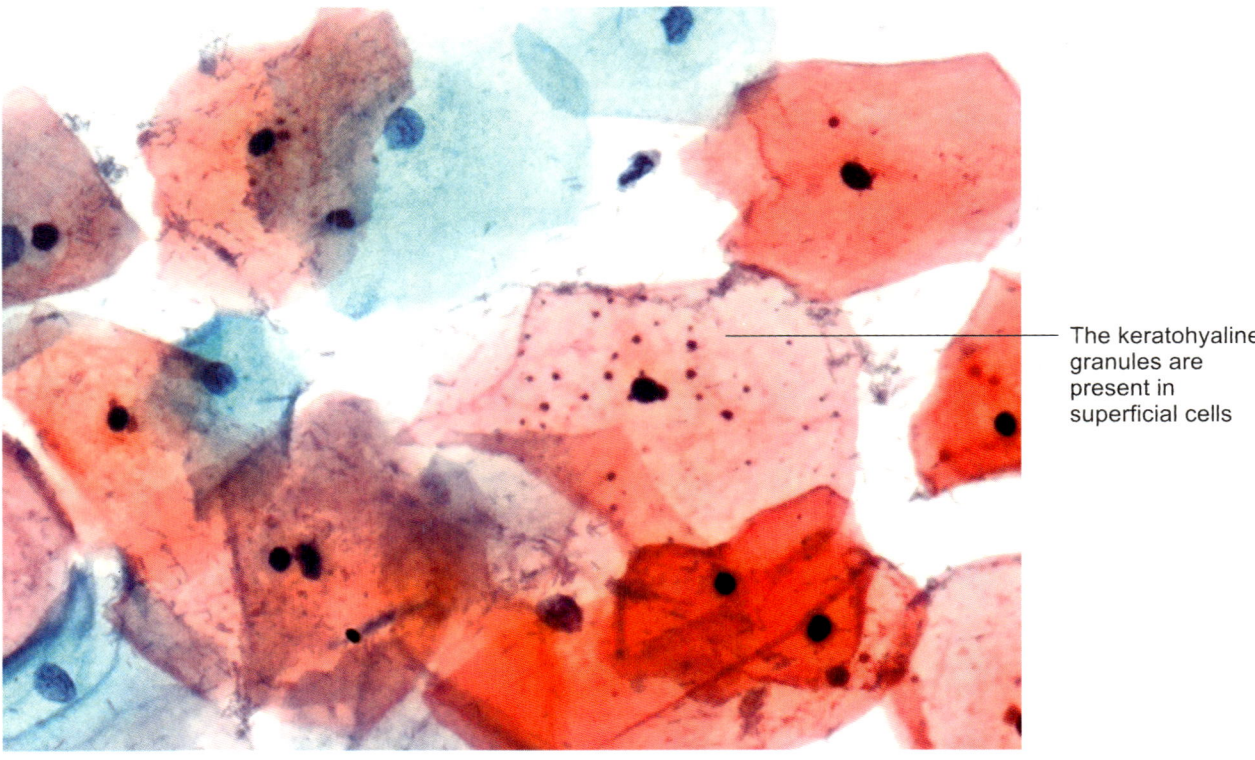

The keratohyaline granules are present in superficial cells

Fig. 9.11

PARABASAL CELLS (Figs 9.12 and 9.13)

Parabasal cells are found just above the basal cells and are smaller than intermediate cells. They are only seen when the epithelium does not mature into intermediate cells in the absence of hormonal stimulation during menopause, when parabasal cells are present at the surface being sampled in cytology.

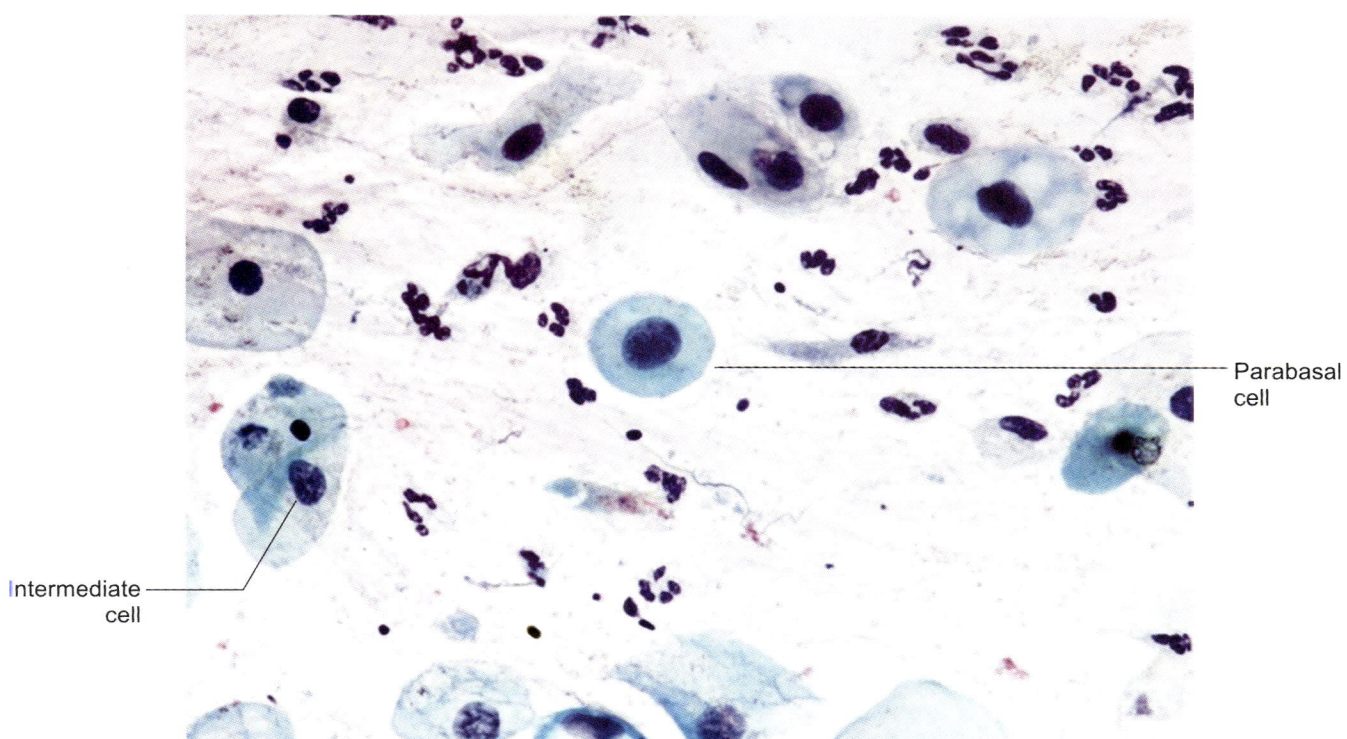

Parabasal cell

Intermediate cell

Fig. 9.12

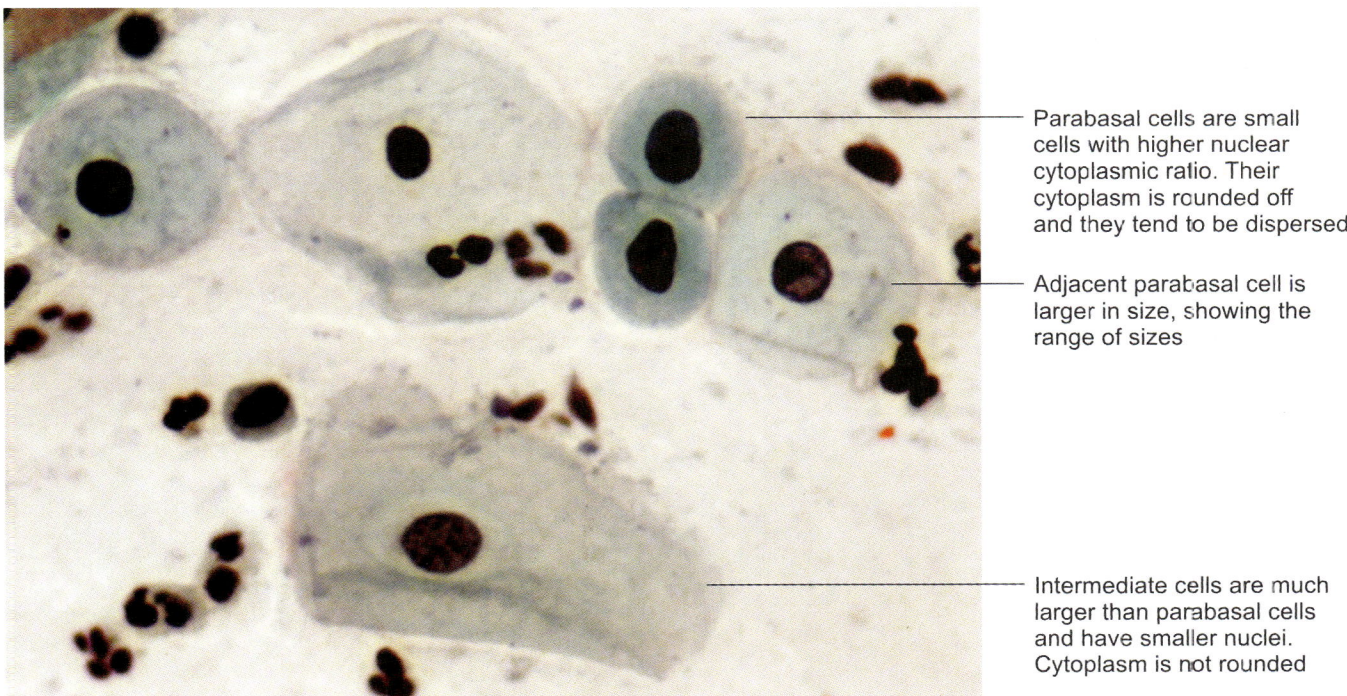

Parabasal cells are small cells with higher nuclear cytoplasmic ratio. Their cytoplasm is rounded off and they tend to be dispersed

Adjacent parabasal cell is larger in size, showing the range of sizes

Intermediate cells are much larger than parabasal cells and have smaller nuclei. Cytoplasm is not rounded

Fig. 9.13

The endocervix (Figs 9.14 to 9.16) is lined by columnar epithelium. The nucleus is basally placed over the basement membrane. Cell is tall and has apically placed mucin vacuole. Nuclei lie at one level.

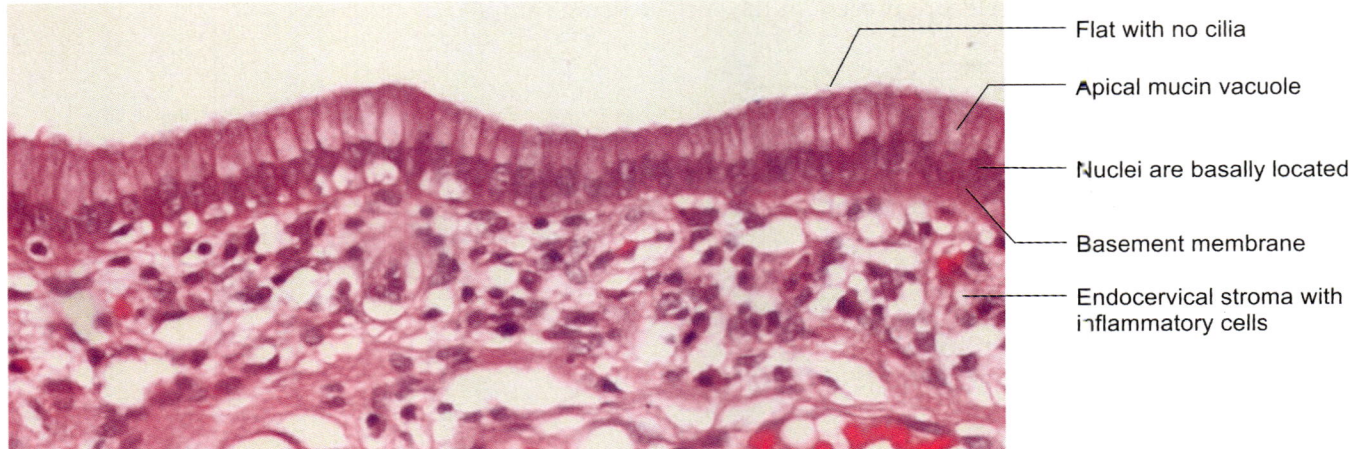

Flat with no cilia

Apical mucin vacuole

Nuclei are basally located

Basement membrane

Endocervical stroma with inflammatory cells

Fig. 9.14

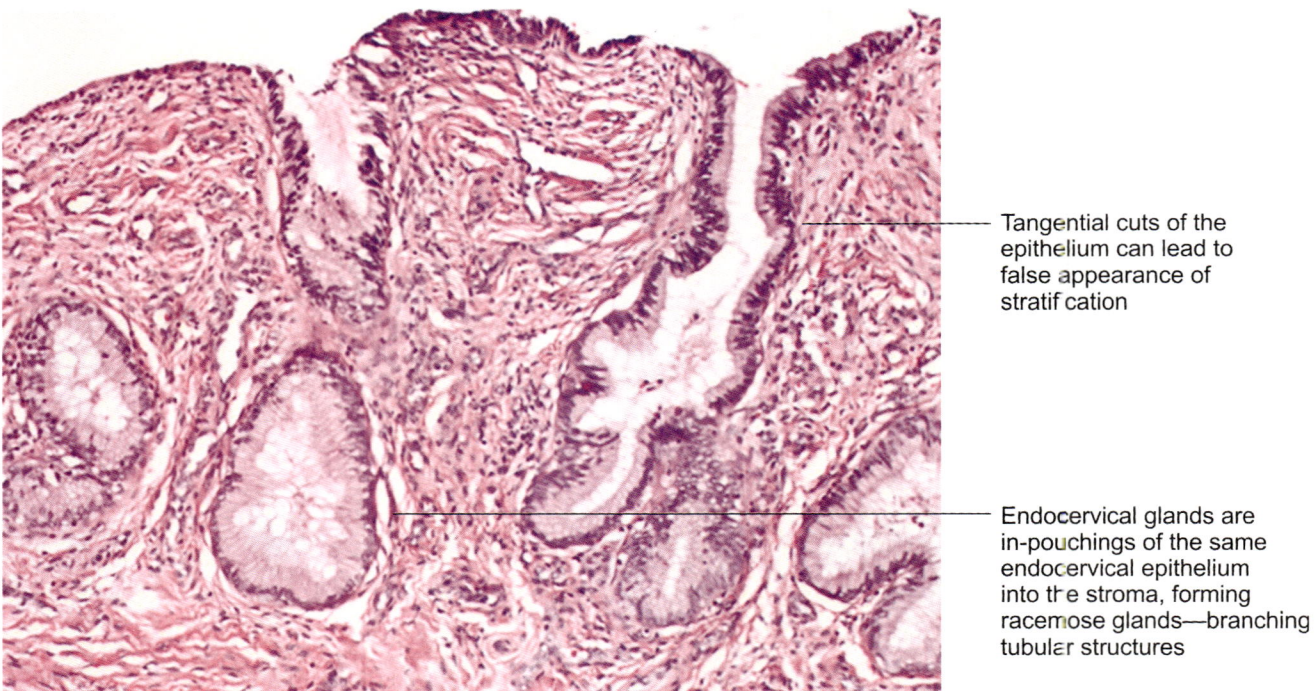

Tangential cuts of the epithelium can lead to false appearance of stratification

Endocervical glands are in-pouchings of the same endocervical epithelium into the stroma, forming racemose glands—branching tubular structures

Fig. 9.15

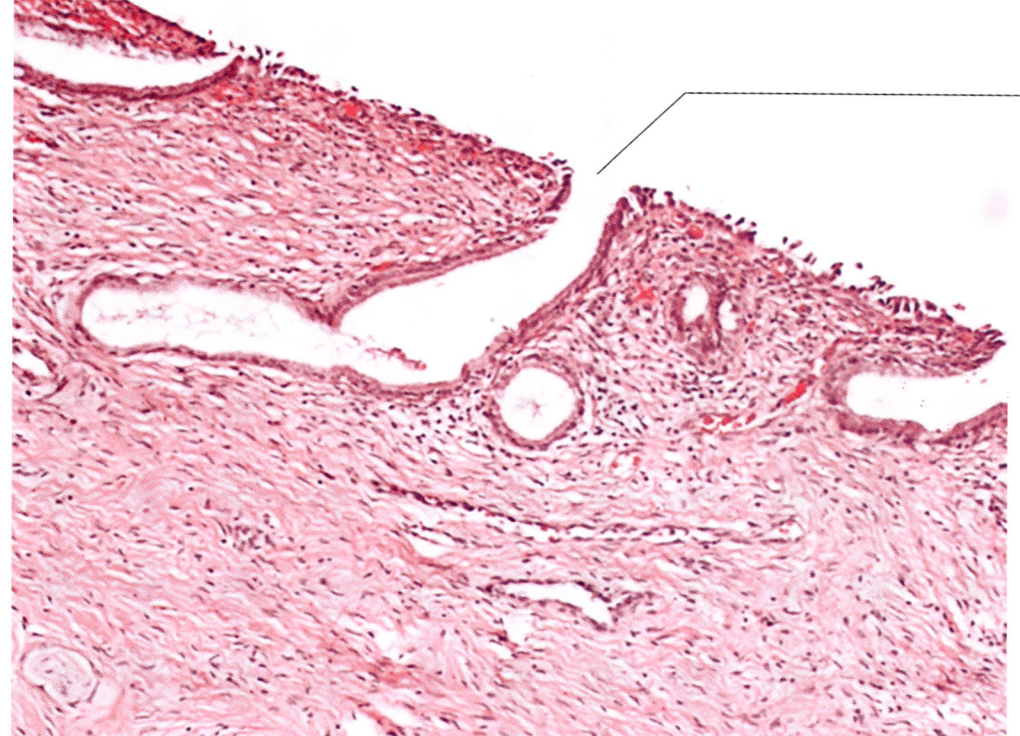

Endocervical glands
can be smaller and
more basic at places
and frequently can be
ulcerated because of
endocervicitis

Fig. 9.16

CYTOLOGY OF ENDOCERVIX

The endocervical epithelium is commonly avulsed in sheets. Individual columnar cells are embedded vertically within the sheet (Figs 9.17 to 9.19).

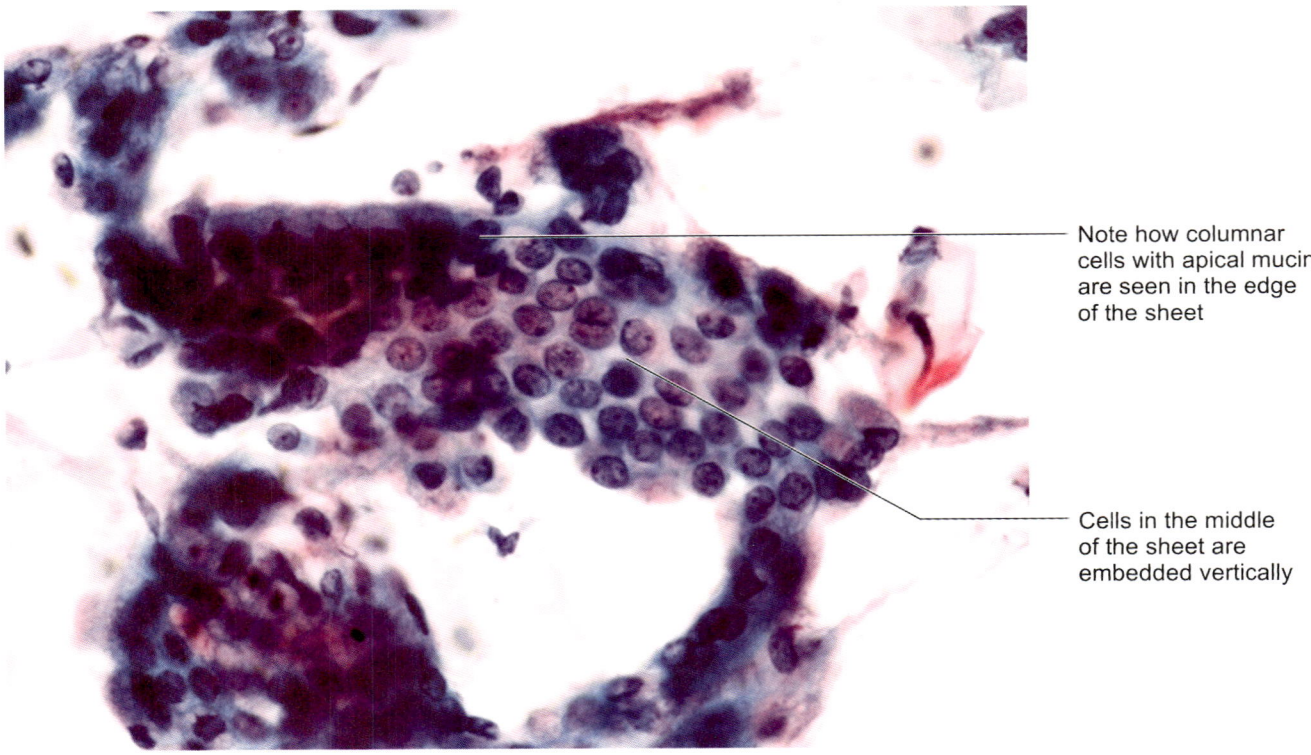

Note how columnar cells with apical mucin are seen in the edge of the sheet

Cells in the middle of the sheet are embedded vertically

Fig. 9.17

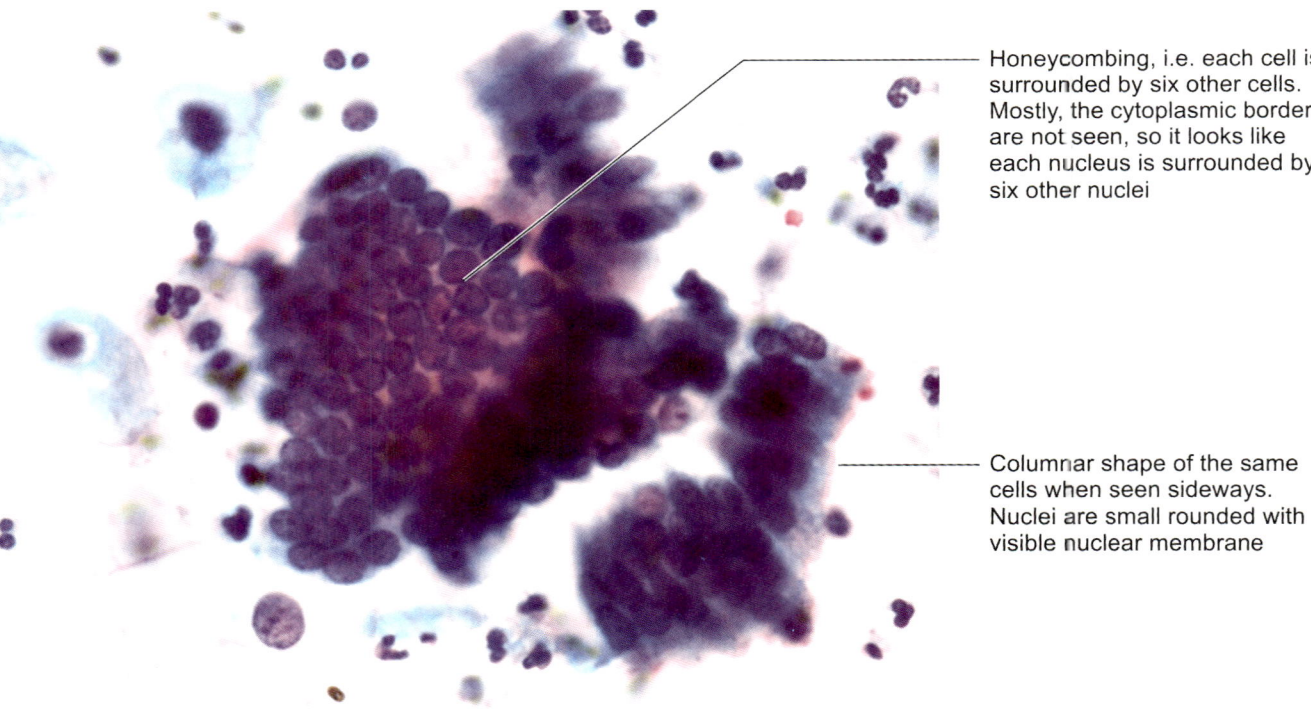

Honeycombing, i.e. each cell is surrounded by six other cells. Mostly, the cytoplasmic borders are not seen, so it looks like each nucleus is surrounded by six other nuclei

Columnar shape of the same cells when seen sideways. Nuclei are small rounded with visible nuclear membrane

Fig. 9.18

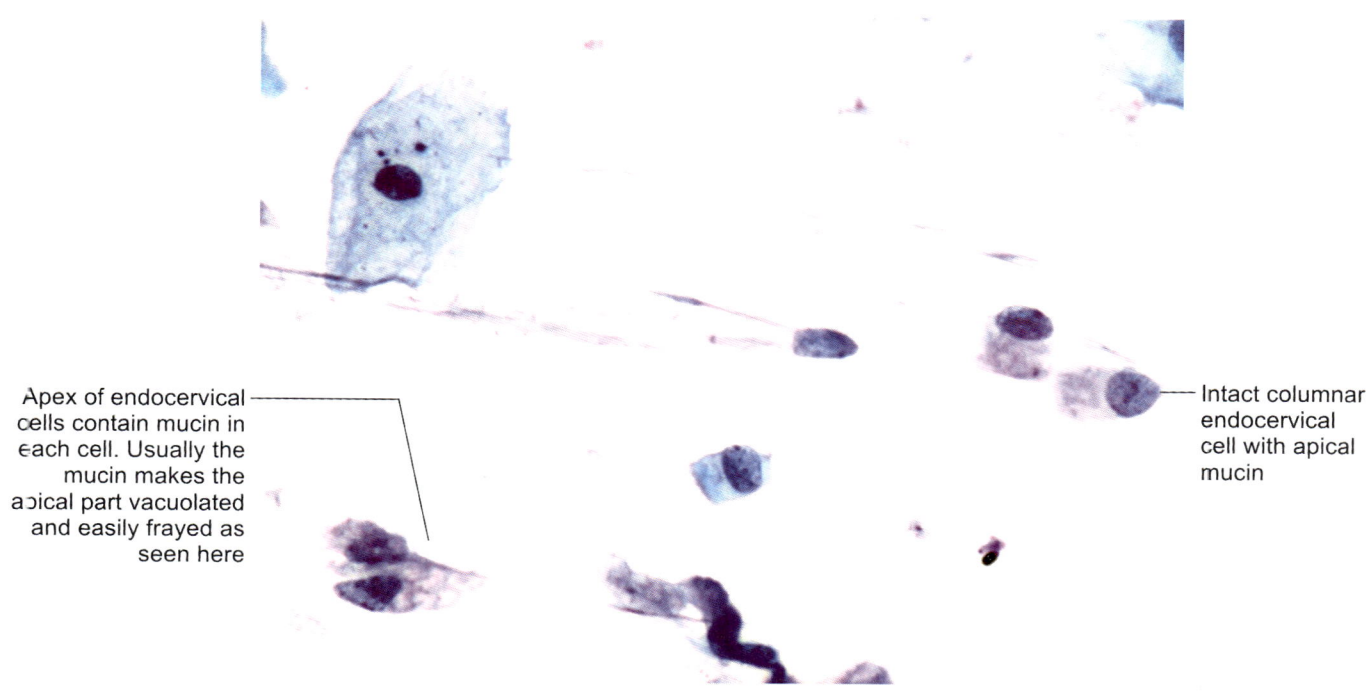

Apex of endocervical cells contain mucin in each cell. Usually the mucin makes the apical part vacuolated and easily frayed as seen here

Intact columnar endocervical cell with apical mucin

Fig. 9.19

Benign Changes: Histology and Cytology

REPAIR OF STRATIFIED SQUAMOUS EPITHELIUM

Normal squamous cells are created by reserve cells in the basal layer of the squamous epithelium. This is a different process from metaplasia. It is best exemplified by healing process when a defect is produced and the body heals it. Similar to healing by first intention, the reserve cells in the basal layer of the stratified squamous epithelium bridge the gap by dividing to create a monolayer of cuboidal cells lining the defect. After the gap is bridged, the monolayer now continues to divide creating heaping up of cells above the monolayer. The initial monolayer turns into the basal cells. The cells heaping up above the basal layer turn into keratinocytes. At the end of this process, mature squamous epithelium is regenerated above the defect (Figs 10.1a to c).

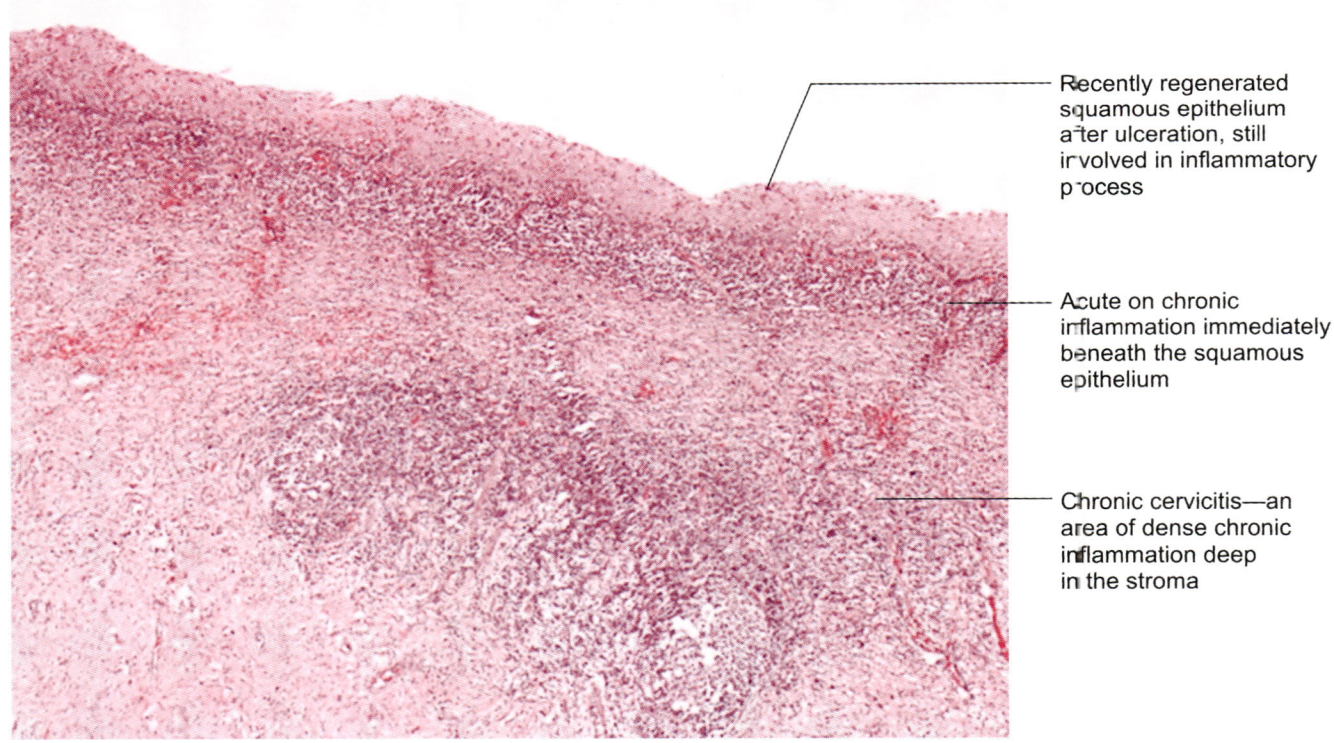

Recently regenerated squamous epithelium after ulceration, still involved in inflammatory process

Acute on chronic inflammation immediately beneath the squamous epithelium

Chronic cervicitis—an area of dense chronic inflammation deep in the stroma

Fig. 10.1a

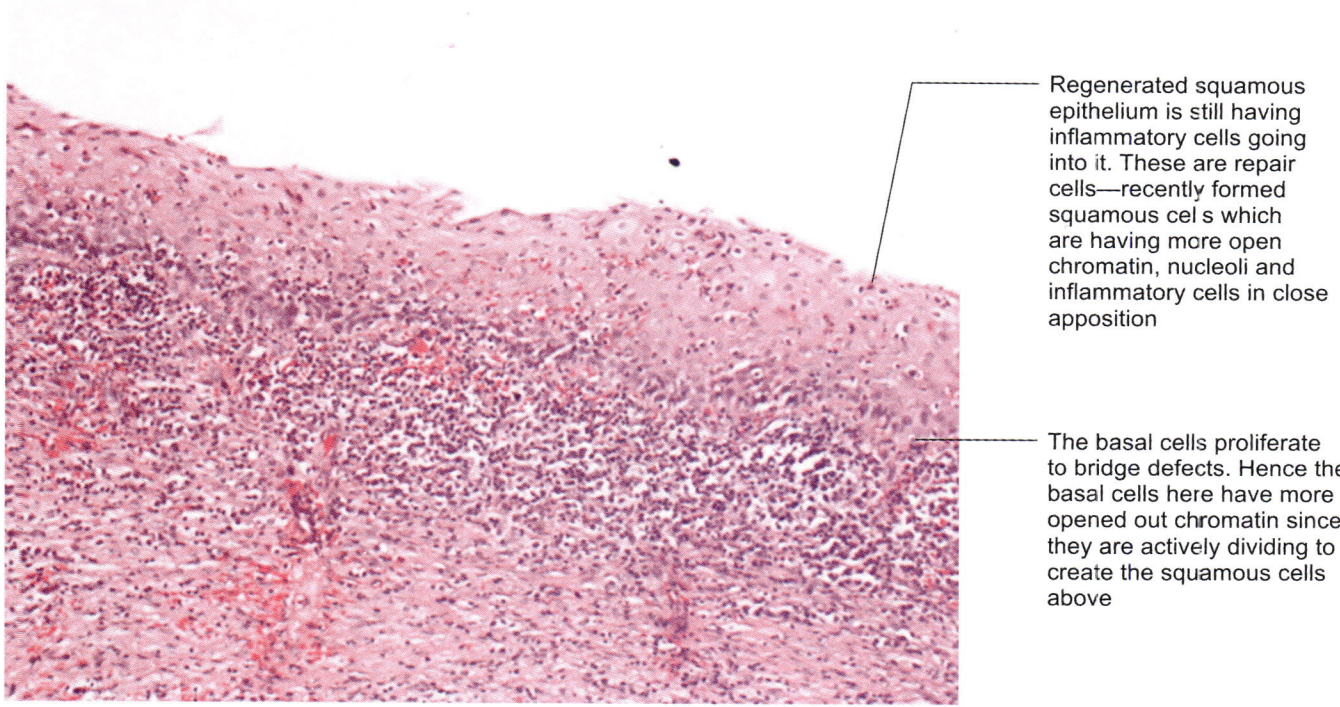

Regenerated squamous epithelium is still having inflammatory cells going into it. These are repair cells—recently formed squamous cel s which are having more open chromatin, nucleoli and inflammatory cells in close apposition

The basal cells proliferate to bridge defects. Hence the basal cells here have more opened out chromatin since they are actively dividing to create the squamous cells above

Fig. 10.1b

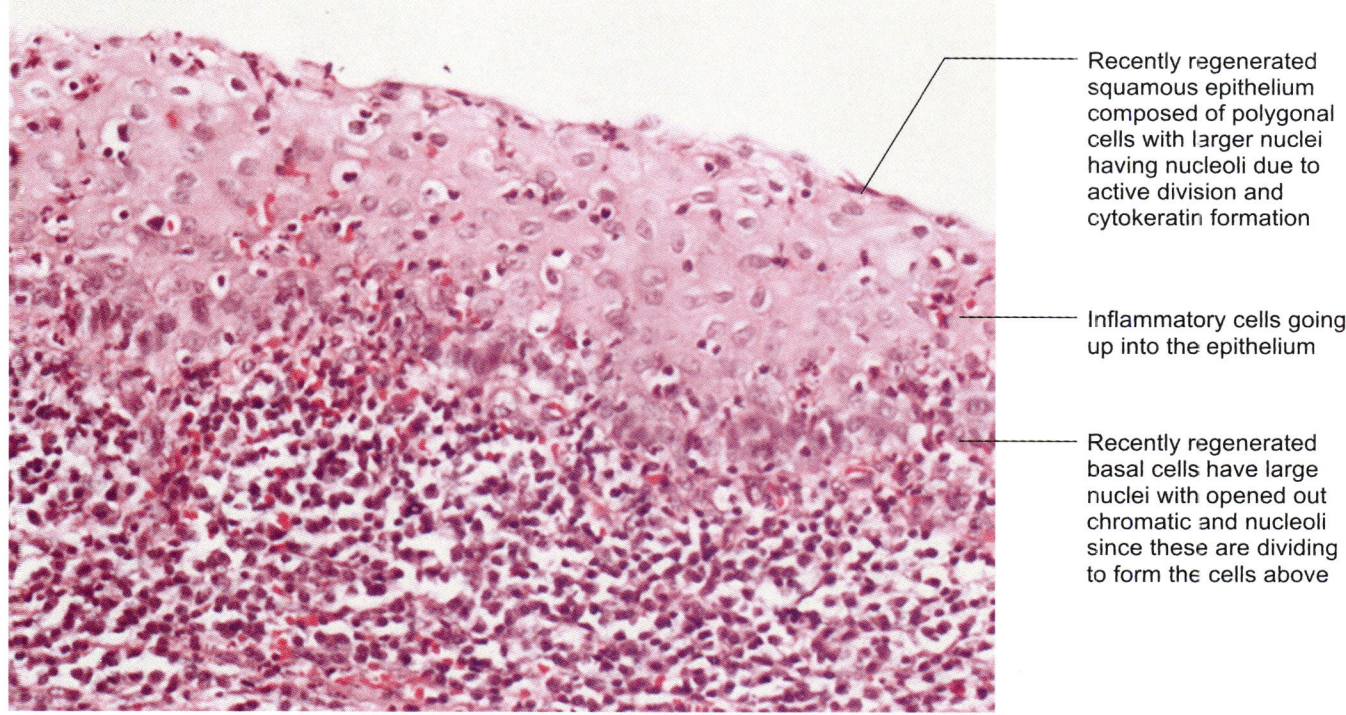

Recently regenerated squamous epithelium composed of polygonal cells with larger nuclei having nucleoli due to active division and cytokeratin formation

Inflammatory cells going up into the epithelium

Recently regenerated basal cells have large nuclei with opened out chromatic and nucleoli since these are dividing to form the cells above

Fig. 10.1c

CYTOLOGY OF REPAIR (Figs 10.2a to c)

During repair, the denuded squamous lining is bridged by the basal cells. Division of the basal cells creates stratified layers of parabasal cells. These are seen in the smears as sheets of parabasal cells.

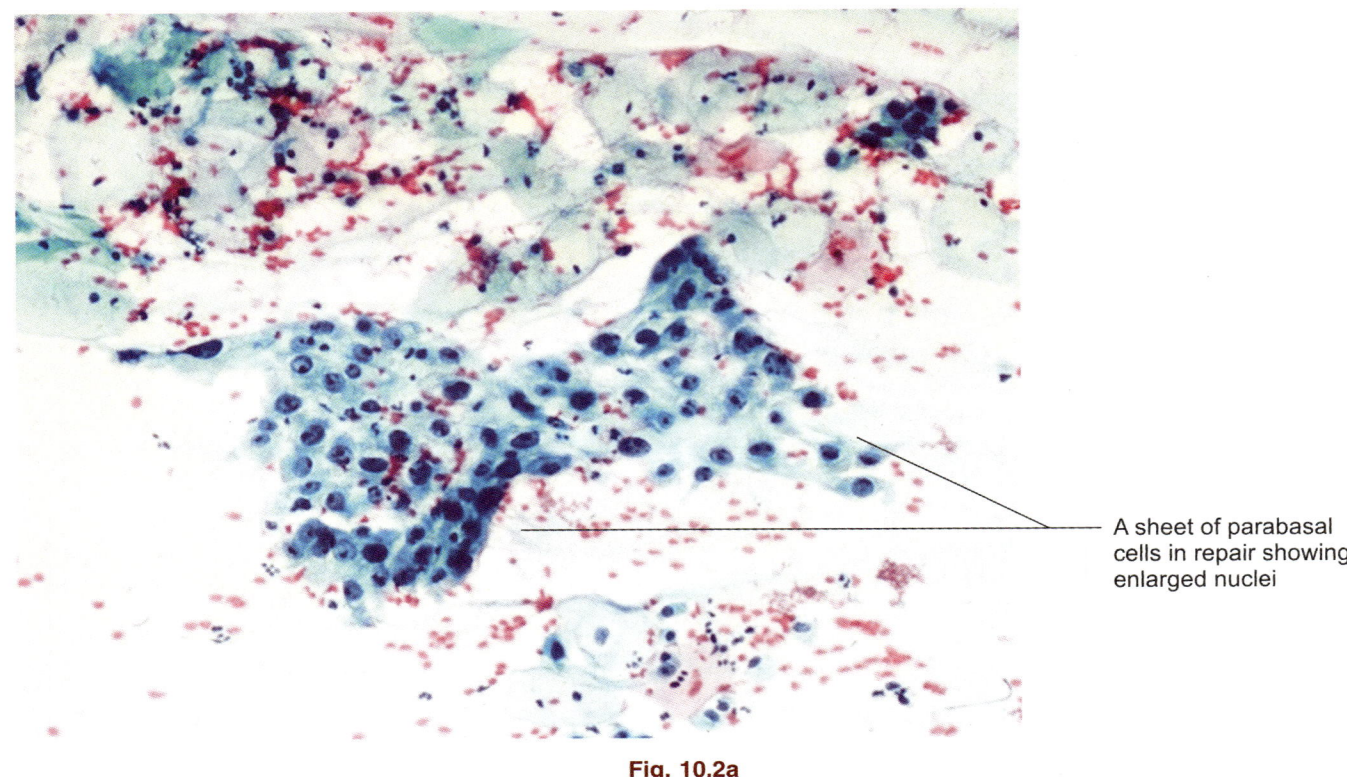

A sheet of parabasal cells in repair showing enlarged nuclei

Fig. 10.2a

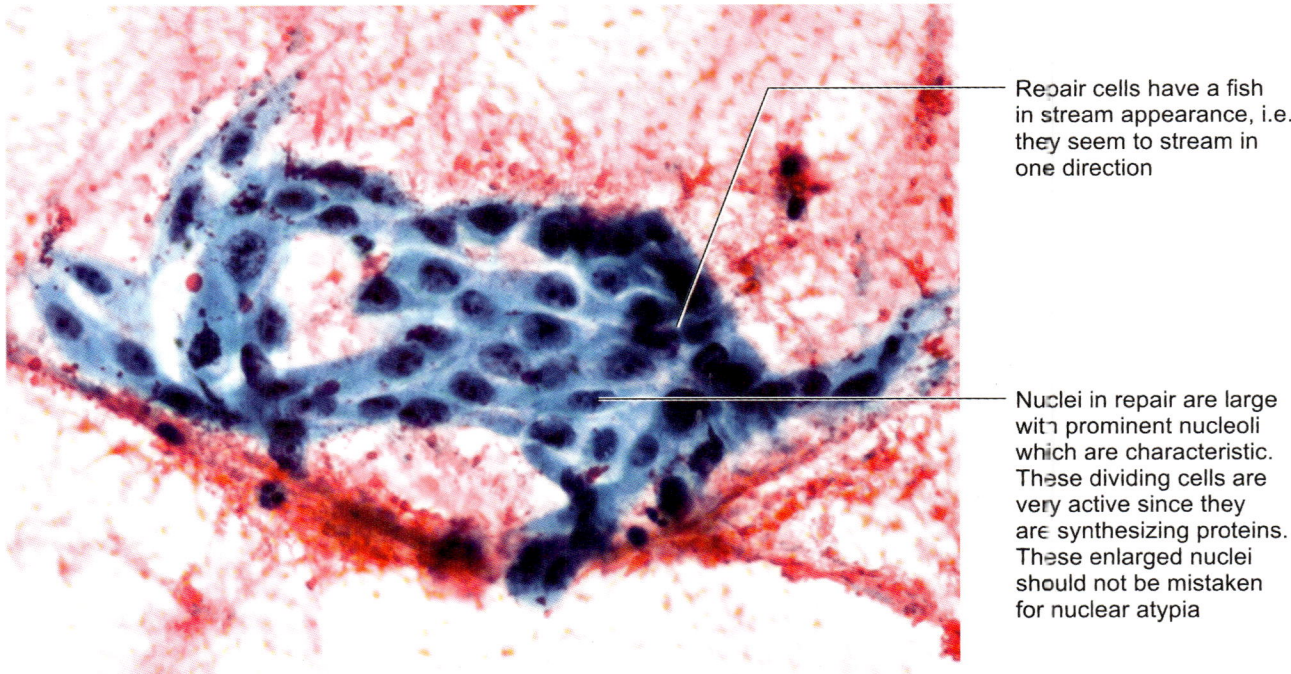

Repair cells have a fish in stream appearance, i.e. they seem to stream in one direction

Nuclei in repair are large with prominent nucleoli which are characteristic. These dividing cells are very active since they are synthesizing proteins. These enlarged nuclei should not be mistaken for nuclear atypia

Fig. 10.2b

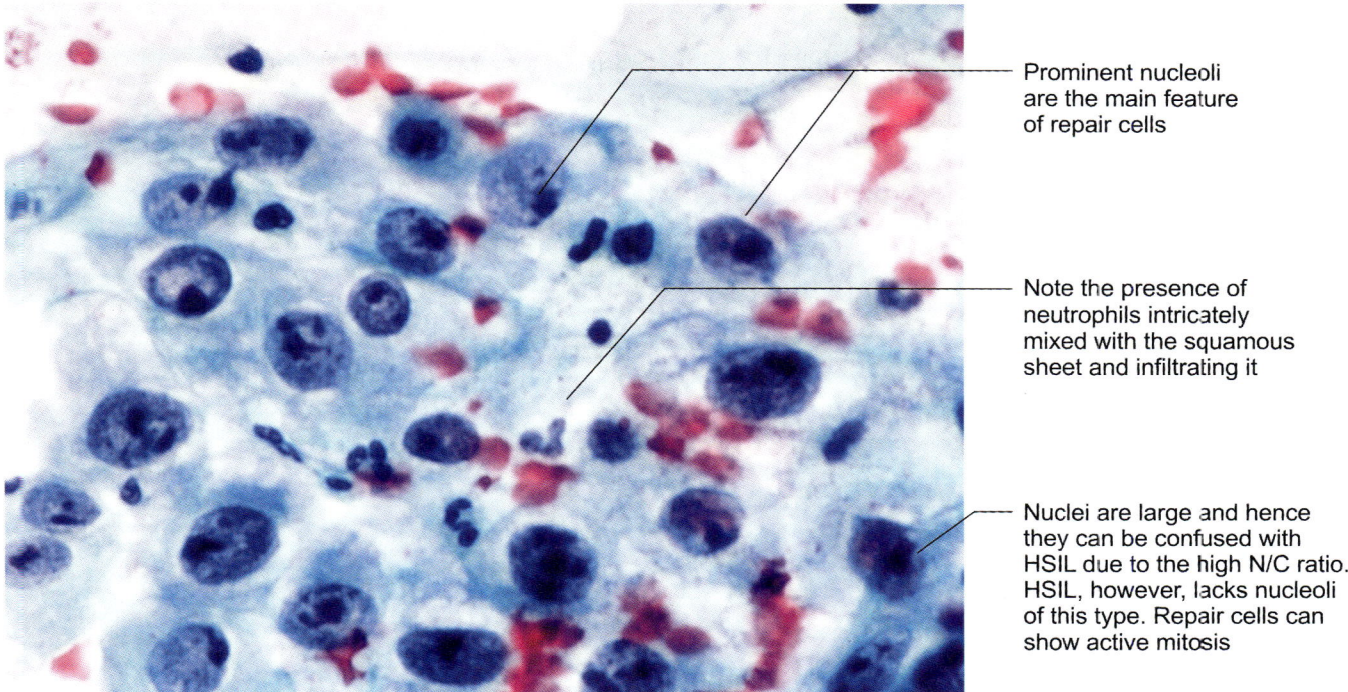

Prominent nucleoli
are the main feature
of repair cells

Note the presence of
neutrophils intricately
mixed with the squamous
sheet and infiltrating it

Nuclei are large and hence
they can be confused with
HSIL due to the high N/C ratio.
HSIL, however, lacks nucleoli
of this type. Repair cells can
show active mitosis

Fig. 10.2c

SQUAMOUS METAPLASIA (Figs 10.3a to d)

This is the most important process to understand for colposcopists. After birth, the normal cervix remains dormant after the effects of maternal hormones Vane.

Squamous metaplasia occurs after menarche. During this time, the squamocolumnar junction moves outwards, exposing the endocervical epithelium which now is situated over the ectocervix. After exposure, the endocervical epithelium undergoes squamous metaplasia. Sometimes there is no squamous metaplasia and, therefore, endocervical epithelium persists over the ectocervix, termed ectropion.

The reason for movement of cervical squamocolumnar epithelium outwards is the hormone-induced growth of the endocervical glands. Like the endometrial grands, endocervical glands also contain estrogen and progesterone receptors. These cause a menarche linked increased proliferation and permanent increase in thickness and number of endocervical glands.

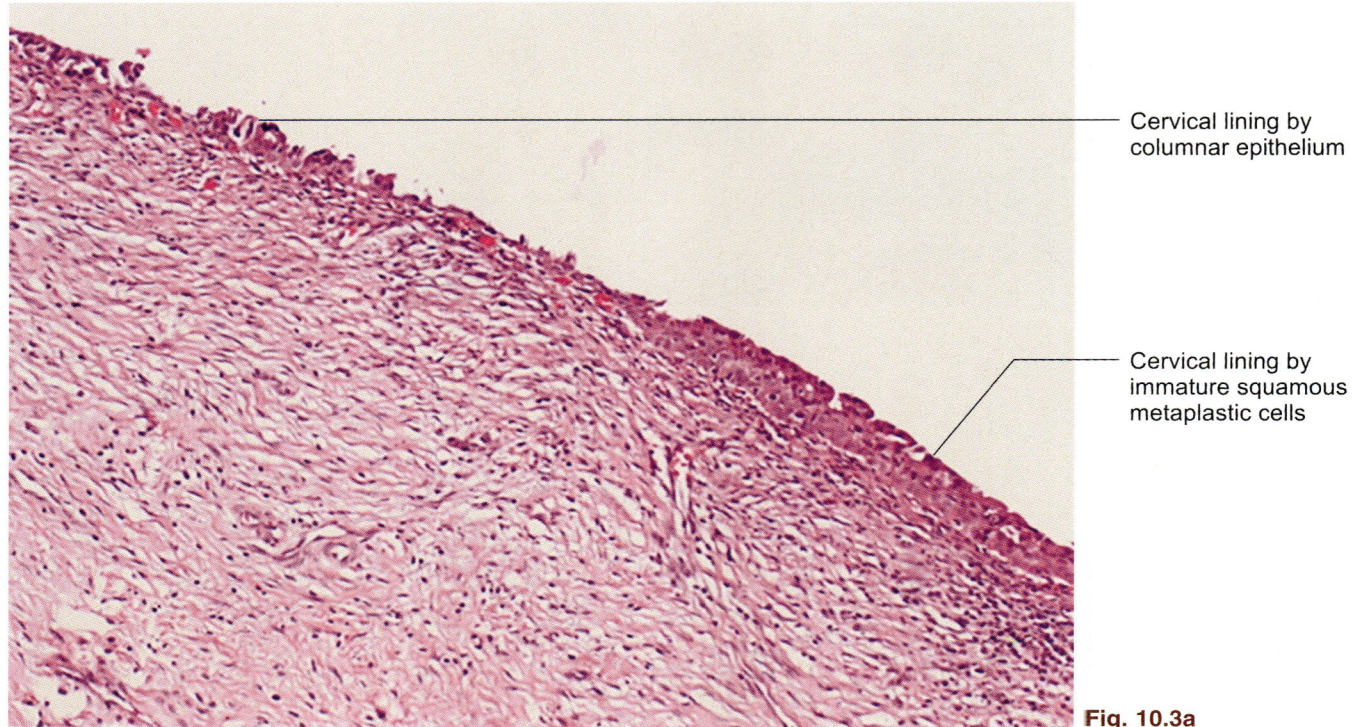

Cervical lining by columnar epithelium

Cervical lining by immature squamous metaplastic cells

Fig. 10.3a

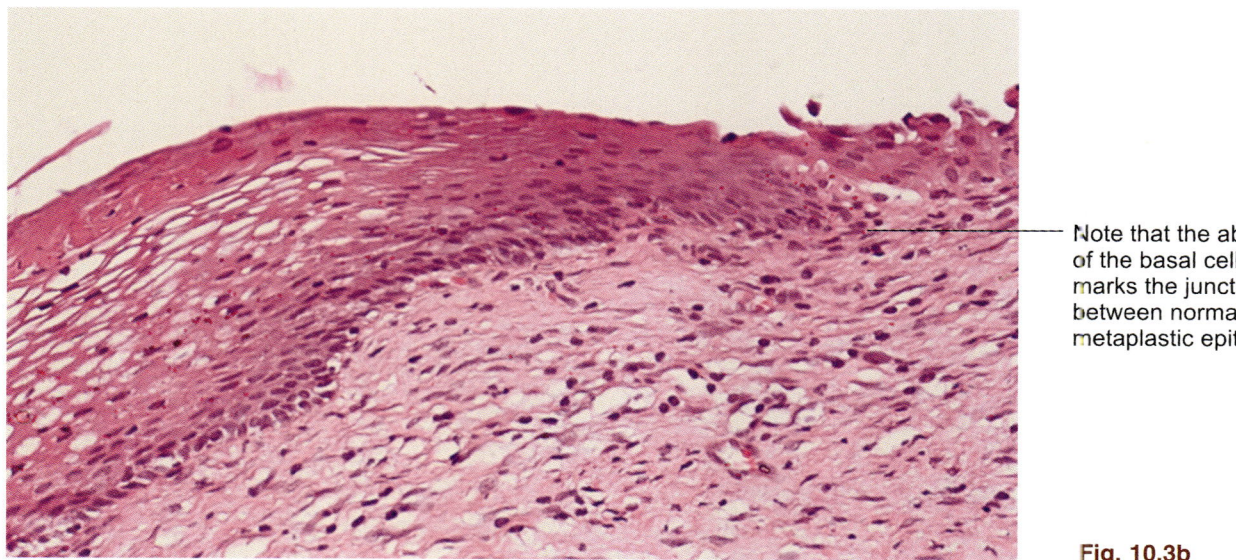

Note that the absence of the basal cell layer marks the junction between normal and metaplastic epithelium

Fig. 10.3b

Subsequently, during the cycles, the production and nature of endocervical mucus is under the control of estrogen and progesterone.

Similarly, during pregnancy and post-pregnancy, the cervix grows and involutes. This changes the number and size of the endocervical glands.

Accordingly, the squamocolumnar junction also moves along with the cervical bulk. At menarche, during the permanent increase in cervical glands, the junction moves outwards. This exposes the endocervical columnar lining to the pH of the vagina and its microflora. To withstand these, the columnar epithelium undergoes metaplasia.

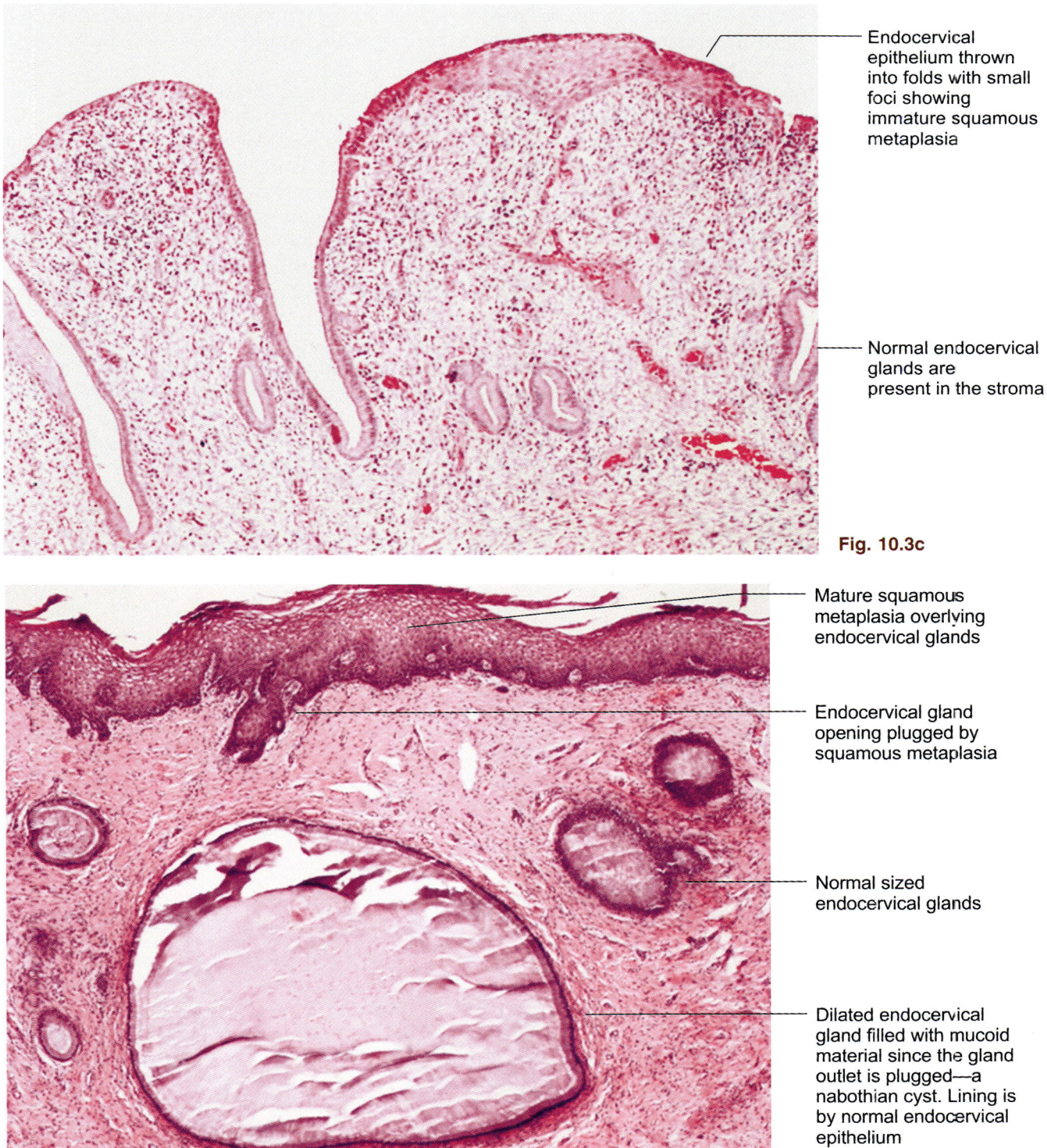

Endocervical epithelium thrown into folds with small foci showing immature squamous metaplasia

Normal endocervical glands are present in the stroma

Fig. 10.3c

Mature squamous metaplasia overlying endocervical glands

Endocervical gland opening plugged by squamous metaplasia

Normal sized endocervical glands

Dilated endocervical gland filled with mucoid material since the gland outlet is plugged—a nabothian cyst. Lining is by normal endocervical epithelium

Fig. 10.3d

IMMATURE SQUAMOUS METAPLASIA (Figs 10.4a and b)

Metaplasia occurs due to reprogramming of reserve cells of the columnar epithelium.

Normally, reserve cells are cells which are stimulated to replace lost endocervical columnar cells with more columnar cells. Reserve cells are a type of committed stem cells which only divide when required to do so. Like other stem cells, they can generate more of themselves as well as the differentiated cells needed. Thus when a reserve cell starts dividing, it creates as many columnar cells as are needed to replace the defect and also reserve cells to remain quiescent until needed again to replace lost columnar cells.

In metaplasia, these reserve cells are reprogrammed to create squamous cells. When any reserve cell divides, it makes a cuboidal cell which then differentiates. The differentiation process is altered in metaplasia so that instead of columnar cells, it changes into squamous cells.

When reserve cells of columnar epithelium are creating the squamous epithelium, the process is different from that described above for repair of stratified squamous epithelium, both on colposcopy and on histology. First, the reserve cells proliferate to create a layer of dividing cells underneath the columnar cells. For a while, the columnar cells containing apical mucin continue to remain in position. After a while, they fall off and only the cuboidal cells which have proliferated from the reserve cells are seen. This type of epithelium is called immature squamous metaplasia. They are composed of cuboidal cells derived from reserve cell proliferation which are slowly acquiring cytokeratins. As more and more cytokeratin proteins accumulate, they start resembling keratinocytes more and more. Unlike for stratified squamous epithelium, there is no basal layer or differentiated layers above, no intermediate and superficial cells. Only cuboidal cells which undergo keratinocyte differentiation without forming well-formed layers.

On histology, these immature metaplastic epithelia look different. They lack the normal basal layer and keratinocyte layers. From basement membrane above, a single type of cuboidal epithelium is present. The more superficial layers are composed of cells which more closely resemble keratinocytes. But none of them looks like mature stratified squamous epithelium. They are smaller cells with larger nuclei (resembling endocervical nuclei) than normal keratinocytes. They have denser cytoplasm which is packed with cytokeratins, of a different type and nature from mature stratified squamous epithelium. They lack the function of glycogen production which is present in mature stratified squamous epithelium.

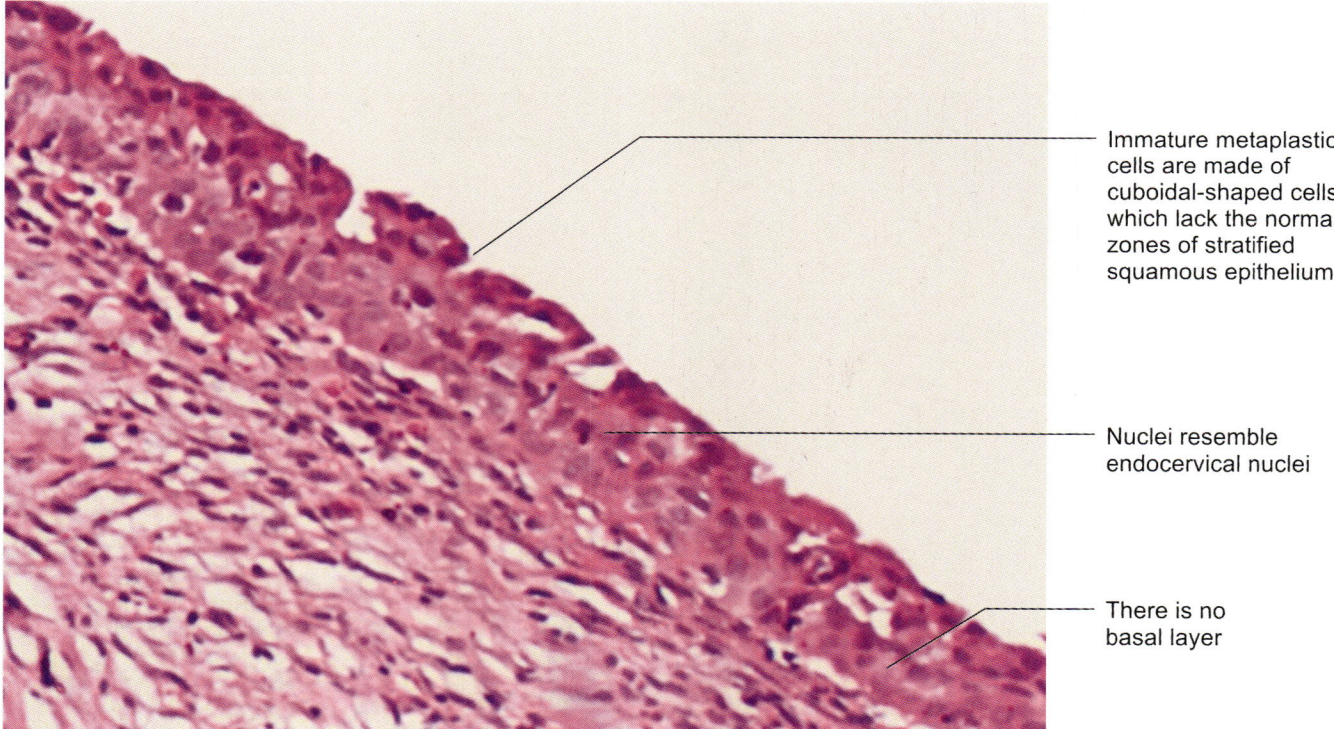

Immature metaplastic cells are made of cuboidal-shaped cells which lack the normal zones of stratified squamous epithelium

Nuclei resemble endocervical nuclei

There is no basal layer

Fig. 10.4a

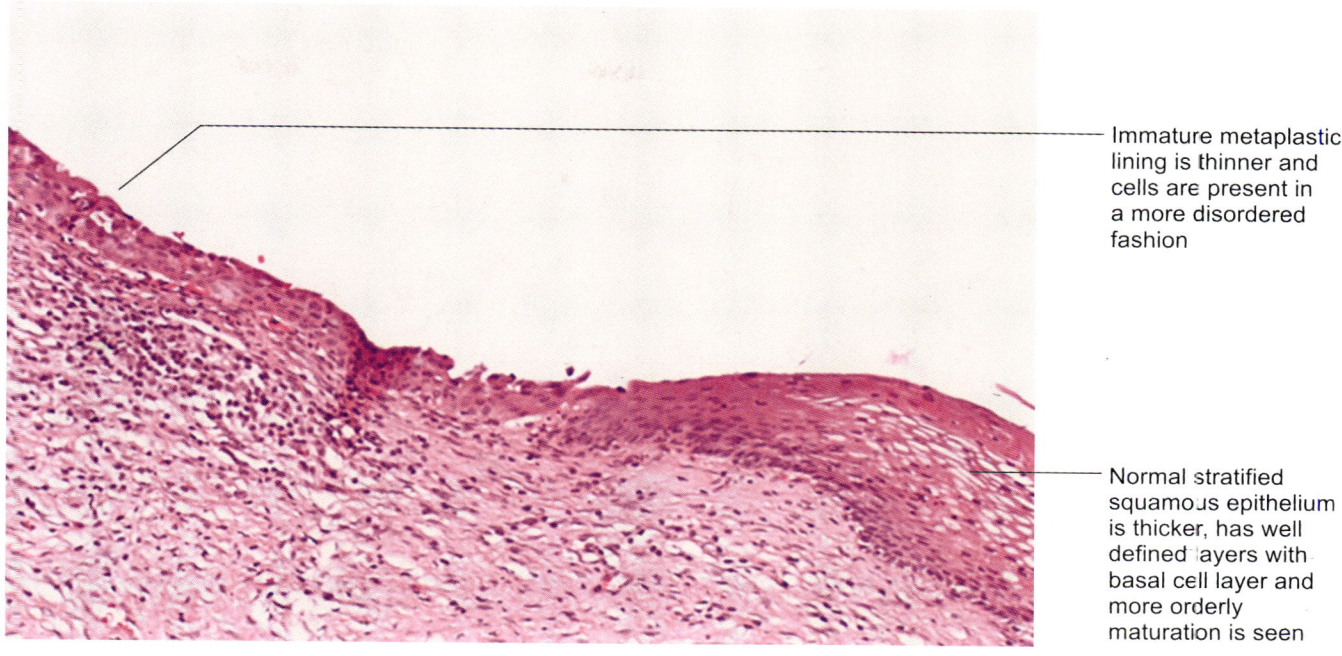

Immature metaplastic lining is thinner and cells are present in a more disordered fashion

Normal stratified squamous epithelium is thicker, has well defined layers with basal cell layer and more orderly maturation is seen

Fig. 10.4b

CYTOLOGY OF SQUAMOUS METAPLASIA (Figs 10.5a to c)

Only cells of immature squamous metaplasia can be recognised on cytology. Mature squamous metaplasia cells look like normal intermediate and superficial cells.

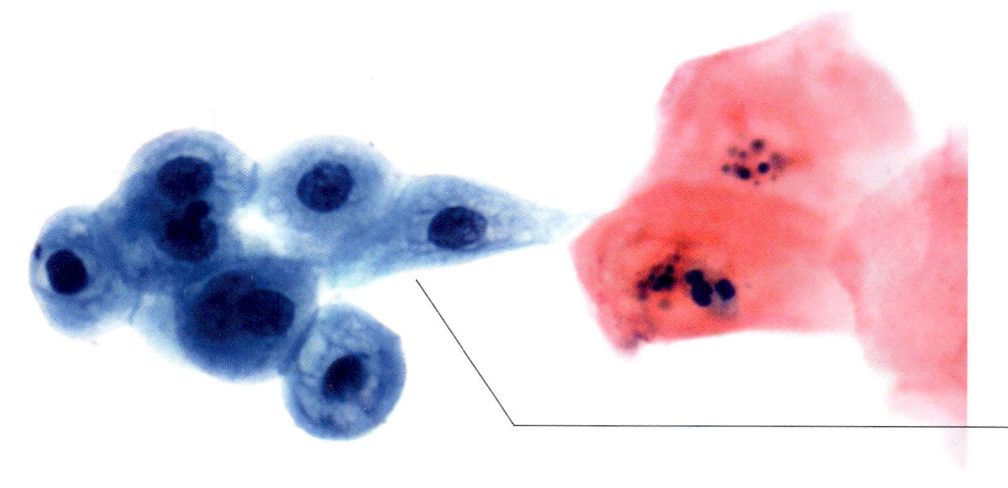

Metaplastic cells are of the same size as parabasal cells but have a very dense and intensely green cytoplasm

Fig. 10.5a

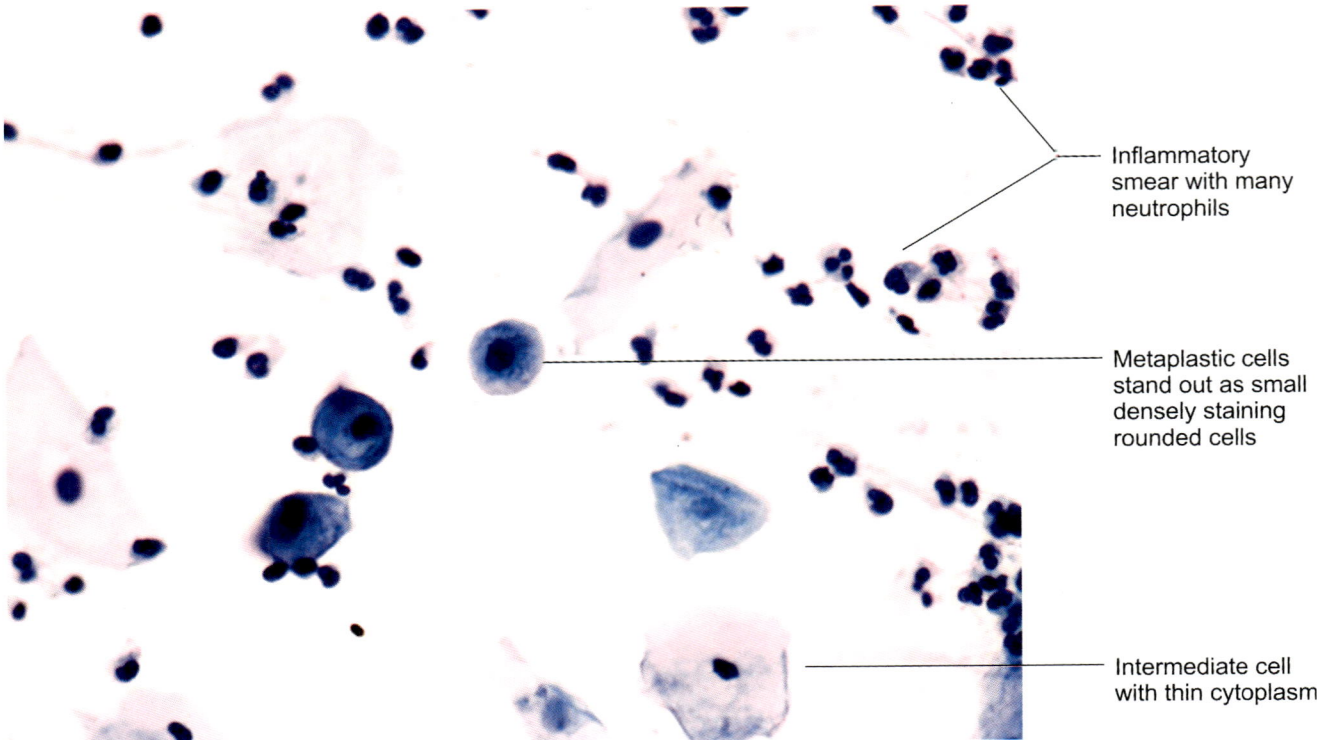

Inflammatory smear with many neutrophils

Metaplastic cells stand out as small densely staining rounded cells

Intermediate cell with thin cytoplasm

Fig. 10.5b

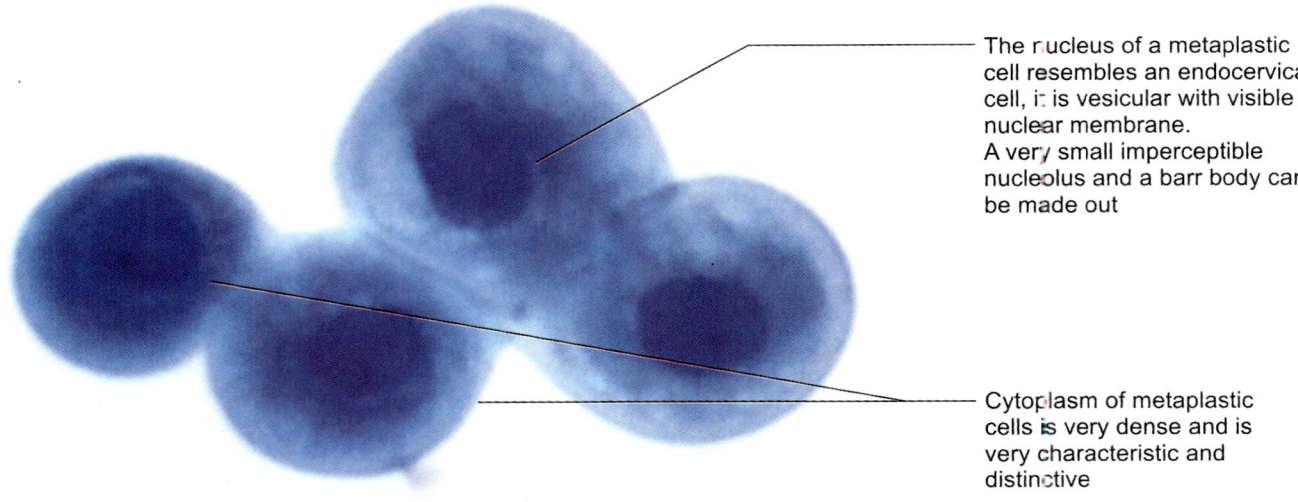

The nucleus of a metaplastic cell resembles an endocervical cell, it is vesicular with visible nuclear membrane.
A very small imperceptible nucleolus and a barr body can be made out

Cytoplasm of metaplastic cells is very dense and is very characteristic and distinctive

Fig. 10.5c

SQUAMOUS METAPLASIA WITH CYTOPLASMIC VACUOLATION (Figs 10.6a to c)

Vacuolation of metaplastic cells due to degenerative changes and cytoplasmic glycogenation as it transformed to mature metaplasia is very common and must not be mistaken for cytopathic changes of HPV in LSIL.

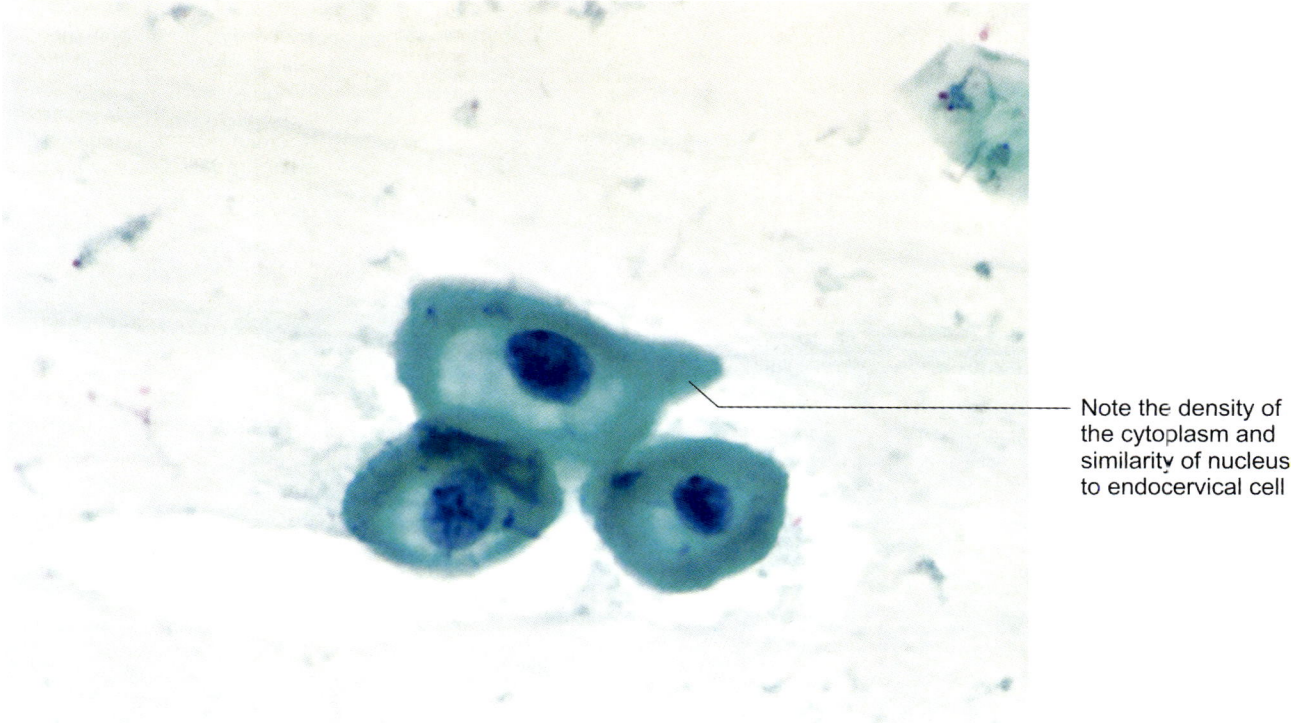

Note the density of the cytoplasm and similarity of nucleus to endocervical cell

Fig. 10.6a

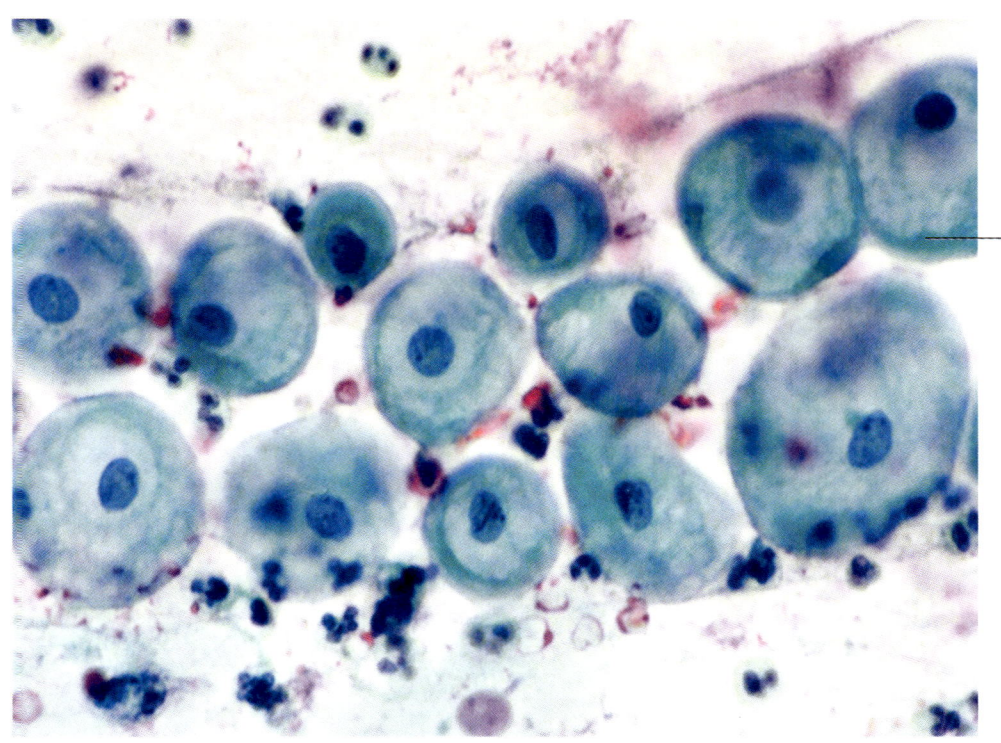

Sometimes the vacuolation can be quite extensive and can make the cell look like a parabasal cell. Seen in a woman in the reproductive age group, the focality and density of cytoplasm helps in identification. Nuclei of metaplastic cells can vary widely

Fig. 10.6b

This group of metaplastic cells is coming close to the changes seen in LSIL. Cytoplasm is, however, dense. Nuclei are darker and more elongated and focally truncated than usual metaplastic cells. However, they are not enlarged to warrant a diagnosis of LSIL and are not sufficiently hyperchromatic or atypical enough. In view of cytoplasmic features, it is better to term the nuclear changes as ASCUS. Such atypical squamous metaplastic cells are a common finding

Fig. 10.6c

ATROPHIC SMEAR (Figs 10.7a to c)

Without hormonal stimulation, epithelium regresses to be made up of mostly parabasal and a few intermediate cells, termed as atrophic smears. Inflammation frequently accompanies atrophy.

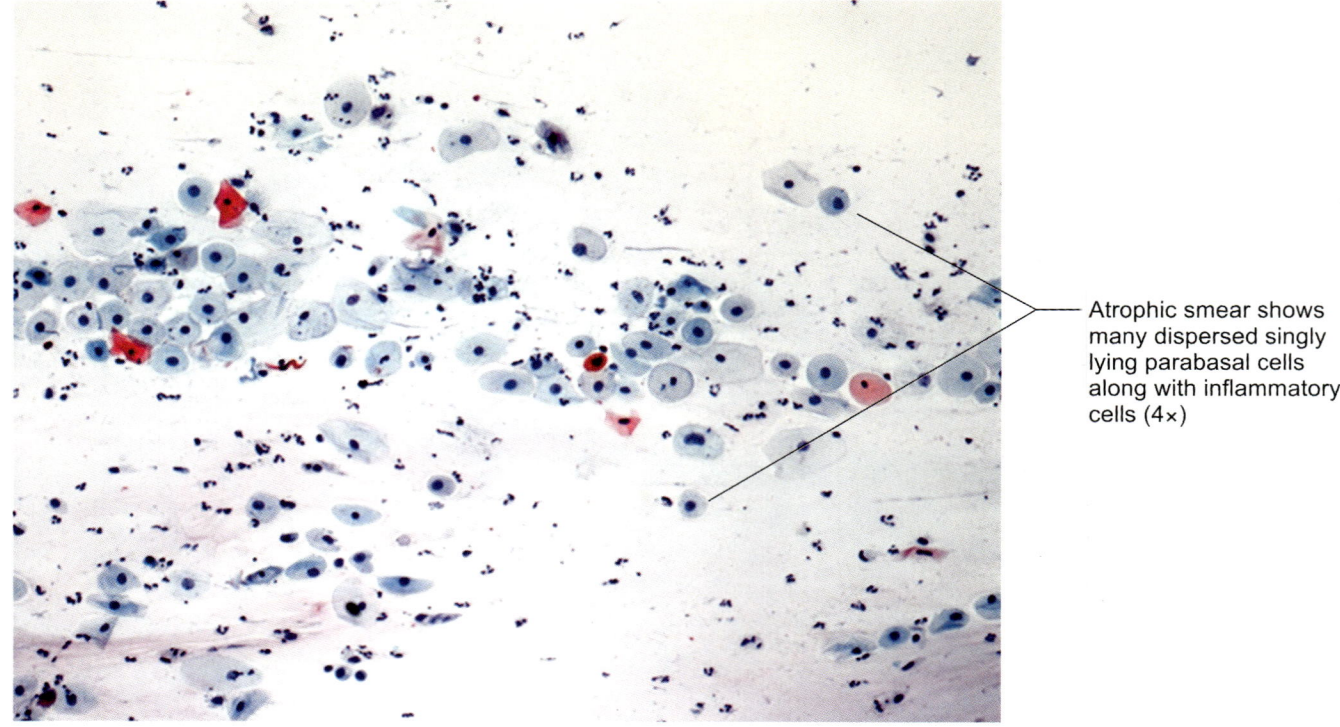

Atrophic smear shows many dispersed singly lying parabasal cells along with inflammatory cells (4×)

Fig. 10.7a

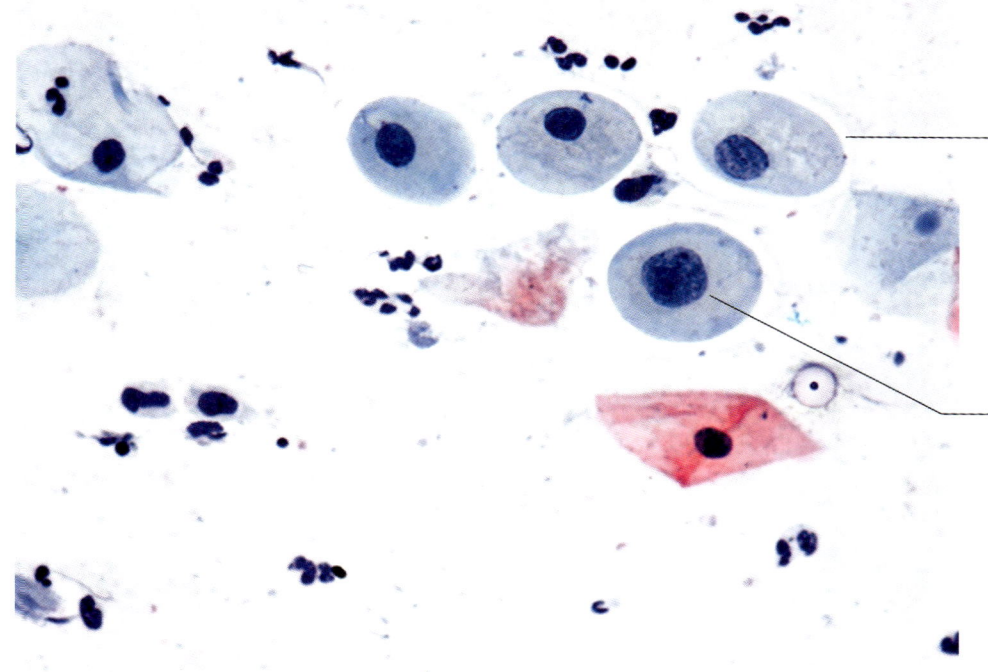

Parabasal cells have less cytoplasm than intermediate cells, are more rounded and show nuclei which are enlarged and also might be slightly more hyperchromatic (10×)

Sometimes the nuclei can be significantly enlarged and hence mistaken for SIL especially since the N/C ratio is altered

Fig. 10.7b

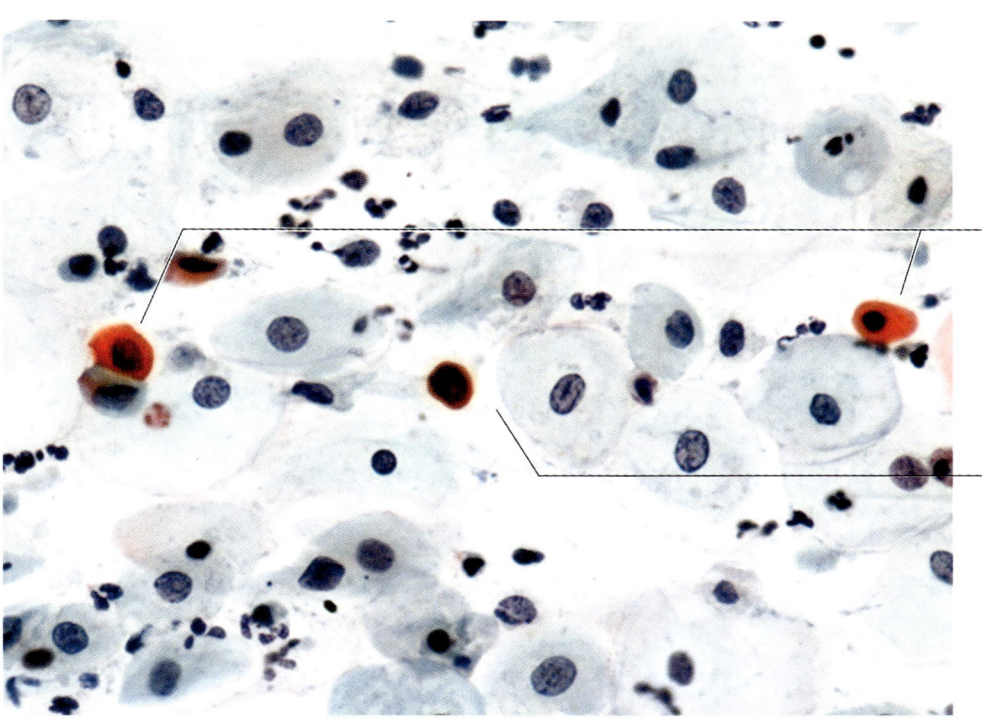

Red atrophy is when there is abrupt keratinization of parabasal cells, which stains orange with the orange G of Pap stain

Red atrophy along with nuclear enlargement of parabasal cells commonly cause a misdiagnosis of HSIL, ASC-H and squamous cell carcinoma in elderly. Senile vaginitis causes inflammation which should not be mistaken for tumor diathesis

Fig. 10.7c

HYPERESTRIN SMEAR (Figs 10.8a to c)

Patients with excess of estrogen throughout the cycle can show features seen in proliferative phase of the endometrium throughout the cycle.

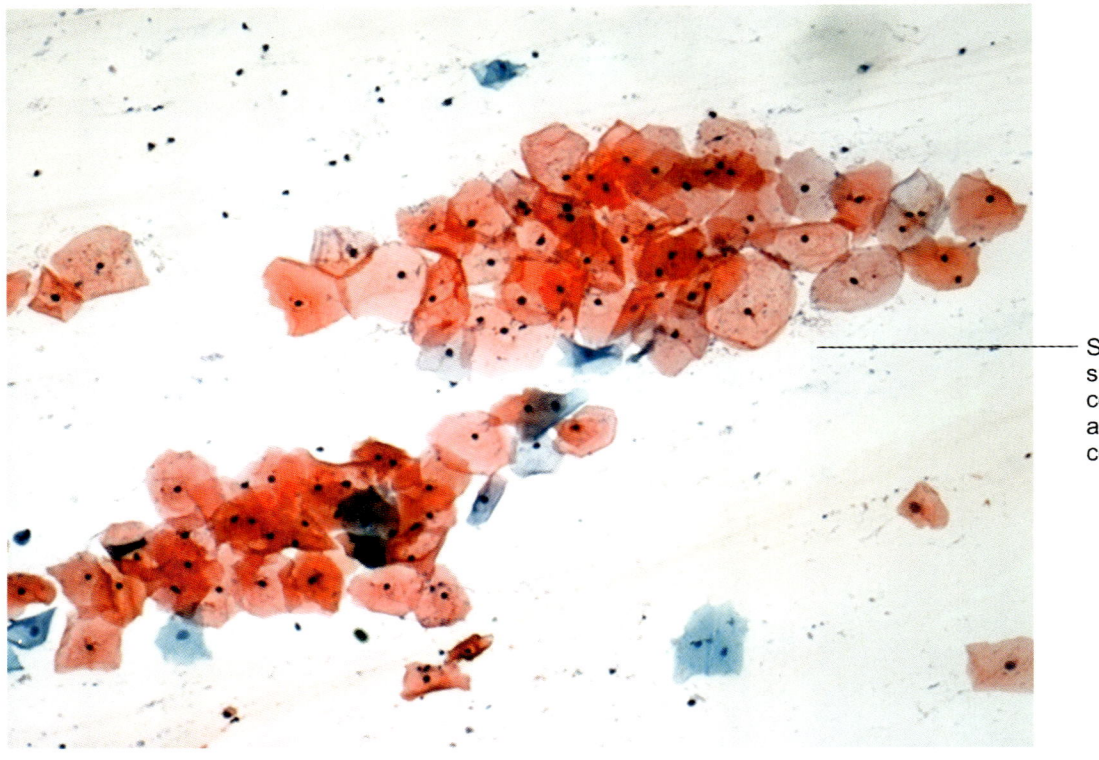

Smear shows mainly superficial cells. Most cells are eosinophilic and are superficial cells

Fig. 10.8a

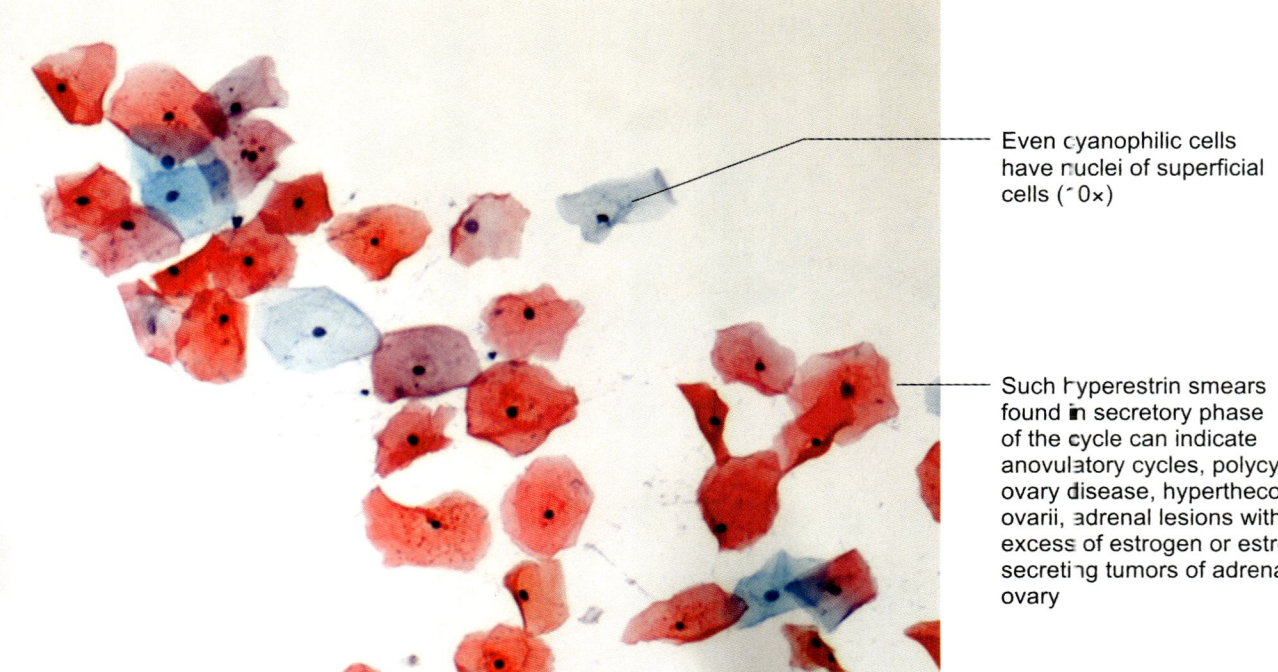

Even cyanophilic cells have nuclei of superficial cells (10x)

Such hyperestrin smears found in secretory phase of the cycle can indicate anovulatory cycles, polycystic ovary disease, hyperthecosis ovarii, adrenal lesions with excess of estrogen or estrogen secreting tumors of adrenal or ovary

Fig. 10.8b

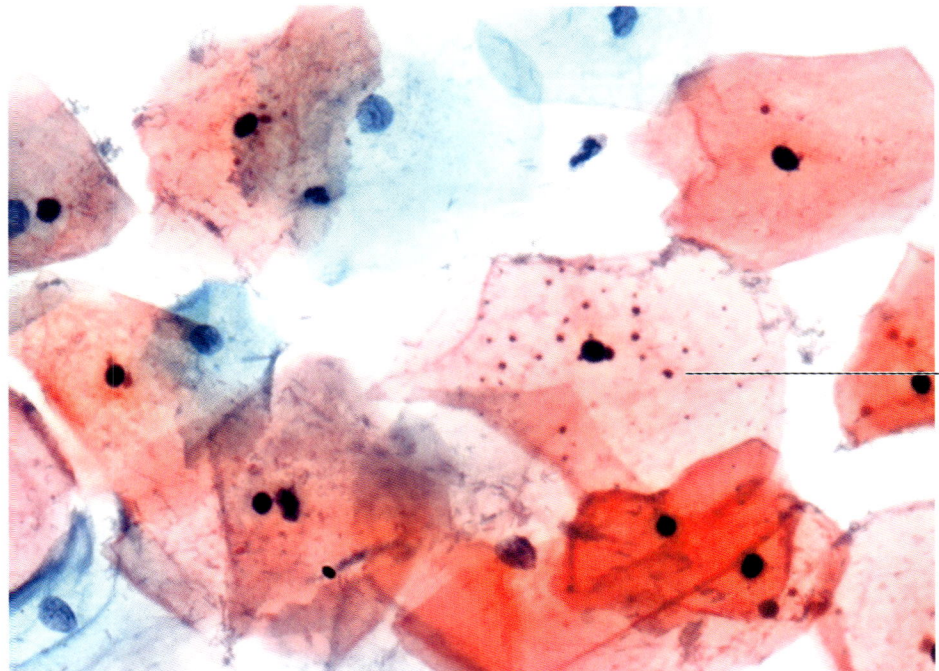

Keratohyaline granules can be seen in superficial cells. While keratohyaline granules are a common feature of LSIL with parakeratosis, they are not specific since they can be seen in any hyperestrin smear which has a lot of superficial cells or even in normal smears and in smears with keratinization due to epidermidization

Fig. 10.8c

EPIDERMIDIZATION (Figs 10.9a to c)

Some smears showing an excess of eosinophilic cells might indicate prolapse with epidermidization of cervix, i.e. presence of keratinized epithelium over the cervix.

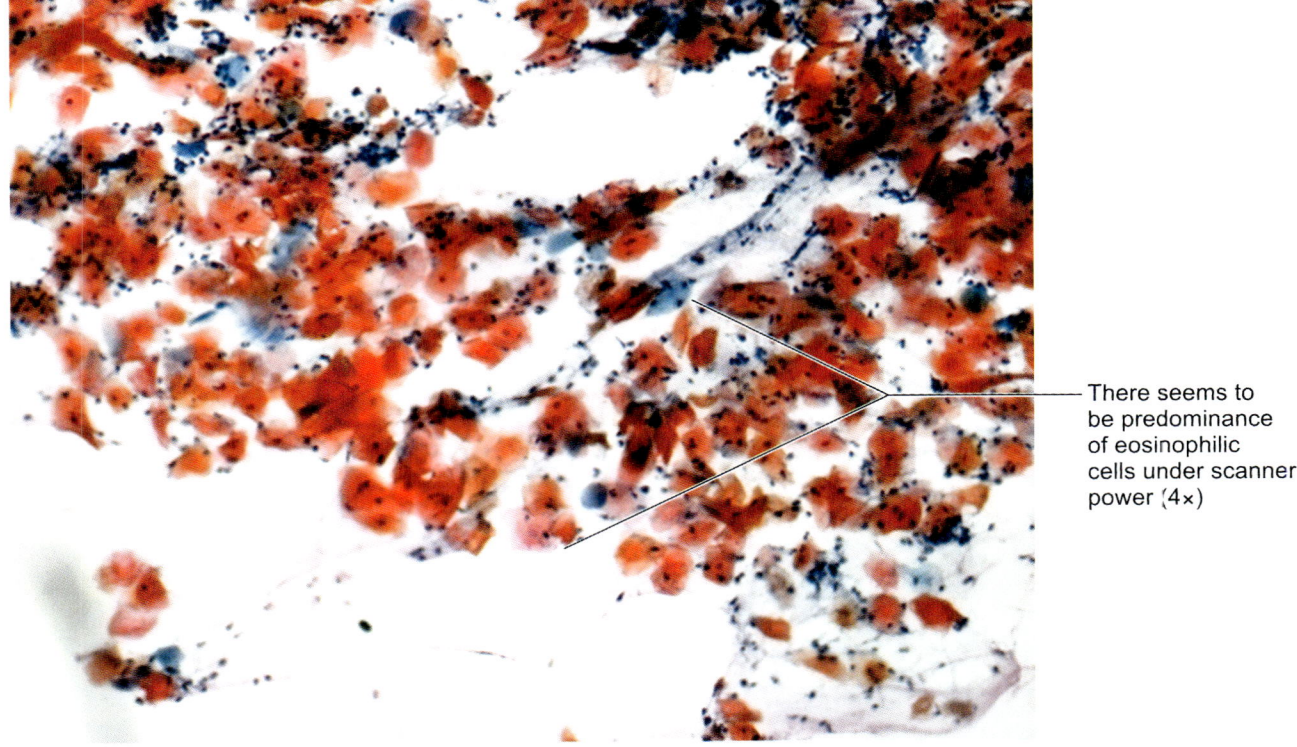

There seems to be predominance of eosinophilic cells under scanner power (4×)

Fig. 10.9a

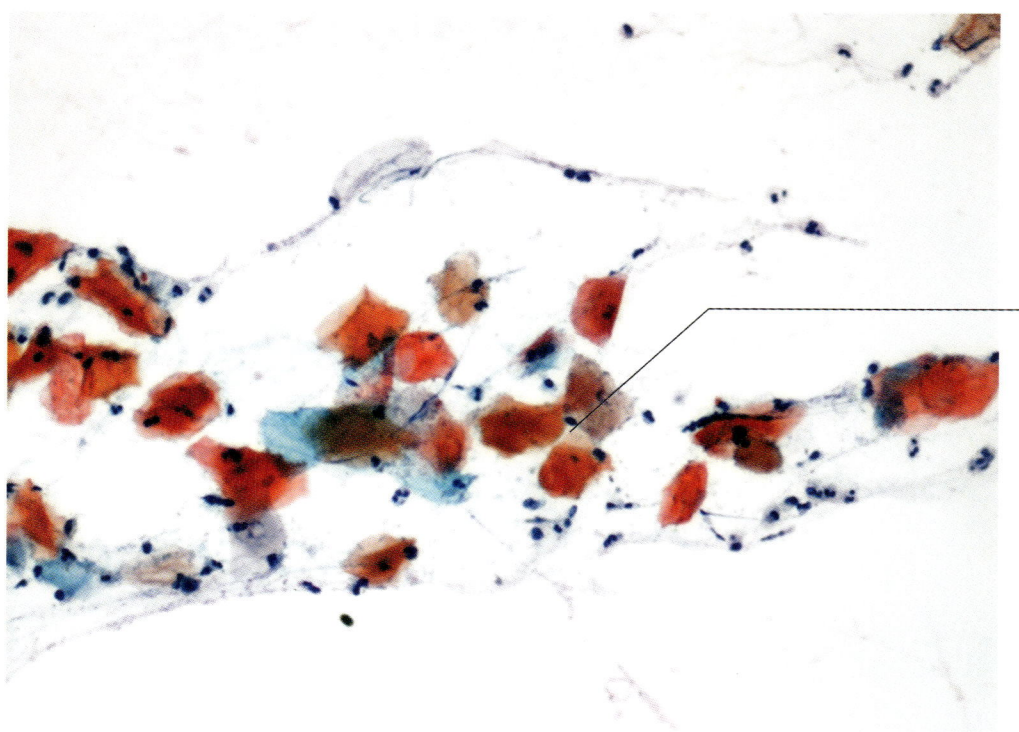

Under low power, one can see that there is orange G staining rather than eosin staining of the cytoplasm. Orange G stains mature keratin when a stratum of keratinized epithelium gets deposited on the surface of the epithelium

Fig. 10.9b

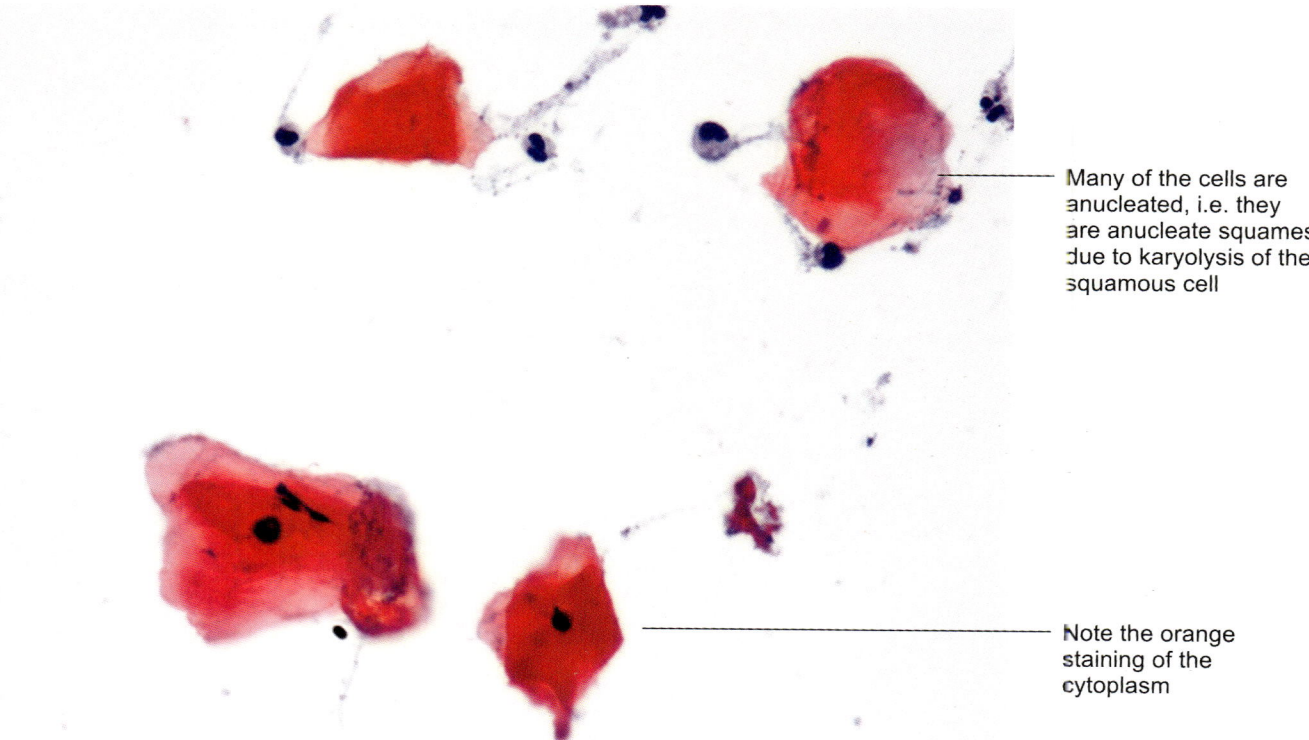

Many of the cells are anucleated, i.e. they are anucleate squames due to karyolysis of the squamous cell

Note the orange staining of the cytoplasm

Fig. 10.9c

Cytology of Infections

Some infections can be identified on cytology smears. The most common are *Trichomonas* and *Candida* which are seen in a background of inflammation. The organisms are easily identified in Pap smears as illustrated below. Rarely one can see herpes simplex or *Actinomycetes*.

CANDIDA INFECTION (Figs 11.1a and b)

Candida infection can be by yeast, pseudohyphae or both.

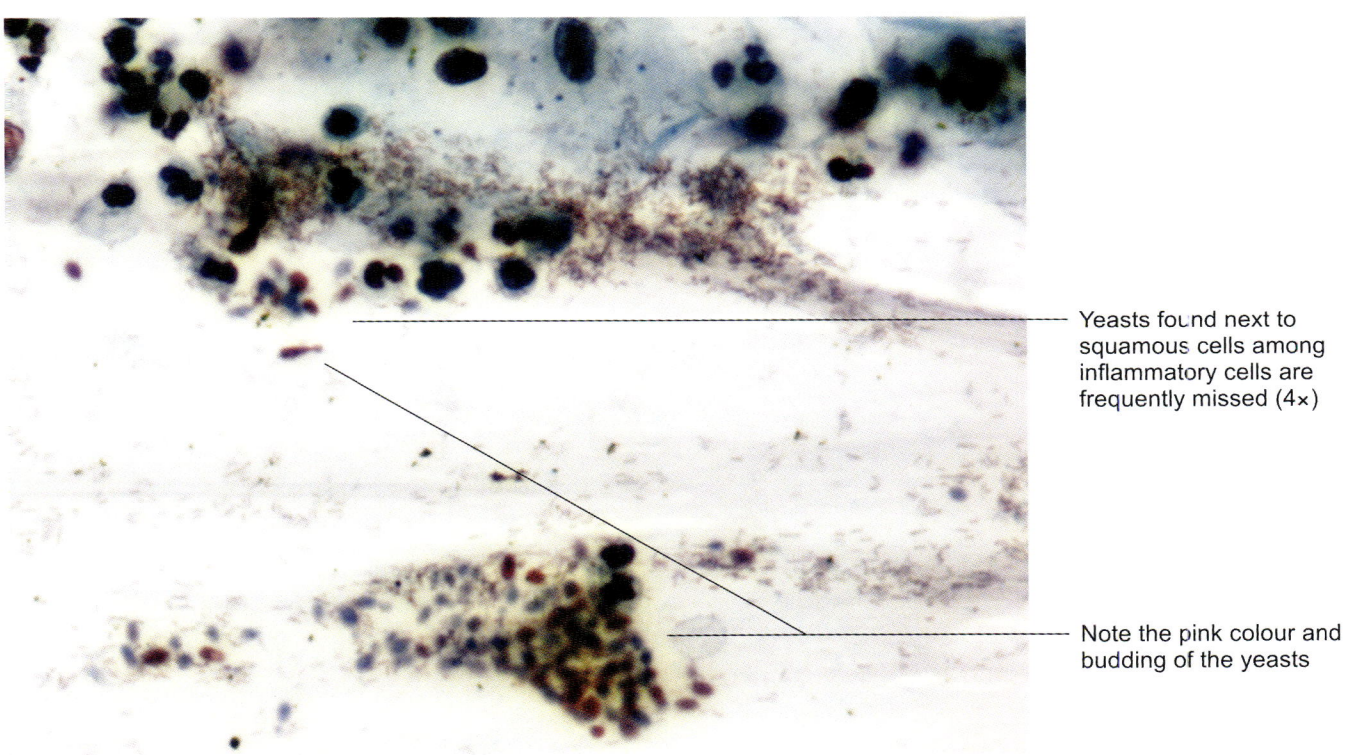

Yeasts found next to squamous cells among inflammatory cells are frequently missed (4×)

Note the pink colour and budding of the yeasts

Fig. 11.1a

Note the yeast form which is budding and continuous with the pseudohyphae

Hyphae of Candida typically are adherent to groups of epithelial cells leading to a Shish Kebab appearance. These are pseudohyphae and can sometimes branch and be present along with and in yeast forms

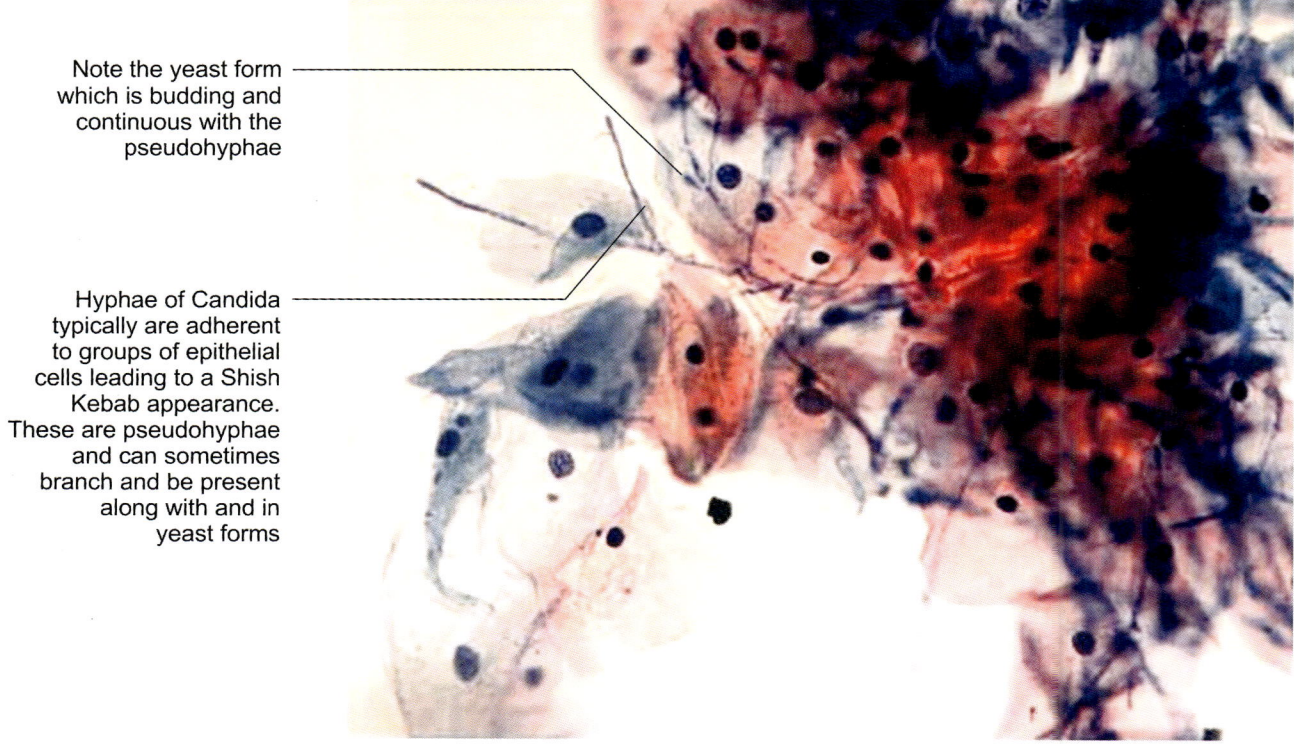

Fig. 11.1b

TRICHOMONAS INFECTION (Fig. 11.2a to c)

Trichomonas infection is typically found in inflammatory smears. *Trichomonas vaginalis* is a pear-shaped protozoal parasite.

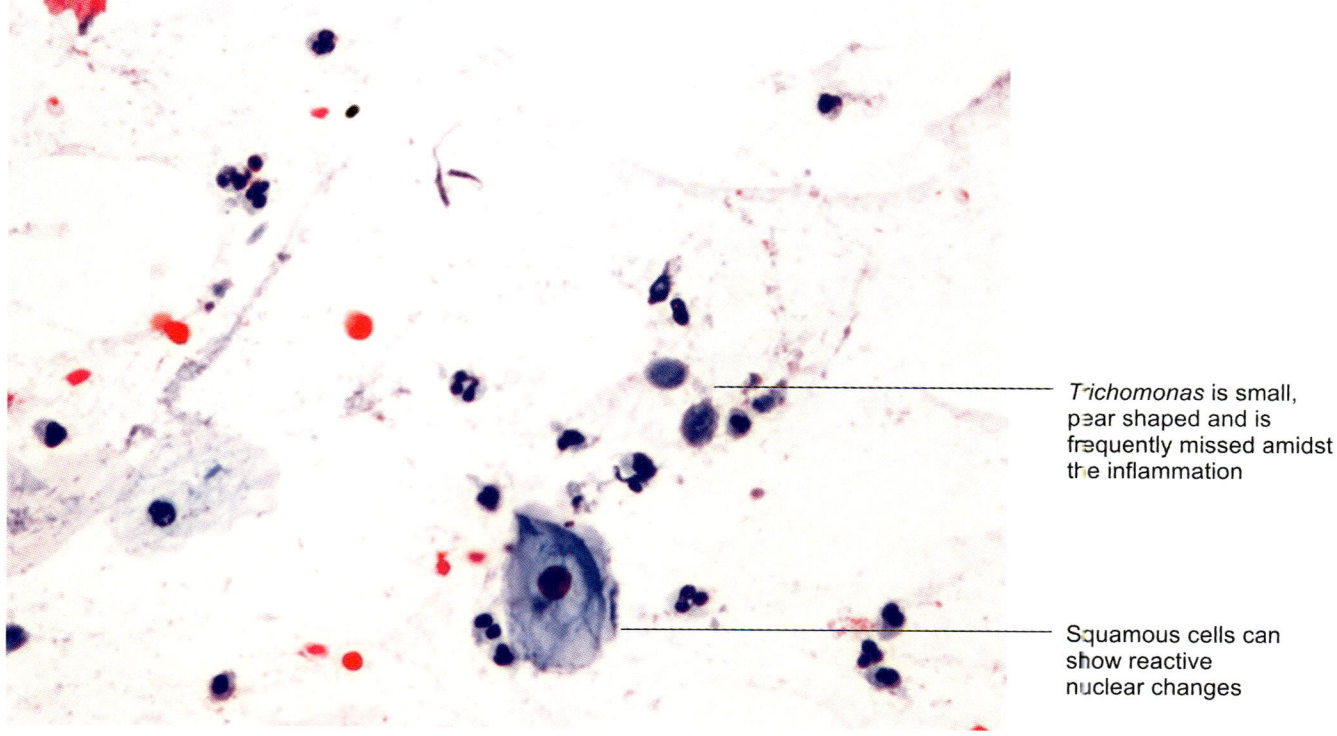

Trichomonas is small, pear shaped and is frequently missed amidst the inflammation

Squamous cells can show reactive nuclear changes

Fig. 11.2a

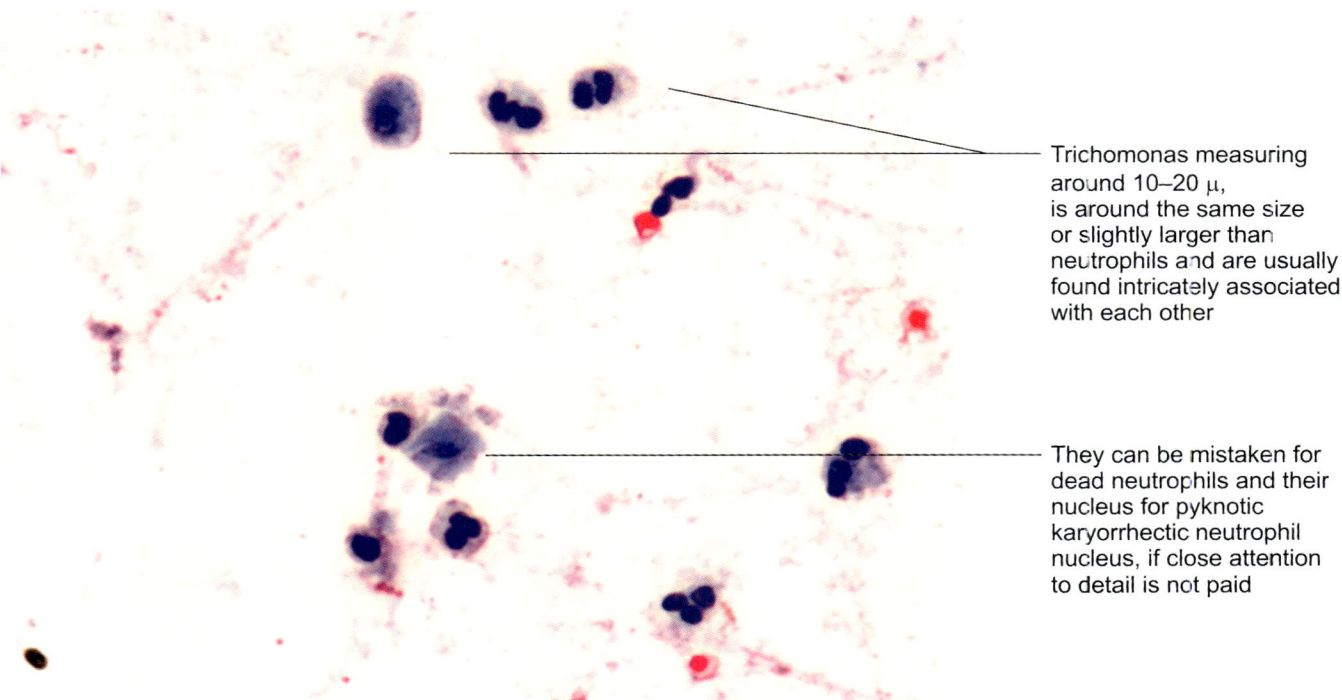

Trichomonas measuring around 10–20 μ, is around the same size or slightly larger than neutrophils and are usually found intricately associated with each other

They can be mistaken for dead neutrophils and their nucleus for pyknotic karyorrhectic neutrophil nucleus, if close attention to detail is not paid

Fig. 11.2b

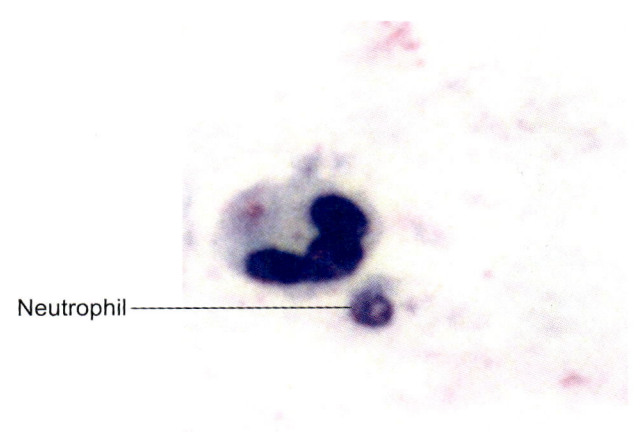

Neutrophil

Fig. 11.2c

HERPES SIMPLEX TYPE 2 INFECTION (Figs 11.3a to c)

Giant cells with multiple nuclei showing a washed out chromatin pattern are seen in herpes infection, formed by fusion of epithelial cells.

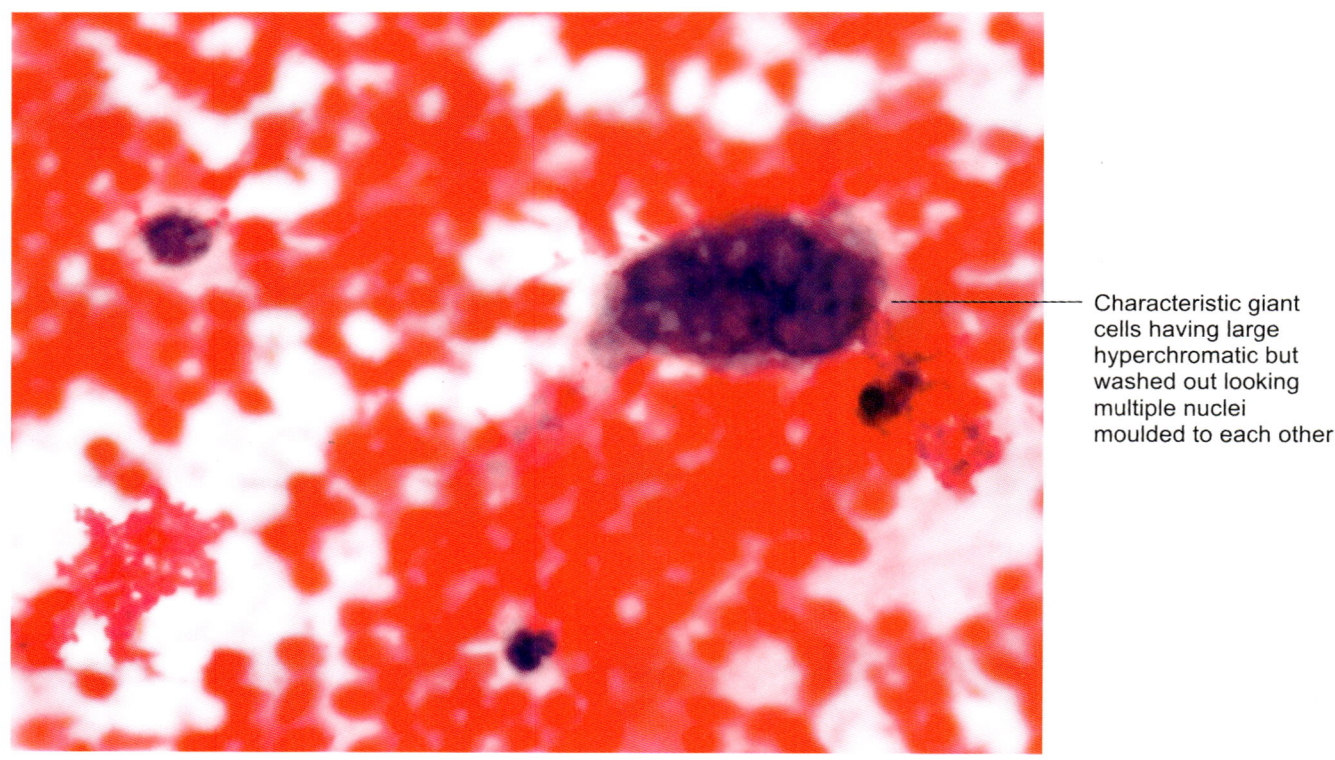

Characteristic giant cells having large hyperchromatic but washed out looking multiple nuclei moulded to each other

Fig. 11.3a

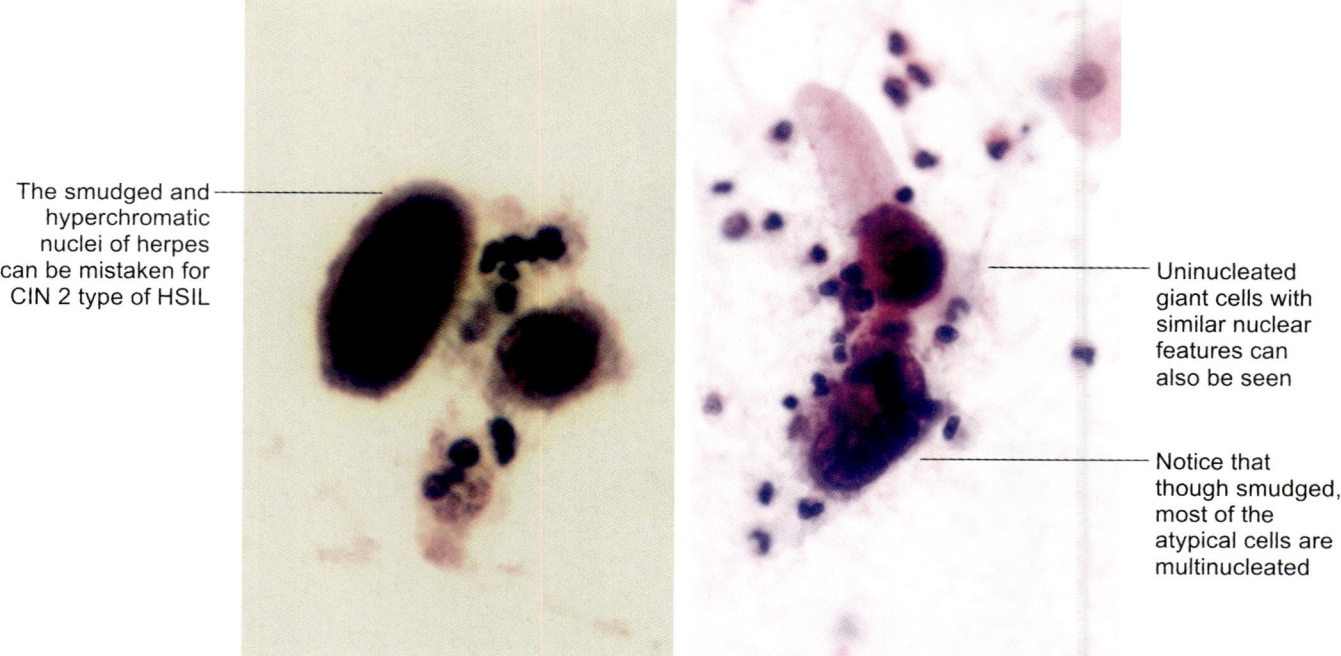

The smudged and hyperchromatic nuclei of herpes can be mistaken for CIN 2 type of HSIL

Uninucleated giant cells with similar nuclear features can also be seen

Notice that though smudged, most of the atypical cells are multinucleated

Fig. 11.3b

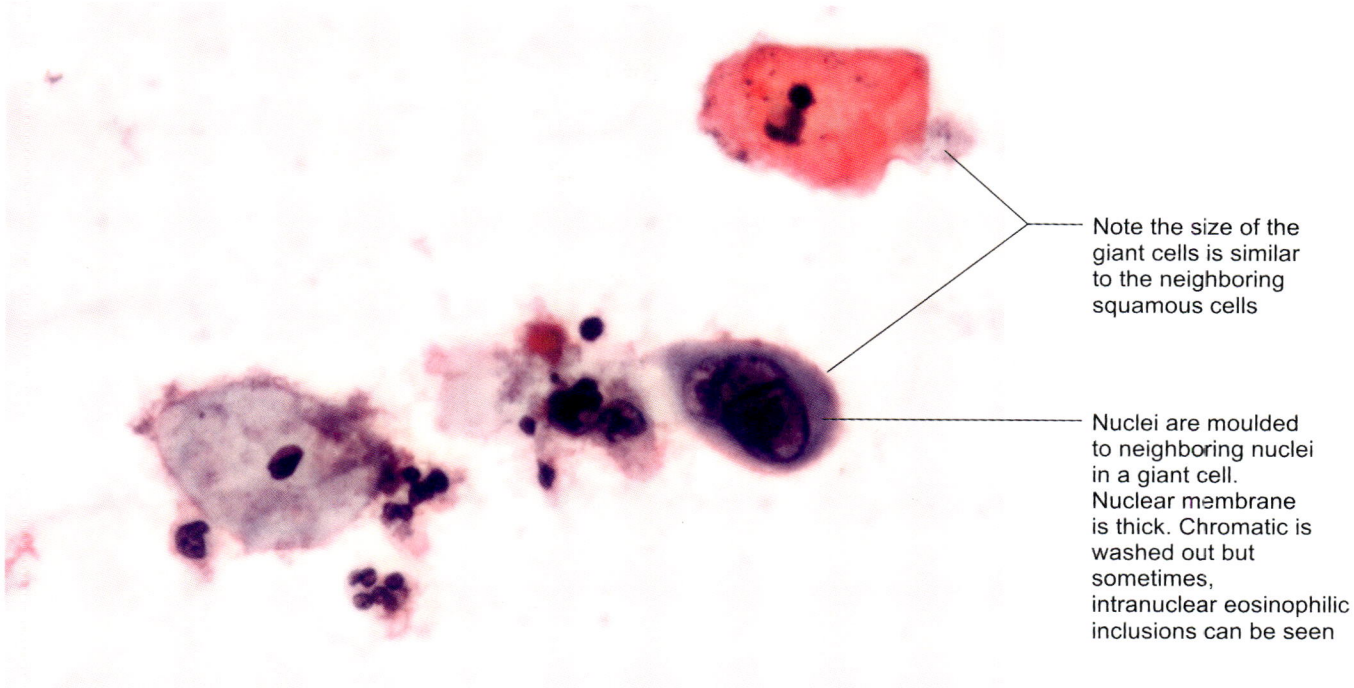

Note the size of the giant cells is similar to the neighboring squamous cells

Nuclei are moulded to neighboring nuclei in a giant cell. Nuclear membrane is thick. Chromatic is washed out but sometimes, intranuclear eosinophilic inclusions can be seen

Fig. 11.3c

ALTERED VAGINAL FLORA (Figs 11.4a and b)

Coccobacilli are very small bacteria which are not round cocci but instead extremely short rod shapes. Coccobacilli include *Gardnerella vaginalis*, *Mobiluncus*, and anaerobic bacteria.

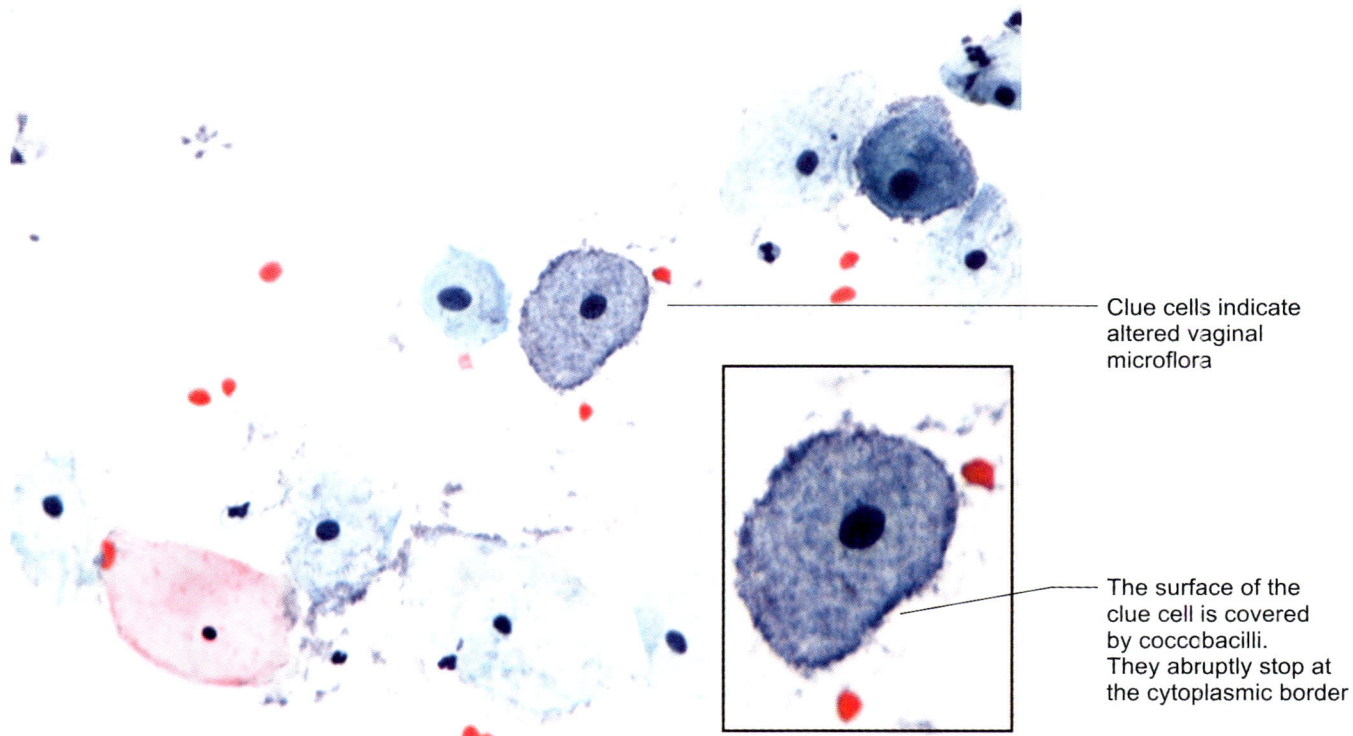

Clue cells indicate altered vaginal microflora

The surface of the clue cell is covered by cocccbacilli. They abruptly stop at the cytoplasmic border

Fig. 11.4a

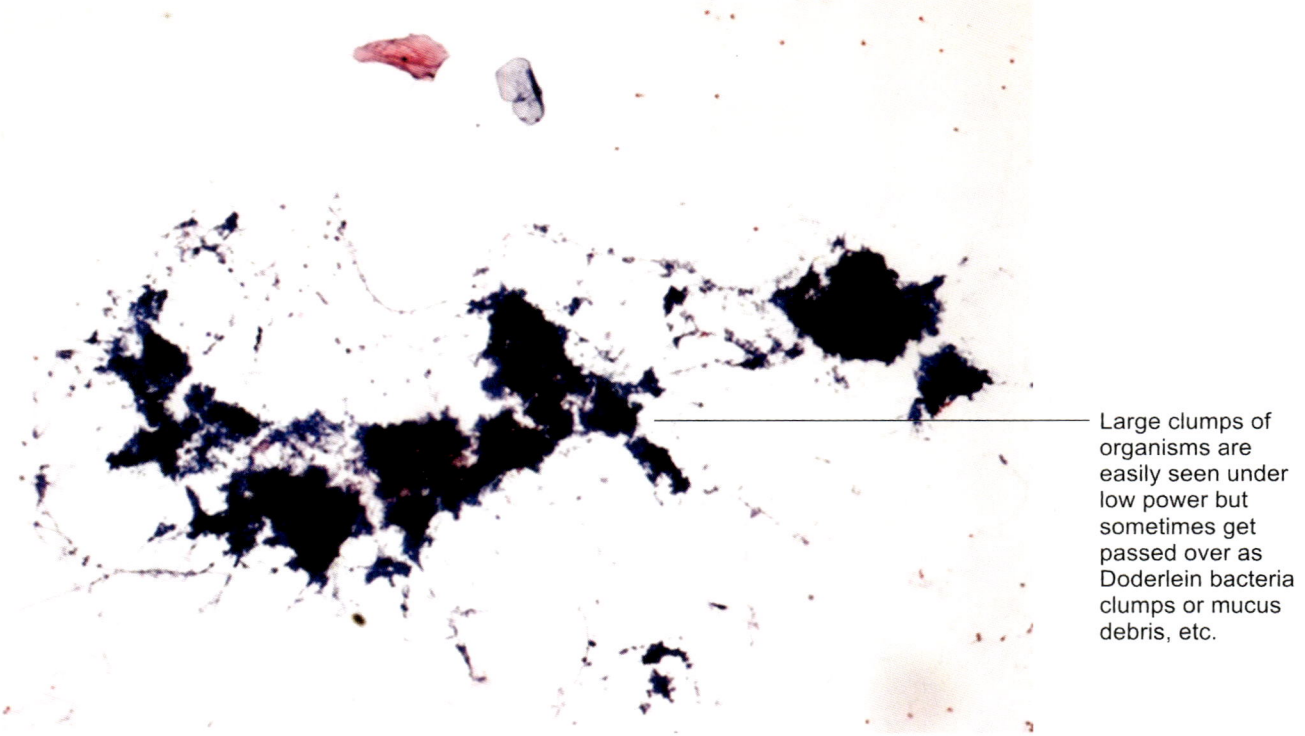

Large numbers of coccobacilli are seen in this slide. They are both stuck to the cytoplasm and forming masses

Fig. 11.4b

ACTINOMYCES INFECTION (Figs 11.5a to c)

Actinomycosis is seen with intrauterine contraceptive use or in a proportion of patients with pelvic inflammatory disease.

Large clumps of organisms are easily seen under low power but sometimes get passed over as Doderlein bacteria clumps or mucus debris, etc.

Fig. 11.5a

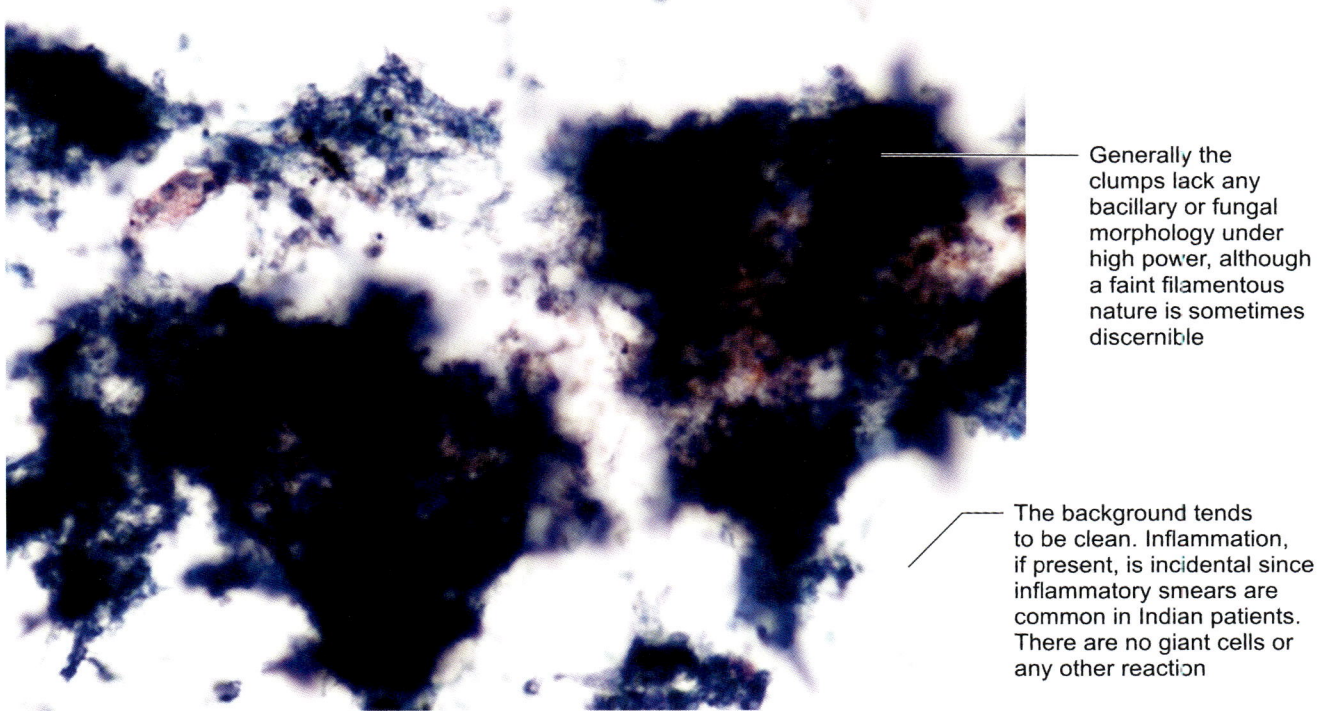

Generally the clumps lack any bacillary or fungal morphology under high power, although a faint filamentous nature is sometimes discernible

The background tends to be clean. Inflammation, if present, is incidental since inflammatory smears are common in Indian patients. There are no giant cells or any other reaction

Fig. 11.5b

Dense center and a lighter periphery where a very vague filamentous appearance is sometimes visible. Note absence of clear filaments, bacillary appearance or cocci-like appearance—the diagnosis is made at low power and not under high power where the clumps take on an amorphous or structureless appearance in the majority

Fig. 11.5c

TUBERCULOSIS (Figs 11.6a to c)

It is very rare to encounter tuberculosis in the cervical smear. When giant cells are seen, which happens sometimes, tuberculosis is a differential diagnosis.

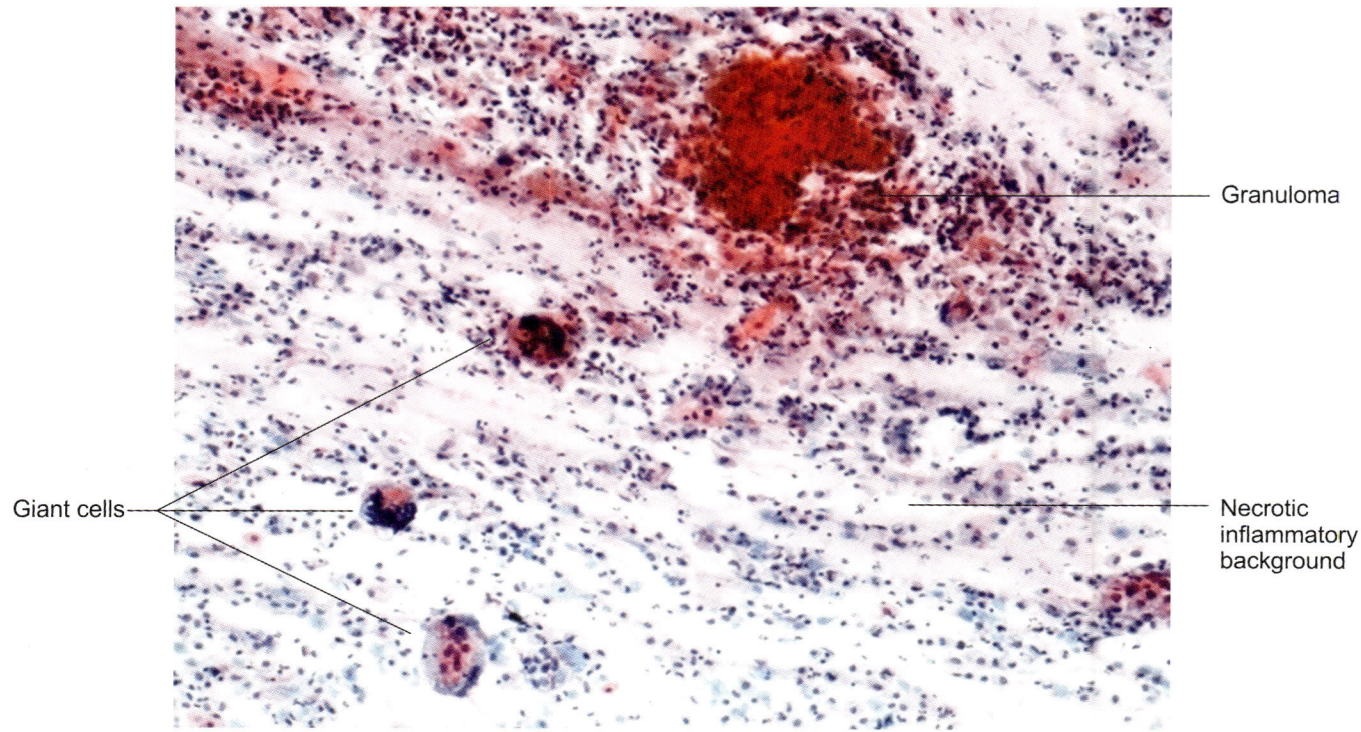

Granuloma

Giant cells

Necrotic inflammatory background

Fig. 11.6a

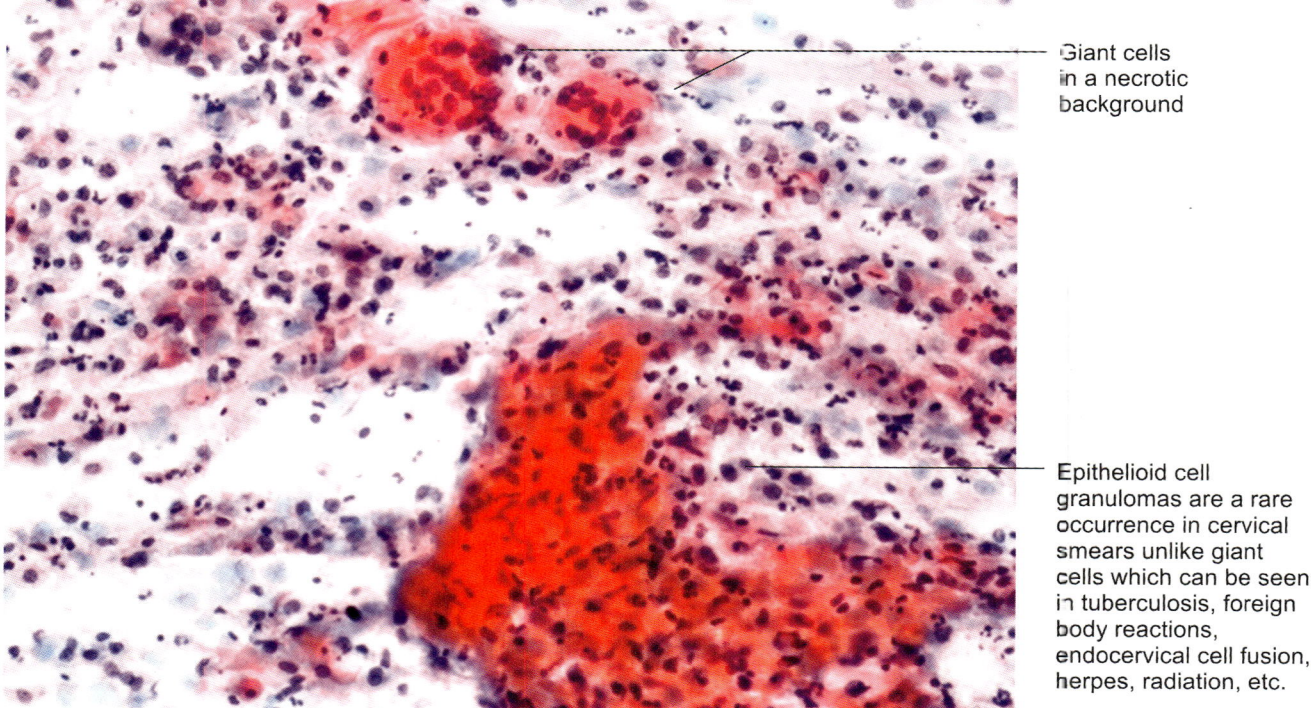

Giant cells in a necrotic background

Epithelioid cell granulomas are a rare occurrence in cervical smears unlike giant cells which can be seen in tuberculosis, foreign body reactions, endocervical cell fusion, herpes, radiation, etc.

Fig. 11.6b

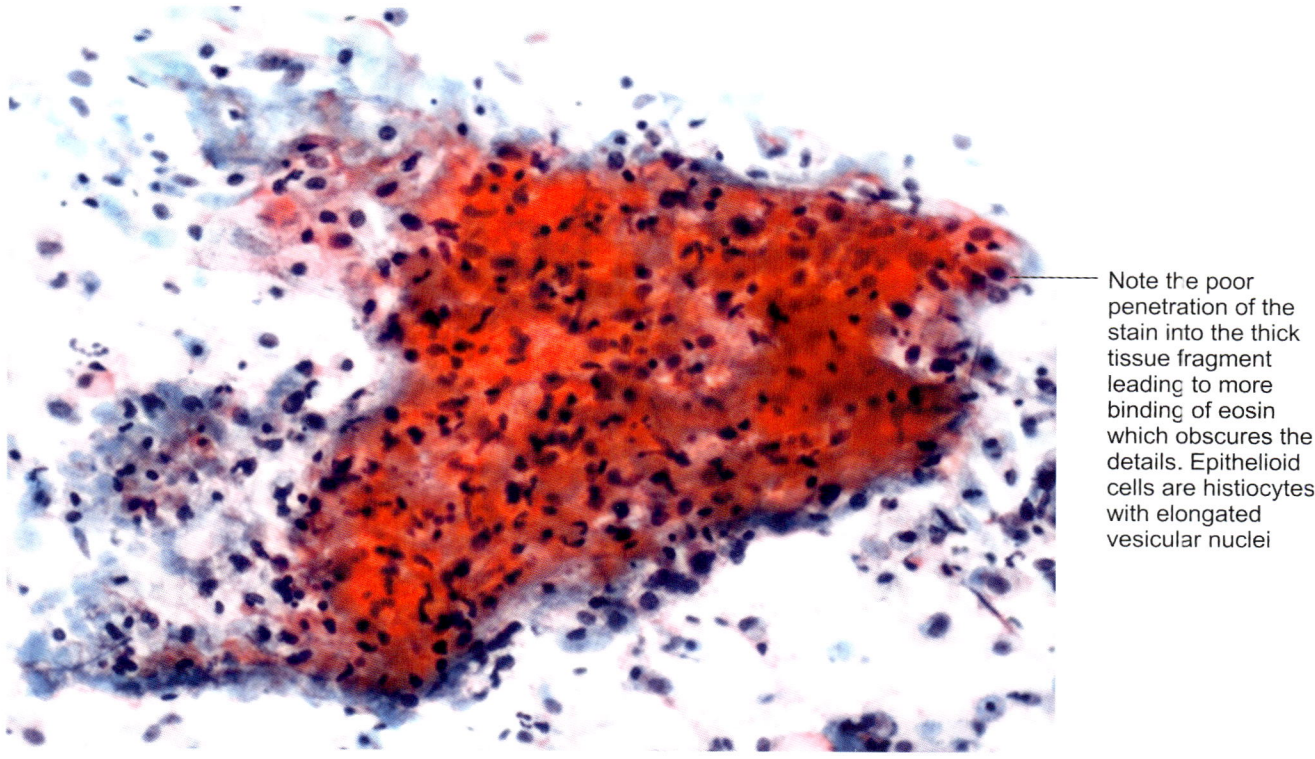

Note the poor penetration of the stain into the thick tissue fragment leading to more binding of eosin which obscures the details. Epithelioid cells are histiocytes with elongated vesicular nuclei

Fig. 11.6c

FOLLICULAR CERVICITIS (Figs 11.7a to c)

In follicular cervicitis, lymphoid follicles are present under the epithelium and are sampled in the cytology.

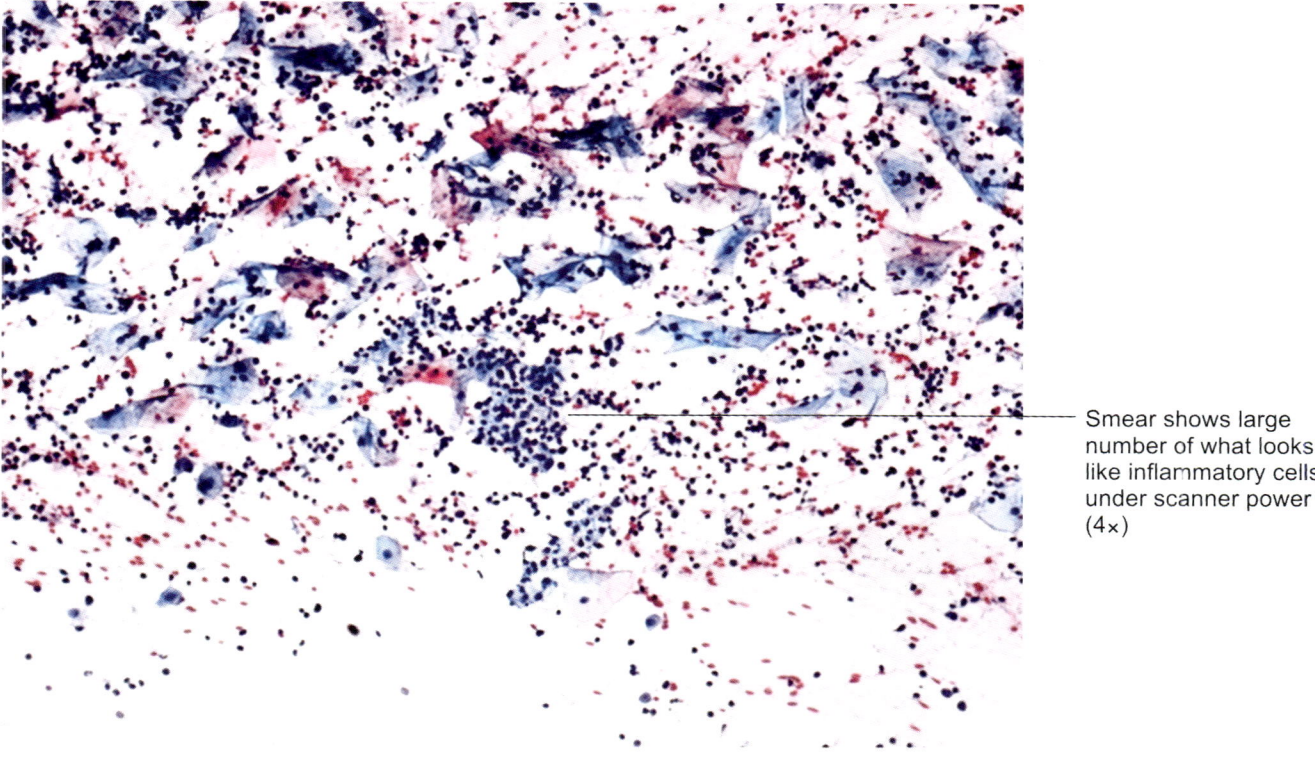

Smear shows large number of what looks like inflammatory cells under scanner power (4×)

Fig. 11.7a

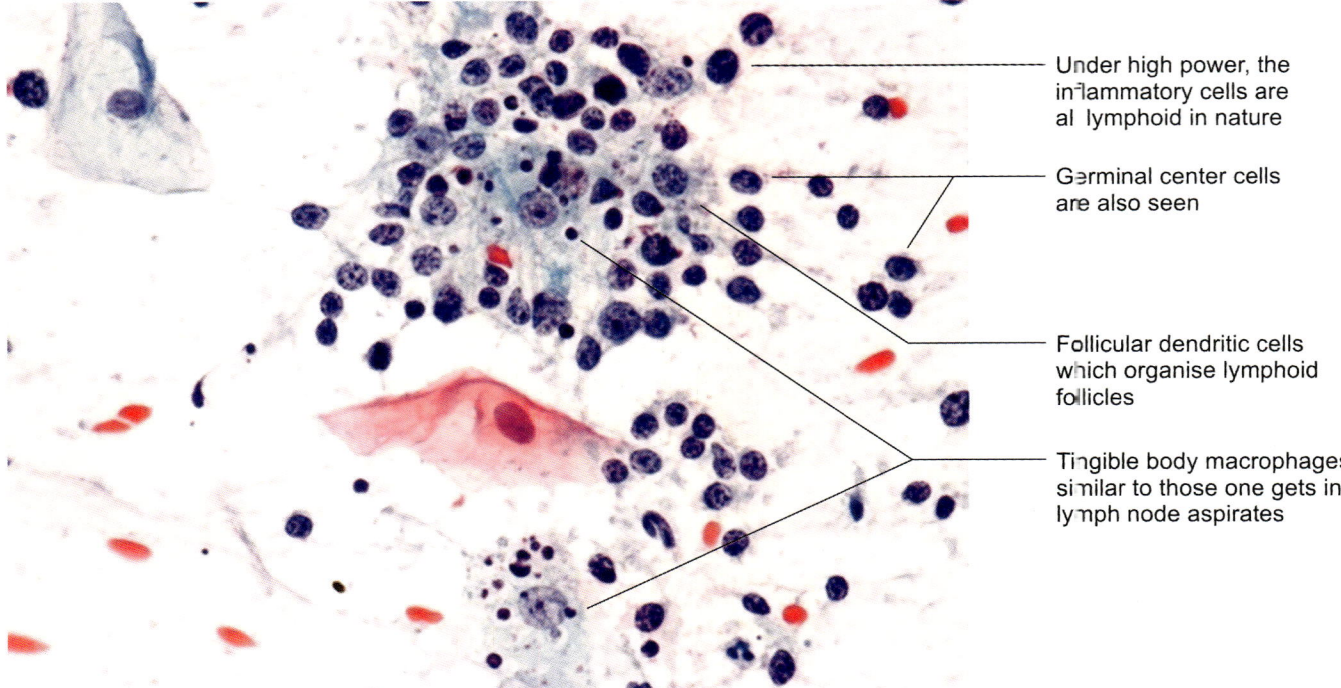

Under high power, the inflammatory cells are al lymphoid in nature

Germinal center cells are also seen

Follicular dendritic cells which organise lymphoid follicles

Tingible body macrophages similar to those one gets in lymph node aspirates

Fig. 11.7b

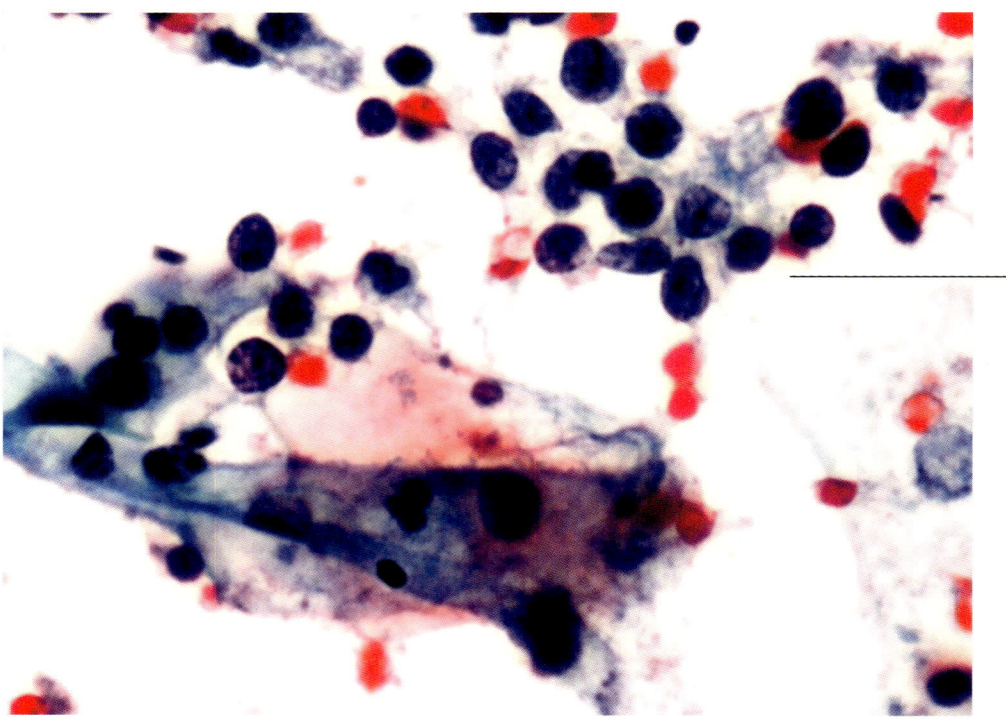

Lymphoid cells from germinal center cells being larger than lymphocytes, one can mistake these hyperchromatic cells with scant cytoplasm as cells from a CIN 3 type of HSIL. Not every case will show tingible body macrophages or follicular dendritic cells and under a darker Pap stain, follicular cervicitis is a known pitfall where a misdiagnosis of HSIL takes place

Fig. 11.7c

Understanding Histopathology of HPV Infection

The human papillomavirus (HPV) gains entry to the basal layers of the squamous epithelium. Typically this happens at the transformation zone at the junction between the columnar and squamous epithelia. HPV, especially HPV type 18, can also enter the columnar epithelial cells and produce squamous metaplasia resulting in a squamous lesion despite initiation over columnar epithelium. Once the virus gains entry into the basal epithelial cells, it can produce different types of lesions as described below.

Virologically, three different types of HPV infection are present. There are:
- Latent infections
- Productive infections
- Integrative infections

Latent HPV Infection

In this condition, the viral genome is present in the squamous epithelium, as detected using highly sensitive detection tests like PCR, hybrid capture, etc. However, the virus is producing no detectable morphological lesion. Either the viral episomes are present in small numbers in basal and suprabasal cells of the squamous epithelium or it is producing very small-sized lesions which are invisible on colposcopy and not sampled on biopsy. Latent infections are the vast majority of HPV infections and account for 6 to 14% of the general population tested for HPV, depending on the geographical location of the population. In India, around 6 to 8% of the general population have HPV coming positive, the vast majority of which are latent HPV infections. The copy number of the HPV episomes tend to be low titre positive on HPV tests in which a titre is generated. However, a few cases might also have higher titres and might correspond to smaller sized productive infections where the lesion is too small to be visible on colposcopy and so small that biopsies and cytology miss the lesion.

Productive HPV Infection

In this condition, the virus is actively replicating in the epithelium producing larger sized lesions which are visible on colposcopy and found on biopsy to have characteristic features. The virus is actively replicating to make numerous copies of itself. The replication occurs in the nucleus where the normal replicating apparatus of the squamous cell is used for viral DNA synthesis. As numerous copies of its genome accumulate in the nucleus, it results in the nuclear changes becoming visible on light microscopy. Nuclei become much larger and hyperchromatic. Viral DNA keeps on increasing as one moves higher and higher up the epithelium. As the nucleus is packed with viral genome, it changes the chromatin character which shifts from being normally vesicular to becoming dyskaryotic with diffuse powdery hyperchromasia. Nuclear membrane becomes altered with thick nuclear membrane which might be thrown into folds, causing tulip or raisin-shaped nuclear outlines. Nuclear elongation, truncation and even bizarrely enlarged nuclei stuffed with viral DNA are seen. The viral genome moves out from the nucleus to the cytoplasm where the complete virions are generated.

As the virions accumulate in the cytoplasm, variable extents of cytopathic changes are produced in the form of perinuclear cytoplasmic clearing with peripheral rim of cytoplasm, resulting in a sharply punched out margin between the rim of cytoplasm and the clearing. These cytopathic changes are seen higher up in the epithelium away from the basement membrane. Parakeratosis, i.e. abnormal keratinization of the superficial cells, is a common finding due to the stimulation of keratin production by the virus. As part of the cytopathic changes, the cells might undergo apoptosis or mitonecrosis. In apoptosis, the cell rounds up and becomes hypereosinophilic with pyknotic nucleus. In mitonecrosis, there is a mitotic catastrophy causing cells to undergo death in division. There is karyolysis of the mitotic nucleus and the cell loses its nucleus.

The virus gains entry to the basal layer. Therefore, it has the lowest copy number. As part of its cycle, the E6 and E7 proteins of the virus have the function of increasing the mitotic rate of the squamous epithelium. As the cell division becomes more and more, driven by the viral E6 and E7 proteins, the replication of the virus which utilizes the host machinery is also increased. Because of its effect on the cell cycle, the number of mitotic figures increases and also the mitotic figures are seen higher up in the epithelium than is seen normally. Under ordinary circumstances, the squamous epithelium shows mitotic activity only in the basal layer. In addition to increasing mitotic rates, the actively proliferating cells acquire a smaller cytoplasm and a larger more opened out chromatic structure in the parabasal layers, producing a visible change in the lower one-third of the epithelium. In view of increased mitosis much in excess of needs, the epithelium can get thrown into folds producing a papillomatosis.

Despite all these morphological changes, the epithelium is not transformed—the visible changes are due to the activity of the virus and its usual processes within the host cell. The cells are not clonal in nature. The changes of productive HPV infection described above are essentially common to all the types of HPV including the low risk 6 and 11 as well as the high risk 16, 18, etc. The extent of cytopathic change and papillomatosis tends to be higher in low-risk types 6 and 11. Cytopathy is less often seen in the high-risk HPV 16, 18, etc. which more frequently are flat lesions. However, in any individual papillary or flat lesion, it is impossible to say whether it is caused by low-risk or high-risk types since there is considerable overlap.

The changes described above are similar to the changes of non-cervical HPV infections like viral warts, plantar warts caused by all types of HPV.

Integrative HPV Infections

In this condition, some of the viral DNA integrates in different sites of the host genome in such a way that it brings about a transformative change in the cell. It only happens with high-risk HPV types like 16, 18, etc. This is because of loss of E2 control over E6 and E7 function and only occurs with the high-risk types of these viral proteins. As a result of this transformation, the cells become premalignant, i.e. changes in the genome have occurred sufficient to cause an *in situ* carcinoma which, however, is not yet capable of invasion. The etiology of this change is accumulation of mutations in the actively replicating cells driven by the HPV infection as explained above. Premalignant clones emerge and these clones selectively overgrow the normal clones and occupy the full thickness of the epithelium. The nature of these mutations varies and hence morphologically the changes are diverse. All are characterized by replacement of the basal and parabasal zones of the epithelium by transformed cells. Changes seen in the higher layers of the epithelium can vary. In some, the cells are small; while in others, the cells are large. In some, the higher layers show the expected keratinocytic differentiation; while in others, the normal process of keratinization is lost.

Despite the morphological differences with productive HPV, these integrative HPV infections can continue to be very actively productive as well. Hence, in addition to the changes of integrative infection, the morphologic changes described for productive HPV infections can also be seen in within these integrative infections. Hence, superficial layers can show koilocyte production in large numbers with all the nuclear and cytoplasmic cytopathic changes.

Fate of HPV Infection

Regardless of the kind of HPV infection occurring as detailed above, the body mounts an immune response which attempt to clear the epithelium of HPV infection. There is a robust antibody response which eliminates cell-to-cell transmission. Latent, productive and integrative infections are all capable of being eliminated based on the immune response.

Latent infections are cleared due to brisk immune response and the virus is eliminated without producing any morphological lesion in the patient. Most of these infections are cleared by 9 months and after 1 year virtually all the patients become negative on HPV testing. However, the immunity is type specific and hence after clearing one type of HPV, the patient can become re-infected by another type of HPV. Depending on the immunity to the new HPV type, patient can again get either latent, productive or integrative infections regardless of what type of infection was seen with the previous HPV type.

Productive infections are cleared in around 98% of the patients within one year. As the body mounts an immune response, the lesions regress in size and if effective immunity is generated, the lesion vanishes completely. All the changes described above reverse and the epithelium becomes indistinguishable from normal epithelium. Both low-risk and high-risk productive infections can be eliminated by the body in the vast majority. However, in 2%

of the productive infections, there is persistence of the infection beyond one year. This persistence can be seen in both low-risk and high-risk HPV types. Large papillary lesions (condylomas) produced by low-risk HPV types can persist and can also spread to new sites in the vulva, vagina and cervix. Rarely these condylomas can also be caused by high-risk HPV types. Flat lesions caused by both low-risk and high-risk HPV types can persist. Rate of persistence of flat lesions caused by high-risk HPV types is higher. Persistence implies that the body is not able to mount an effective immune response or it is slower and less effective. Over a period of time, persistent infections are also cleared slowly.

Integrative infections tend to occur mainly in persistent infections. As the body fails to eliminate the infection, the active proliferation produced by the productive infection continues unabated. This provides a good milieu for the integration of viral genome into the host DNA. This integration can alter the control of viral proteins E6 and E7 by the viral protein E2, usually because of break in the viral genome in this region. The proliferation in such integrative infections is much greater and in this background of uncontrolled proliferation, mutations accumulate. Once a sufficiency of mutations arises, the cell becomes transformed into a premalignant clone.

Despite such transformation, the body can eliminate the infection, if immune response improves. In about 30% of these integrative infections, the premalignant lesion transforms into malignancy as more mutations capable of giving the ability to invade the basement membrane accumulate. If left untreated, around 30%, therefore, progress to invasive cancer. However, in about 20%, the changes are completely reversed in the absence of treatment. Since currently all such lesions are treated, these observations are based on historical studies where patients were not treated. In the remaining 50% of the cases, the premalignant integrative infection persists indefinitely, i.e. it neither progresses to invasive cancer nor does it revert to normal. However, a small number continue to become malignant each year, if left untreated.

Now that the underlying virology is understood, it becomes easier to understand the histopathology of these lesions.

A. LOW GRADE SQUAMOUS INTRAEPITHELIAL LESION (LSIL)

Normal epithelium: This is seen in uninfected or latent infections. There is no morphological change.

Low grade squamous intraepithelial lesion (LSIL) or CIN 1 (mild dysplasia): Cervical intraepithelial neoplasia grade 1 of the Richart classification corresponds to a productive HPV infection. It was previously called mild dysplasia. It is important to understand that though commonly thought to affect the lower one-third of the epithelium, it does not mean that the upper two-thirds are normal—rather, the upper two-thirds show the changes of productive HPV infection and hence are not normal.

The lower one-third of the epithelium shows changes related to high proliferation. Hence, there is nuclear enlargement and decreased cytoplasm resulting in mild change in nuclear cytoplasmic ratio when compared to normal. Mitotic figures are increased and can be present in cells a few layers higher than basal cells. Such changes can also be seen in hyperplastic epithelium unrelated to HPV infection. Therefore, finding the characteristic changes in the upper two-thirds of the epithelium is essential before the diagnosis of CIN 1 can be made.

The top two-thirds of the epithelium shows nuclear enlargement with diffuse powdery hyperchromasia. There is nuclear elongation and truncation with increased frequency of binucleation. Nuclear membrane is thrown into folds and the nuclear margins are thickened. Apoptosis, mitonecrosis and bizarre enlarged nuclei are seen. These nuclear changes are essential to make a diagnosis of CIN 1. Cytoplasm shows variable changes and are not essential for making the diagnosis of CIN 1. The cytoplasm is enlarged, i.e. cytomegaly. In this common condition, since both nuclei and cytoplasm are enlarged, the nuclear cytoplasmic ratio may not be altered. Perinuclear cytoplasmic clearing with sharply defined margin with the normal cytoplasm may be present. The combination of nuclear changes with cytoplasmic clearing is commonly referred to as koilocytic atypia or koilocytic change. It is also commonly called features suggestive of HPV infection although the above discussion would have made it clear that even in the absence of cytoplasmic clearing, these changes of CIN 1 indicate HPV infection of productive type. There can be no CIN 1 in the absence of HPV infection.

The top one-third or the most superficial layers of the epithelium can, in addition, show parakeratosis, i.e. presence of keratinization with the presence of nucleated keratinized superficial cells. This is usually accompanied by presence of keratohyaline granules in squamous cells below the parakeratosis. If parakeratosis is present, then the "koilocytic atypia", i.e. cytoplasmic clearing is present focally in the middle third of the epithelium only.

CIN 1 can be present with or without papillomatosis. Usually, flat lesions with CIN 1 are called CIN 1 only while papillary lesions with CIN 1 may be variably called CIN 1 or condyloma or wart or HPV infection. Regardless of any of these terms being used, they are all CIN 1.

Differential Diagnosis

Hyperplastic epithelia are frequently misdiagnosed as CIN 1 because the lower one-third of the epithelium has changes similar to productive HPV infections. However, upper two-thirds of hyperplastic epithelium lack the characteristic changes described above for CIN 1.

Hyperplastic epithelium with cytoplasmic glycogenation is frequently mistaken for CIN 1 with koilocytic atypia. Glycogen vacuoles are, however, not sharply punched out from the peripheral rim of cytoplasm unlike CIN 1 with cytopathic vacuolation. More importantly, glycogenation is not accompanied by the characteristic nuclear changes which are essential for diagnosis of CIN 1.

Papillary lesions can be misdiagnosed as condyloma which in current understanding automatically implies a diagnosis of CIN 1 even if not mentioned. Papillary lesions lack the typical nuclear and cytoplasmic changes associated with HPV infection described above.

CIN 1 with bizarre nuclear changes can be misdiagnosed as CIN 2. Please see the discussion below.

Biopsies with CIN 1 need to be carefully examined to ensure that foci with CIN 2 or CIN 3 are not present. It is possible for some areas to show changes of CIN 1 and others to show changes of CIN 2 or CIN 3.

HISTOLOGY OF LSIL (Figs 12.1a to h)

LSIL lesions can also be termed as flat condyloma—they represent HPV infection of productive type. The epithelium is of normal thickness or slightly thicker and is not thrown into folds.

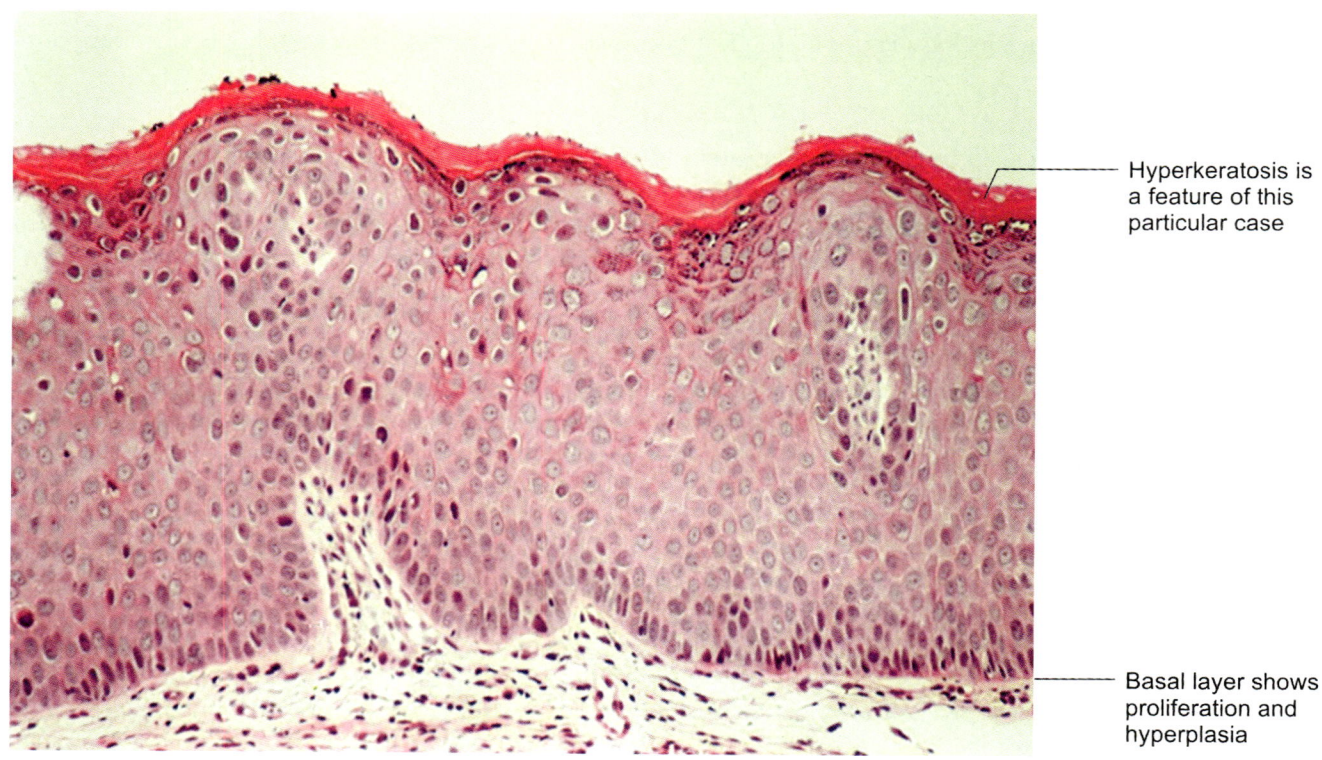

Hyperkeratosis is a feature of this particular case

Basal layer shows proliferation and hyperplasia

Fig. 12.1a

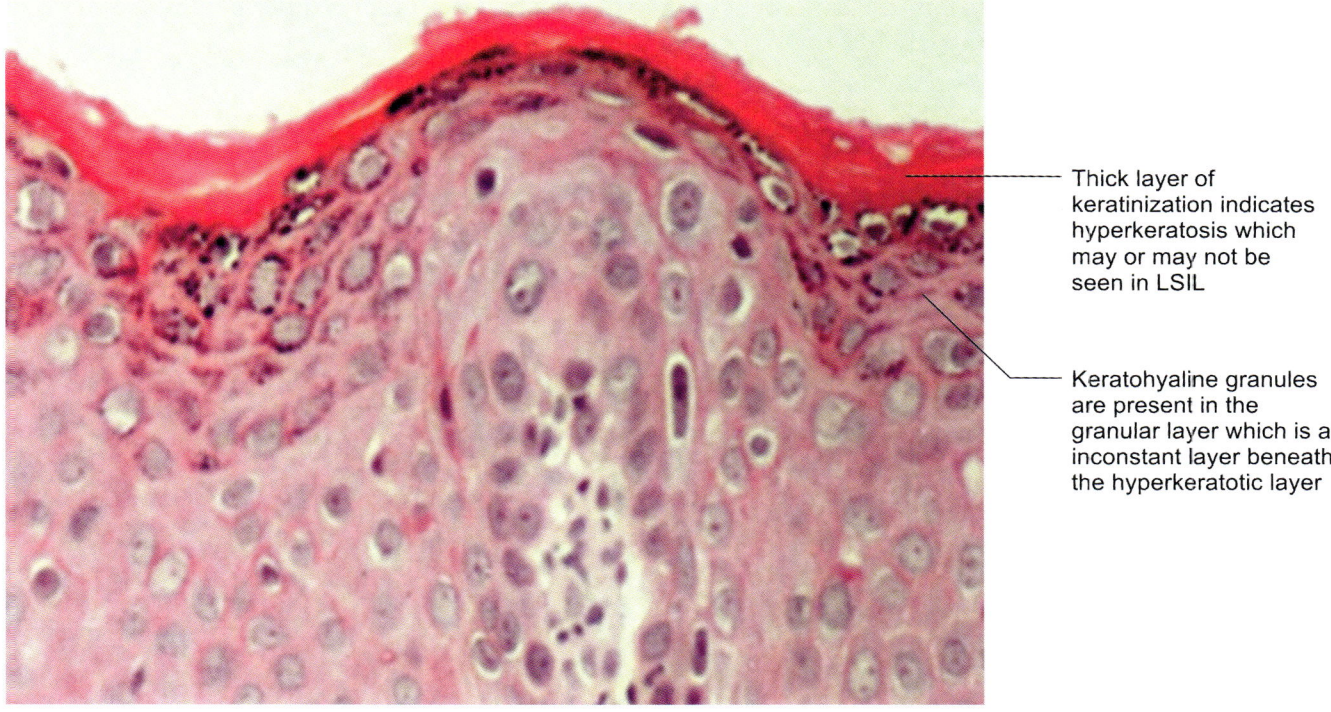

Thick layer of keratinization indicates hyperkeratosis which may or may not be seen in LSIL

Keratohyaline granules are present in the granular layer which is an inconstant layer beneath the hyperkeratotic layer

Fig. 12.1b

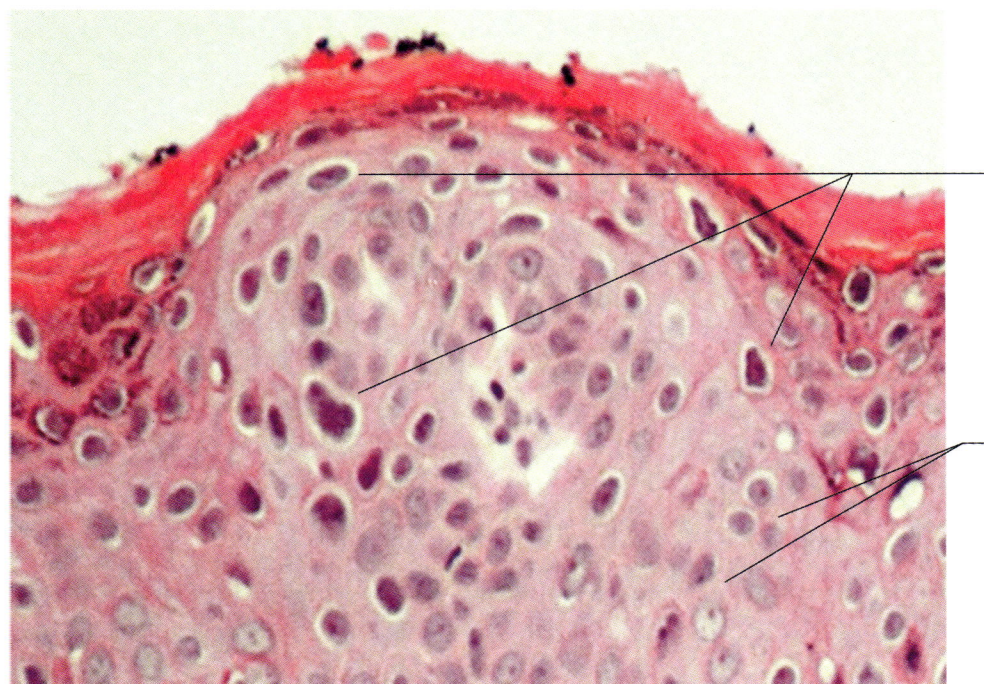

The nuclei of squamous cells in this superficial part are enlarged and very darkly stained because they are packed with the DNA of the HPV virus

Nuclei in the deeper part of the epithelium are less darkly hyperchromatic because the virus has proliferated less and hence making the nucleus less dark as compared to the nuclei higher up in the epithelium

Fig. 12.1c

Koilocytes are described based on nuclear features rather than on cytoplasmic vacuolation. However, it is a prominent feature of productive HPV infection.

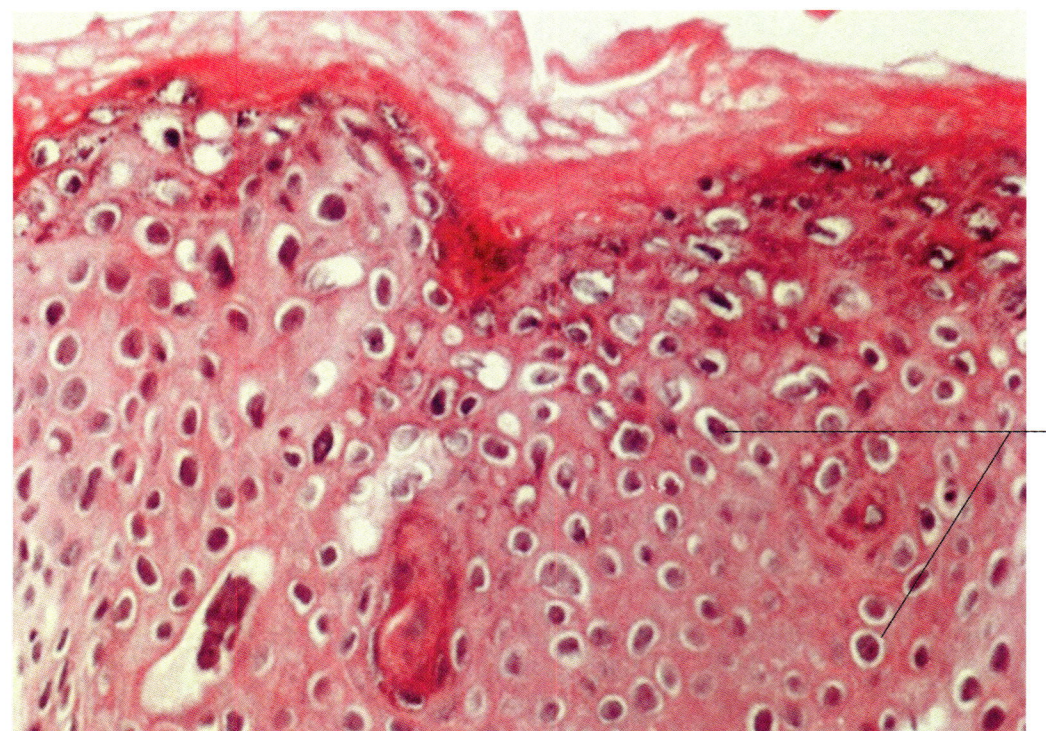

The presence of encapsulated virions in the cytoplasm causes a cytopathic change resulting in clear vacuoles surrounding the nucleus

Fig. 12.1d

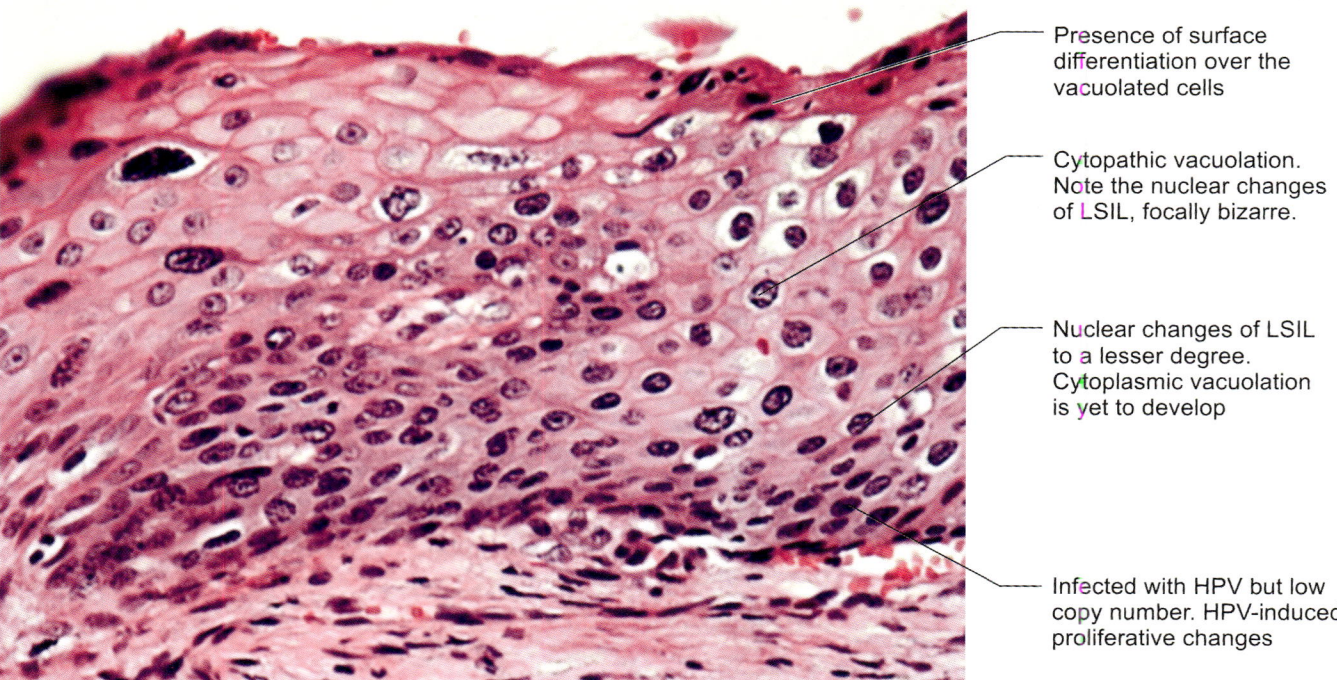

Presence of surface differentiation over the vacuolated cells

Cytopathic vacuolation. Note the nuclear changes of LSIL, focally bizarre.

Nuclear changes of LSIL to a lesser degree. Cytoplasmic vacuolation is yet to develop

Infected with HPV but low copy number. HPV-induced proliferative changes

Fig. 12.1e

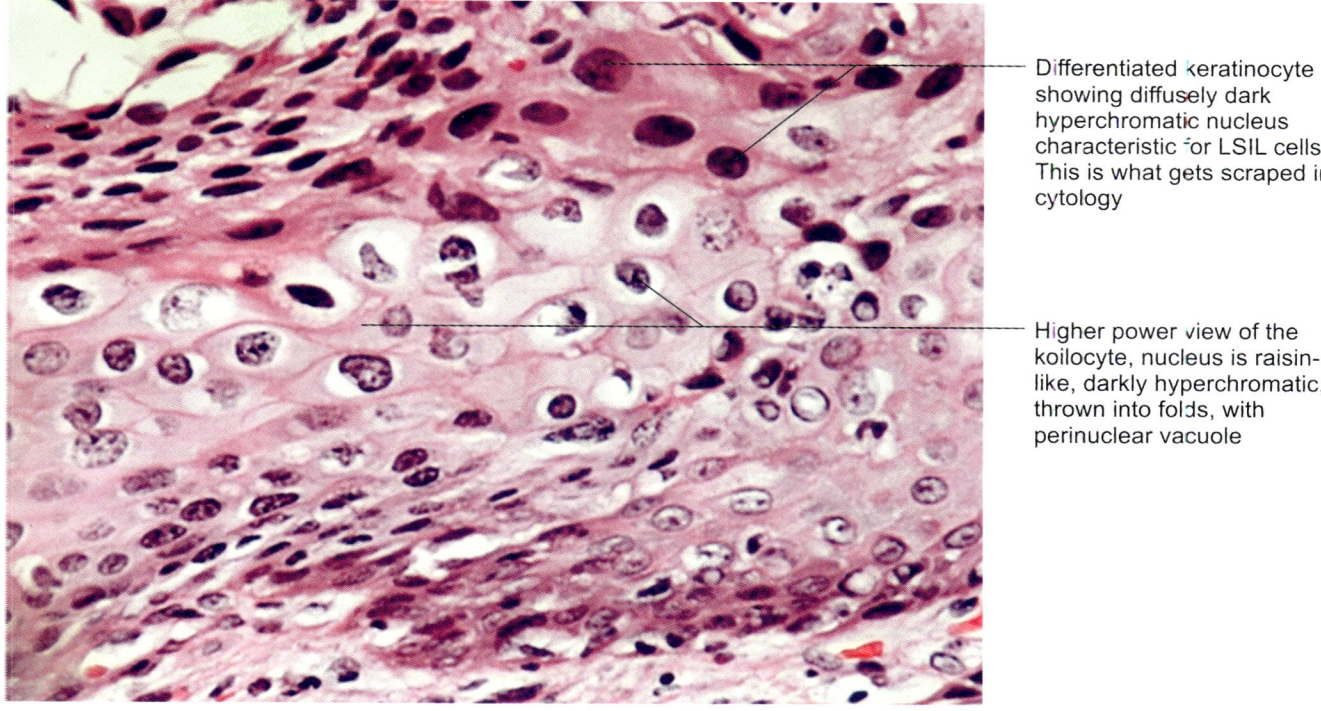

Differentiated keratinocyte showing diffusely dark hyperchromatic nucleus characteristic for LSIL cells. This is what gets scraped in cytology

Higher power view of the koilocyte, nucleus is raisin-like, darkly hyperchromatic, thrown into folds, with perinuclear vacuole

Fig. 12.1f

Nuclei of LSIL show characteristic membrane folds, elongation, truncation, tulip or raisin-like appearance and binucleation.

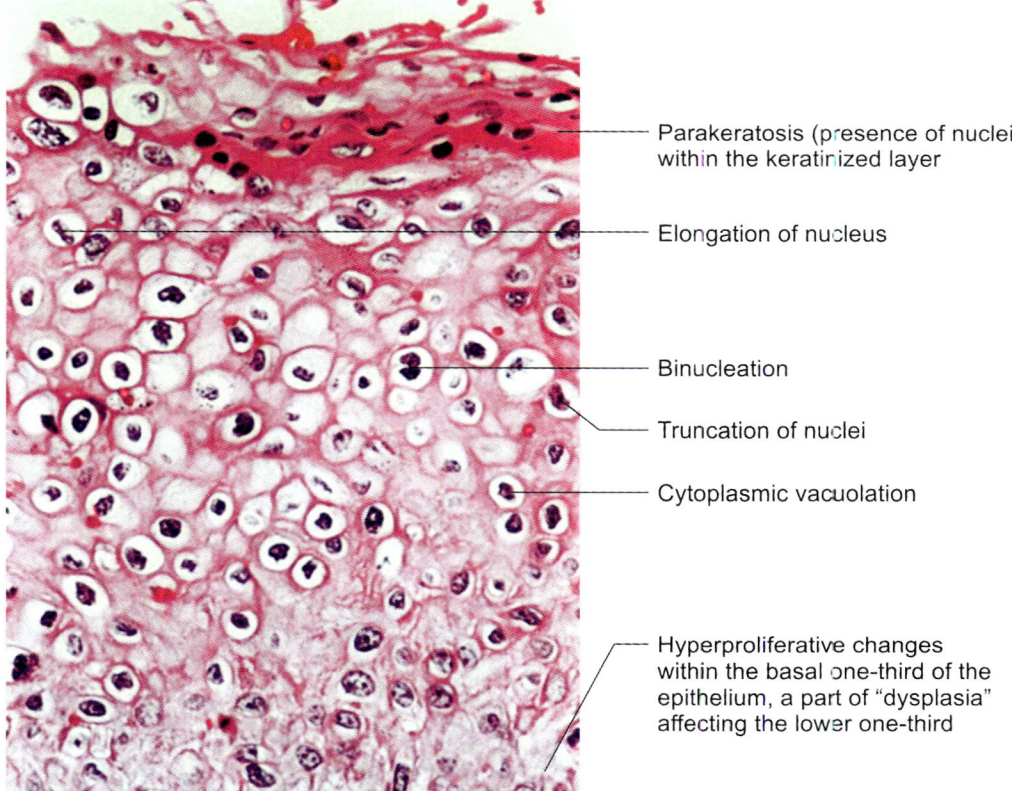

Parakeratosis (presence of nuclei within the keratinized layer

Elongation of nucleus

Binucleation

Truncation of nuclei

Cytoplasmic vacuolation

Hyperproliferative changes within the basal one-third of the epithelium, a part of "dysplasia" affecting the lower one-third

Fig. 12.1g

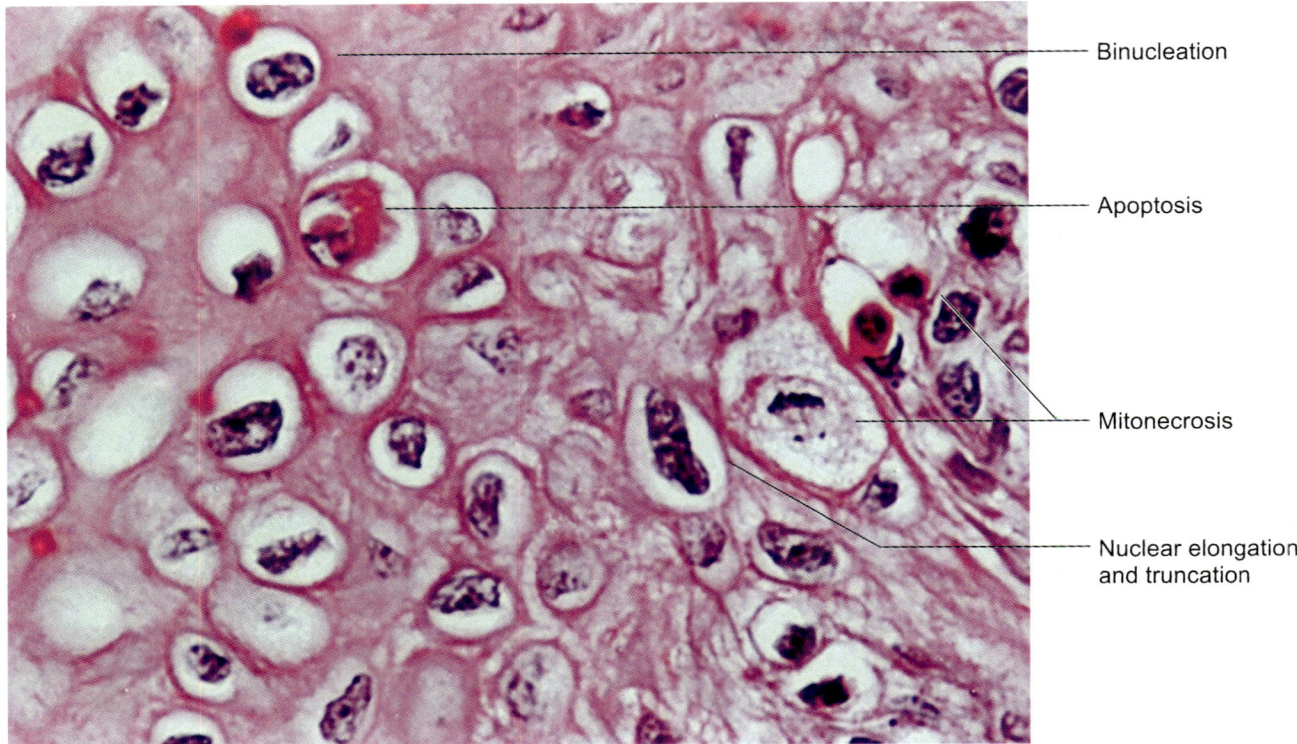

Binucleation

Apoptosis

Mitonecrosis

Nuclear elongation and truncation

Fig. 12.1h

CYTOLOGY OF LSIL (Figs 12.2a to k)

Cells shed from LSIL are intermediate-sized cells with nuclei enlarged to over three times the normal sized nuclei of intermediate cells.

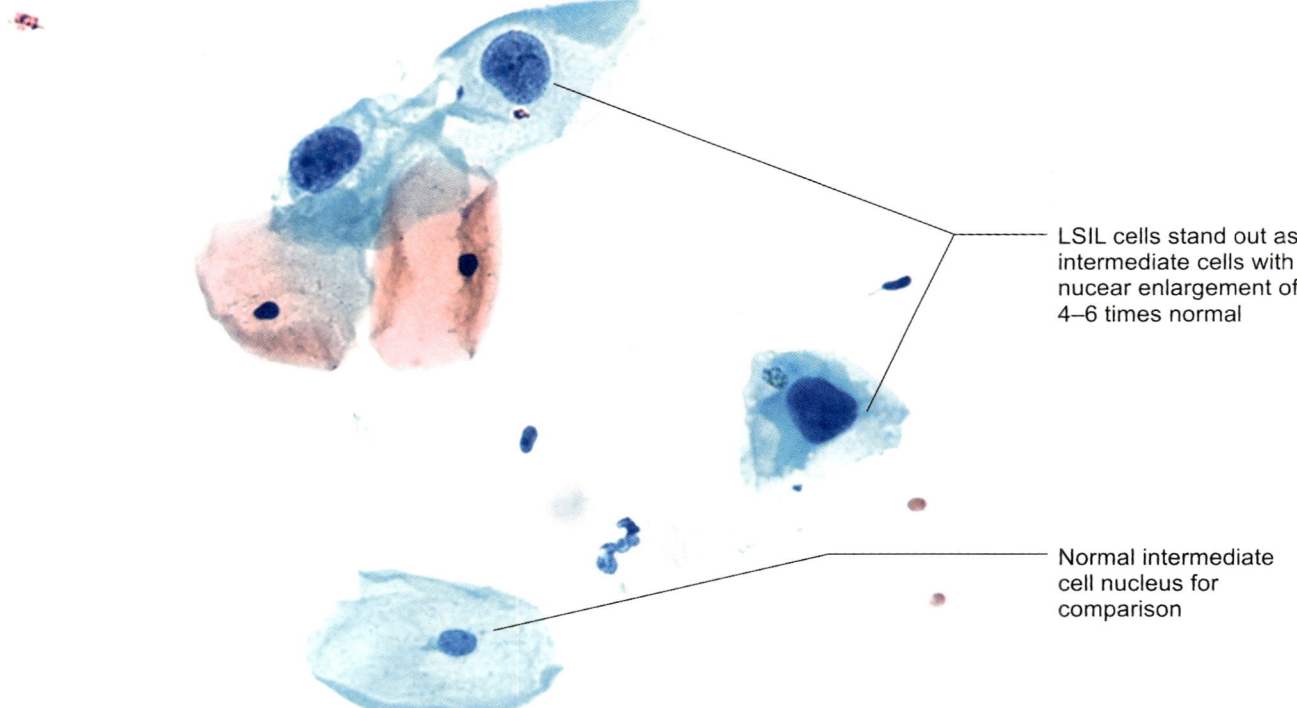

LSIL cells stand out as intermediate cells with nucear enlargement of 4–6 times normal

Normal intermediate cell nucleus for comparison

Fig. 12.2a

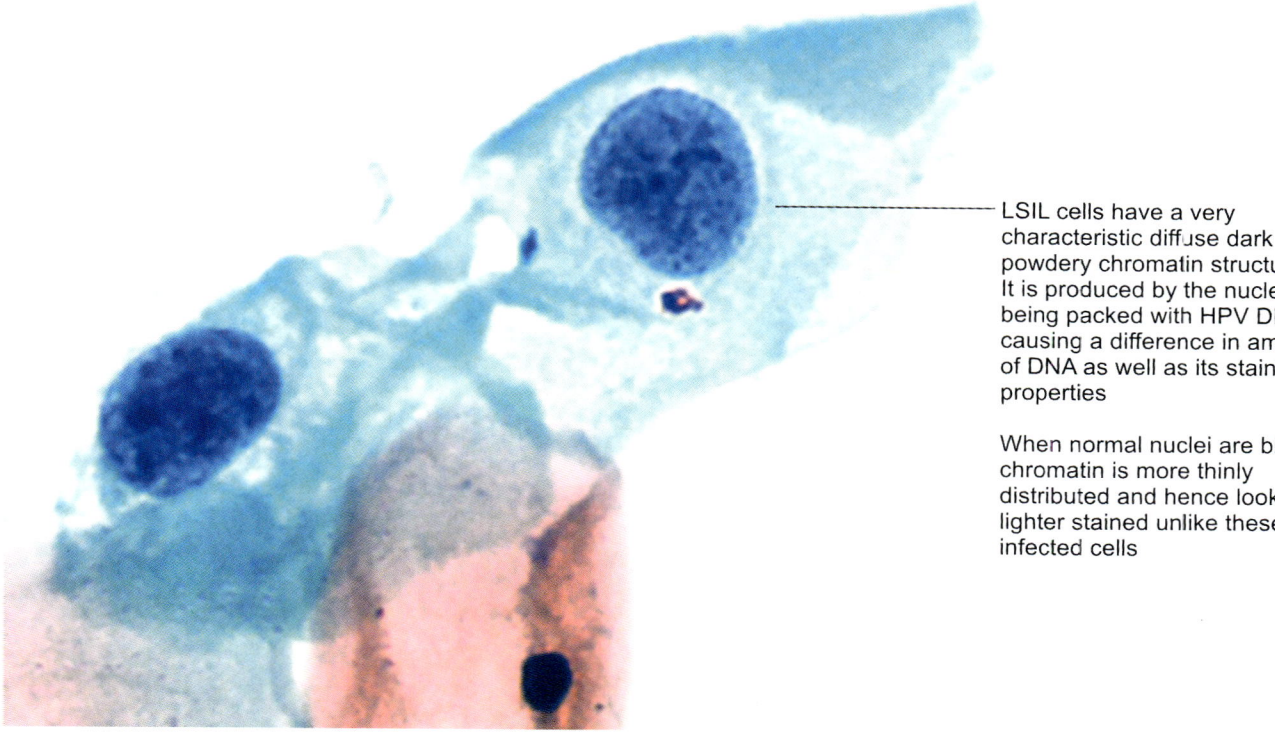

LSIL cells have a very characteristic diffuse dark powdery chromatin structure. It is produced by the nucleus being packed with HPV DNA causing a difference in amount of DNA as well as its staining properties

When normal nuclei are big, the chromatin is more thinly distributed and hence looks lighter stained unlike these HPV infected cells

Fig. 12.2b

Normal intermediate cells

Intermediate cells with LSIL nuclei—dark, hyperchromatic, enlarged to over three times the size of normal intermediate cells

Nuclear groove

Fig. 12.2c

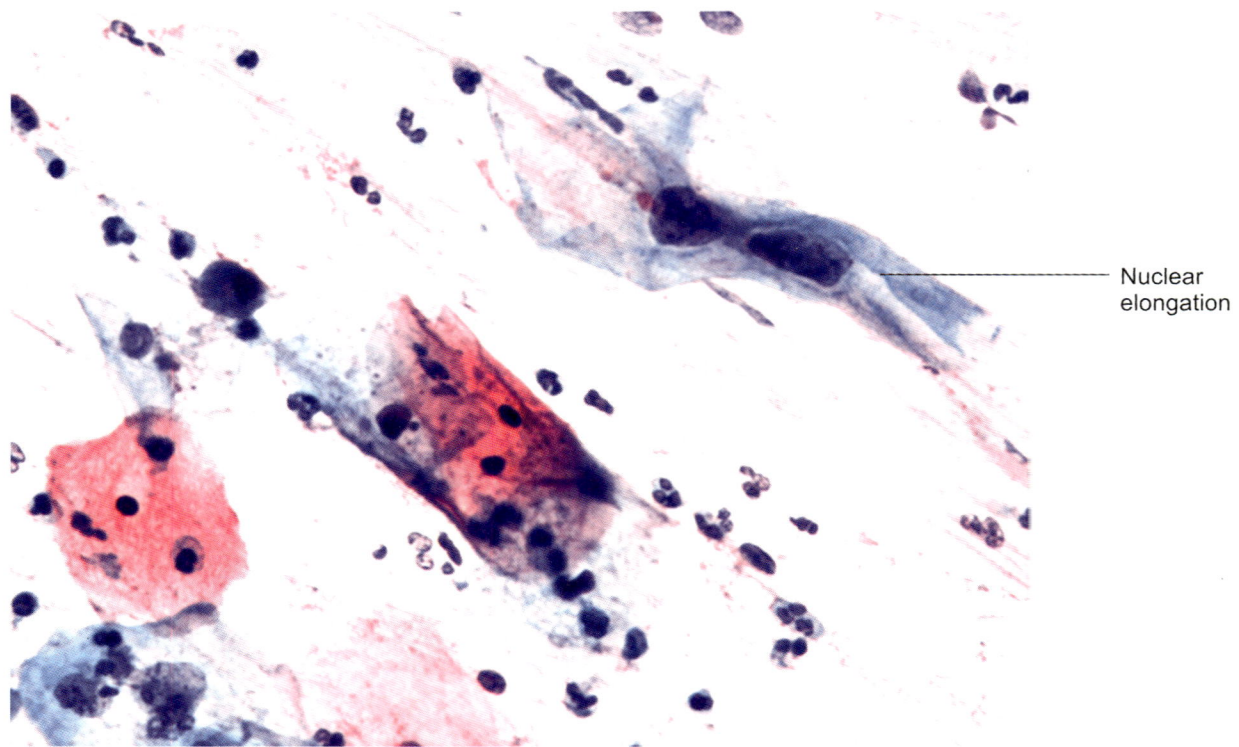

Nuclear
elongation

Fig. 12.2d

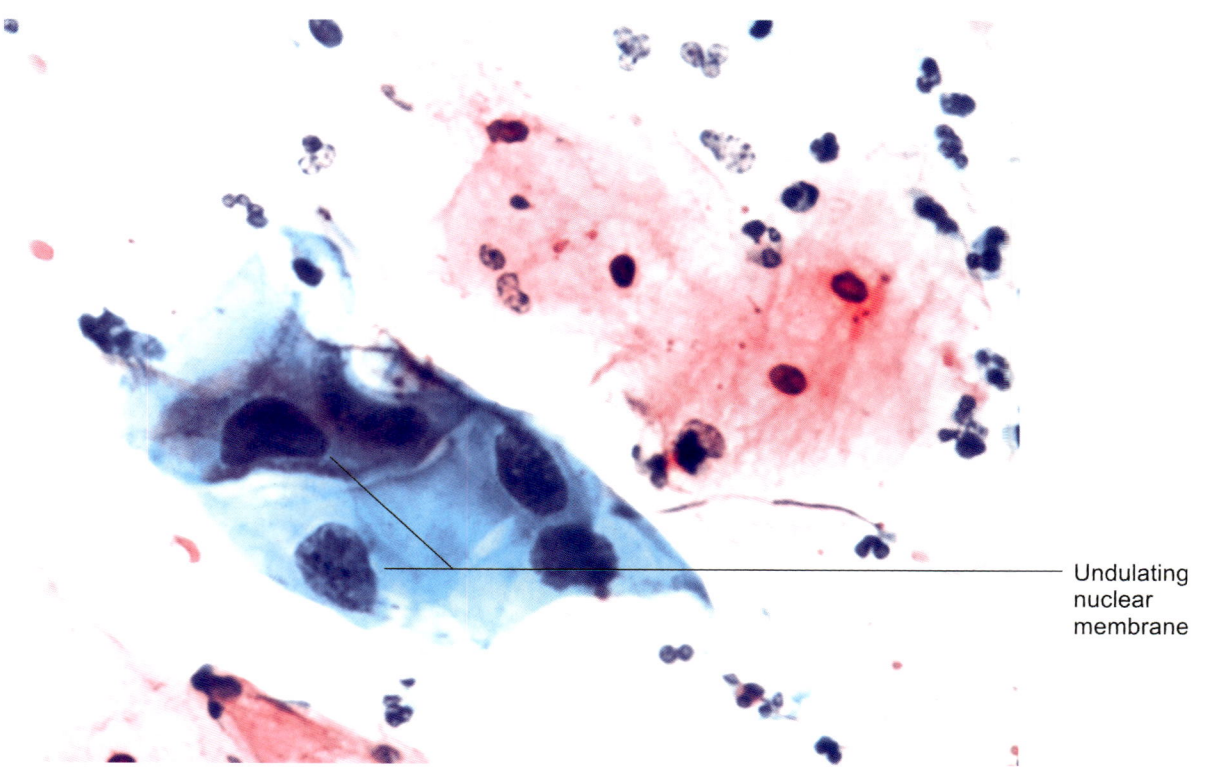

Undulating
nuclear
membrane

Fig. 12.2e

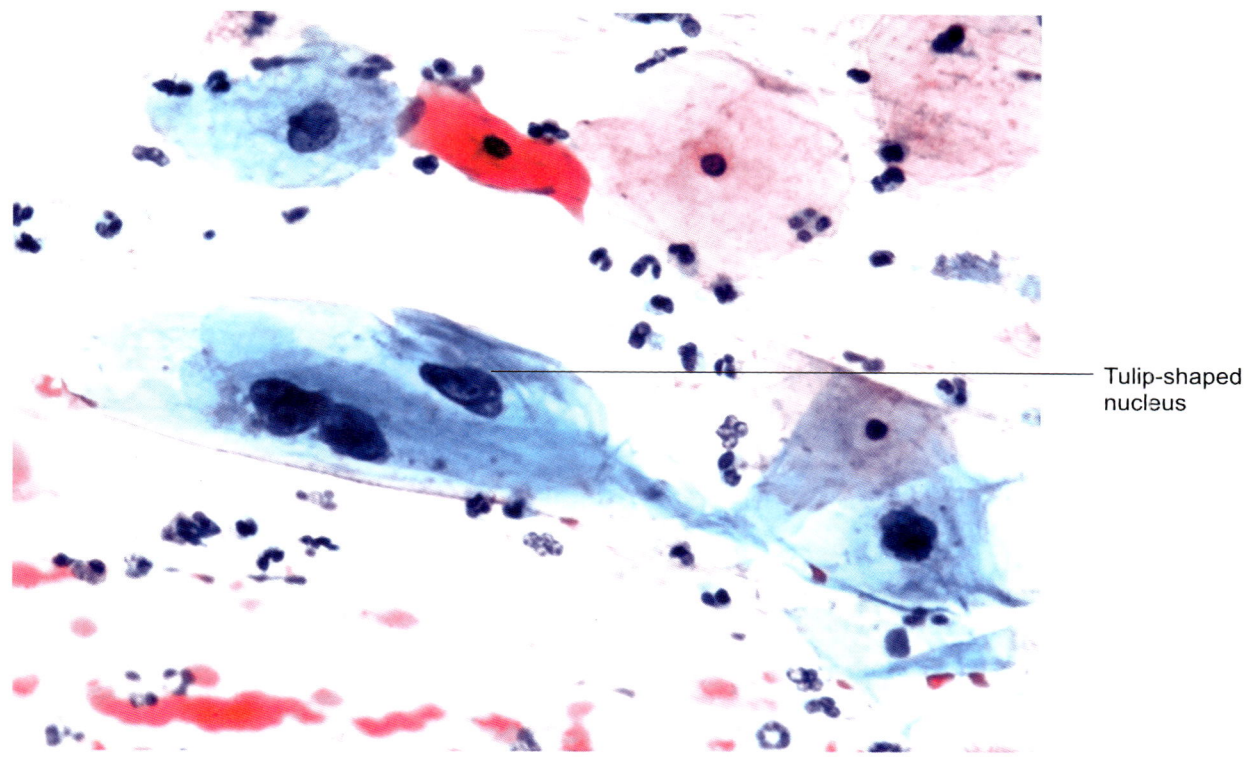

Tulip-shaped
nucleus

Fig. 12.2f

Nuclear membrane
irregularity and early
cytopathic changes in
the immediate
perinuclear viscinity

Enlarged nucleus
with characteristic
nuclear chromatin
pattern

Fig. 12.2g

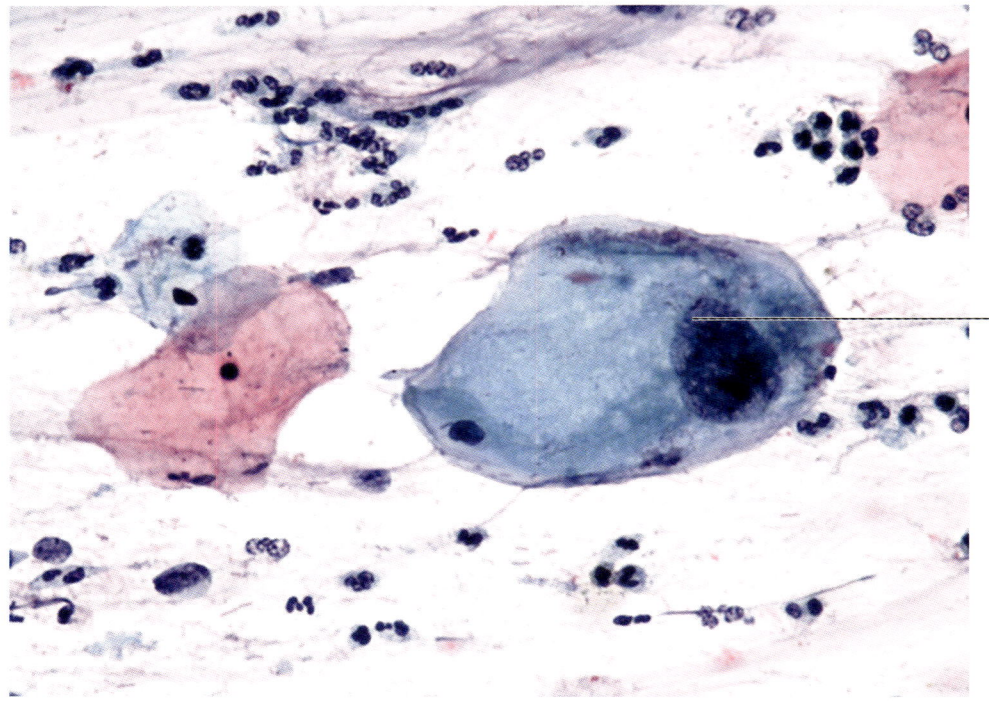

This cell from LSIL is almost double the size of the neighboring superficial cells. Ncleus is almost ten times the size of an intermediate cell nucleus (bizarre nucleus) but since the cytoplasm is correspondingly increased, the nuclear cytoplasmic ratio is appropriate for CIN 1 rather than CIN 2 since the latter has scant cytoplasm resulting in high nuclear cytoplasmic ratio

Fig. 12.2h

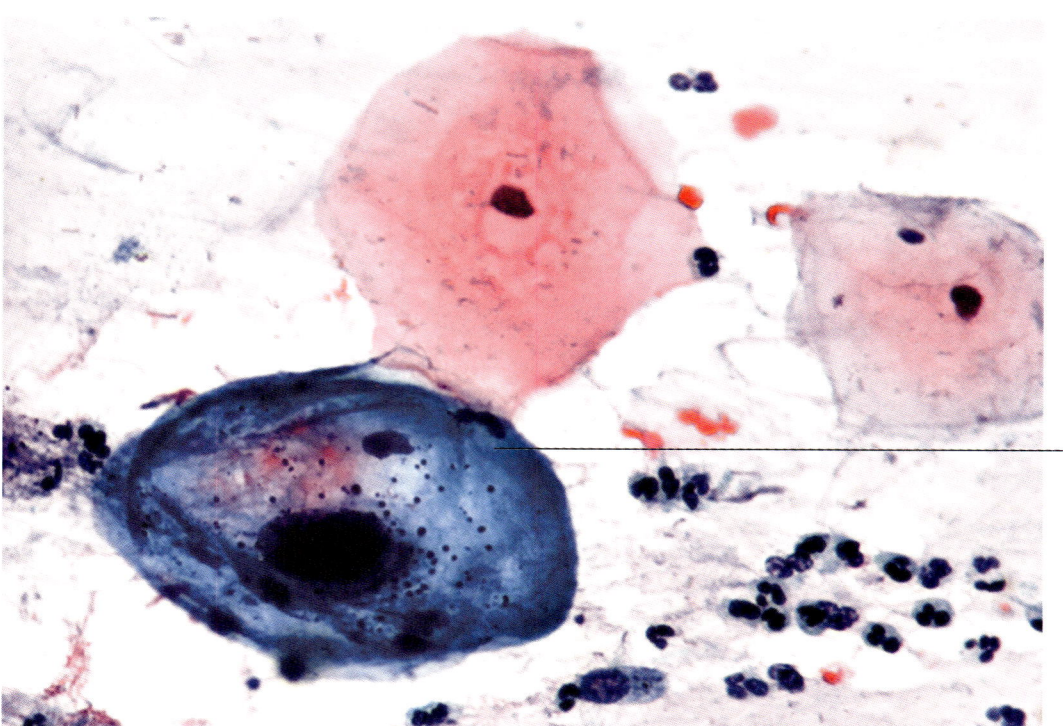

Cell from LSIL with keratohyaline granules in the cytoplasm

Fig. 12.2i

Cytoplasmic vacuolation around the nucleus is a common cytopathic change in LSIL. Cells of LSIL do not necessarily have vacuolation though.

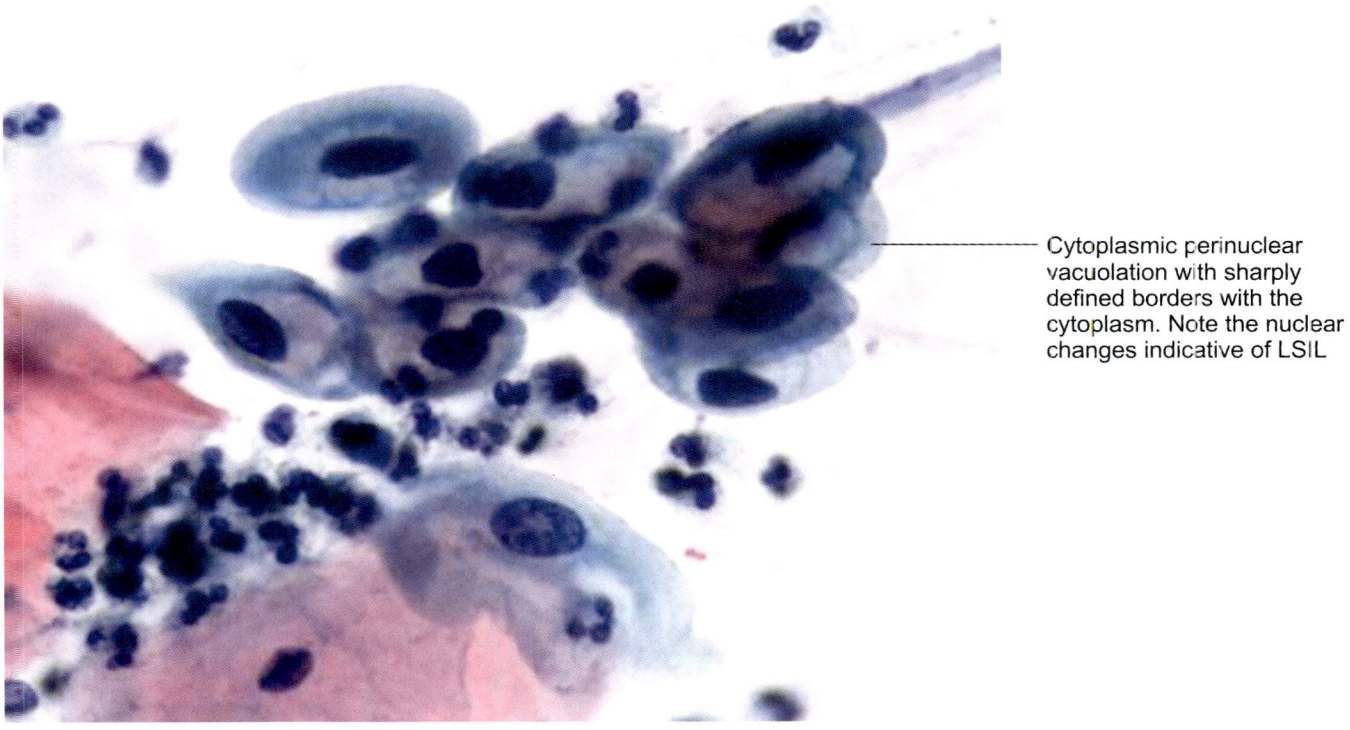

Cytoplasmic perinuclear vacuolation with sharply defined borders with the cytoplasm. Note the nuclear changes indicative of LSIL

Fig. 12.2j

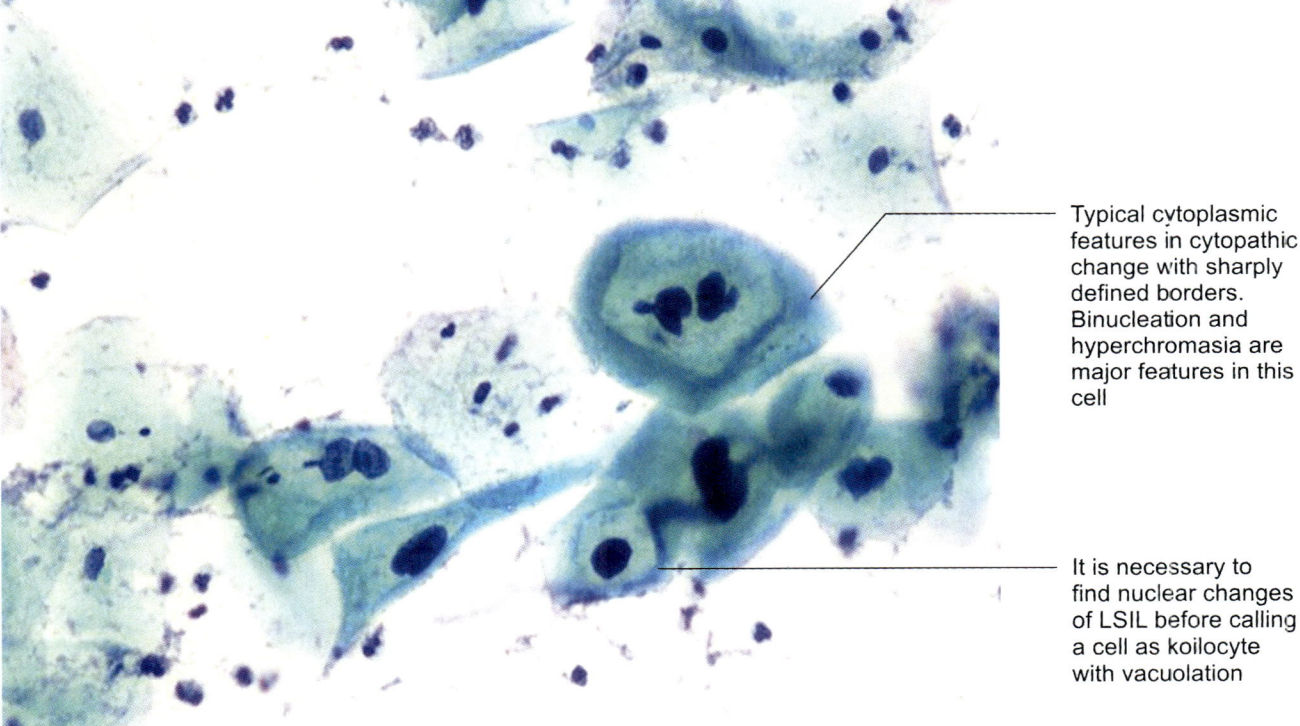

Typical cytoplasmic features in cytopathic change with sharply defined borders. Binucleation and hyperchromasia are major features in this cell

It is necessary to find nuclear changes of LSIL before calling a cell as koilocyte with vacuolation

Fig. 12.2k

ASCUS (Fig. 12.3)

Changes suggestive but nor diagnostic for LSIL are called ASCUS. Nuclei are not larger than three times of an intermediate cell nucleus and do not show characteristic hyperchromasia.

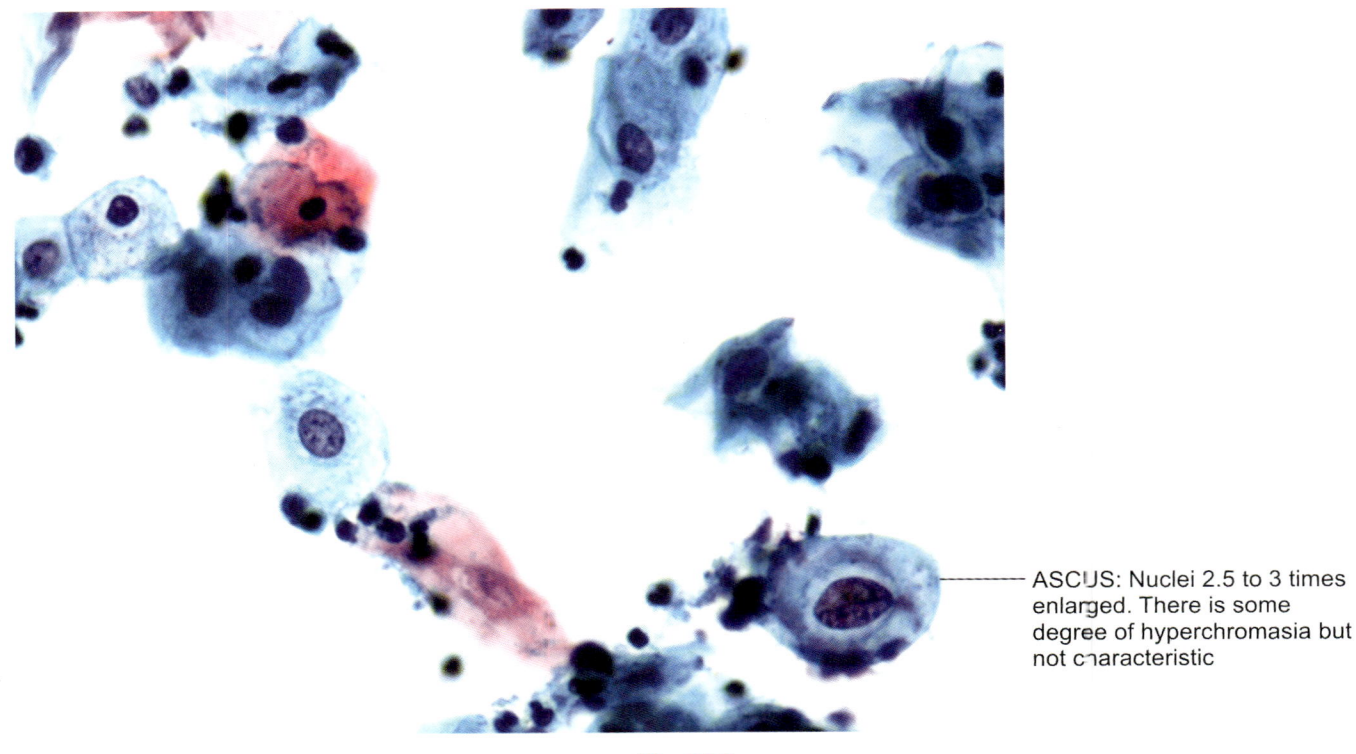

ASCUS: Nuclei 2.5 to 3 times enlarged. There is some degree of hyperchromasia but not characteristic

Fig. 12.3

B. HIGH GRADE SQUAMOUS INTRAEPITHELIAL LESION

CIN 2

These are integrative HPV infections with transformation of squamous cells, composed of large-sized cells with superficial layers of the epithelium showing keratinocytic differentiation. Since the upper one-third of the epithelium shows differentiation, therefore, it is considered that CIN 2 involves the lower two-thirds of the squamous epithelium. Note that despite differentiation, the upper third of the epithelium is still composed of transformed epithelial cells which are clonally derived from the transformed cells present in the lower two-thirds of the epithelium.

In contrast to CIN 1, the basal layers of CIN 2 show enlarged nuclei with coarse clumping of chromatin and very high nuclear cytoplasmic ratio. The cell junctions are haphazard leading to a disordered look. Since nuclei and cytoplasm of basal cells are both much larger than those seen in CIN 1, this is a useful feature for identification. Cells in the middle third of the epithelium are also large with very hyperchromatic nuclei having coarse clumping of chromatin and sharply angulated nuclear membrane which is irregular and clumped. Cytoplasm is moderate to abundant and hence, despite very large nuclei, the nuclear cytoplasmic ratio is not as high as the nuclear features might lead one to expect. The upper one-third shows squamous cells with keratinocytic differentiation in the form of cell junctions and progressive flattening of the epithelial cells. Cytoplasm, therefore, becomes abundant. Nuclei, however, continue to show the same changes described for the middle third of the epithelium for CIN 2. Mitotic figures are present in much higher layers of the epithelium including in the middle third of the epithelium. Number of mitotic figures are increased and it is also possible to identify atypical mitotic figures.

Focally, it is possible to identify cytopathic vacuolation of the cytoplasm in CIN 2 similar to productive HPV infection, but this is not common. Note that even if the cytoplasm shows vacuolation, the nuclear changes are indicative of CIN 2, i.e. coarse clumping of chromatic and sharply angulated nuclear margins are present. In some lesions, some of the epithelium shows changes of CIN 2 while other areas show changes of CIN 1, i.e. both are present adjacent to each other.

Differential Diagnosis

CIN 1 with bizarre cells can be misdiagnosed as CIN 2. Bizarre cells of CIN 1 are usually present isolated and in the upper one-third of the epithelium. Rest of the epithelium does not show coarse clumping of the chromatin. Atypical mitotic figures are absent in CIN 1. This is an important distinction since CIN 2 requires ablation whereas CIN 1 does not.

CIN 3 might show superficial most layer (10% or less) with flattening or keratinocytic differentiation.

Some cases of CIN 3 might be composed of larger cells which might approach cell sizes of CIN 2. These differences are, however, better viewed as a continuum.

CIN 2 and CIN 3 are both transformative lesions which require ablation and hence some people prefer to use the cytopathological term of high grade squamous intraepithelial lesion for histopathology also in which CIN 2 and CIN 3 are clubbed together.

CIN 3

These are transformative HPV infections composed of small-sized cells which are present in the full thickness of the epithelium with superficial layers not showing any evidence of keratinocyte differentiation.

The cell size is usually much smaller than CIN 2 and may be half or even less than half the size of the cells in CIN 2. The reason for small size is very scant cytoplasm, whereas CIN 2 has moderate to abundant cytoplasm depending on the position of the cell in the layer. In CIN 3, the cells in even superficial layers are composed of cells with scant cytoplasm lacking keratinocyte differentiation. In some cases, the cell size is a little larger but not as large as CIN 2. Some cases might show minimal flattening and keratinocytic differentiation in the top most layer, i.e. superficial 10% of the cells. Inner 90%, however, does not show keratinocyte differentiation and hence does not fall into the definition of CIN 2. Nuclei of CIN 3 are larger than normal or hyperplastic nuclei with coarse clumping of chromatin. This clumping is accompanied by less degrees of hyperchromasia than in CIN 2. Nuclei tend to be more rounded than CIN 2 without the sharply angulated nuclear membranes. Despite these differences from CIN 2, nuclei of CIN 3 are significantly more malignant looking than cells of CIN 1 in terms of irregular clumping and membrane irregularities. Mitotic figures are increased and might be present even in upper third of the epithelium. Atypical mitotic figures might be found. Cytopathic vacuolation due to HPV are much rarer than with CIN 2. However, lesions of CIN 1 might be present adjacent to lesions of CIN 3.

Differential Diagnosis

Some CIN 3 lesions showing superficial flattening or larger cell size can be difficult to distinguish from CIN 2.

Atrophic squamous epithelium is composed of parabasal cells in all the different layers of the epithelium. Since parabasal cells have larger nuclei and scant to moderate cytoplasm, they can mimic CIN 3 on casual inspection due to the high cell density within the epithelium with single cell type in all layers. This is a common misdiagnosis in older women.

HSIL

HSIL from earlier system of classification is divided into CIN 2 and CIN 3. Although conceptually, it is attractive to combine CIN 2 and CIN 3 into a single group of HSIL, there are significant differences between CIN 2 and CIN 3 on morphology, both on histology and cytology. Hence, the distinction is still being retained.

Both CIN 2 and CIN 3 are technically full thickness abnormalities but in CIN 2, there is retention of the superficial keratinocyte differentiation. Thus, in CIN 2, the lower two-thirds is fully abnormal and the upper third, though abnormal, shows flattening and differentiation. Therefore, the lesion is considered to involve the lower two-thirds. However, it is important to realise that the nuclei of the upper one-third are just as abnormal as the lower two-thirds. Only cytoplasm shows differentiation.

CIN 3, there is no such understanding required. It involves the full thickness and cells are the same throughout the epithelium to look at. However, it is important to appreciate the other feature of CIN 3—it is composed of smaller sized cells than CIN 2. Thus the two main features used to distinguish CIN 2 and CIN 3 are the presence of superficial keratinocyte differentiation and the cell size.

This distinction is more important in cytology screening. CIN 2 cells are big and easily identified on cytology smears. CIN 3 cells, on the other hand, are easily missed due to their small size.

From the clinical point of view, it is more important to distinguish CIN 1 or LSIL from HSIL which includes both the above. CIN 1 nuclei are hyperchromatic but smooth textured. CIN 2 and CIN 3 nuclei show coarse clumping of chromatin. Nuclear membrane in CIN 1 is thrown into smooth folds but in CIN 2 and CIN 3 the membrane shows thickening and sharp angular abnormalities. To a pathologist, the nuclei of CIN 2 and CIN 3 look malignant. In CIN 1, the nuclei are peculiar but not malignant looking.

Conceptually, both CIN 2 and CIN 3 have undergone malignant transformation but have yet not acquired the ability to invade.

HISTOLOGY OF HSIL (Figs 12.4a to e)

When entire thickness of the epithelium is composed of abnormal cells, it is HSIL. Nuclei show coarse clumped chromatin and this indicates neoplastic tranformation.

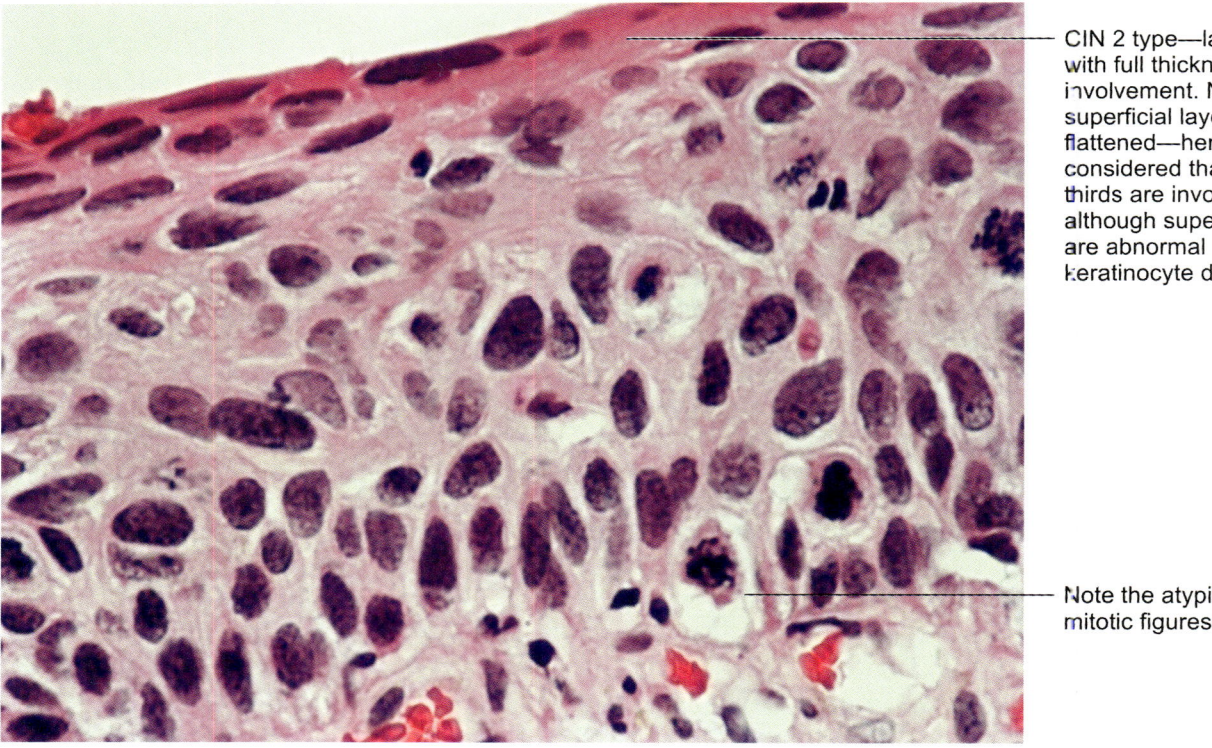

CIN 2 type—large cells with full thickness involvement. Note how superficial layers are flattened—hence considered that lower two-thirds are involved, although superficial layers are abnormal despite keratinocyte differentiation

Note the atypical mitotic figures

Fig. 12.4a

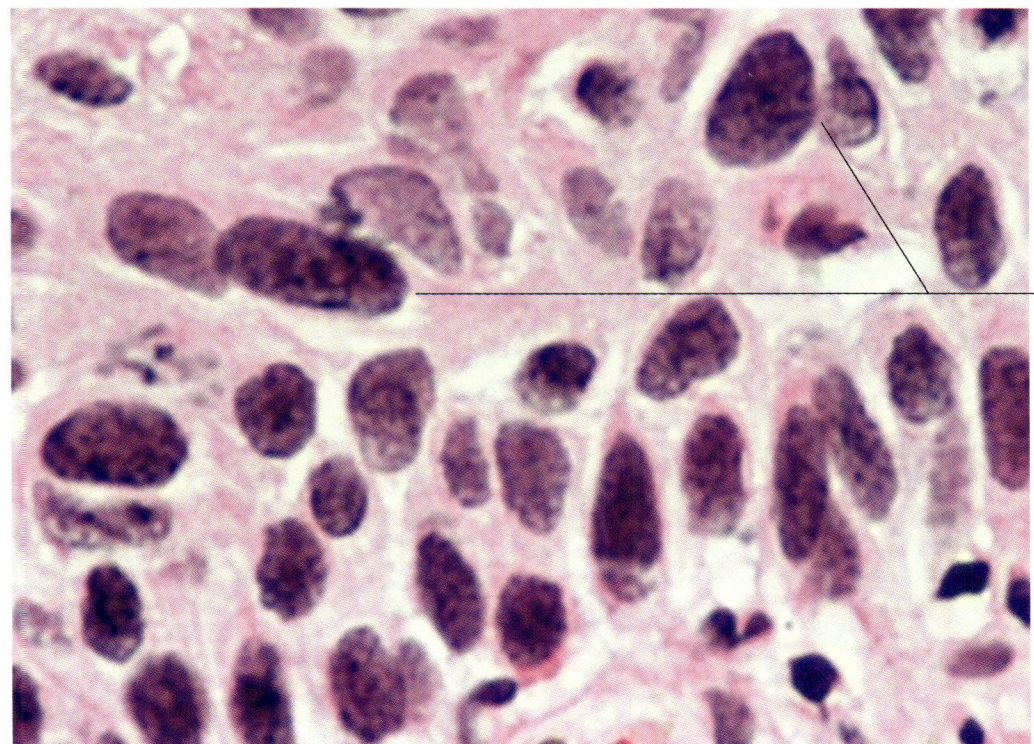

Note how abnormal the nuclear chromatic texture and shapes are in CIN 2. The nuclei are the same from deepest to upper layers—shapes are irregular and there is marked hyperchromasia

Fig. 12.4b

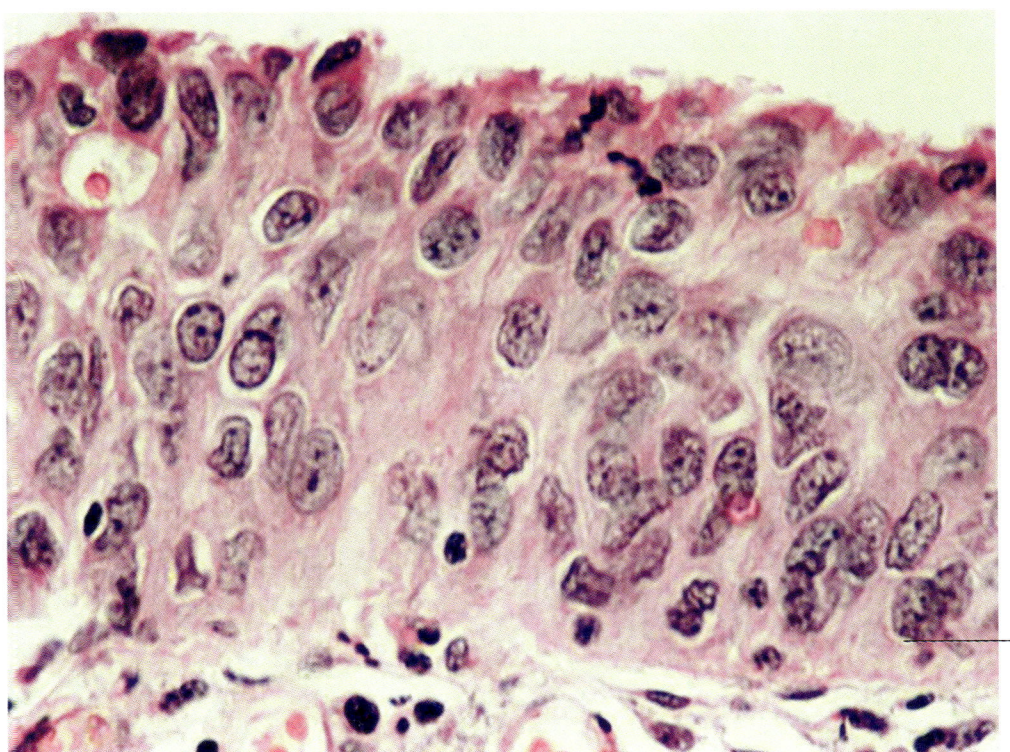

Another example of CIN 2—large cells with full thickness involvement. Note how superficial layers are less flattened here—thus the size of cells is also an important criterion to use between CIN 2 and CIN 3. Nowadays, most people combine these into HSIL even on histology

Note the abnormal nuclear texture and the clumping into coarse granules

Fig. 12.4c

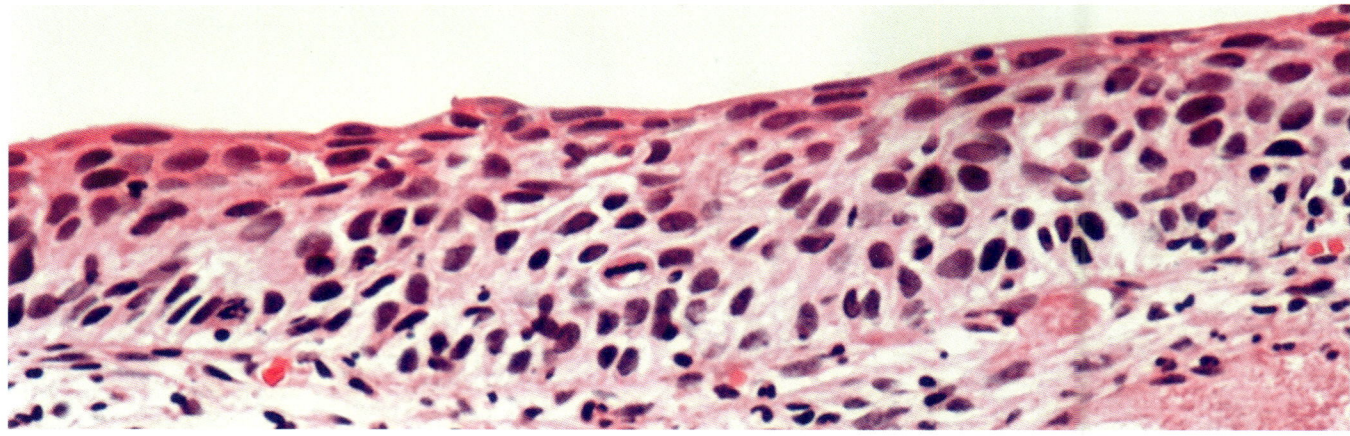

A strip of squamous epithelium showing changes of CIN 2, since the upper most layers are flattened showing keratinocytic differentiation and because cell size is large. Marked nuclear hyperchromasia with very dark nuclei.

Fig. 12.4d

A strip of squamous epithelium showing changes of CIN 2 on the right, transitioning into normal ectocervical epithelium on the left. Note how a few of the CIN 2 cells seem to be invading the neighboring epithelium—this kind of migration is common but is not considered invasion since there is no basement membrane breach

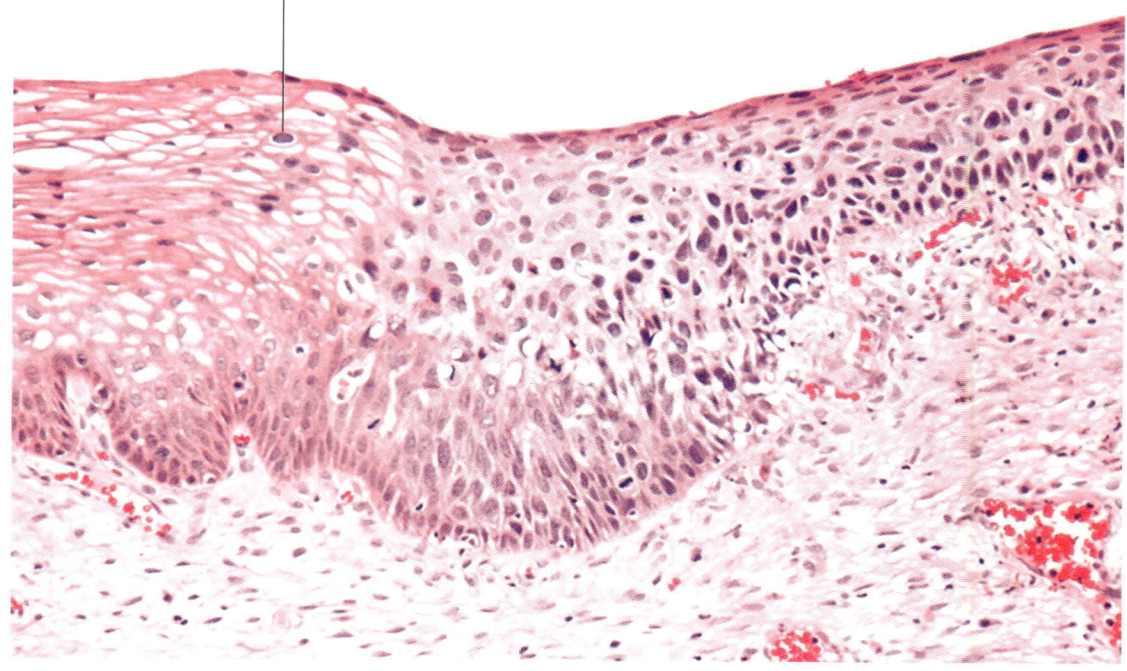

Fig. 12.4e

CYTOLOGY OF CIN 2 (Fig. 12.5)

CIN 2 cells are large intermediate-sized cells and have very large nuclei making them stand out during screening. In comparison to CIN 1 cells, cytoplasm is less and hence nuclear cytoplasm is much less than CIN 1.

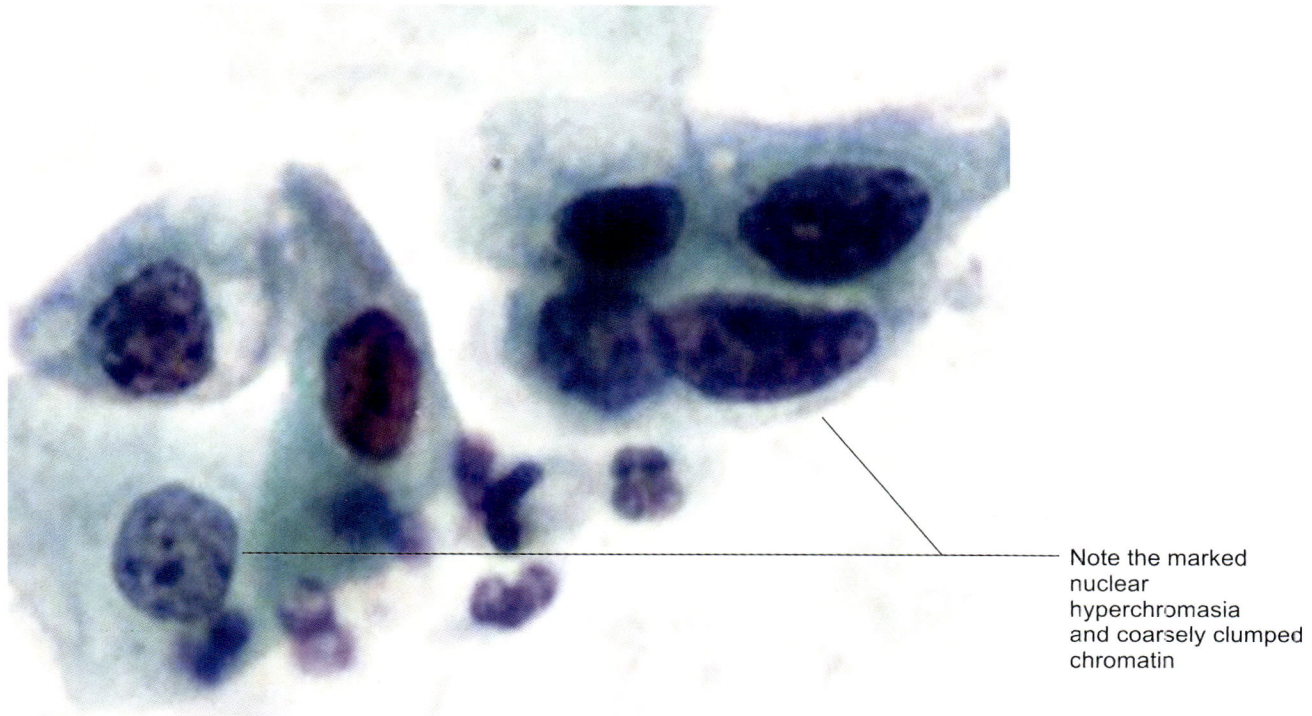

Note the marked nuclear hyperchromasia and coarsely clumped chromatin

Fig. 12.5

HISTOLOGY OF CIN 3 (Figs 12.6a to f)

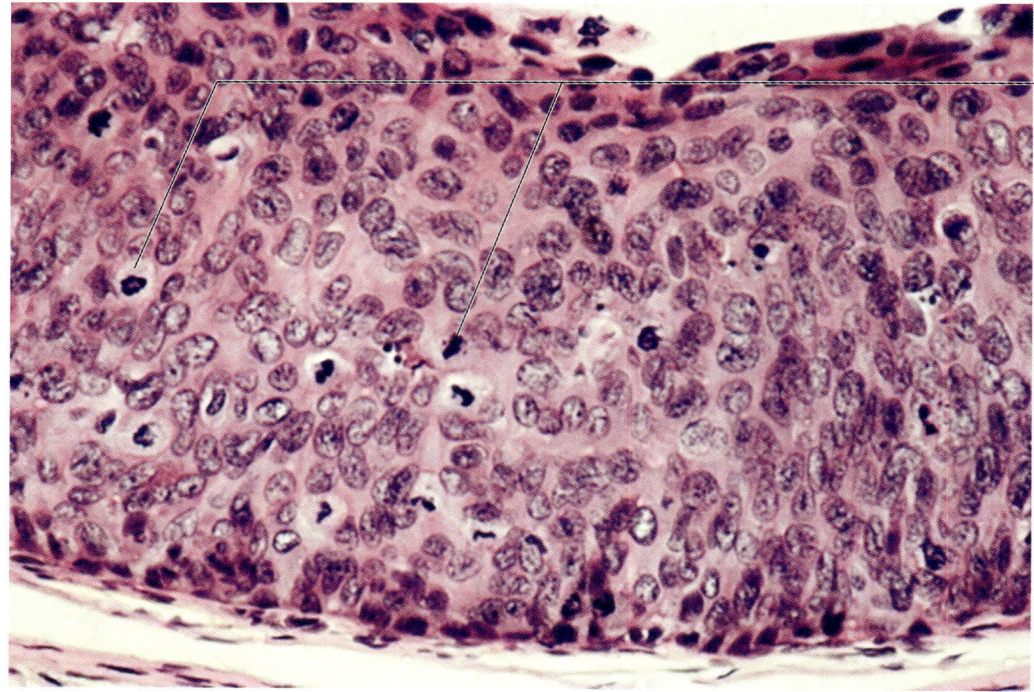

Note the numerous mitotic figures

CIN 3 lesions also show full thickness involvement but are composed of smaller cells than CIN 2 and show no keratinocyte differentiation. Hence superficial layers are not flattened though in this example, there is some minimal flattening of around upper tenth. Note how many more cells are present in CIN 3 than CIN 2, since the cells are small and pack the full thickness

Fig. 12.6a

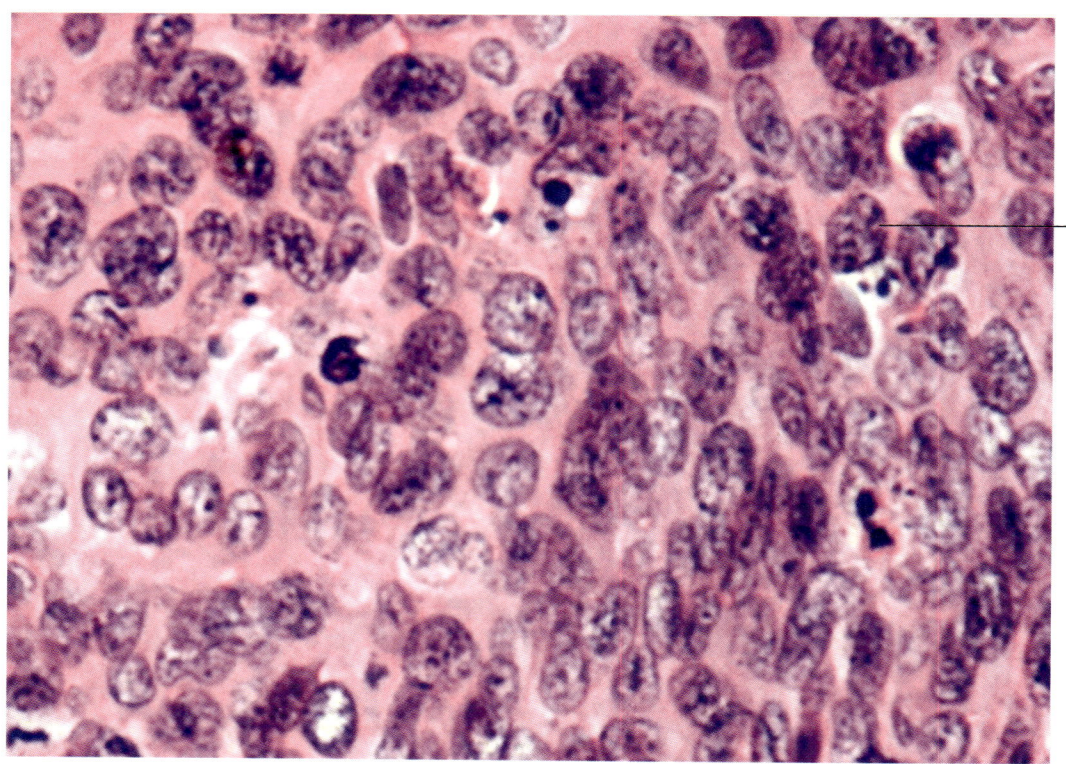

Under high power, CIN 3 cells show marked nuclear hyperchromasia and clumped chromatin. These are highly abnormal nuclei though small in size

Fig. 12.6b

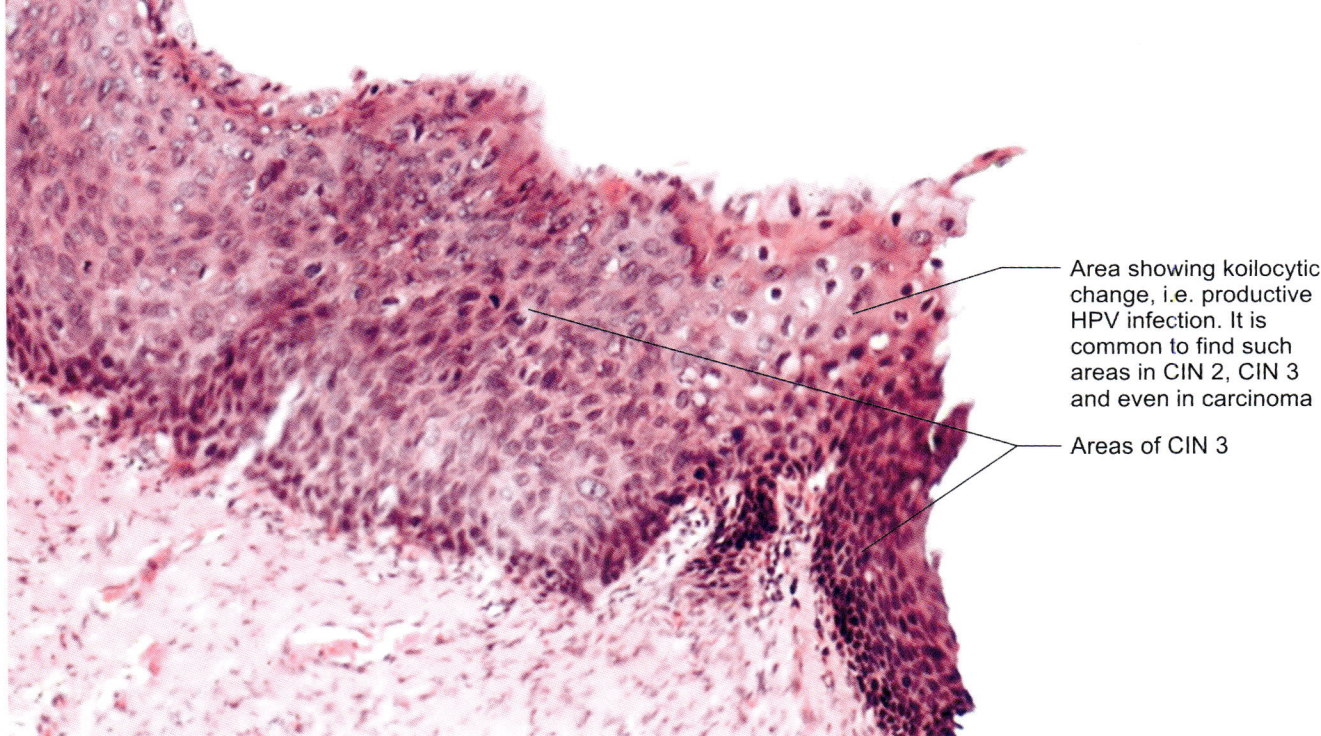

Area showing koilocytic change, i.e. productive HPV infection. It is common to find such areas in CIN 2, CIN 3 and even in carcinoma

Areas of CIN 3

Fig. 12.6c

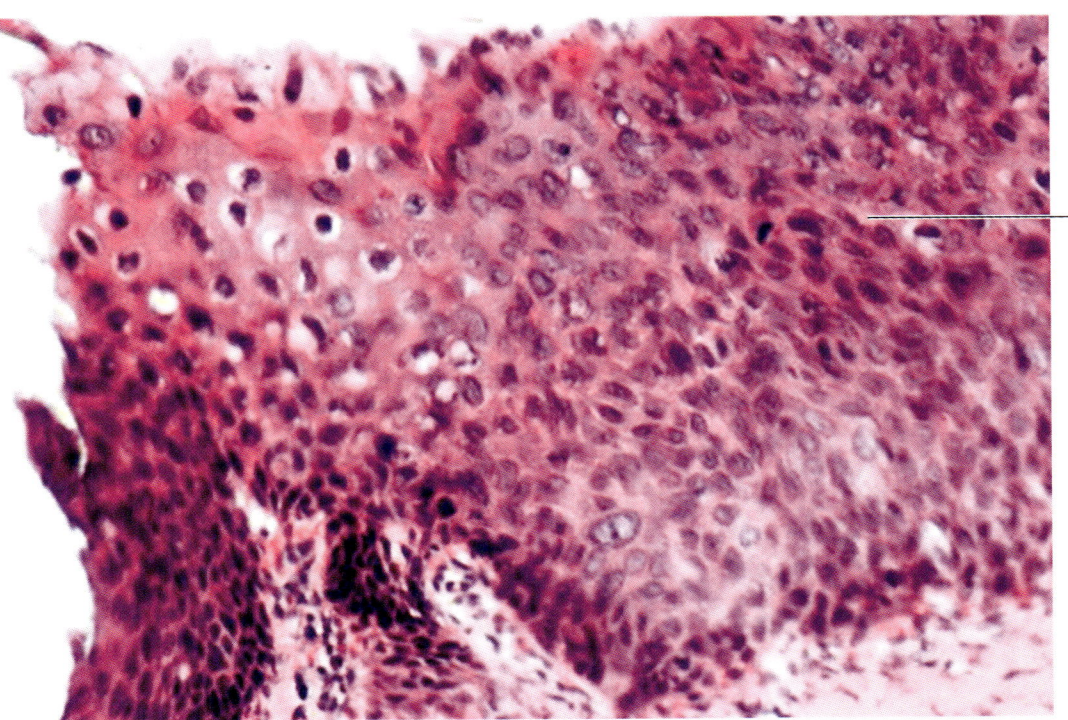

Note the small-sized cells with marked nuclear abnormalities making this a CIN 3 and not CIN 1 as one might mistake it for based on the koilocytic changes

Fig. 12.6d

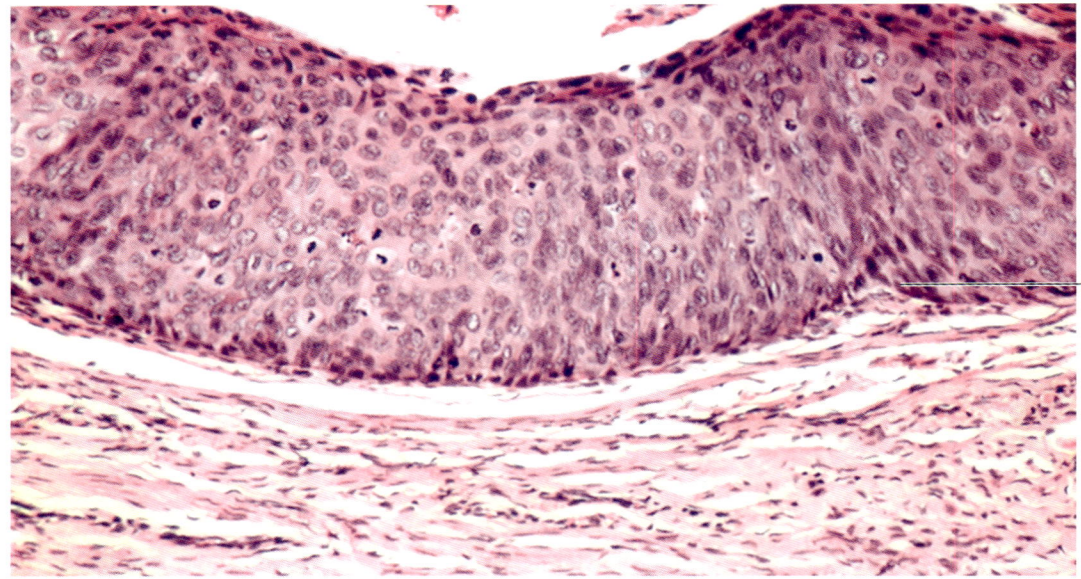

CIN 3 changes—small atypical cells packing the epithelium in full thickness

Fig. 12.6e

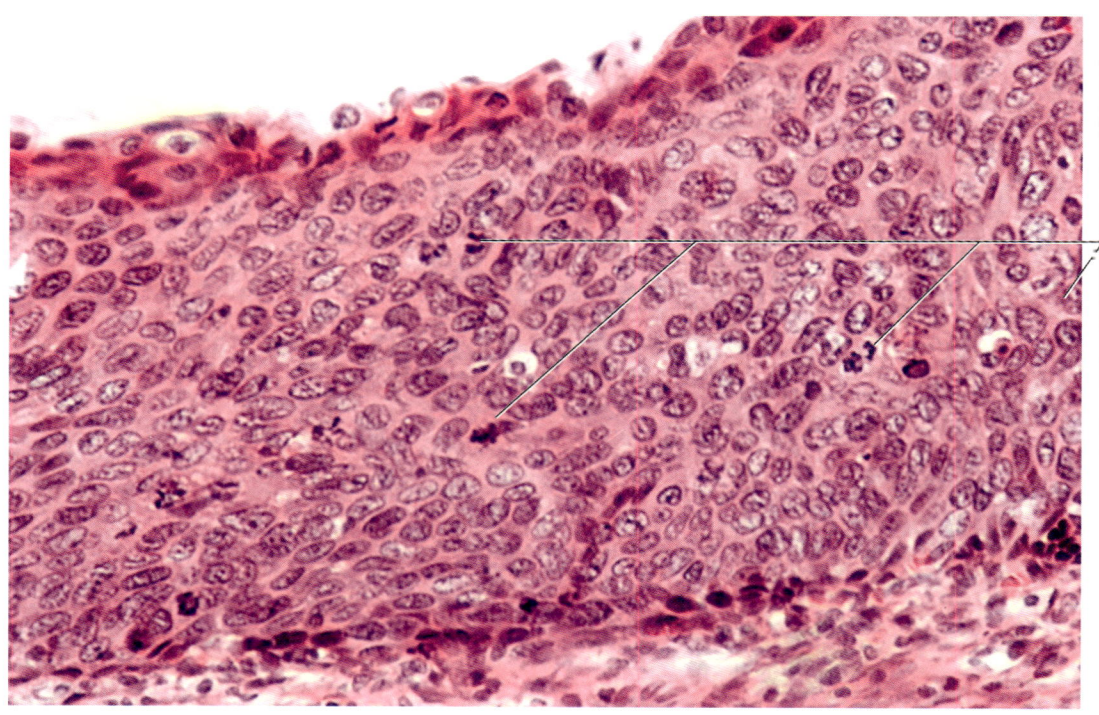

CIN 3 cells—note the numerous small atypical cells packing the epithelium in full thickness

Fig. 12.6f

CYTOLOGY OF CIN 3 (Figs 12.7a to e)

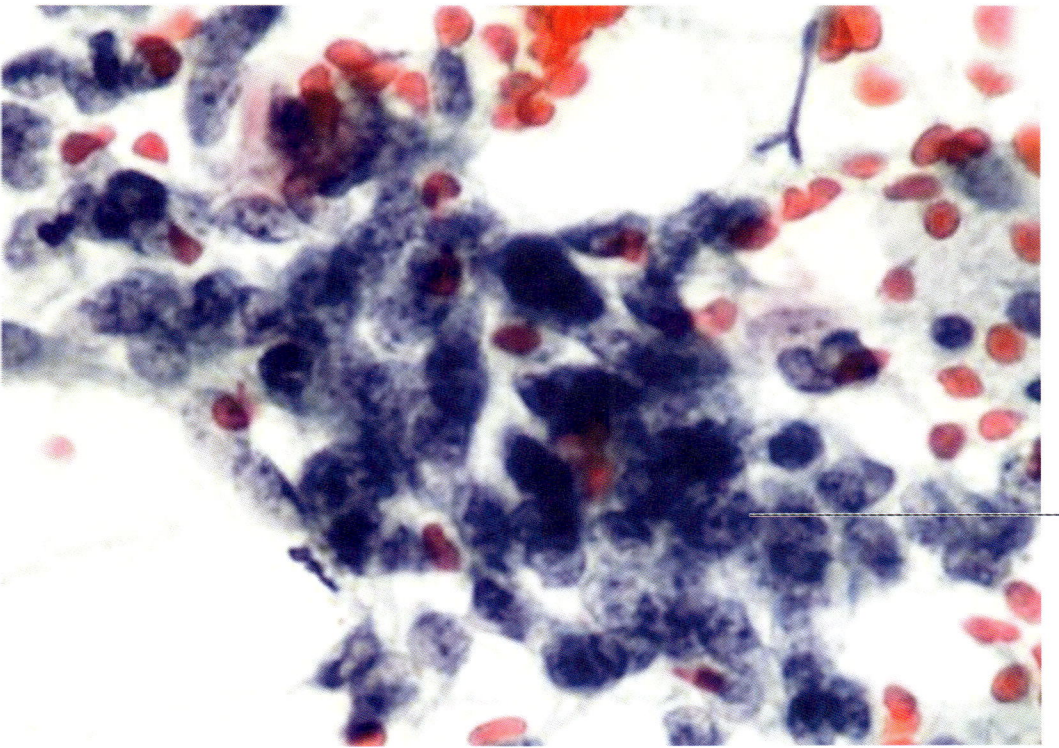

CIN 3 on cytology comes as small cells with dark nuclei having high nuclear cytoplasmic ratio. Under low power, these can be missed as endocervical cells unless carefully examined under high power

Note the coarse texture of the chromatin, similar to the histology above

Fig. 12.7a

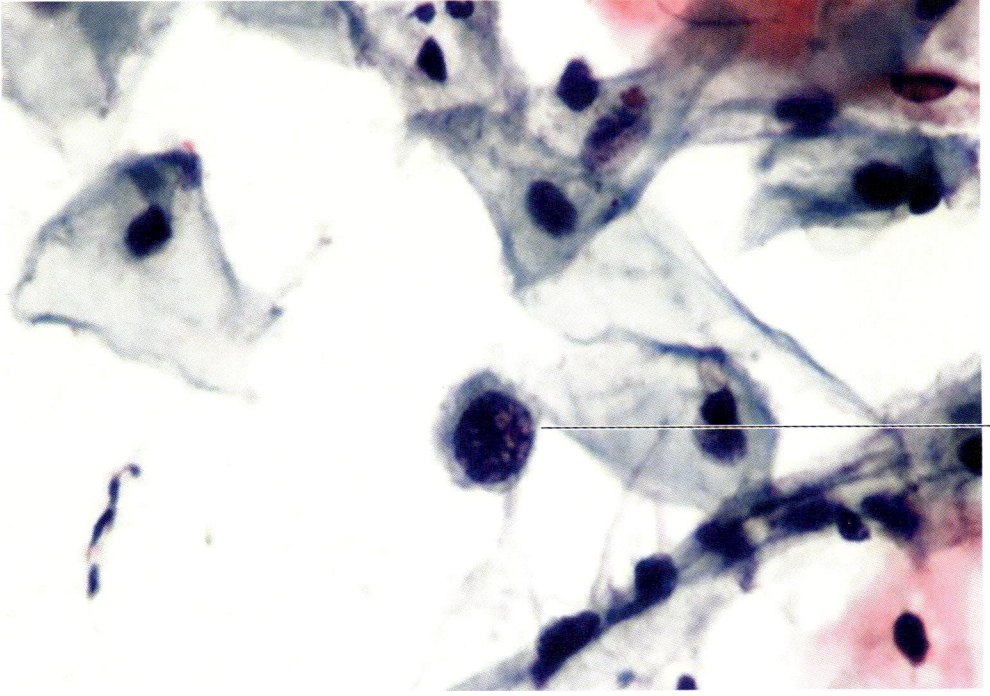

CIN 3 cells can also be shed singly and hence can be missed. This is more common in liquid based cytology

Note the highly abnormal chromatic pattern with coarse clumping. Cytoplasm is so scant it is difficult to say it is squamous. One can pass it off as a histiocyte unless carefully evaluated under high power.

Fig. 12.7b

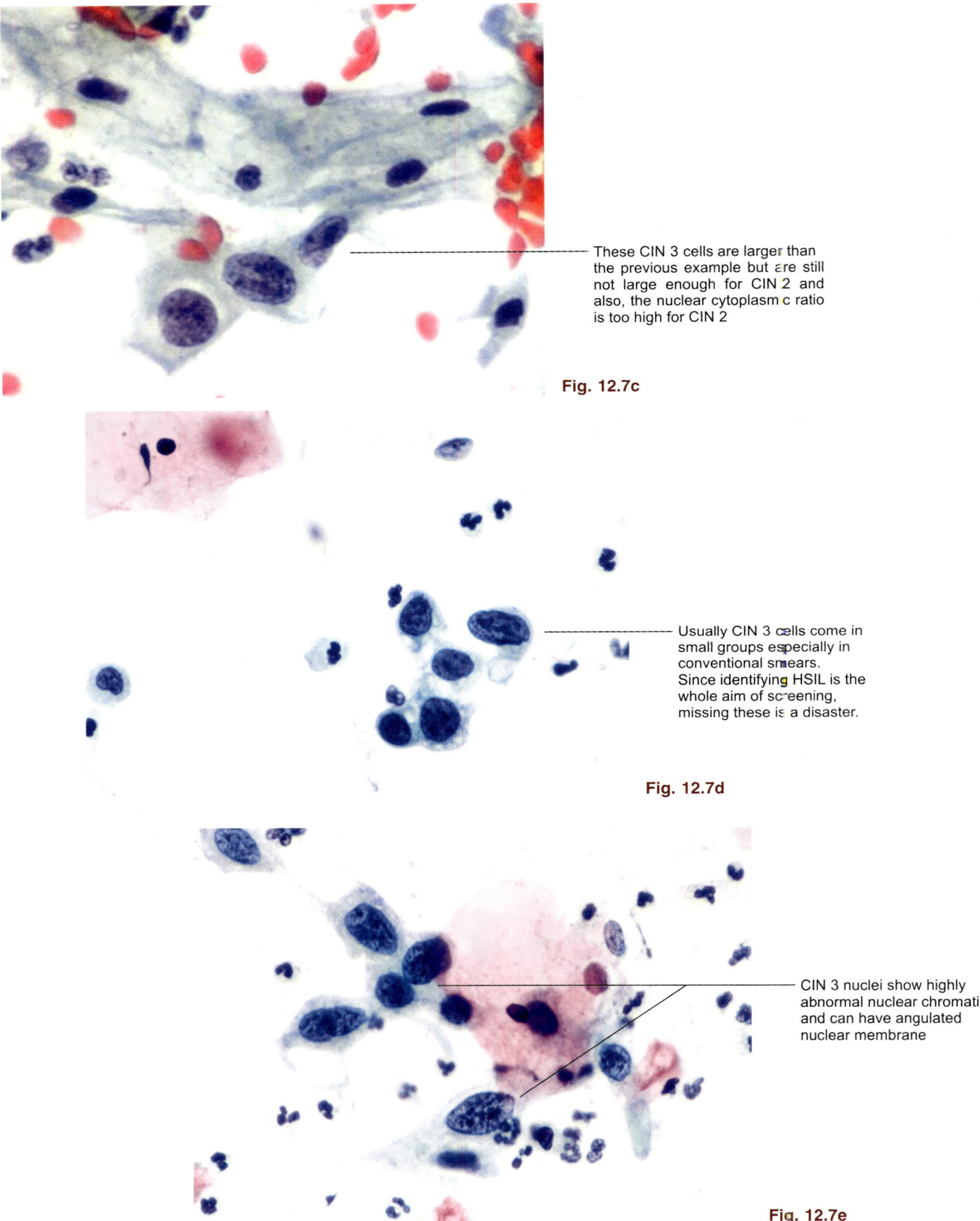

These CIN 3 cells are larger than the previous example but are still not large enough for CIN 2 and also, the nuclear cytoplasmic ratio is too high for CIN 2

Fig. 12.7c

Usually CIN 3 cells come in small groups especially in conventional smears. Since identifying HSIL is the whole aim of screening, missing these is a disaster.

Fig. 12.7d

CIN 3 nuclei show highly abnormal nuclear chromatin and can have angulated nuclear membrane

Fig. 12.7e

CYTOLOGY OF CIN 3 IN LIQUID-BASED CYTOLOGY (Figs 12.8a to c)

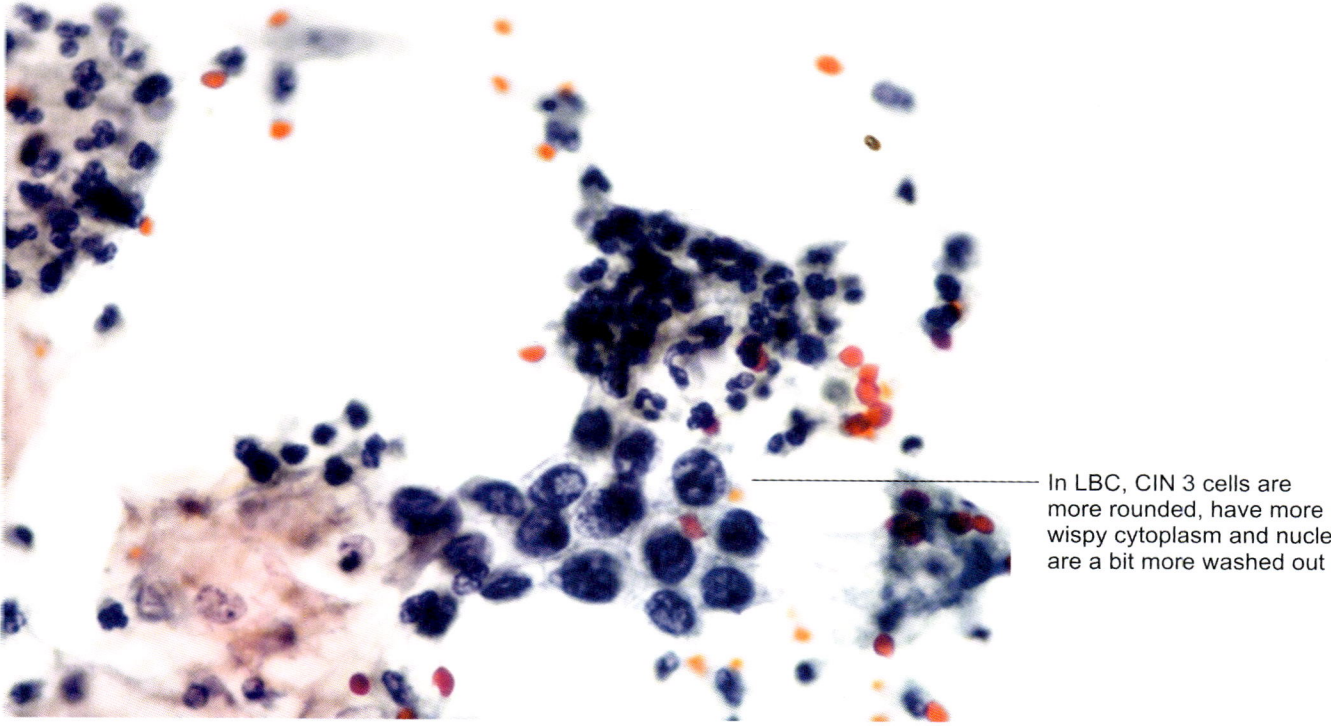

In LBC, CIN 3 cells are more rounded, have more wispy cytoplasm and nuclei are a bit more washed out

Fig. 12.8a

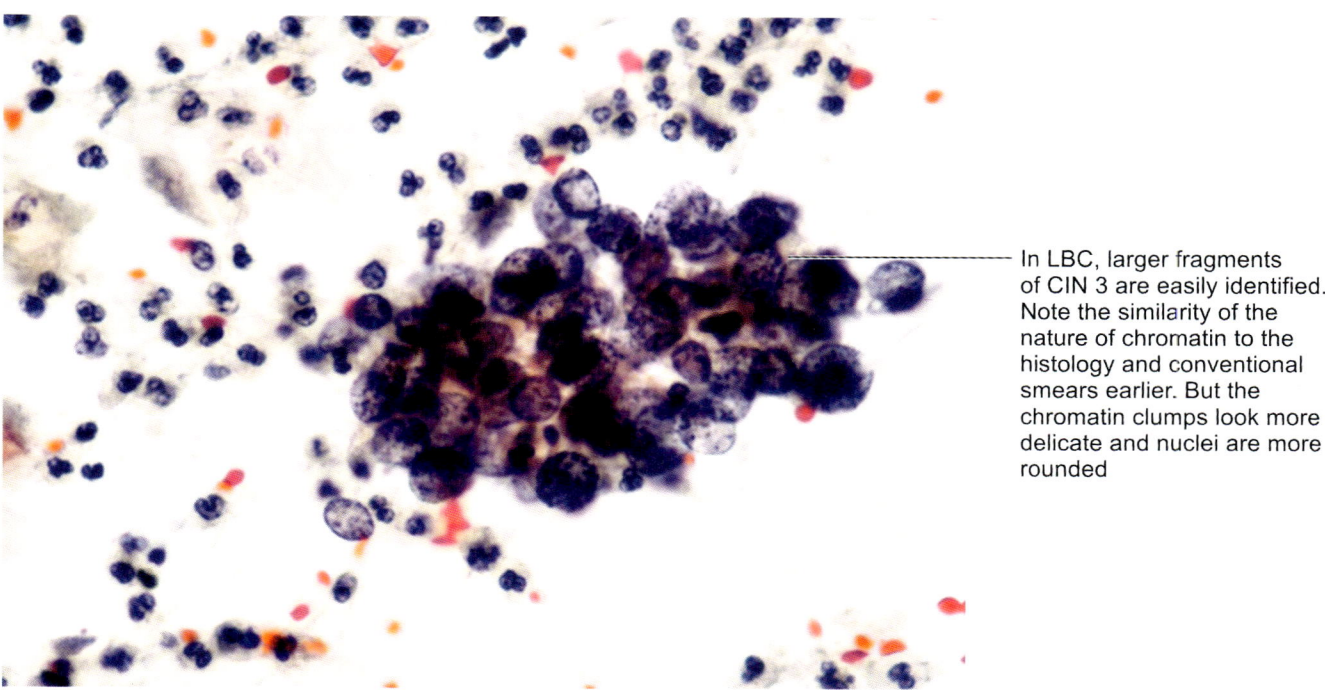

In LBC, larger fragments of CIN 3 are easily identified. Note the similarity of the nature of chromatin to the histology and conventional smears earlier. But the chromatin clumps look more delicate and nuclei are more rounded

Fig. 12.8b

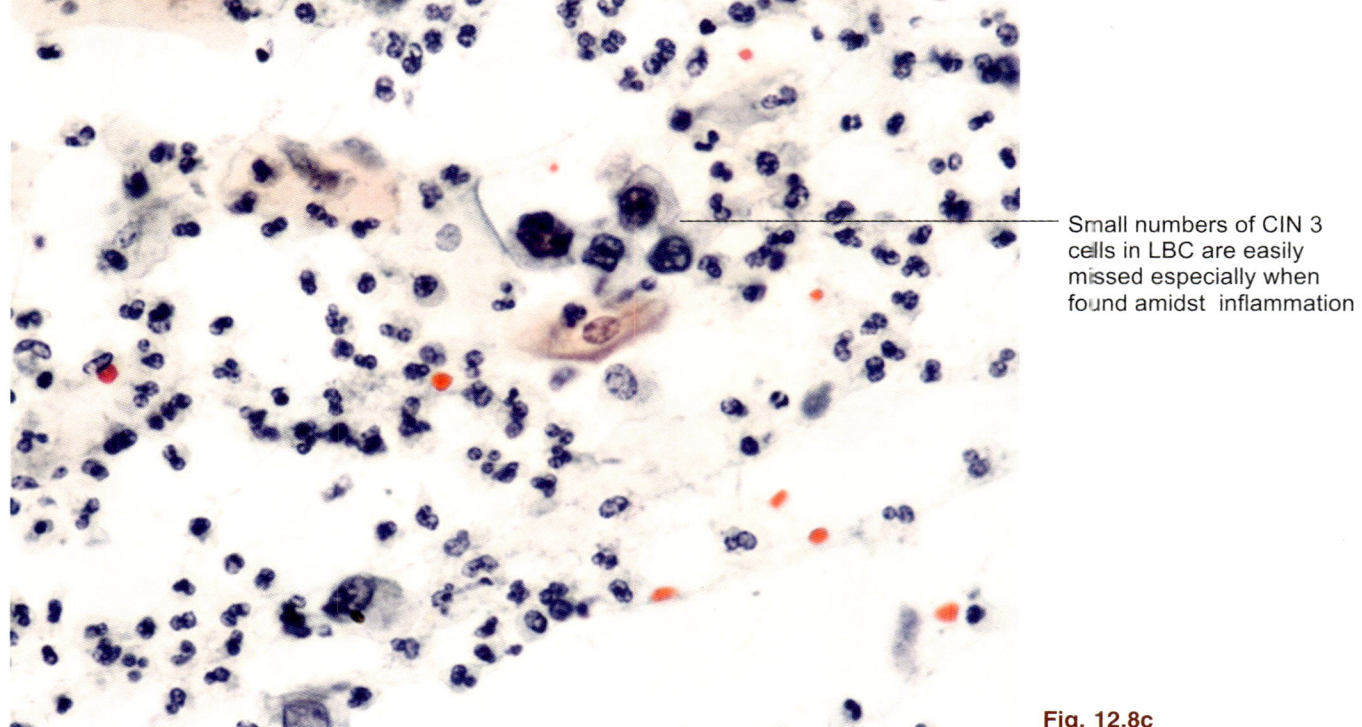

Small numbers of CIN 3 cells in LBC are easily missed especially when found amidst inflammation

Fig. 12.8c

CONDYLOMA (Fig. 12.9)

A condyloma is a low grade lesion of the cervix which is thrown into multiple papillary folds, making it look like a wart. Any warty lesion of the cervix is called a condyloma, those caused by the HPV infection being called condyloma accuminata. Many times, the changes of viral infection are only focally identified in some of the papillae and not everywhere.

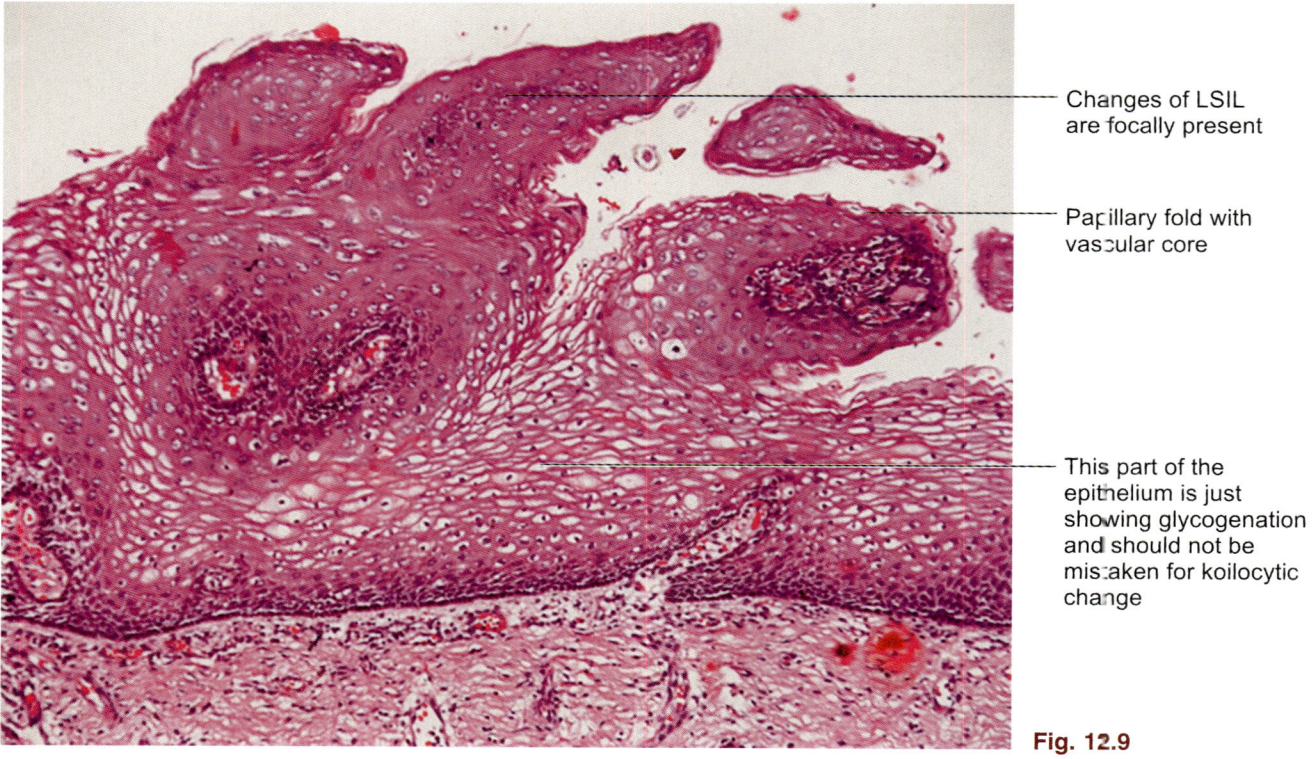

Changes of LSIL are focally present

Papillary fold with vascular core

This part of the epithelium is just showing glycogenation and should not be mistaken for koilocytic change

Fig. 12.9

Squamous Cell Carcinoma

HISTOLOGY OF SQUAMOUS CELL CARCINOMA (Figs 13.1a and b)

Squamous cell carcinoma is made up of cells similar to CIN 2 or CIN 3 but they are piled up and invading. Their proliferation potential is much more than in HSIL and hence it folds up the basement membrane to throw it into folds, making it seem thicker even in places where no basement membrane breach is identified.

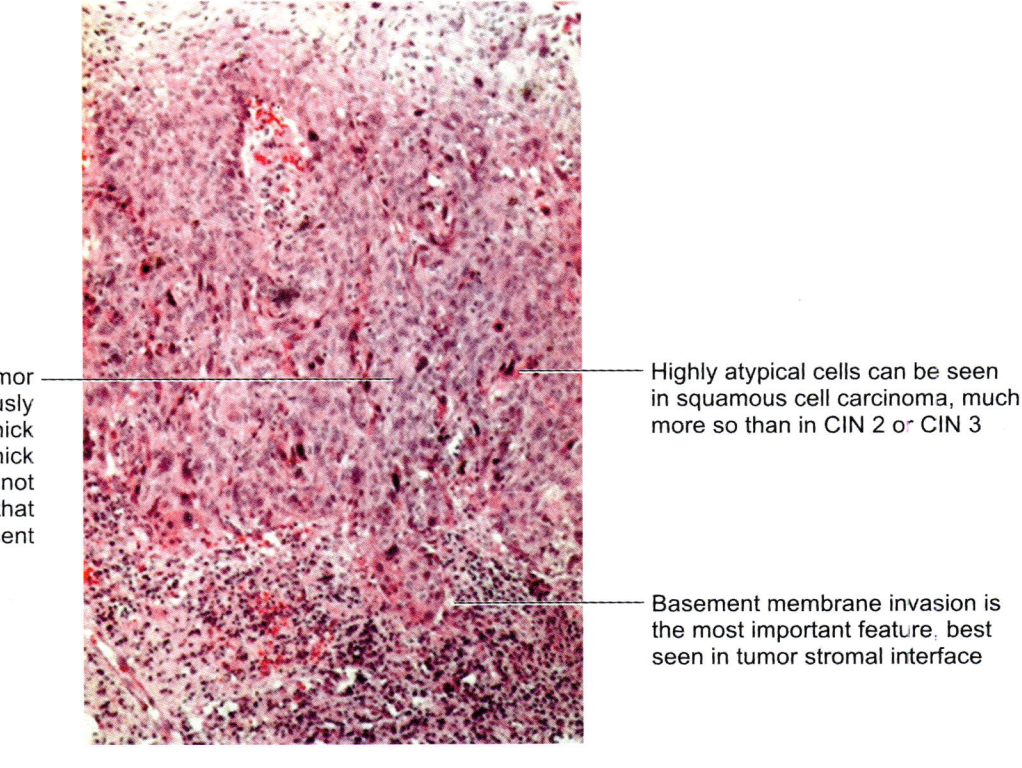

These thick areas of tumor are made of previously invaded cells growing thick and dense to form a thick layer where there is not enough stroma to tell that invasion is present

Highly atypical cells can be seen in squamous cell carcinoma, much more so than in CIN 2 or CIN 3

Basement membrane invasion is the most important feature, best seen in tumor stromal interface

Fig. 13.1a

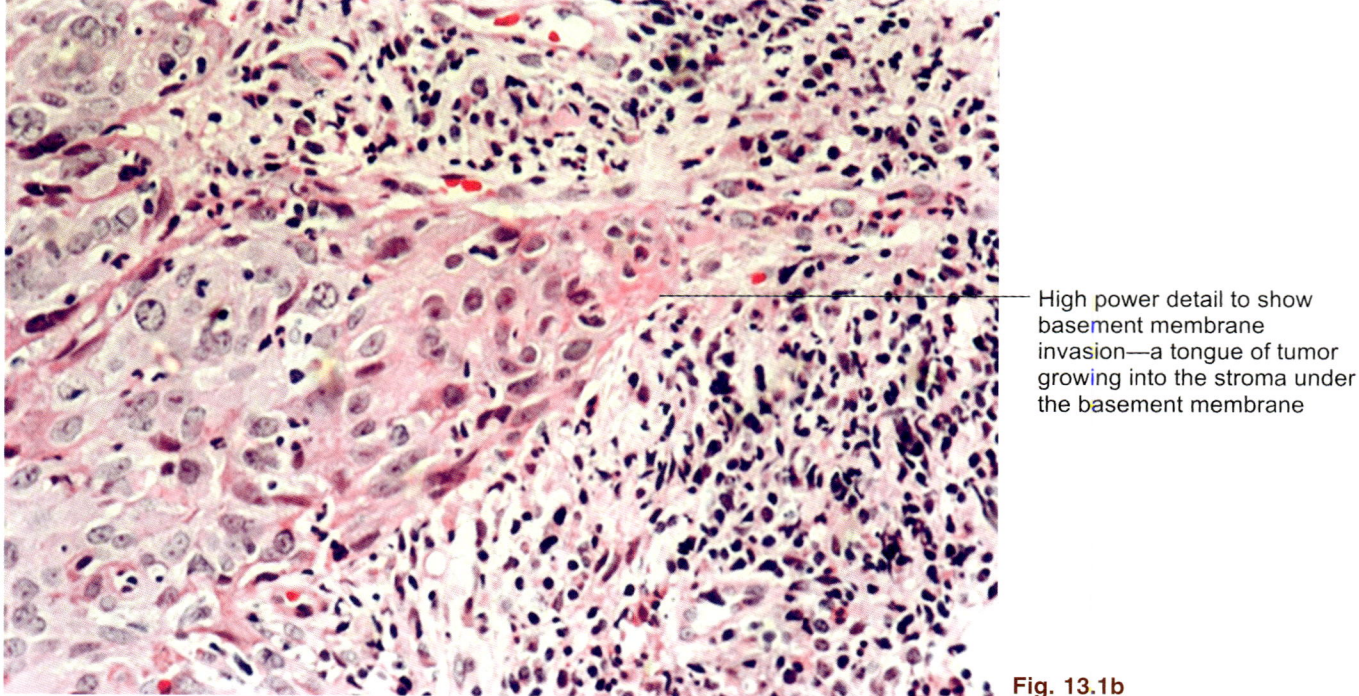

High power detail to show basement membrane invasion—a tongue of tumor growing into the stroma under the basement membrane

Fig. 13.1b

HISTOLOGY OF KERATINIZING SQUAMOUS CELL CARCINOMA
(Fig. 13.2)

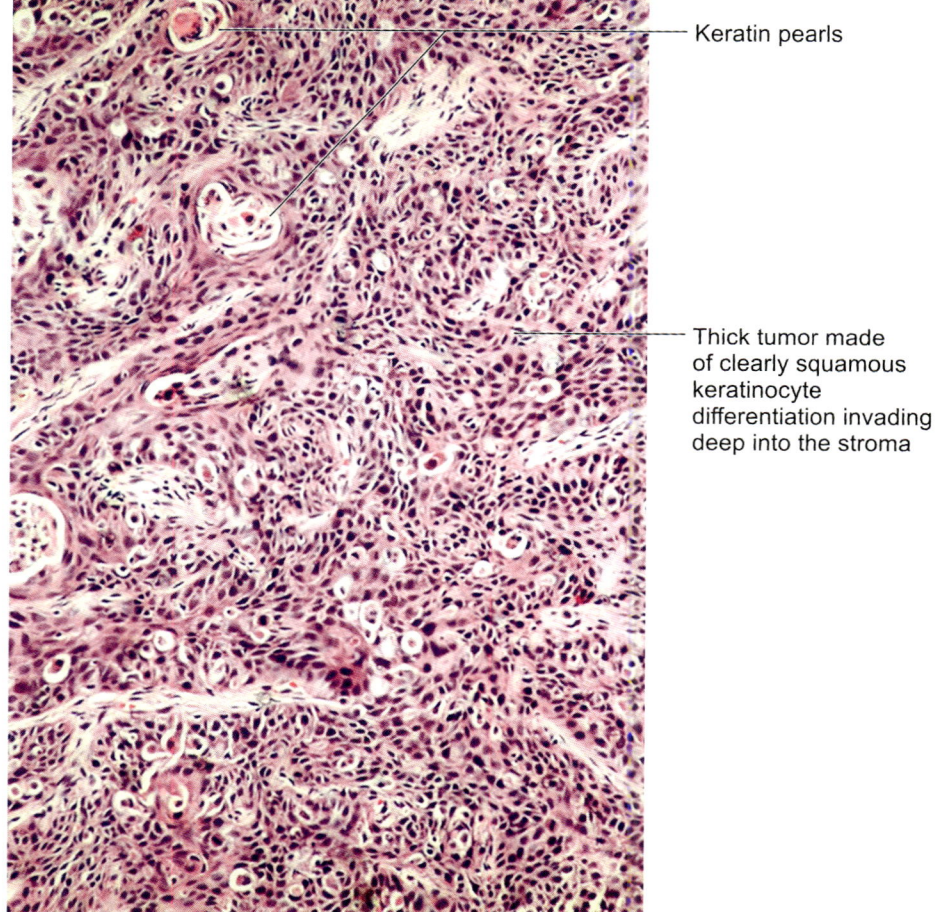

Keratin pearls

Thick tumor made of clearly squamous keratinocyte differentiation invading deep into the stroma

Fig. 13.2

CYTOLOGY OF SQUAMOUS CELL CARCINOMA (Fig. 13.3)

Frank squamous cell carcinoma usually shows large number of cells. Cytoplasmic abnormalities like tadpole cells or strap cells are pesent. Both keratinizing and non-keratinizing suqmous cell carcinoma show keratinized cells in cytology. Nuclei are very abnormal much more than in CIN 2 and CIN 3 and are seen in profusion.

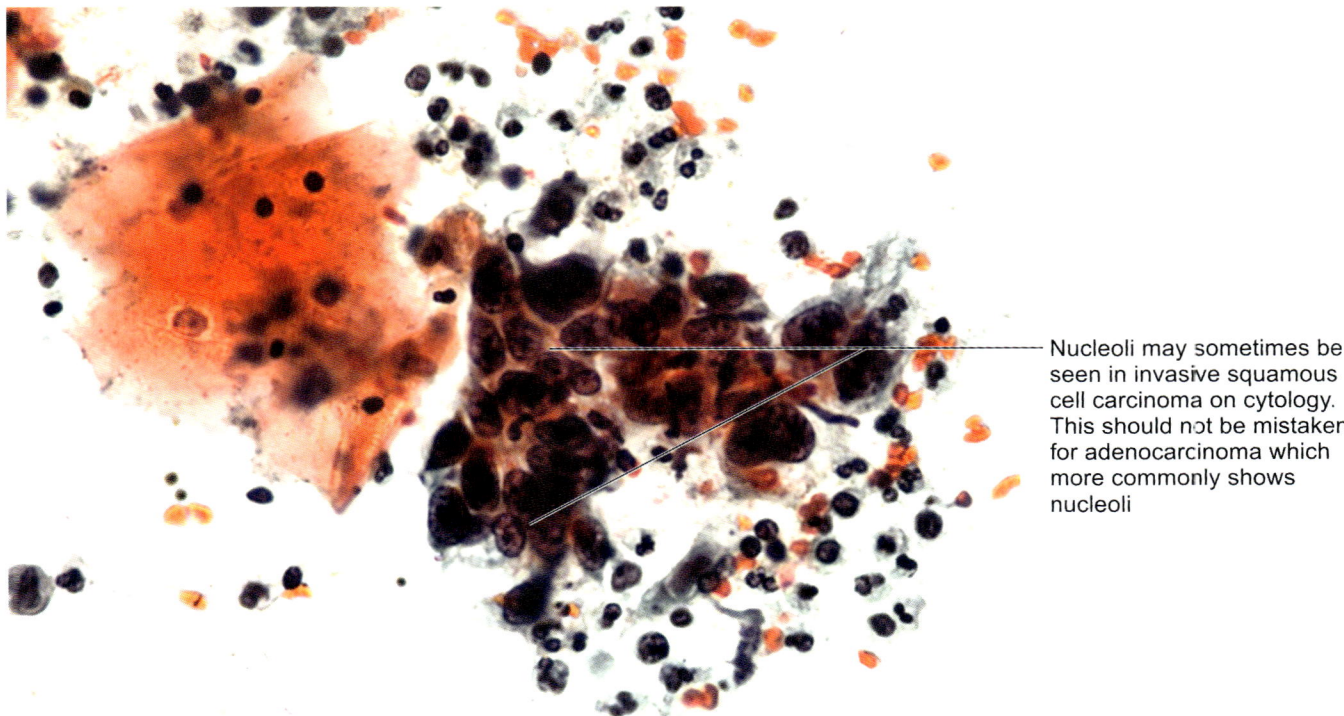

Nucleoli may sometimes be seen in invasive squamous cell carcinoma on cytology. This should not be mistaken for adenocarcinoma which more commonly shows nucleoli

Fig. 13.3

TUMOR DIATHESIS ON CYTOLOGY (Figs 13.4a–c)

Tumor diathesis is a very important feature to recognise in frank invasive squamous cell carcinoma. It indicates sampling of the necrotic bleeding tumor surface. Hence tumor cells are few. The term encompasses three things— necrotic cells, inflammatory cells and red blood cells. Despite finding small numbers of atypical cells, which is a feature otherwise in favour of HSIL, the presence of tumor diathesis suggests carcinoma and hence biopsy confirmation has to be done immediately.

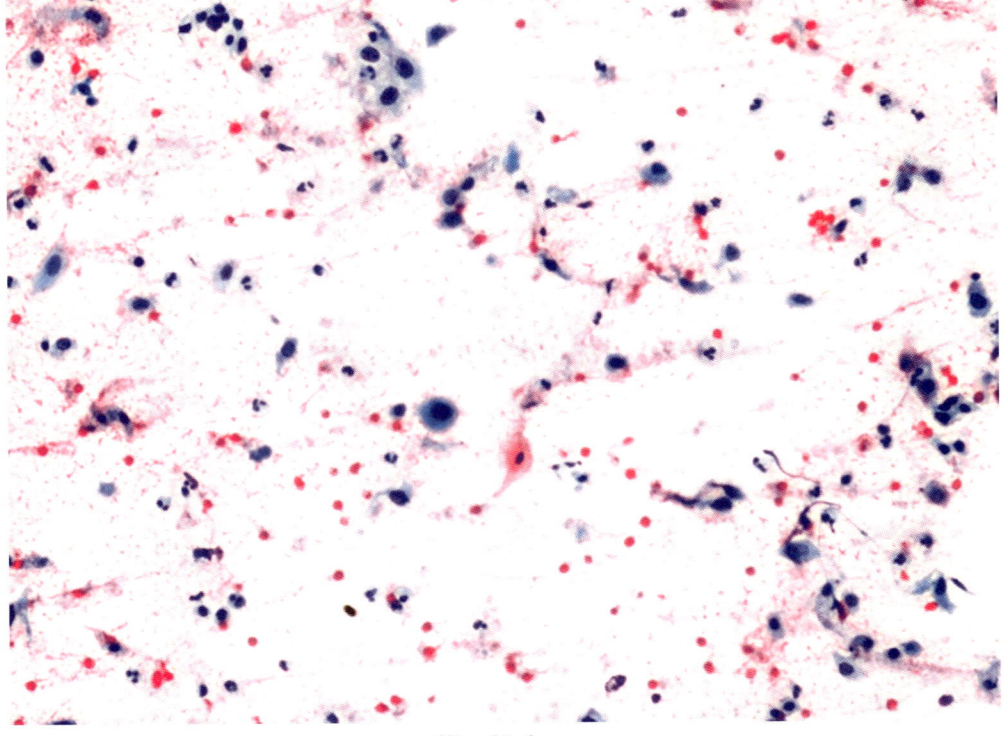

Fig. 13.4a

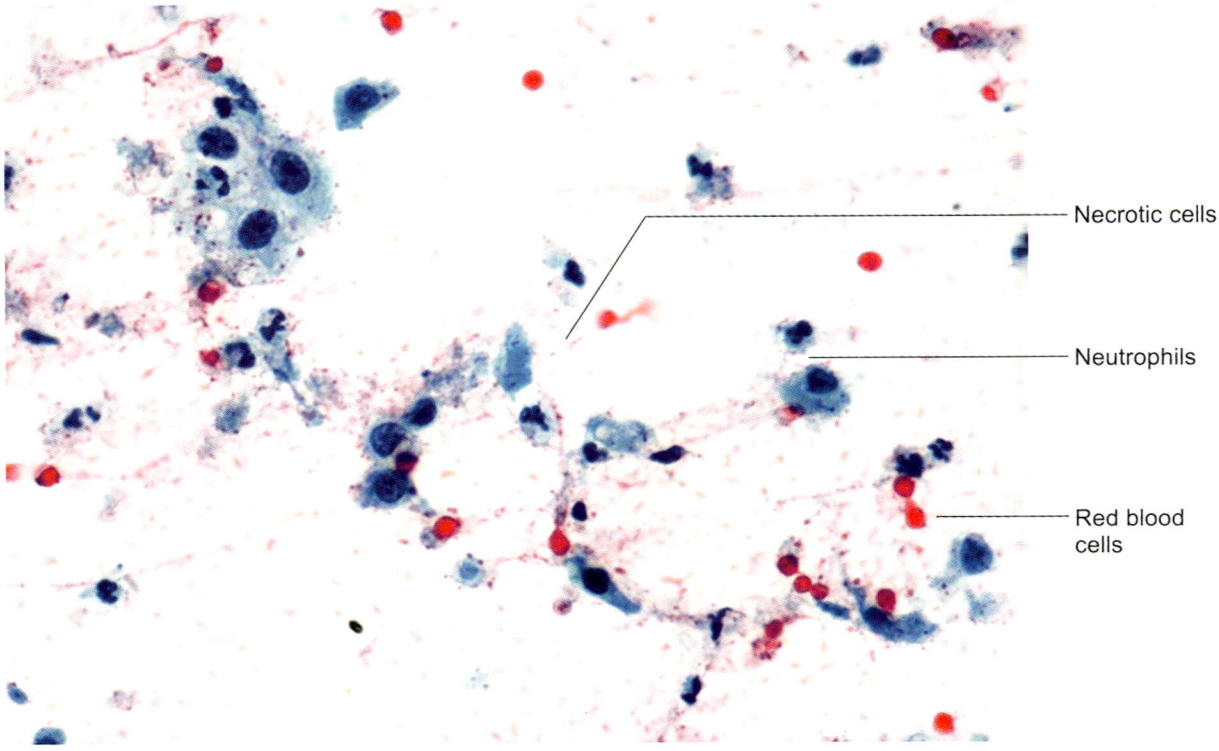

Necrotic cells

Neutrophils

Red blood cells

Fig. 13.4b

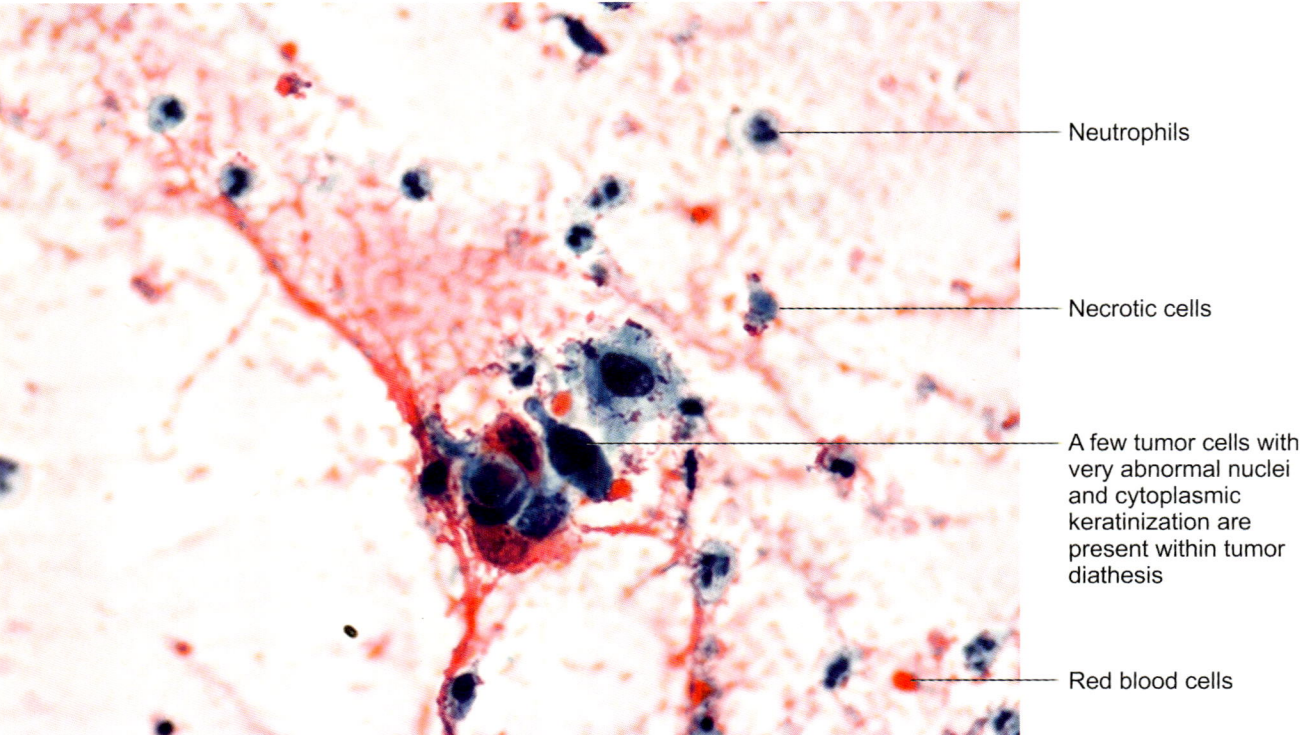

Neutrophils

Necrotic cells

A few tumor cells with very abnormal nuclei and cytoplasmic keratinization are present within tumor diathesis

Red blood cells

Fig. 13.4c

Adenocarcinoma

HISTOLOGY OF ADENOCARCINOMA (Fig. 14.1)

Adenocarcinoma of cervix is much less common than squamous cell carcinoma but is also caused by HPV infection. On histology, however, there is no feature of HPV infection visible. Instead it looks like any other adenocarcinoma. However, the test for HPV comes strongly positive in the tumor.

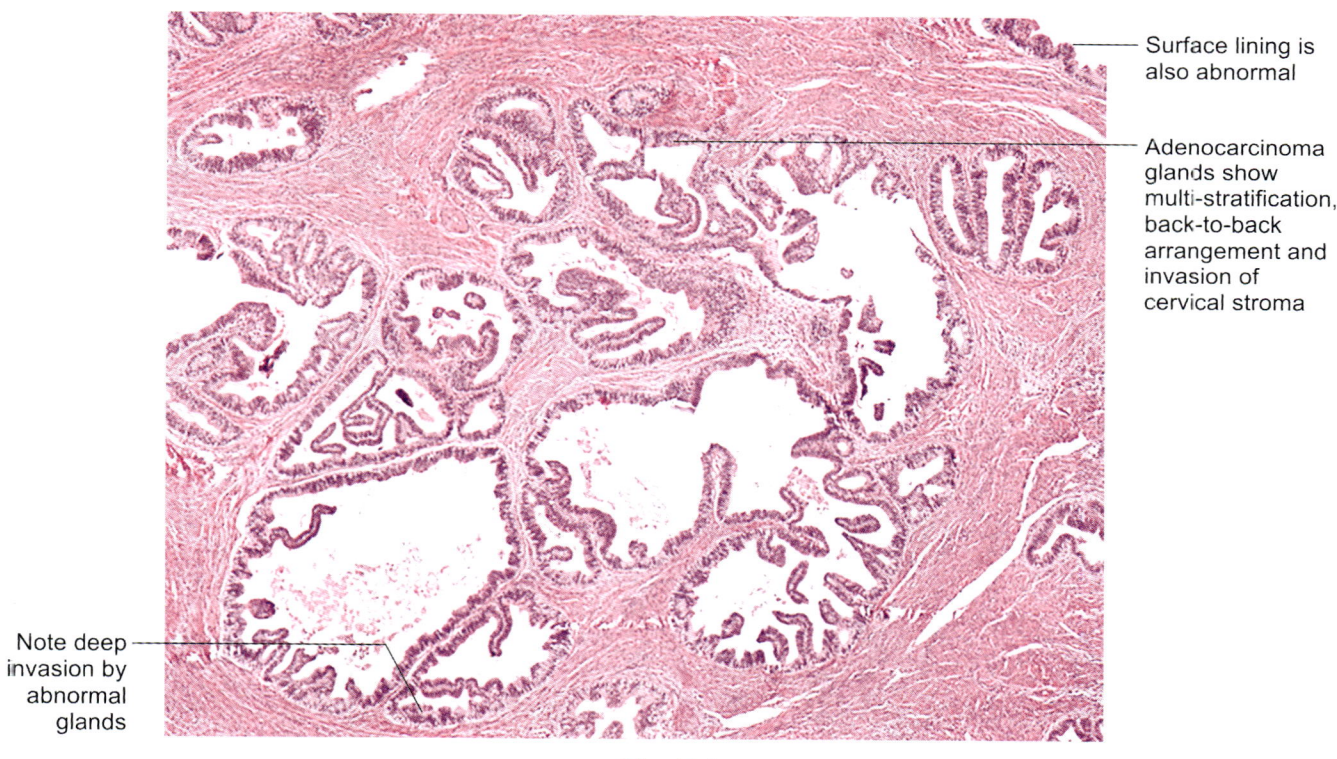

Surface lining is also abnormal

Adenocarcinoma glands show multi-stratification, back-to-back arrangement and invasion of cervical stroma

Note deep invasion by abnormal glands

Fig. 14.1

CYTOLOGY OF ADENOCARCINOMA (Figs 14.2a and b)

Adenocarcinoma cells typically lack the coarse chromatin of squamous carcinomas but are instead more vesicular and have nucleoli.

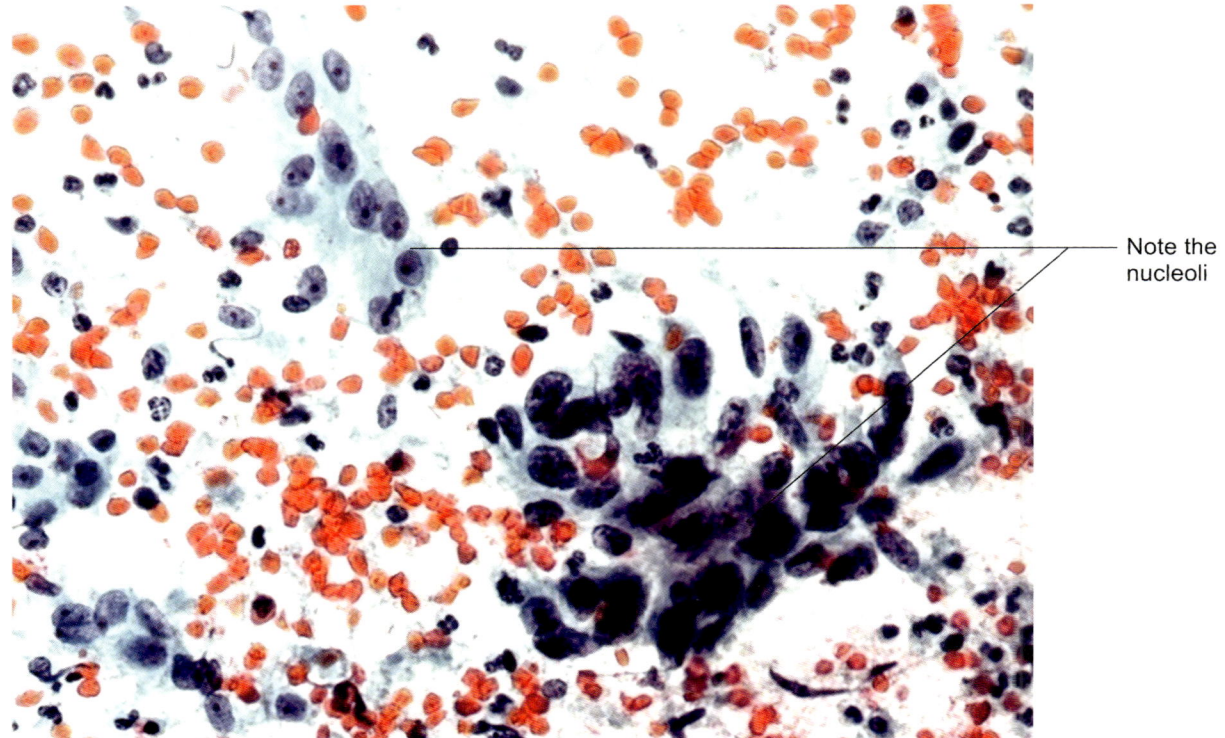

Note the nucleoli

Fig. 14.2a

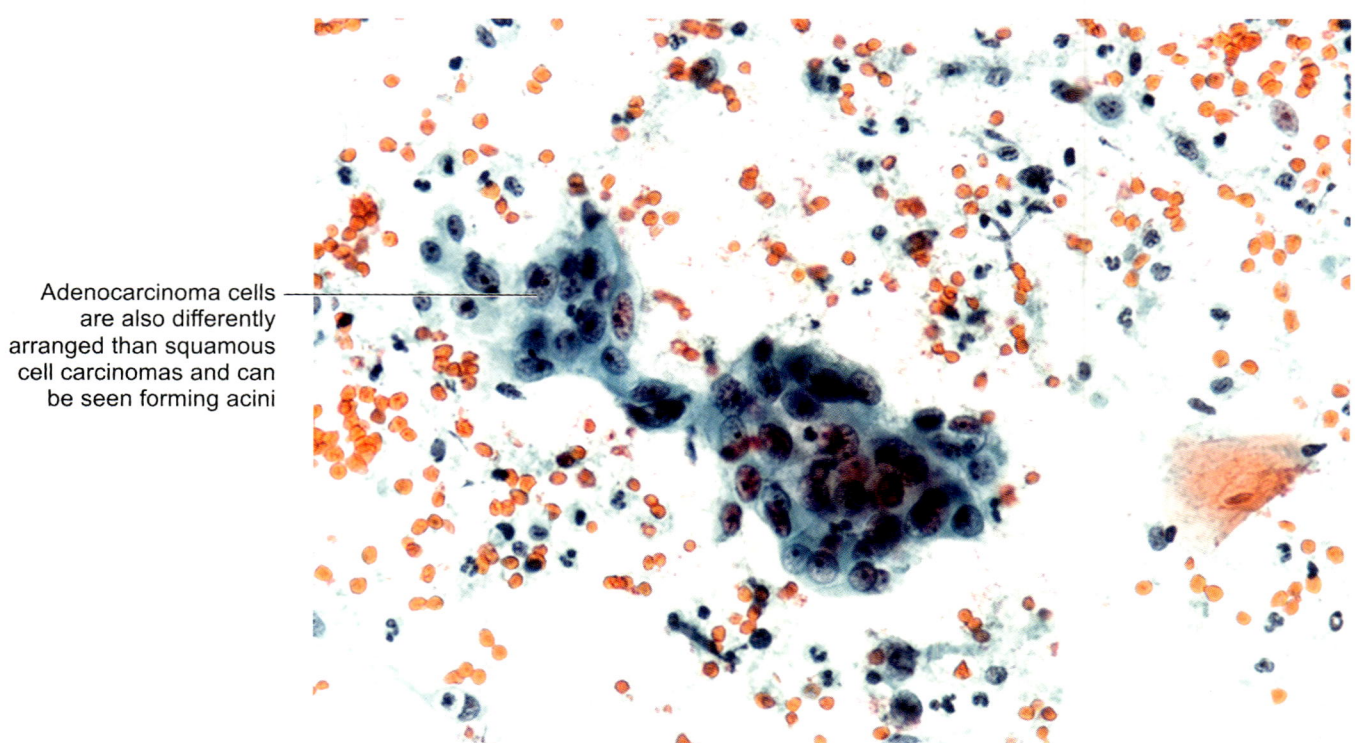

Adenocarcinoma cells are also differently arranged than squamous cell carcinomas and can be seen forming acini

Fig. 14.2b

CYTOLOGY OF ADENOCARCINOMA *IN SITU* (Fig. 14.3)

Adenocarcinoma *in situ* is very rare, forming perhaps one in ten thousand women—about a hundred times less common than HSIL. But it is important to recognise them because they progress to invasive adenocarcinomas very silently.

To identify AIS, one needs to look carefully at the endocervical cells. On cytology, AIS cells form clusters of cells with acinar arrangement instead of the honeycombing—a useful feature to pick up clusters on low power. With acini in the center, nuclei tend to come out at the other side, sheared from basement membrane—a feature termed as feathering. Snake egg appearance is also seen—snake (i.e. long columnar cell) swallowing the egg (nucleus).

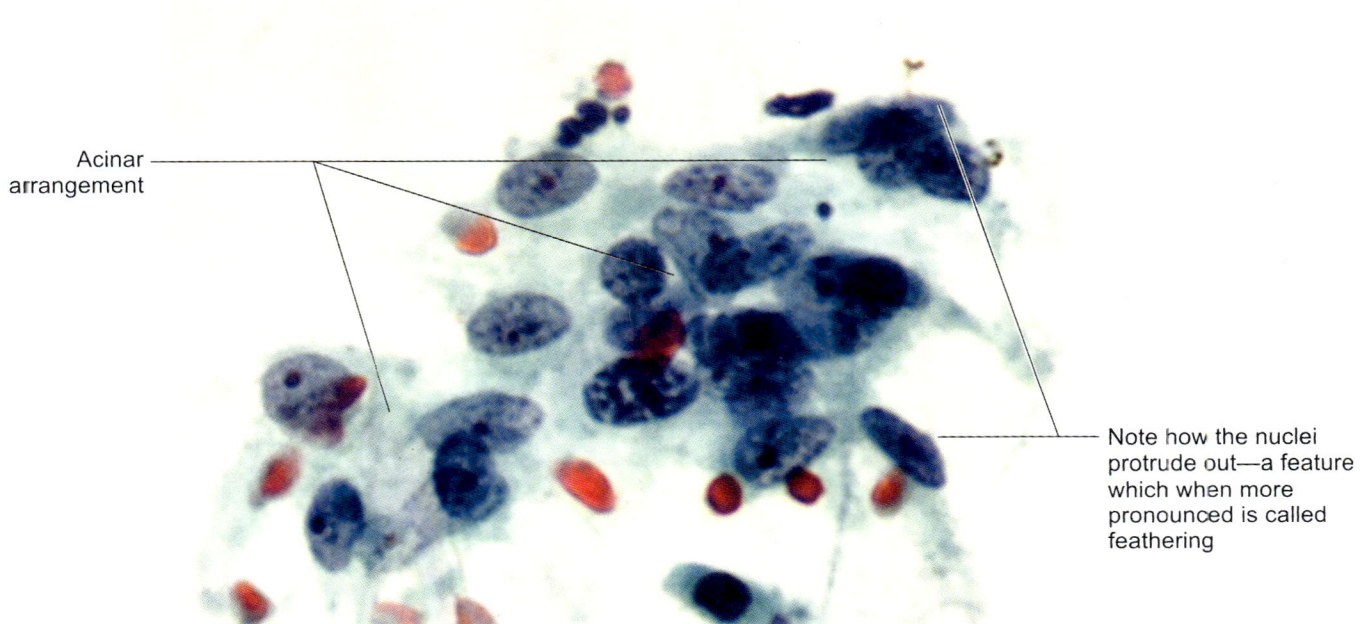

Acinar arrangement

Note how the nuclei protrude out—a feature which when more pronounced is called feathering

Fig. 14.3

CYTOLOGY OF PAPILLARY ADENOCARCINOMA (Figs 14.4a and b)

Finding a profusion of abnormally architectures but honeycombed cells should alert one to the possibility of papillary adenocarcinoma.

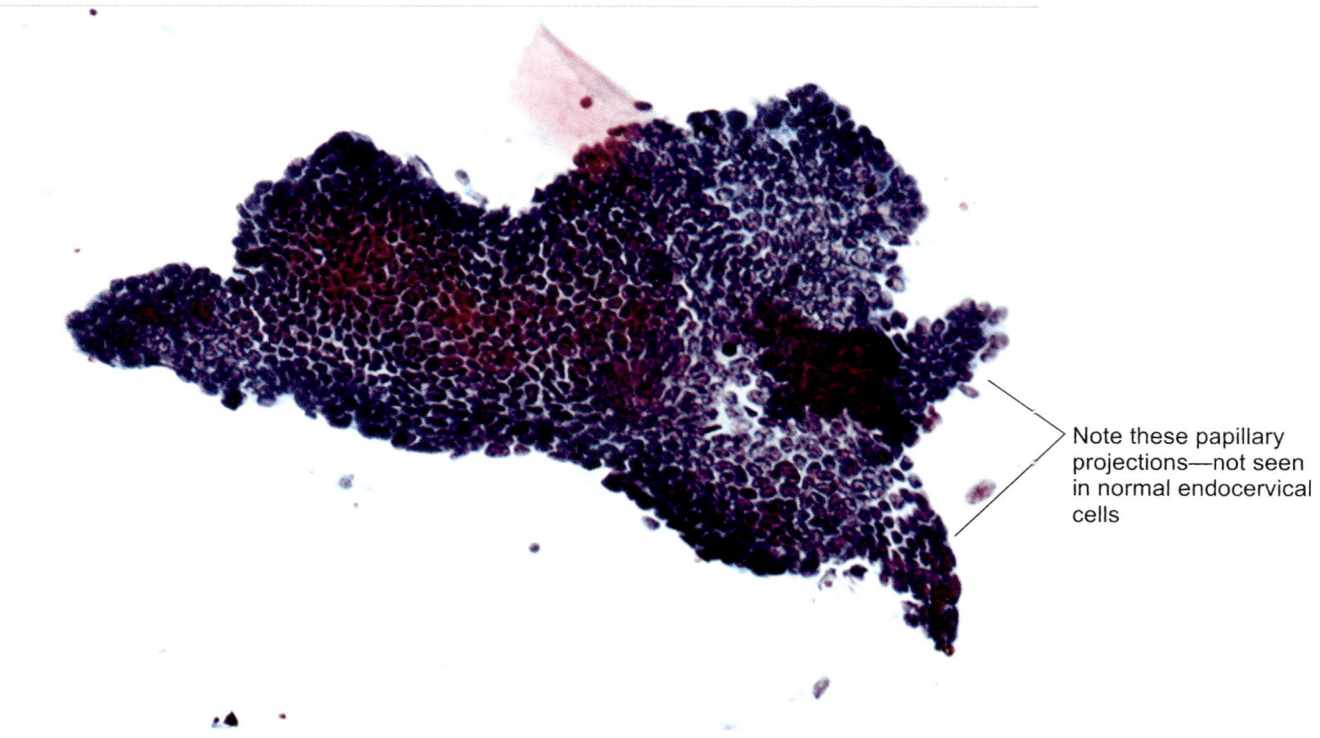

Note these papillary projections—not seen in normal endocervical cells

Fig. 14.4a

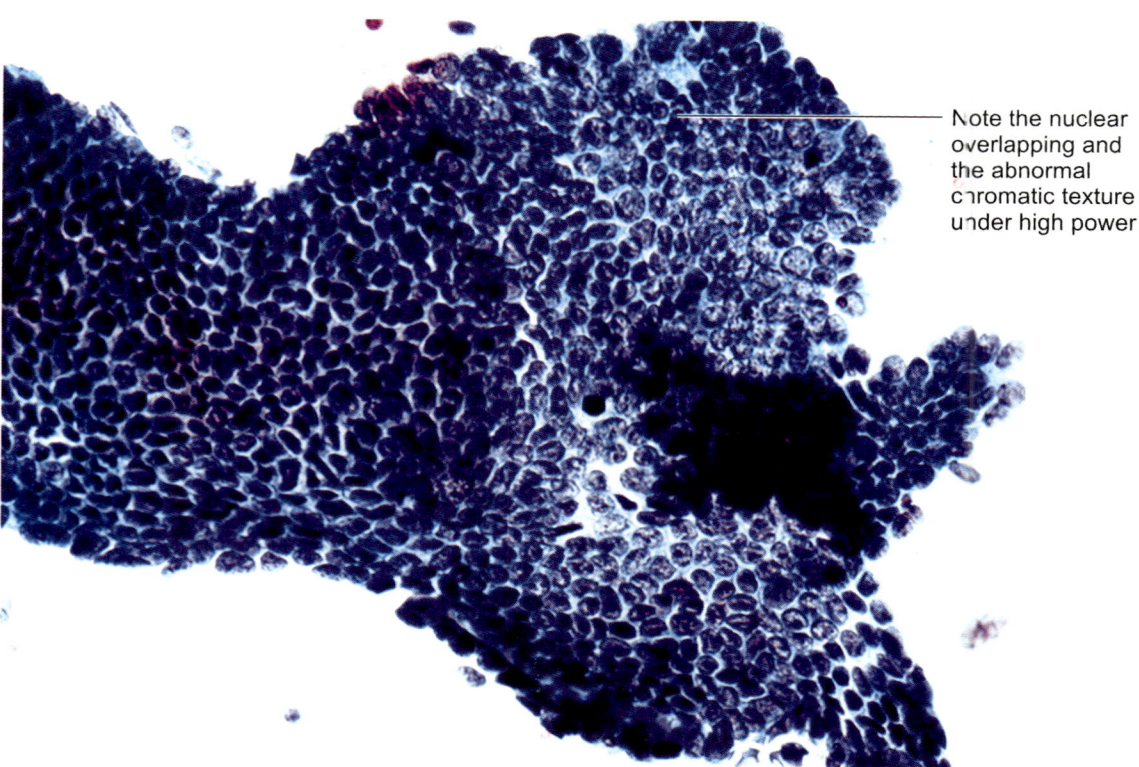

Note the nuclear overlapping and the abnormal chromatic texture under high power

Fig. 14.4b

Miscellaneous Conditions

VAGINAL INTRAEPITHELIAL NEOPLASIA (Fig. 15.1)

Vaginal intraepithelial neoplasia is also caused by HPV infection and is very similar to the cervical counterpart. It is also known to progress to squamous cell carcinoma. High grade VIN is almost identical to the HSIL of the cervix.

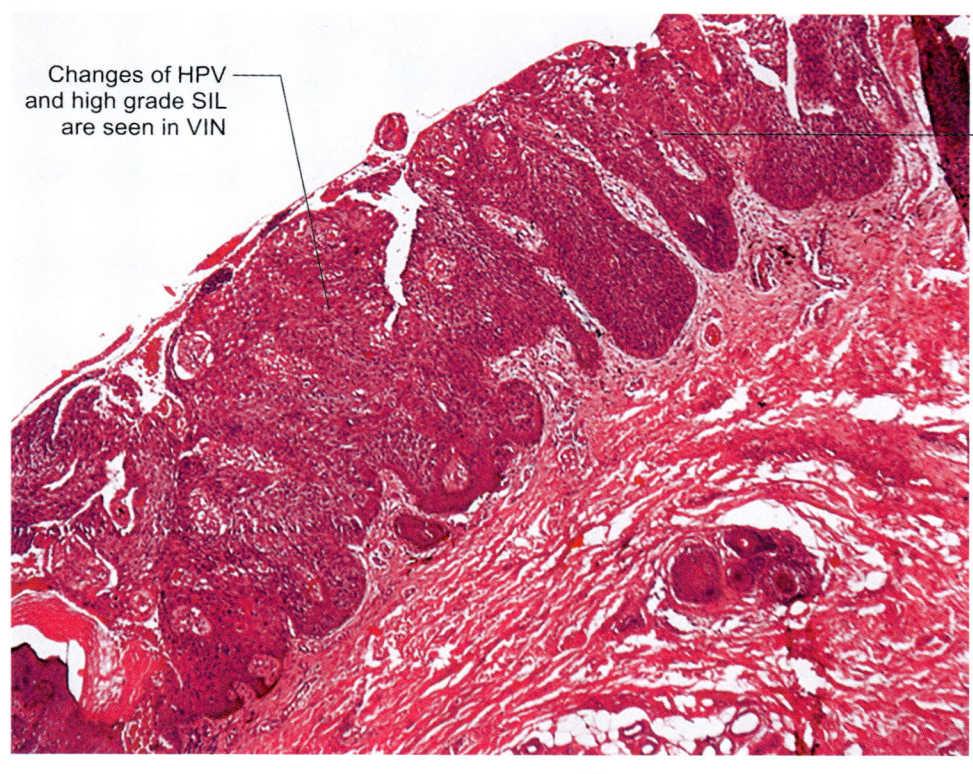

Changes of HPV and high grade SIL are seen in VIN

Marked papillomatous downward prolongation of rete ridges

Fig. 15.1

CYTOLOGY OF ENDOMETRIAL CELLS IN PAP SMEARS (Figs 15.2a to c)

Endometrial gland fragments are seen in early menstrual phase. Gland cells can surround the stroma leading to a top hat appearance.

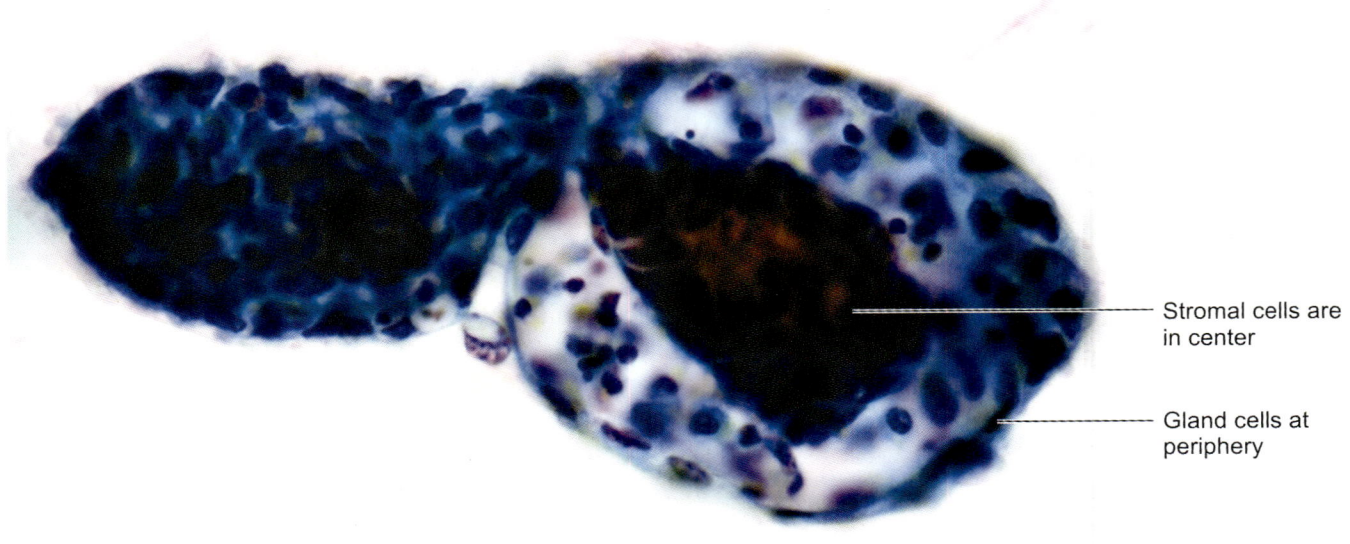

Stromal cells are in center

Gland cells at periphery

Fig. 15.2a

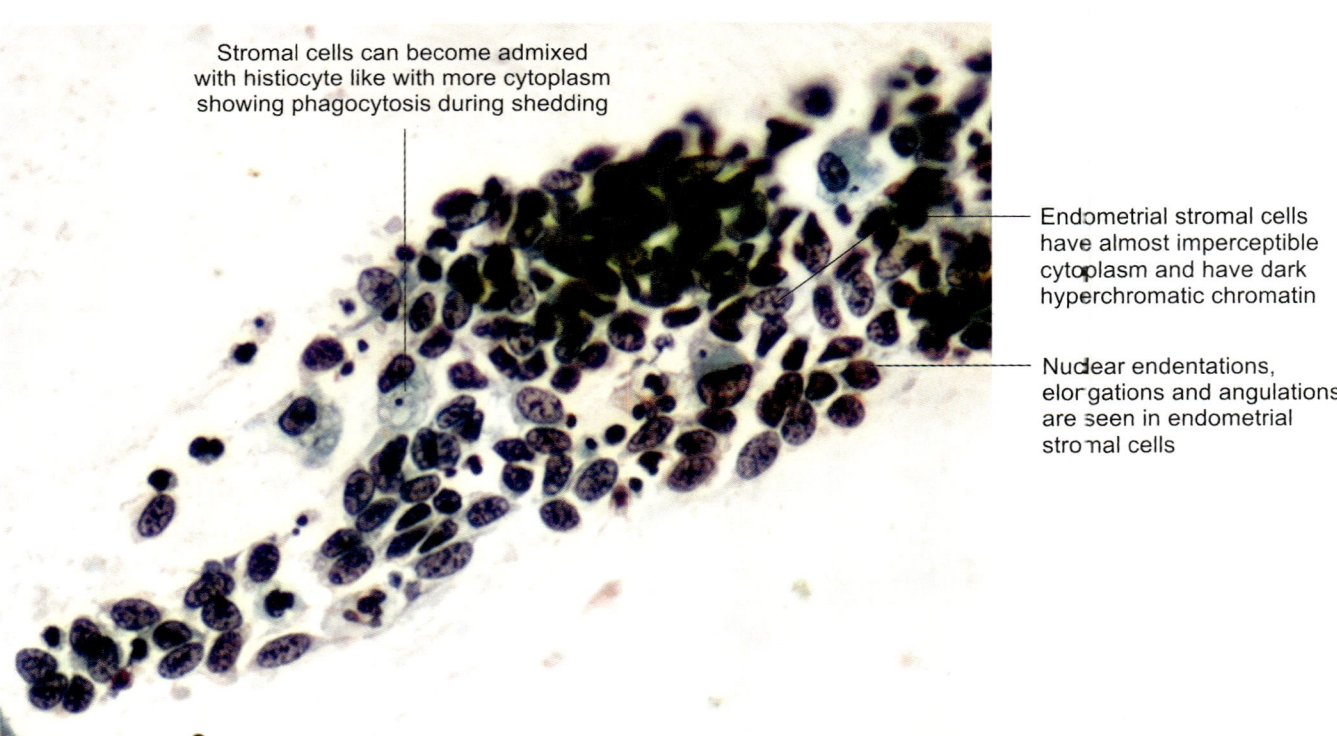

Stromal cells can become admixed with histiocyte like with more cytoplasm showing phagocytosis during shedding

Endometrial stromal cells have almost imperceptible cytoplasm and have dark hyperchromatic chromatin

Nuclear endentations, elongations and angulations are seen in endometrial stromal cells

Fig. 15.2b

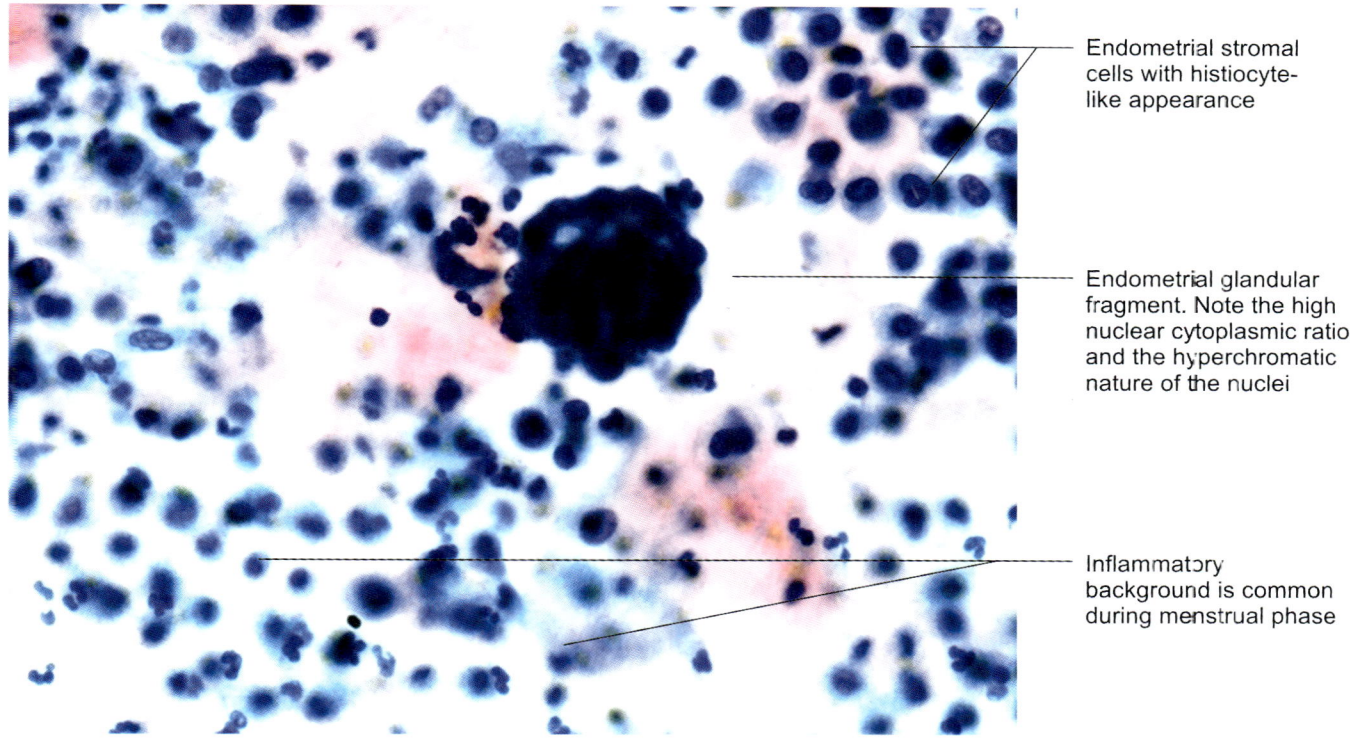

Endometrial stromal cells with histiocyte-like appearance

Endometrial glandular fragment. Note the high nuclear cytoplasmic ratio and the hyperchromatic nature of the nuclei

Inflammatory background is common during menstrual phase

Fig. 15.2c

HISTIOCYTES AND ENDOMETRIAL STROMAL CELLS (Figs 15.3a to c)

In the later part of menstrual cycle and in earliest proliferative phase, the endometrium sheds large numbers of histiocytes which can be seen in cervical smears. Ideally cervical smear should not be taken at this time.

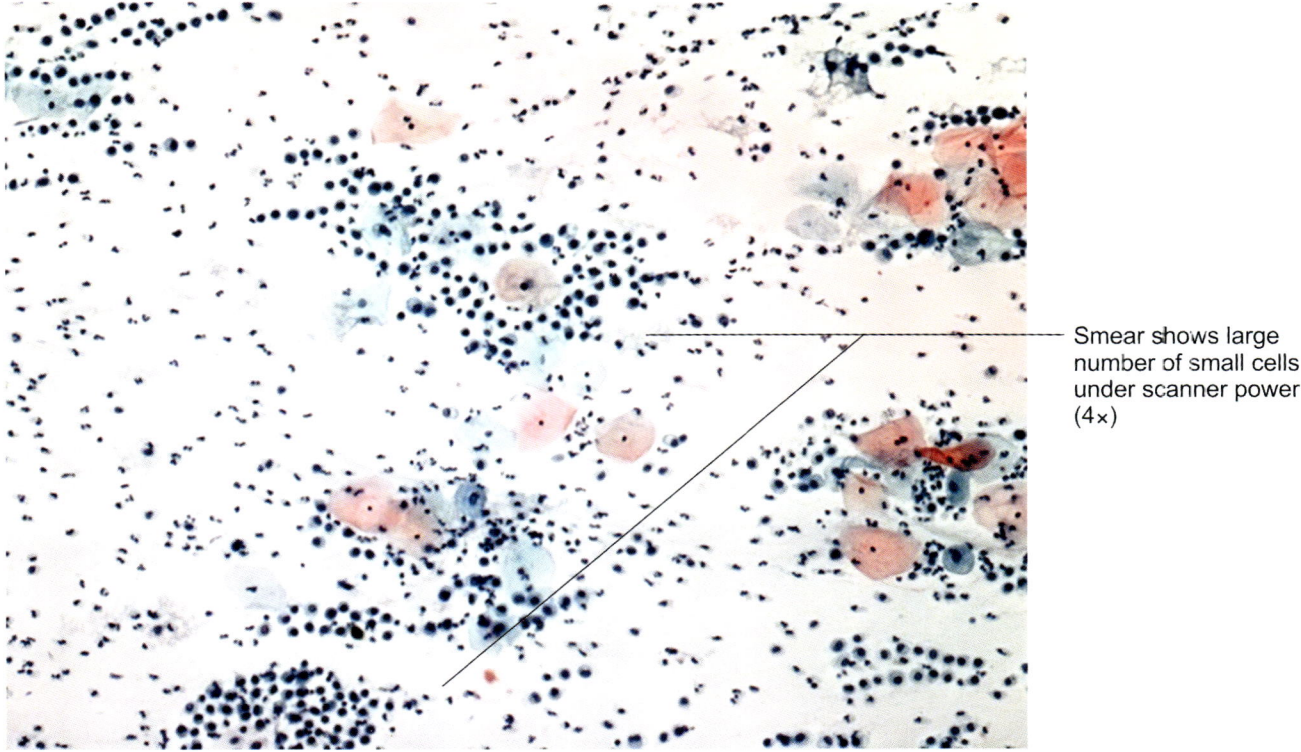

Smear shows large number of small cells under scanner power (4×)

Fig. 15.3a

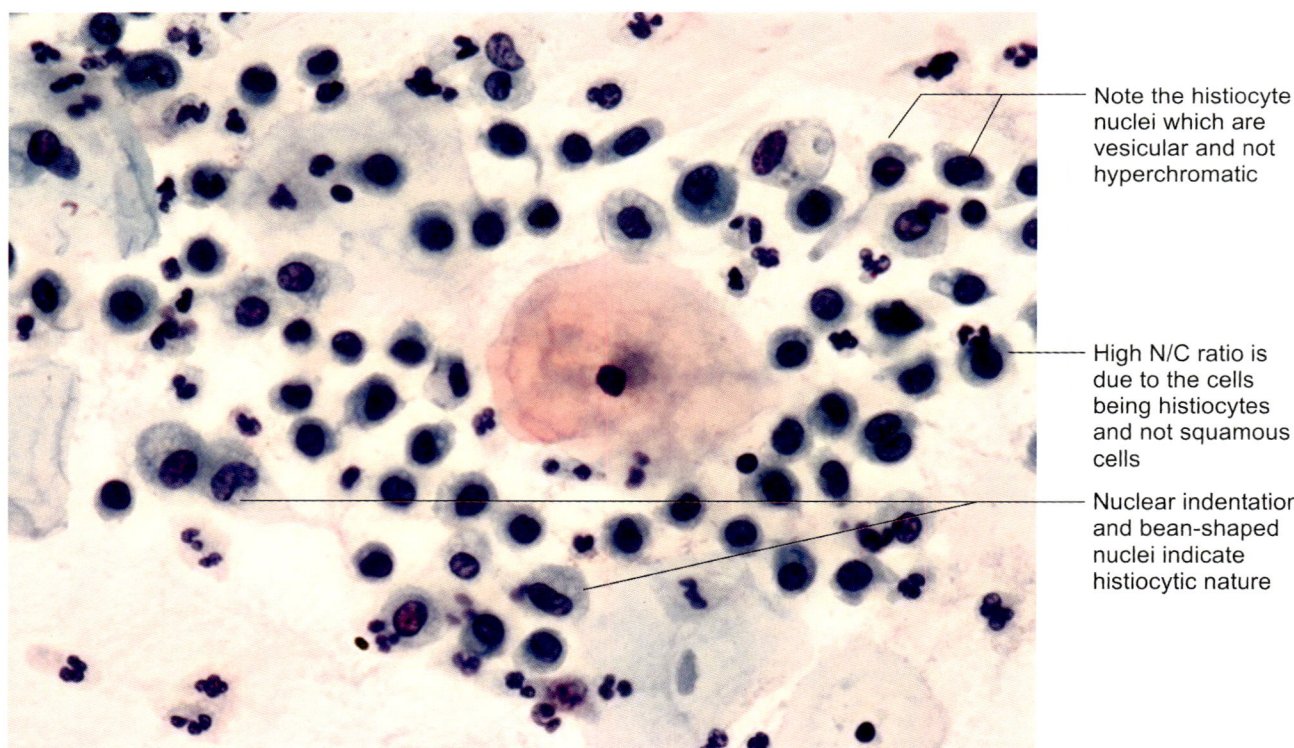

Small cells with dark nuclei having high nuclear cytoplasmic ratio mimic high grade SIL on low power examination (10×)

Cytoscreener has to go down under high power to evaluate all such cell groups to rule out SIL or ASC-H which is a common misdiagnosis

Fig. 15.3b

Note the histiocyte nuclei which are vesicular and not hyperchromatic

High N/C ratio is due to the cells being histiocytes and not squamous cells

Nuclear indentation and bean-shaped nuclei indicate histiocytic nature

Fig. 15.3c

ATYPICAL GLANDULAR CELLS
(Fig. 15.4)

A group of cells showing acinar arrangement and abnormal nuclear chromatin for glandular cells. These could be atypical endometrial or atypical endocervical cells. It is not possible to be certain. These must be reported and patient needs an endometrial aspiration and encocervical curettage.

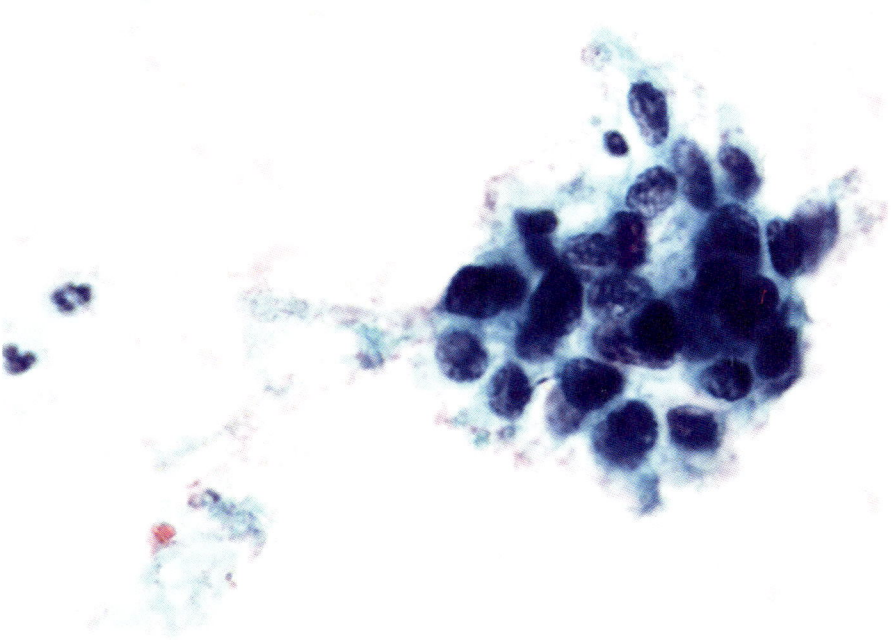

Fig. 15.4

TUBAL METAPLASIA (Figs 15.5a to c)

Tubal metaplastic cells can be mistaken for atypical glandular cells on cytology, because of darker and multilayered nuclei. However, the presence of cilia indicates their true nature.

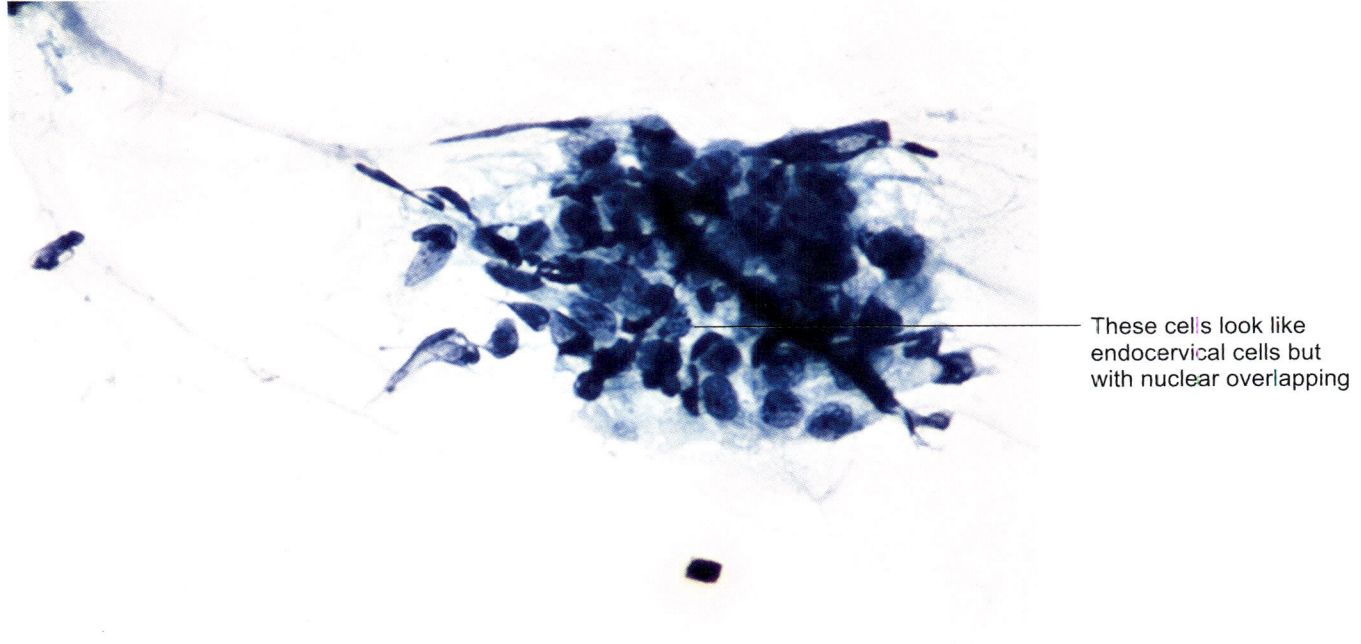

These cells look like endocervical cells but with nuclear overlapping

Fig. 15.5a

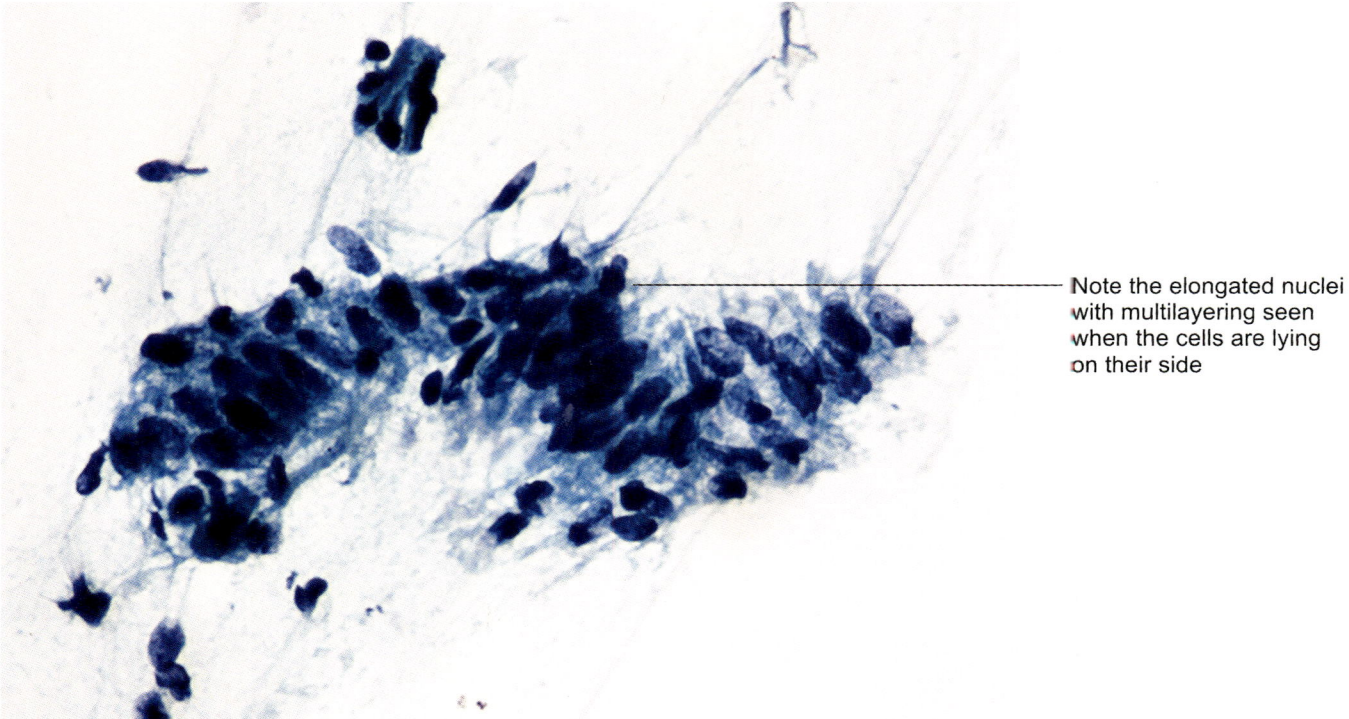

Note the elongated nuclei with multilayering seen when the cells are lying on their side

Fig. 15.5b

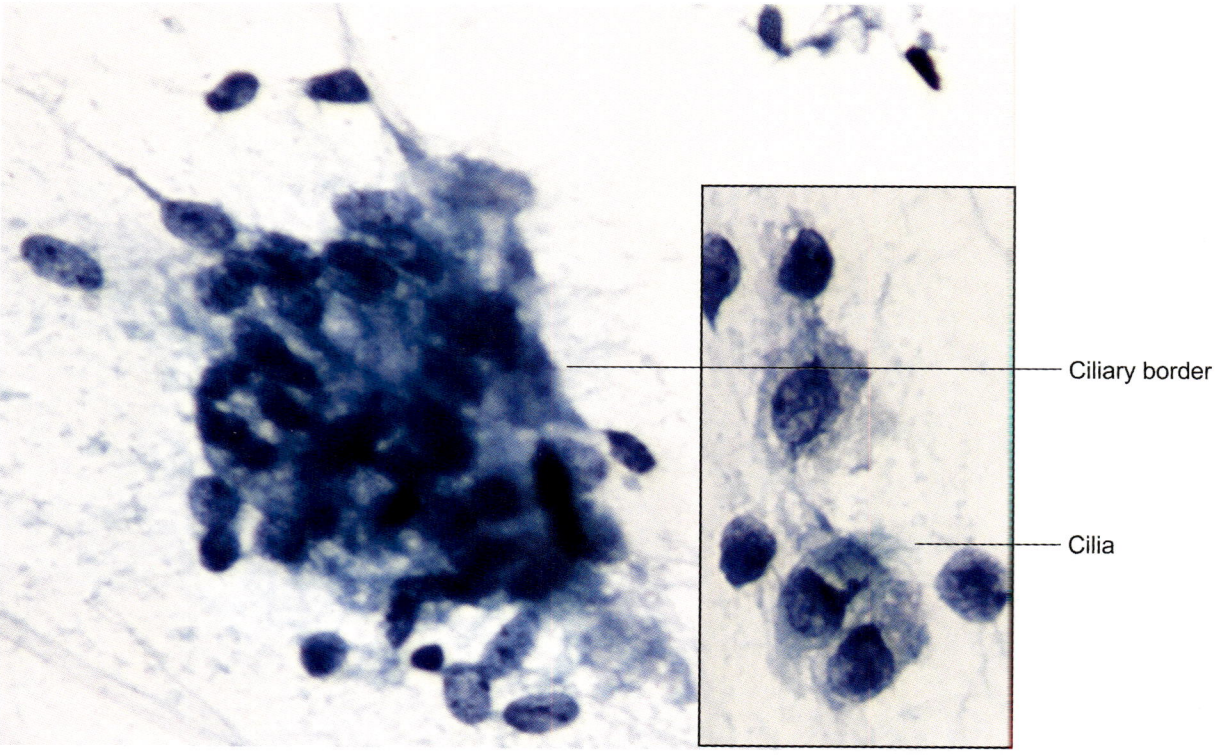

Ciliary border

Cilia

Fig. 15.5c

HANDLING OF HISTOPATHOLOGY SAMPLES

Cervical Punch Biopsy

These need to be properly embedded to get the surface epithelium oriented appropriately. Serial sections need to be examined in every case. If epithelium is not present lining the tissue sample, it can represent improper orientation—hence tissue in the block needs to be re-embedded and serial sectioned. It is very common for CIN 2 and CIN 3 to have ulceration and avulsion of the squamous epithelium away from the subepithelial tissue. Hence, all tissues need careful processing.

Endocervical Curettage

This needs to be done in cases where squamocolumnar junction is not visible on colposcopy or in cases where HPV or cytology is positive but colposcopy shows no lesion. It is a common mistake to mainly take out mucus and fragmented glands. Nice strips of squamous epithelium should be visible on gross evaluation to be confident that a good sampling has been achieved. Grossing of these tissues should be done using Whatman filter paper so that all the tiny strips are adequately sampled. Alternatively, a cell block processing similar to cytology samples can be done, if tissue is very scant. Serial sectioning to exhaust all tissue should be done in these samples to avoid missing small or focal lesions. Many CIN 2 or CIN 3 lesions might shed the epithelium by ulceration and finding small strips of atypical epithelium is needed for diagnosis.

LEEP Excision

This is a curative ablation procedure to remove a lesion previously biopsy confirmed to be CIN 2 or CIN 3. The sample needs to be tagged with sutures for the margins and properly separately labeled, if taken out in more than one piece. If in multiple pieces, each piece is marked with suture for margin. Margin marked with suture needs to be marked with ink prior to embedding. The tissue needs serial sectioning using scalpel blade keeping margin to margin slices in separate cassettes to finish all the tissue. Confirmation of the diagnosis as CIN 2 or CIN 3 and presence of any focus of invasion is noted. Margin of normal squamous epithelium should ideally be identified on both ends if possible but due to cautery effects usually the edge of the tissue is burnt and hence margins may not be always evaluable. Sometimes the epithelium ulcerates or separates during sectioning and hence serial sections are needed.

Cone Biopsy

It is important that the cone biopsy should be unrolled before fixation. If the cone is fixed in closed position, it becomes difficult or impossible to open up later after fixation is complete and the epithelium cracks. Upper and lower margins as well as the 12 O'clock and 3 O'clock positions need to be marked with different types of suture. Grossing is done after painting the margins with India Ink and by serial sections going from upper margin to lower margin. One section for each O'clock position needs to be taken. Microscopy confirms the diagnosis of CIN 2 or CIN 3 as given in the prior punch biopsy. Each section has an upper and a lower margin and it is essential to confirm that these margins are free of the CIN 2 or CIN 3 lesion as the case might be. If the margins are positive, then the exact focus needs to be identified and re-excised from appropriate location.

CONCLUSION

It can be seen from the above discussion that two-tier system as used in virology and cytology is also applicable to histopathology. Mild dysplasia, CIN 1 and productive viral infection are all the same lesions corresponding to low grade squamous intraepithelial lesion. These lesions are reversible in the vast majority and hence need no treatment except follow up.

The terms CIN 2 and CIN 3, also termed moderate dysplasia, severe dysplasia and carcinoma *in situ* are all different names for a single category of lesions where HPV integration has produced a transformation. All of these can be grouped together into a single term-high grade squamous intraepithelial lesion. Separation of CIN 2 and CIN 3 is only done because they have significant morphological differences with each other. All of these lesions require treatment in the form of ablation using various techniques.

Early diagnosis and treatment of high grade squamous intraepithelial lesion before it progresses into carcinoma is the aim of cervical cancer screening. Biopsy confirmation of all lesions is, however, essential prior to ablation. Margin evaluation to ensure that no island of transformed premalignant cells are left behind is vital to get a curative ablation.